HEALTH CARE INFORMATICS

AN INTERDISCIPLINARY APPROACH

HEALTH CARE INFORMATICS

AN INTERDISCIPLINARY APPROACH

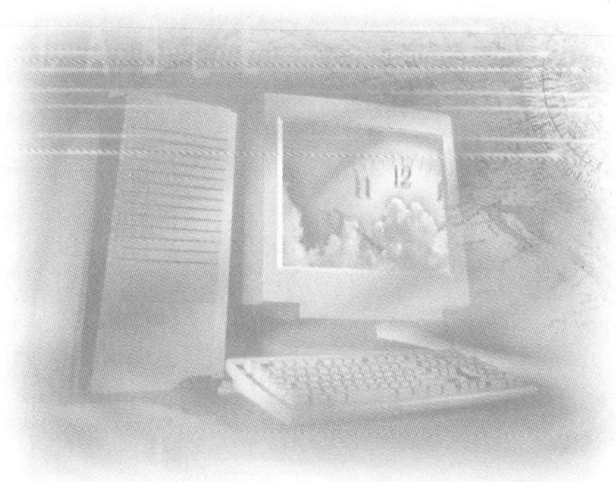

Sheila P. Englebardt, PhD, RN, CNA
Director, Center for Instructional Technology and Educational Support
Clinical Associate Professor
School of Nursing
The University of North Carolina at Chapel Hill
Chapel Hill, North Carolina

Ramona Nelson, PhD, RN, BC
Professor
Co-Director, Health Care Informatics Program
Slippery Rock University
Slippery Rock, Pennsylvania

Illustrated

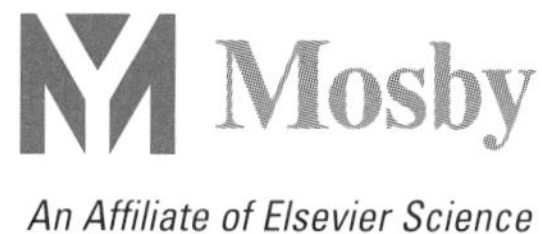

An Affiliate of Elsevier Science

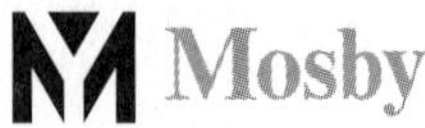

An Affiliate of Elsevier Science

Vice President and Publishing Director, Nursing Division: Sally Schrefer
Executive Editor: June D. Thompson
Managing Editor: Linda Caldwell
Project Manager: Deborah L. Vogel
Production Editor: Deon Lee
Book Design Manager: Judi Lang
Cover Design: Michael Warrell

Mosby, Inc.
11830 Westline Industrial Drive
St. Louis, Missouri 63146

Printed in the United States of America

International Standard Book Number 0-323-01423-2

03 04 05 TG/FF 9 8 7 6 5 4 3 2

ABOUT THE AUTHORS

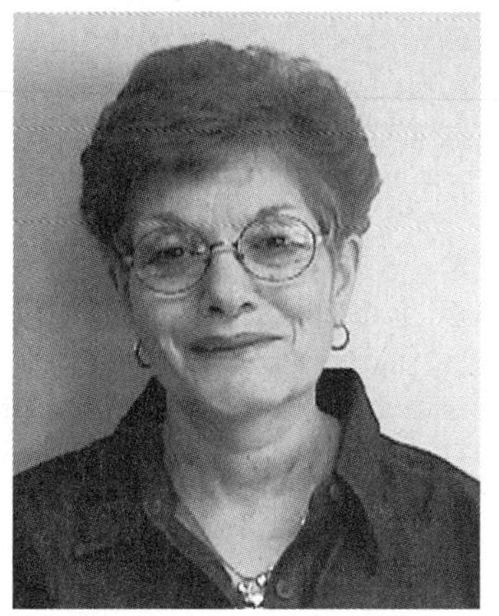

Sheila P. Englebardt

Sheila Englebardt is an Associate Clinical Professor in the School of Nursing at the University of North Carolina at Chapel Hill. Sheila received her baccalaureate degree in nursing from New York University–Bellevue Hospital Center. She holds a master's degree in education with a focus in curriculum and instruction from the University of North Carolina at Charlotte. In addition, she completed a postgraduate certificate program in health care financial management at the University of Colorado. Her doctorate is in nursing from the Virginia Commonwealth University. She is board certified by the American Nurses Credentialing Center as a nurse administrator.

Sheila teaches Health Care Informatics in the Health Care Systems master's program. Her Web-based informatics course was the first completely online course in the School of Nursing. Sheila is the Director of the Center for Instructional Technology and Educational Support (CITES) at the School of Nursing, which is responsible for developing Web-based course materials and technology-derived professional presentations. She has particular interest in the diffusion of technology in education and in the development of evaluation standards for Web-based education.

Sheila is a well-known speaker in the area of instructional technology with a focus on using interactive communication tools in Web-based courses. She is an active member of the American Nurses Association, the Council on Nursing Informatics of the North Carolina Nurses Association, and the American Medical Informatics Association and is an appraiser for the Magnet Nursing Services Recognition Program of the American Nurses Credentialing Center. In addition, Sheila is the Editor in Charge of Nursing Administration and Instructional Technology for the *Online Journal of Nursing Informatics*.

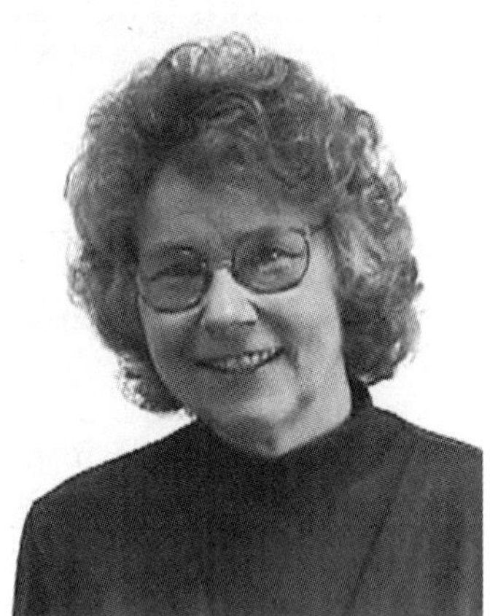

Ramona Nelson

Ramona Nelson is a professor in the nursing department at Slippery Rock University (SRU). She teaches courses on introductory and advanced health care informatics as well as managed care and community health. All of these courses are offered via Web-based distance education technology. In addition to teaching, Ramona is currently Co-Primary Investigator and Project Director for the Pennsylvania State System of Higher Education Program Initiative Grant to expand the SRU Web-based RN → BSN program within Pennsylvania. In addition, Ramona codirects the Health Care Informatics Program at SRU. Ramona's research interests focus on health care informatics and distance education. Current research projects involve consumer informatics and assessment processes in distance education.

Ramona holds a doctorate in higher education, as well as two master's degrees from the University of Pittsburgh. She holds a master's degree in nursing with a clinical focus on cardiovascular nursing and an emphasis on education, as well as a Master's of Science in Information Science with an emphasis on systems design. In addition, Ramona completed a postdoctorate program in nursing informatics at the University of Utah School of Nursing and is board certified by the American Nurses Credentialing Center as an informatics nurse. Before completing these degrees, she received her baccalaureate degree in nursing from Duquesne University.

Ramona is an active member of the American Nurses Association, the American Medical Informatics Association, the National League for Nursing, and the Healthcare Information and Management Systems Society. She recently served as a member of the American Nurses Association's task force responsible for revising the standards and scope of practice for nursing informatics. She has chaired the National League for Nursing (NLN) Council for Nursing Informatics and in this position coordinated the first Web broadcast offered by the NLN. Ramona is a distinguished lecturer for Sigma Theta Tau, speaking on both health care informatics and distance education.

REVIEWERS

Connie Delaney, PhD, RN, FAAN
Associate Professor
University of Iowa
Iowa City, Iowa

Ricardo Martinez, PhD
President
Medicolegal Consultants
San Antonio, Texas

Katharine West, MSN, RN, MPH
Instructor
School of Nursing
Azusa Pacific University
Azusa, California

CONTRIBUTORS

Patricia A. Abbott, PhD, RNC
Assistant Professor and Coordinator, Graduate Programs in Nursing Informatics
Adjunct Assistant Professor
School of Nursing
University of Maryland
Baltimore, Maryland
Chapter 5, Supporting Clinical Decision Making

W. Holt Anderson, BA
Executive Director
North Carolina Healthcare Information & Communications Alliance, Inc.
Research Triangle Park, North Carolina
Chapter 20, Protection of Health Care Information

Donna W. Bailey, PhD, MN, RN
School of Nursing
University of North Carolina at Chapel Hill
Chapel Hill, North Carolina
Chapter 19, The Implications of Accreditation and Governmental Regulations for Health Care Informatics
Chapter 20, Protection of Health Care Information

Carol J. Bickford, PhD(c), MS, RN,C
Senior Policy Fellow
American Nurses Association
Washington, DC
Chapter 18, Professional Health Care Informatics Standards

June Blalock Craig, BSN, MEd, PhD
Product Manager and Developer
Cerner Corporation
Kansas City, Missouri
Chapter 9, The Life Cycle of a Health Care Information System

Jacqueline Dienemann, PhD, RN, CNAA, FAAN
Clinical Associate Professor
School of Nursing and Health Studies
Georgetown University
Washington, DC
Chapter 14, The Impact of Health Care Informatics on the Organization

Marina Douglas, RN, MS
Clinical Practice Director
SAIC
Falls Church, Virginia
Chapter 8, Strategic and Tactical Planning for Health Care Information Systems

Sheila P. Englebardt, PhD, RN, CNA
Director, Center for Instructional Technology and Educational Support
Clinical Associate Professor
School of Nursing
University of North Carolina at Chapel Hill
Chapel Hill, North Carolina
Chapter 12, Technology and Distributed Education
Chapter 23, Future Directions in Health Care Informatics

William Scott Erdley, DNS, RN
Clinical Assistant Professor
Nurse Anesthesia Program
School of Nursing
University at Buffalo
Buffalo, New York
Chapter 21, The History of Health Care Informatics

Margaret M. Hassett, MS, RN,C
ICU Project Manager, Boston Children's Hospital
Boston, Massachusetts
Adjunct Faculty, University of Maryland School of Nursing
Lecturer, Johns Hopkins University School of Nursing
Baltimore, Maryland
Chapter 7, Applications for Health Care Information Systems

Robert G. Henshaw, MS, BA
Computing Consultant, Academic Technology and Networks
Adjunct Instructor, School of Information and Library Science
University of North Carolina at Chapel Hill
Chapel Hill, North Carolina
Chapter 11, Technological Approaches to Communication

Kathleen Milholland Hunter, PhD, RN
Independent Practice in Informatics
Visiting Research Associate Professor
School of Nursing
University of Maryland
Baltimore, Maryland
Chapter 10, Electronic Health Records

Michael H. Kennedy, PhD, MHA
Associate Professor
Health Services Administration Program
Slippery Rock University
Slippery Rock, Pennsylvania
Chapter 4, Supporting Administrative Decision Making

David C. Kibbe, MD, MBA
Chairman and Cofounder, Canopy Systems, Inc.
Adjunct Assistant Professor
School of Public Health
University of North Carolina at Chapel Hill
Chapel Hill, North Carolina
Chapter 13, eHealth Trends and Technologies: The Impact of the Internet on Health Care Providers and Patients

Kay S. Lytle, MSN, RN,C
Director, Nursing Informatics
University of North Carolina Hospitals
Chapel Hill, North Carolina
Chapter 19, The Implications of Accreditation and Governmental Regulations for Health Care Informatics

Kathleen A. McGraw, MA, MLS
Information Services Coordinator
Health Sciences Library
University of North Carolina at Chapel Hill
Chapel Hill, North Carolina
Chapter 2, Computer, Information, and Health Care Informatics Literacy

Margaret Eilene Moore, AMLS, MPH
User Services Department Head
Health Sciences Library
University of North Carolina at Chapel Hill
Chapel Hill, North Carolina
Chapter 2, Computer, Information, and Health Care Informatics Literacy

Ramona Nelson, PhD, RN, BC
Professor
Co-Director, Health Care Informatics Program
Slippery Rock University
Slippery Rock, Pennsylvania
Chapter 1, Major Theories Supporting Health Care Informatics
Chapter 23, Future Directions in Health Care Informatics

Charles Oleson, EdD, CISA
Technical Practice Director
Cerner Corporation
Kansas City, Missouri
Chapter 6, The Purpose, Structure, and Functions of Health Care Information Departments

Kay M. Sackett, EdD, RN
Clinical Assistant Professor
School of Nursing
University at Buffalo
Buffalo, New York
Chapter 21, The History of Health Care Informatics

Julia R. Shaw-Kokot, MSLS
Education Services Coordinator
Health Sciences Library
University of North Carolina at Chapel Hill
Chapel Hill, North Carolina
Chapter 2, Computer, Information, and Health Care Informatics Literacy

Kathleen Smith, MScEd, RN,C
Project Director, Nursing Informatics
Richard S. Carson and Associates, Inc.
Falls Church, Virginia
Chapter 17, Technical Standards Used in Health Care Informatics

Nancy Staggers, PhD, RN, FAAN
Associate CIO, Information Technology Services
Health Sciences Center
University of Utah
Salt Lake City, Utah
Chapter 15, Human-Computer Interaction in Health Care Organizations

Linda Q. Thede, PhD, RN,C
Informatics Consultant
Aurora, Ohio
Chapter 3, Understanding Databases

Joan E. Thiele, PhD, RN
Professor of Nursing
Intercollegiate Center for Nursing Education
College of Nursing
Washington State University
Spokane, Washington
Chapter 16, The Implications of Information Technology for Research

James P. Turley, PhD, RN
Vice Chairman, Department of Health Informatics
School of Allied Health Sciences
University of Texas
Houston, Texas
Chapter 22, The Future of Health Care Informatics Education

Barbara Van de Castle, MSN, RNC, CS
Instructor
School of Nursing
Johns Hopkins University
Baltimore, Maryland
Chapter 14, The Impact of Health Care Informatics on the Organization

Marianela E. Zytkowski, BSN
Graduate Assistant in Nursing Informatics
School of Nursing
University of Maryland
Baltimore, Maryland
Chapter 5, Supporting Clinical Decision Making

FOREWORD

Imagine a time when the network is the world and the world is the network. A time when networked devices and mechanisms are so deeply embedded into daily lives that the only time they may ever be noticed is when they are not working.
D. Crawford (2001, p. 29)

In March 2001, the Association of Computing Machinery (ACM) hosted a "futuristic conference to educate and enlighten the public and the profession on life in the new millennium" (Crawford, 2001, p. 5). The goal of the conference was to explore "how computing will influence, even determine, the future directions of biology, oceanography, astrophysics, life sciences, social sciences and education" (Crawford, 2001, p. 5). An accompanying issue of its journal, *Communications of the ACM,* contained essays by leading experts on their expectations in the great digital beyond. These essays project trends in networked technologies, cyberwear, virtual beings, ubiquitous user-aware software, and a host of other futuristic tools and technologies. These are intertwined with essays warning of potential dangers, abuses, and unintended consequences. In my reading of this issue, four observations stand out. First, the world of computing and communications will undoubtedly affect every facet of our lives. Second, trends in computing power, information infrastructure, and human connections will provide a dynamic platform for the growth of emerging technologies. Third, health care was noticeably absent, with only one essay dealing with medicine and another mentioning health care. Fourth, we cannot realize the hopes and dreams of the future unless we strengthen our educational endeavors and ensure that education is the source from which our future advances. These observations provide a framework for highlighting the strengths of this text.

FIRST OBSERVATION: TRANSFORMATIONS

Scientific advances in computing and communications technologies are transforming every facet of our lives. These technologies have transformed and will continue to transform the way we live, work, and interact with one another. Technology surrounds us—people checking their calendars on their personal digital assistants (PDAs), beaming their business cards to colleagues, reading eMail on their cell phones, and using global positioning systems to find the location of a restaurant. Each year staggering numbers of new eMail, Internet, and mobile communication users are reported. Information and knowledge are now freely and easily accessible at all times (on a 24/7/365 basis). Bastions of higher education, such as the Massachusetts Institute of Technology, are now extending their knowledge by offering Web-based courses accessible to the public. Wearable computers such as smart socks and digital jewelry and even smart pets are now being interwoven into the fabric of our lives. Information and communication technologies are truly becoming ubiquitous and pervasive in our society. As you read this text, you will be able to observe how information technologies will change the way health care is practiced and delivered. You will be exposed to the newest technologies and learn about their impact on health care professionals, consumers, clients and their families, as well as the health care system.

In health care, these transformations will influence the way health care is delivered and the relationship between the health care provider and the consumer. Concurrent trends in health care such as evidence-based practice, consumerism, and managed care are also precipitating necessary changes in the practice arena. All contribute to the exciting possibilities of new practice methods. As you read this book, think about these five technology challenges that will influence the next decade:

- Data-driven decisions will alter the practice of health care
- Health care professionals will need to rethink the structure and dynamics of human relationships in terms of communication and collaboration
- Health care professionals will need to learn how to create a sense of presence regardless of location
- Emerging technologies will democratize information and augment human capabilities to manipulate, manage, synthesize, and create knowledge
- Health care professionals will need to reshape legal, ethical, and political frameworks to support computer-mediated health care (Skiba, 1999, p. 26)

SECOND OBSERVATION: EMERGING TECHNOLOGIES PLATFORM

The platform that serves as the backbone of these emerging technologies interconnects three important components: computing power, information infrastructure, and human connections. Taken together they provide a dynamic platform for the development of emerging technologies. Without the first component, the tremendous increase in computing power and speed, it would be impossible to manipulate and manage the information resources and data sets currently available. The simultaneous increase in storage capacity is also a necessary condition for these emerging technologies. Microprocessing speeds are dramatically increasing, far exceeding Moore's Law of an annual rate of 1.60. Recent technology advances—such as nanotechnology; spintronics; and quantum, molecular, and biocomputing—are pushing the envelope to dramatically increase processing speed. For example, biocomputing, advocated by physicist George Ditto and his colleagues at the Georgia Institute of Technology, combines living nerve cells or neurons with silicon circuits.

The second component, the necessary information infrastructure for the emerging technologies, includes the interconnected networks of computers, devices, and software. The future will be highly dependent on the ability to connect to others' computers, devices, and networks. In terms of connectivity, bandwidth and wireless connections will be the most important infrastructure requirements during the next decade. The explosive growth of the Internet, fueled by the World Wide Web, has increased the demand for bandwidth capacity. Recent advances in communication technologies serve as a catalyst for mobile or wireless communications. In the mobile communications arena, growth has far exceeded projections. To survive in this networked society, we must create devices that are easier to use and smarter so that all can participate in the transformation. Web-based PDAs, information appliances, and smart devices are among the many emerging devices. These emerging devices demand new software protocols and programming languages. The ultimate goal of all these devices is to bring all people into a networked society.

The final and perhaps most important component is the human connection. The development of human-centered systems will greatly facilitate the use of emerging technologies by the masses. Accordingly, human-centered systems enable humans and information infrastructure components to work together more effectively and transparently. Human connection technologies will significantly affect the relationship between humans and their technologies. Intelligent agents, softbots, user-aware software, and perceptual user interfaces are all on the horizon. Many in the human-computer interaction arena believe that we are entering the post-WIMP (windows, icons, menus, and pointing devices) user interface era. In this post-WIMP era, interfaces do not use windows, menus, icons, forms, or toolbars but rely on all senses and natural language processing. This is particularly true as computers become ubiquitous. Small mobile devices, embedded computers in the home, and wearable computers will all demand a different user interface model. These human connections supported by perceptual user interfaces will promote the interactions using more natural and humanlike communications, gestures, and even touch. Human-centered systems will be designed to foster human connections and ensure rapid adoption of these emerging technologies.

As you read, think about how computing power and the information infrastructure influence the expansion and use of information and communication technologies in health care. Pay particular attention to the human connections component because this factor greatly influences the rapid adoption and diffusion of any technology in an organization.

THIRD OBSERVATION: ABSENCE OF HEALTH CARE

Although there was little mention of health care in the *Communications of the ACM* issue, since the 1960s numerous attempts have been made to integrate information technology into the health care arena. Examples of early computer applications included the use of physiological monitors in intensive care units, administrative systems to calculate patient acuity and staffing, and hospital information systems and statistical reporting systems for community health. Most applications focused on data collection (physiological monitoring), data analysis (acuity and staffing, statistical reporting), and data storage (clinical documentation), or what Sandelowski (1993) termed *information-producing applications*. With the emergence of the electronic health (EHR) record, decision support, and expert systems, the health care arena moved to an era of information-managing technologies (Sandelowski, 1993). One of the most significant information-managing technologies, the EHR, allows clinicians, administrators, and researchers to capture, transmit, store, manipulate, and retrieve patient-specific information. In recent years the use of Web-based interfaces for electronic records, wireless connections, and PDAs has expanded the information-management component at the point of care. In the last decade we have shifted to an era of therapeutic technologies (Sandelowski, 1993), where technologies are used as health care interventions. Electronic support groups and other Web-based applications are good examples of therapeutic technologies.

This book provides health care professionals with a wealth of knowledge about the use of databases, clinical and administrative decision support systems, and hospital information systems in health care. Drs. Nelson and Englebardt have assembled a stellar group of health care professionals who provide both a historical and a current perspective of information technologies in the health care arena. The book also addresses many of the new and burgeoning applications in the areas of communication technologies and eHealth.

This book recognizes that without an examination of organizational issues and infrastructure, the growth of emerging technologies in health care would be questionable. These chapters echo the disquieting fact that health care has been late in embracing information and communication technologies. Recent reports have further explicated this concern. This quote from a recent Institute of Medicine (IOM) report, *Crossing the Quality Chasm: A New Health System for the 21st Century,* summarizes the current view of technology in health care (IOM, 2001, p. 3):

> *What is perhaps most disturbing is the absence of real progress toward restructuring health care systems to address both quality and cost concerns, or toward applying advances in information technology to improve administrative and clinical processes.*

As a result of this observation, the IOM report recommended the following (IOM, 2001, p. 5):

> *. . . that purchasers, regulators, health professionals, educational institutions and the Department of Health and Human Services create an environment that fosters and rewards improvement by (1) creating an infrastructure to support evidence-based practice, (2) facilitating the use of information technology, (3) aligning payment incentives, and (4) preparing the workforce to better serve patients in a world of expanding knowledge and rapid change.*

This text represents the first step in addressing this recommendation by setting the stage for the potential use of technologies in health care, the necessary infrastructure to support technologies, and most of all, an interdisciplinary approach to educate the health care workforce about health care informatics.

FOURTH OBSERVATION: EDUCATION

The last recommendation, preparing the workforce to better serve patients, is the essence of this text. If we are to reach the potential of information technologies in health, we must begin the process by educating both the current and future health care workforces. Drs. Nelson and Englebardt have devoted a good portion of their professional careers to providing educational opportunities for health care professionals in the field of health care informatics. The collective knowledge of these assembled authors will undoubtedly inspire and propel the field of health care informatics into the next era.

Diane J. Skiba, PhD
Associate Dean for Informatics
Director, Academic Innovations
School of Nursing
University of Colorado Health Sciences Center

REFERENCES

Crawford, D. (2001). Editorial pointers. *Communications of the Association of Computing Machinery, 44*(3), 5, 29.

Institute of Medicine Committee on Quality of Health Care in America. (2001). *Crossing the quality chasm: A new health system for the 21st century.* Washington, DC: National Academy Press.

Sandelowski, M. (1993). Toward a theory of technology dependency. *Nursing Outlook, 41*(1), 36-42.

Skiba, D. (1999). Shaping the landscape of technology and health care in the 21st century. *Proceedings of the 1999 Emergency Nurses Association's Chaos and Complexity: Writing our Preferred Future.* Des Plaines, IL: Emergency Nurses Association.

PREFACE

Health Care Informatics: An Interdisciplinary Approach provides the reader with an understanding of the theoretical underpinnings of health care informatics as well as a comprehensive overview of health care informatics practice. The first assumption in this book is that the primary goal of health care informatics is the improvement of the health care delivery system for all. This means that health care informatics improves the quality of health care delivered to clients, improves the quality of the professional work world of providers, and assists health care institutions in achieving their missions. Figure 1 presents a model and the related definitions of the groups within the health care delivery system; these groups include the clients, health care providers, professionals who provide support services, and other organizations and professionals who work within the health care delivery environment. In Figure 1, an individual may be employed in a position that includes functions from more than one area.

The boundaries of the areas identified in the diagram are permeable. Positions within each area are not mutually exclusive. An example is a health care informatics specialist who designs and presents health care education over the Internet for a select population. The health care informatics specialist is a health care provider as well as a support service professional in the organization.

All groups within the diagram generate data. Health care data are the basic building blocks of the health care information system. Professionals and clients within health care collect and use data from their own areas as well as from all other areas in Figure 1. These data are often named or classified by their source or users. For example, nursing data may refer to data that are generated by nurses, to data that are used by nurses, or to both. As a result the same data element may be given a different name or may be classified in different ways. For example, hemoglobin levels may be referred to as laboratory data, patient data, medical data, or nursing data. Health care informatics recognizes these various classifications while focusing on the interdisciplinary nature of data elements. Effective planning of health care information systems analyzes the decisions made by the different groups in Figure 1, determines the information needed for effective decision making, and then identifies the data needed to produce required information. Understanding the decision-making process, as a basis for planning health care information systems, is a theme found throughout this book.

Health informatics professionals as support service professionals (Figure 1) work with integrated information systems covering all areas of the diagram. Depending on their specific position, informatics professionals may support the work of personnel in any area of the diagram. As a result, there is some controversy about and a great deal of variation in job titles and reporting structures of health care informatics personnel. One example is the debate about whether nursing informatics specialists should report to nursing services or to information services. The job titles and reporting structures often reflect educational backgrounds or the group being supported (nursing informatics specialist), the type of information systems with which they are working (clinical analysts), or the technical role in the organization (systems analyst). In this book, the term *health care informatics specialist* is used to reflect the roles of health care informatics professionals as opposed to a specific job title.

FIGURE 1 Health Care Delivery Model

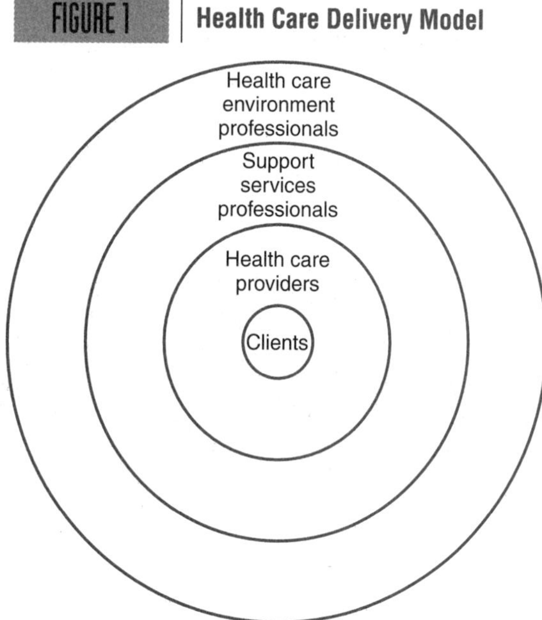

Definitions: *Clients* are individuals (health care consumers or patients), families, groups, communities, and populations. *Support services professionals* are those who hold administrative, education, research, and informatics positions and provide support services to health care providers and others within the health care system (e.g., vice-president for clinical services, chief information officer, health-related university professors, clinical researchers, and nursing informatics specialists). *Health care environment professionals* are those who are not employed by and do not function within the health care system but who do affect its structure, function, and purpose (e.g., legislators, stockholders in publicly traded health-related companies, health-related reporters or publishers, and insurance executives).

FIGURE 2 Health Care Informatics Specialist: Umbrella Model

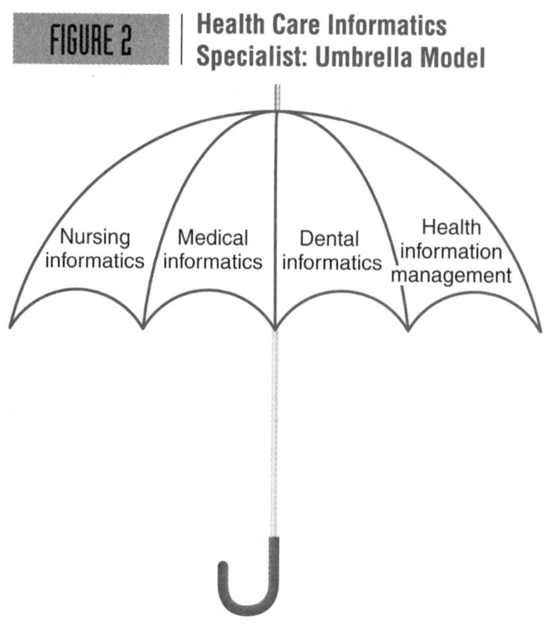

FIGURE 3 Health Care Informatics Specialist: Overlapping Model

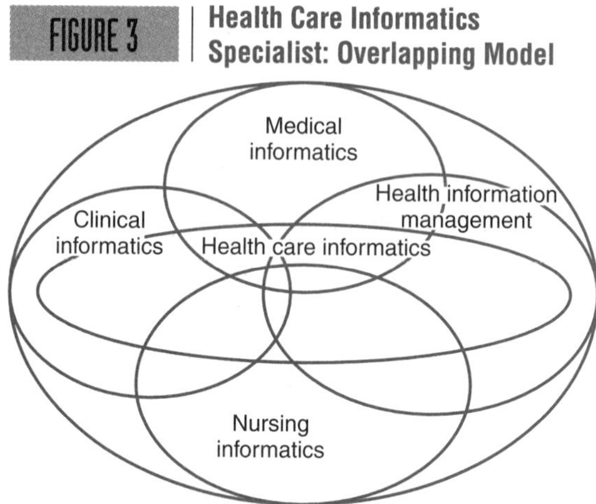

WHAT IS A HEALTH CARE INFORMATICS SPECIALIST?

The term *health care informatics* can be interpreted in two different ways. These interpretations are depicted in Figures 2 and 3. In Figure 2, an umbrella is used to illustrate health care informatics. Each panel of the umbrella represents a different specialty, and the umbrella frame represents health care informatics. If all the panels are removed, only the frame of the umbrella exists. In other words, in this conceptual model health care informatics as a field of study does not exist in itself but is an umbrella term referring to all of the special areas of study that are encompassed by the term. The second conceptual model is represented by Figure 3. In this model, areas of specialization and functional areas overlap. Health care informatics exists in its

Table 1 Educational Programs in Health Care Computing

Level of Education	Health Care Informatics	Medical Informatics	Nursing Informatics	Health Information Management
Postdoctorate				
Doctorate				
Master's				
Certificate				
Postmaster's				
Postbaccalaureate				
Other				
Baccalaureate (major or minor)				
Associate degree (at this level one may see individual courses as opposed to specific programs)				

Table 2 Relationship Between Functional Roles and the Two Models

Clinical	Educational	Research	Administration	Health Policy
Health care informatics specialist	Clinical informatics specialist ↓			
Nursing informatics specialist				
Medical informatics specialist				

own right but at the same time overlaps several other areas in the field of informatics.

In this book both models are acceptable conceptualizations of the field. Health care informatics exists as both an overriding term referring to multidisciplinary health-related informatics specialties and a field of study with its own educational programs. A review of existing educational programs in health care informatics demonstrates the reality of both these models. Each of the cells in Table 1 can be filled in with a specific educational program that can be found by searching the Internet.

Existing professional roles within health care informatics provide support for both models. Table 2 demonstrates the relationship between functional roles and the two models. Note how a professional concerned with health information systems used in clinical settings could be employed as a clinical informatics specialist with a background in health care informatics or nursing informatics or medical informatics. This same concept applies to a person employed in education, research, administration, or health policy. Each type of professional would bring his or her distinct knowledge and skills to the role. For example, a person prepared in medical informatics would approach health care policies from a different perspective than a person with a background in nursing informatics. However, both of these individuals could be well prepared to interpret health policy issues related to health care informatics.

This book accepts both of these models and defines **health care informatics** as the study of how health data, information, knowledge, and wisdom are collected, stored, processed, communicated, and used to support the process of health care delivery to clients and providers, administrators, and organizations involved in health care delivery. This book is written as a textbook and reference for all health care informatics specialists working within either of the two models.

ORGANIZATION OF THE BOOK

Health Care Informatics: An Interdisciplinary Approach consists of six parts. Part One, Foundations of Health Care Informatics, is composed of five chapters. Each chapter presents an aspect of health care informatics that is foundational to the understanding of the total field. These include basic concepts, theories, and models (Chapter 1); information literacy skills (Chapter 2); database concepts (Chapter 3); administrative decision support systems (Chapter 4); and clinical decision support systems (Chapter 5).

The focus of Part Two is on health care information systems. This part includes an introduction to the information systems department (Chapter 6), an overview of the applications used in health care (Chapter 7), an analysis of the planning processes used to manage health care information systems (Chapter 8), and the life cycle of a health care information system (Chapter 9). Part Two concludes with the primary application in health care, the electronic health record (EHR) (Chapter 10).

Part Three, Using Technology to Deliver Health Care and Education, is not an overview of hardware and software used in health care, but rather recognizes how technology is changing health care communication and in turn health care delivery. Chapter 11 provides an overview of the types of technology used in health care communication. Chapter 12 explores how the technology is changing both professional and consumer education. Chapter 13 analyzes the impact of eHealth on the evolving health care system.

Part Four, The Impact of Informatics on the Sociocultural Environment of Health Care, explores how informatics and health care information systems are changing and are being changed by the social and cultural environment of health care. Chapter 14 applies these concepts to the organization, Chapter 15 investigates the relationship between the computer and humans, and Chapter 16 presents what this means for informatics research.

Part Five, Infrastructure to Support Health Care Informatics, examines the professional, governmental, and technical structures that are required for the success of health care information systems. Chapter 17 presents technical standards that are required for the integration of information systems. Chapter 18 contributes the professional standards such as a common language and ethics. Chapter 19 discusses how accreditation and governmental regulations support the development of health care information systems, and Chapter 20 identifies the processes and procedure in place and under development to protect health care information. Without the protection of health care information, automated health care information systems will be unacceptable to society.

Part Six, Yesterday, Today, and Tomorrow, looks at the birth of health care informatics, the current state, and predictions of what might occur in the future. The goal of this part is that by understanding the history, the current status, and the potential future, health care informatics students will better appreciate their ability to help create that future.

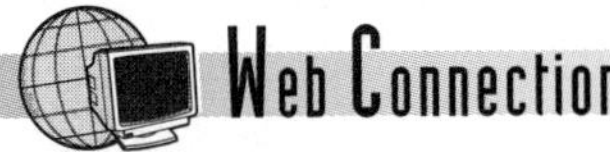

This book, with its focus on the use of technology to facilitate the delivery of health care, examines examples of past, current, and future applications of technology to education, research, and practice. Therefore it is appropriate that we expand the traditional notion of a textbook to a new level; this book has both a time-honored print component and a forward-thinking Web component. The content of the print component was current when the book went into production, but given the nature of the field, changes occur frequently. Therefore this book has an adjunct Web site to enhance the core text and to provide a supplementary learning environment that will continue to be updated with current information as it becomes available. Web site content for each chapter includes links to other Web sites that are congruent with and augment chapter content. In addition to the Web site links, there are interactive exercises that expand chapter content. For instructors there are PowerPoint slides and test questions for each chapter.

The Web site is available at **http://evolve.elsevier.com/Englebardt/.**

Sheila P. Englebardt
Ramona Nelson

ACKNOWLEDGMENTS

A first edition of any book is rarely the product of the authors alone; it is completed only with the assistance, guidance, and kindness of others. We were fortunate to have had the counsel and support of many people. We recognize June Thompson, our Executive Editor, for conceptualizing this book, seeking us as the editors, encouraging us, and mentoring us through the developmental process. We recognize Linda Caldwell, our Managing Editor, for her patience, humor, and intelligent problem solving as we went through the process of reviewing, revising, and rewriting that culminated in a completed manuscript. We thank Deon Lee, our Production Editor, for her clear eye, copyediting expertise, and willingness to work around our busy schedules.

We especially acknowledge the chapter authors, who demonstrated specific expertise in the content of the individual chapters woven together to form the fabric of this book. Our electronic and telephone discussions with many of the chapter authors helped us to formulate our ideas and to consolidate varying thoughts into a cohesive whole. We learned a lot from each of them and thank them for their important contributions to the book.

In writing and editing this book, both editors learned a great deal. The most important lesson learned was that a book of this type—a project of this magnitude—is possible only with the support of family and colleagues.

This book is dedicated to our husbands,
Arthur J. Englebardt and *Glenn M. Nelson*

CONTENTS

PART ONE

Foundations of Health Care Informatics

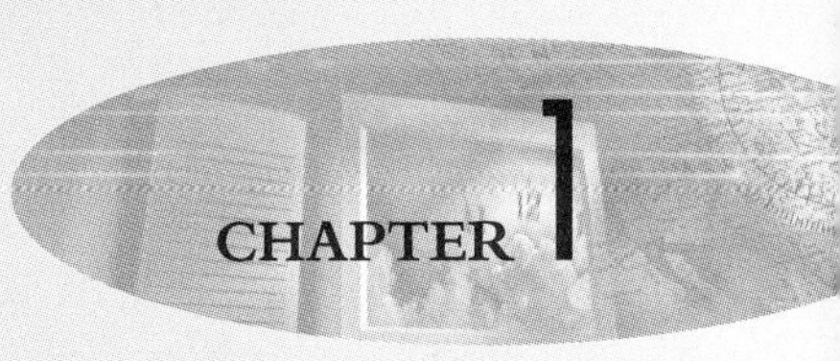

Major Theories Supporting Health Care Informatics

RAMONA NELSON

Learning Objectives

Upon completion of this chapter, the reader will be able to:

1. ***List*** major theories used in health care informatics.
2. ***Describe*** how selected theories and models explain and predict phenomena of importance to health care informatics practitioners.
3. ***Use*** selected theories to analyze problems and challenges encountered when using automation to support health care delivery.

Outline

Key Terms

adult learning theories
andragogy
attributes
automated decision support system
automated expert system
automated information system
behavioral learning theories
boundary
change theories
channel
closed system
cognitive learning theories
concepts
data
diffusion of innovation
dynamic homeostasis
early adopters
early majority
encoder
entropy
equifinality
framework
information
innovators
knowledge
laggards
late majority
lead part
learning
learning styles
model

Key Terms—cont'd

negentropy	reverberation	system
noise	sender	target system
open system	specialization	theoretical model
phenomenon	subsystem	theory
receiver	supersystem	wisdom

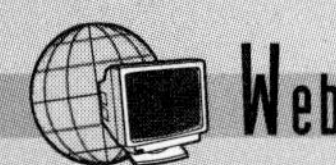

Web Connection

Go to the Web site at http://evolve.elsevier.com/Englebardt/. Here you will find Web links and activities related to major theories supporting health care informatics.

A **theory** explains the process by which certain **phenomena** occur (Hawking, 1988). It begins with an observation of the specific phenomena. An example of a phenomenon is that people frequently resist change. But why and how does this phenomenon occur? A theory related to this phenomenon would explain why people resist change and predict when and how they will demonstrate resistance.

The following is the four-stage process by which most theories develop:

1. A specific phenomenon is noted or observed.
2. An idea is proposed explaining the development of the phenomenon.
3. A model is developed to explain the operation of the phenomenon. Concepts key to explaining the phenomenon are identified, and the processes by which the concepts interact are described.
4. The model is tested, and as supporting evidence accumulates, a theory develops.

There is no single set of consistent criteria that can be applied to decide when a **model** becomes a theory. As a result, the terms are often used interchangeably. In other words, it is possible for one reference to refer to a phenomenon as a theory and for another reference to refer to the same phenomenon as a model. For example, one reference may refer to a communication theory and another reference may refer to a communication model, yet both references may be describing the same phenomenon. In addition, a **theoretical model** is often used to explain a theory. A theoretical model is a description or figure used to help visualize a theory. It includes the concepts and interactions among the concepts operating within the theory.

The building blocks of a theory are called **concepts.** Concepts may be abstract, such as love, or concrete, such as fruit. Concepts provide structure to a theory. For example, in Figure 1-1 the relationship among four concepts is depicted. These four concepts and the location of the concepts in the figure demonstrate the structure of the theory. The interactions among the concepts in a theory explain the function or operations of

FIGURE 1–1 | Open System Interacting With the Environment

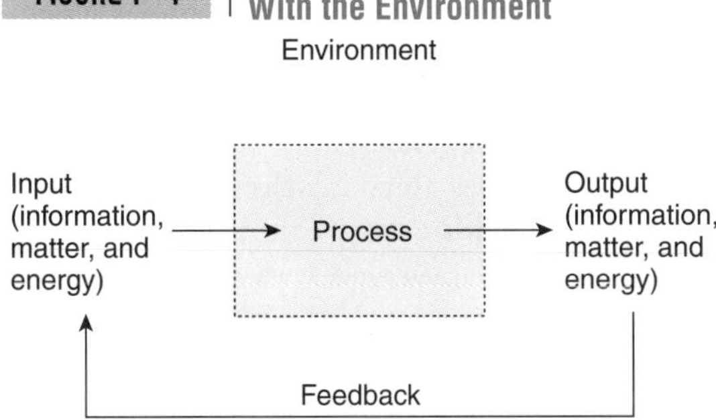

that theory. For example, the electrical system of the heart is a concrete concept. Impulses travel through this system and produce a contraction of the atria and ventricles. The concept of the heart's electrical system and the description of how it functions provide a theory that can be used to explain how the heart beats.

Because a theory explains the what and how of a phenomenon, it can provide direction for planning interventions. Continuing the cardiac example, the cardiac impulse normally begins in the sinoatrial (SA) node in the right atrium and travels across the atrioventricular (AV) node to the ventricles. In atrial fibrillation this normal process is disrupted, and impulses arise at a rapid rate from multiple sites in the atrial muscle. This can result in a fast ventricular response, or tachycardia. Drugs that block or slow the rate of impulse transmission at the AV node can be used to treat tachycardia caused by atrial fibrillation. This is an example of using a theory to understand and manage a problem.

Health care informatics, as an applied field of study, incorporates theories from information science, computer science, and cognitive science, as well as from the wide range of sciences used in the delivery of health care. As a result, health care informatics specialists draw on a wide range of theories to guide their practice. This chapter focuses on selected theories from a variety of disciplines that are of major importance to health care informatics. These theories are key to understanding and managing the challenges faced by health care informatics specialists. In analyzing the selected theories, the reader will discover that understanding these theories presents certain challenges. Some of the theories overlap, different theories are used to explain the same phenomena, and sometimes different theories have the same name. All of these challenges can be found in the theories of information (see the Information Theories section).

The one theory underlying all of the theories used in health care informatics is systems theory. Therefore this is the first theory to be discussed in this chapter.

SYSTEMS THEORY

A **system** is a set of related interacting parts enclosed in a boundary (Von Bertalanffy, 1975). Examples of systems include computer systems, school systems, the health care system, and a person. Systems may be living or nonliving. For example, a person is a living system, whereas a computer is a nonliving system (Joos, Nelson, & Lyness, 1985).

Systems may be either open or closed. **Closed systems** are enclosed in an impermeable boundary and do not interact with the environment. An example of a closed system is a chemical reaction enclosed in a glass structure with no interaction with the environment outside the glass. **Open systems** are enclosed in semipermeable boundaries and do interact with the environment. This chapter focuses on open systems. Open systems can be used to understand technology and the people who interact with the technology. Figure 1-1 demonstrates an open system interacting with the environment. As shown in Figure 1-1, open systems take input (information/matter/energy) from the environment, process the input, and then return output to the environment. The output then becomes feedback to the system. Concepts from systems theory can be applied in understanding the way people work with computers in a health care organization. These concepts can also be used to analyze individual elements, such as software, or the total picture of what happens when systems interact.

A common expression in computer science is "garbage in, garbage out," or "GIGO." GIGO refers to the input-output process. The counter-concept implied from this expression is that quality input is required to achieve quality output. Although this expression usually is used when referring to computer systems, it can apply to any open system. Some examples include the role of a poor diet in the development of health problems or the role of informed, active participants in selecting a health care information system. In these examples "garbage in" can result in "garbage out," or quality data can support quality output. Not only is quality input required for quality output, but also the system must have effective procedures in place for processing these data. Systems theory provides a **framework** for looking at the input into a system, for analyzing how the system processes that input, and for measuring and evaluating the output from the system.

Characteristics of Systems

Open systems have three types of characteristics: purpose, functions, and structure. The purpose is the reason for the system's existence. The purpose of an institution or program is often stated in the mission statement. For example, the purpose of a bachelor of science in nursing (BSN) educational program is to prepare professional nurses. Often computer systems are referred to or classified by their purpose. The purpose of a radiology system is to support the radiology department; the purpose of a laboratory system is to support the laboratory department. A scheduling system is used to schedule either clients or staff.

Purpose

It is possible for a system to have more than one purpose. For example, a family system or a hospital information system may have several different purposes. One of the purposes of a hospital information system is to provide interdepartmental communication. Another purpose is to maintain a census that can be used to bill patients for services rendered.

One of the first steps in selecting a computer system in a health care organization is to identify the purpose(s) for that system. There may be a tendency to minimize this step on the basis of the assumption that everyone already agrees on the purpose of the system. Taking the time to specify the purpose helps to ensure that the representatives from the clinical, administrative, and technology domains agree on the reasons for selecting a system and understand the scope of the project. Purpose answers the question, "Why select a system?"

Functions

Functions, on the other hand, focus on the question, "How will the system achieve its purpose?" Functions are sometimes mistaken for purpose. However, it is important to clarify why a system is needed and then to identify what functions the system will carry out. Functions are activities that a system carries out to achieve its purpose. For example, a hospital information system may achieve the interdepartmental communication purpose by maintaining an eMail program, as well as a program for order entry and results reporting. Each time an order is entered into the system, it is communicated to the appropriate department. Each time a department has results to report, they are communicated back to the clinical unit or appropriate health care provider.

When a computer system is being selected, the functions are carefully identified and defined in writing. These are listed as functional specifications. Functional specifications identify each function and describe how that function will be performed.

Structure

Systems are structured in ways that allow them to perform their functions. Structure follows function. Note how health care teams are organized. The organizational structure varies with the purpose of the organization and the functions that are to be performed. The organization of a nursing staff on a clinical unit demonstrates this concept. They may be organized using the concept of team nursing, primary nursing, or case management. In each case the purpose is to provide patient care. The staff is structured to ensure that the functions necessary for nursing care are completed.

Structure Conceptualization Two different models can be used to conceptualize the structure of a system. These are hierarchical and web. Both models are in operation at the same time. The first model discussed is the hierarchical model. Figure 1-2 demonstrates this model. In this figure each computer is part of a local area network (LAN). The LANs join together to form a wide area network (WAN) that is connected to the mainframe computer. The mainframe is the lead computer, or **lead part.**

In an analysis of the hierarchical model, the term *system* may refer to any level of the structure. In Figure 1-2 an individual computer may be referred to as a system, or the whole diagram may be considered a system. Three terms are used to indicate the level of reference. These are subsystem, target system, and supersystem. A **subsystem** is any system within the **target system.** For example, if the target system is an LAN, each computer is a subsystem. The **supersystem** is the overall structure in which the target system exists. If the target system is an LAN, then Figure 1-2 represents a supersystem.

The second model for analyzing the structure of a system is the web model. The interrelationships among the different LANs function like a web. Laboratory data may be sent to the pharmacy, and at the same time the clinical unit data collected by nursing, such as weight and height, may be sent to each department needing these data. The web model can also be applied to living systems. Note the processes whereby various body systems interact with each other. In health care informatics much of the work is accomplished in task groups corresponding to body systems. Although someone is in charge of the task group, the relationships and communication among the members of the group flow in a web pattern. As these examples demonstrate, a system includes structural elements from both the web and the hierarchical model.

Structure Characterization **Boundary, attributes,** and environment are three concepts used to characterize structure. The boundary of a system forms the demarcation between the target system and the environment of the system. Input flows into the system by moving across the boundary, and output flows into the environment across this boundary. Understanding boundary concepts assists in the development of health care information systems. For example, one of the techniques used in developing health care information systems is to divide the health care delivery system into modules or subsystems. This process helps to establish the boundaries of a project. In Figure 1-2 each LAN is a target system. Each computer in the diagram represents a subsystem that can be automated. For example, a health care institution may be planning for a new pharmacy information system. The new pharmacy system becomes the target system. However, the pharmacy system interacts with other subsystems within the total system. As the task group goes about the work of selecting the new pharmacy system, it will need to identify the functional specifications needed to automate the pharmacy and the functional specifications needed for the pharmacy system to interact with the other systems in the environment. Clearly specifying the target system and the other systems in the environment will assist in defining the scope of the project. By defining the scope of the project, it becomes possible to focus on the task at hand while planning for the integration of this computer system with other systems in the institution.

FIGURE 1–2 | Hierarchical Information System Model

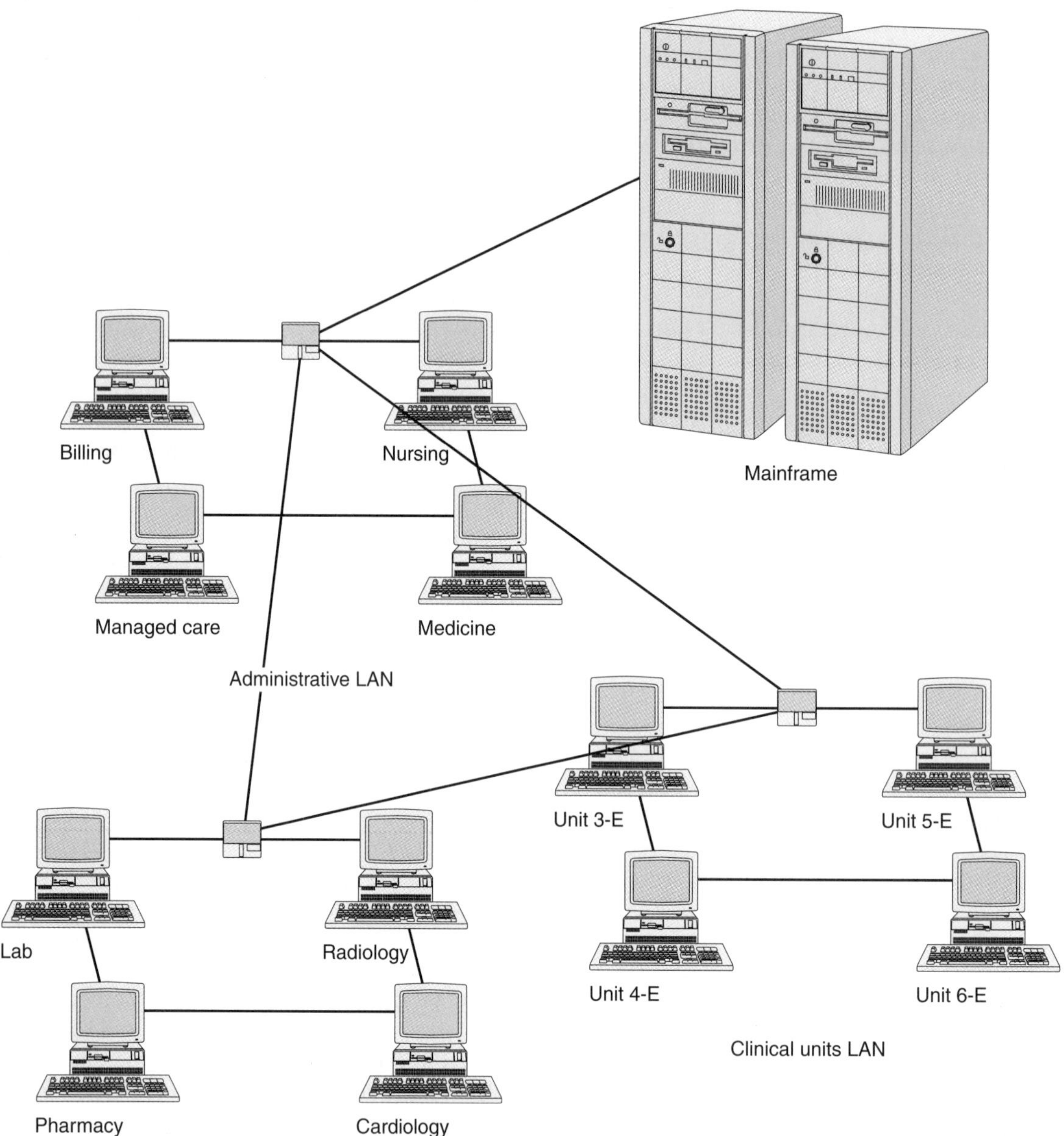

When health care information systems are being planned, attributes of the system must be identified. Attributes are the properties of the parts or components of the system. They are the terms used to describe a system. For example, the attributes of a person include hair color, weight, and intelligence quotient (IQ). Computer hardware attributes are usually referred to as specifications. An excellent example of a list of attributes or specifications can be seen in advertisements or the owner's manual for computer hardware. These include such things as the amount of random access memory (RAM), the size of the hard drive, and even the size of the case covering the computer. Another example of a list of attributes can be seen on an intake or patient assessment form for a health care setting. The form lists the attributes of interest. A completed form describes the individual patient's expression of these attributes.

Attributes and the expression of those attributes play a major role in the development of databases. Field names are a list of the attributes of interest for a specific system. The datum in each cell is the individual system's expression of that attribute. A record lists the attributes for each individual system. The record can also be seen as a subsystem of the total database system. A complete discussion of databases can be found in Chapter 3.

Systems and the Change Process

Both living and nonliving systems are constantly in a process of change. Six concepts are helpful in understanding the change process. These are dynamic homeostasis, entropy, negentropy, specialization, reverberation, and equifinality. **Dynamic homeostasis** refers to the processes used by a system to maintain a steady state or balance. An excellent example is the fluctuations seen in normal body chemistry. Blood levels of normal blood elements begin the drift down or up. Through a feedback loop the body begins to produce more of the decreasing elements and eliminate the excess elements. As the blood level changes, the feedback loop kicks in to reverse the process.

Chapter 10 discusses the life cycle of an information system. One of the stages in this life cycle is maintenance. Maintenance includes a number of activities that function to keep the system operating. Organizations that experience rapid or extensive change experience increased stress because the dynamic homeostasis of the organization is challenged. People working within changing organizations will attempt to maintain a steady state. The result can be seen as resistance to change. An informatics example is the introduction of automation or the introduction of a new computer system that stresses the dynamic homeostasis of the organization. Managing change and thereby decreasing the stress experienced by individual users, as well as the stress experienced by the organization as a whole, is a major piece of the work accomplished by the health care informatics specialist.

Entropy is the tendency of all systems to break down into their simplest parts. As they break down, the systems becomes increasingly disorganized or random. In data transmission, entropy measures the loss of information when a signal is transmitted. Entropy is demonstrated in the tendency of all systems to wear out. It is the tendency of all living systems to reach the point of death. Even with maintenance, a health care information system will reach a point where it must be replaced.

Negentropy is the opposite of entropy. This is the tendency of living systems to grow and become more complex. This is demonstrated in the growth and development of an infant, as well as in the increased size and complexity of today's health care system. With the increased growth and complexity of the health care system there has been an increase in the size and complexity of health care information systems.

As systems grow and become more complex, they divide into subsystems and then subsubsystems. This is the process of differentiation and

specialization. Note how the human body begins as a single cell and then differentiates into different body systems, each with specialized purposes, structures, and functions. This same process occurs with health care delivery systems, as well as with health care information systems. As this process occurs, a lead part emerges. The lead part is at the top of the hierarchy. Lead parts play primary roles in organizing and maintaining vertical and horizontal data/information flow. Changes to the lead part can have a major impact across the total system. For example, if the chief information officer leaves the organization, the impact is much more significant than if a beginning-level systems analyst moves to another organization. If the mainframe in Figure 1-2 were to stop functioning, the impact would be much more significant than if an individual computer on one of the LANs were to stop functioning. Understanding the role of the lead part can be key to developing the security and disaster plan for a health care information system.

Change within any part of the system will be reflected across the total system. This is referred to as **reverberation.** Reverberation is reflected in the intended and unintended consequences of system change. When planning for a new health care information system, the team will attempt to identify the intended consequences or expected benefits to be achieved. Although it is often impossible to identify a comprehensive list of unintended consequences, it is important for the team to consider the reality of unintended consequences. The potential for unintended consequences should be discussed during the planning stage; however, these consequences will be more evident during the testing stage that precedes implementation, or "go live." Often, unintended consequences are not considered until after go live, when they become obvious. For example, eMail may be successfully introduced to improve communication in an organization. However an unintended consequence can be an increased workload resulting from irrelevant eMail messages.

Equifinality refers to the ability of open systems to reach the same end state by starting at different initial states and by using different means. For example, several hospitals may be implementing new hospital information systems. The staff in the various hospitals may or may not be experienced in using this type of software. The hospitals may select from several different approaches for training the staff. Some may use clinical staff and develop superusers. Others may hire outside consultants to do all the training. Others may use information technology or staff development personnel to do the training. No matter what the initial knowledge level of the personnel or the training approach used, each of these hospitals has the potential to effectively train staff and experience a successful implementation. In other words, there is no one correct way to manage many of the challenges inherent in health care informatics.

All systems change and in the process interact with the environment. This interaction is shown in Figure 1-1. Input into the system consists of energy, information, and matter. This input is then processed and results in output. Understanding this process as it applies to informatics involves an understanding of information theories.

INFORMATION THEORIES

The term *information* has several different meanings (Information, 2000). An example of this can be seen in Box 1-1. Just as the term *information* has more than one meaning, the term *information theory* refers to more than one theory. This chapter examines two theoretical models of information theories: Shannon and Weaver's information-communication model and Blum's model.

Shannon and Weaver's Information-Communication Model

Information theory as a formal theory was born in 1948 with the publication by Claude Shannon of the landmark paper "A Mathematical Theory of Communication" (Shannon, 1948).

The concepts in this model are presented in Figure 1-3. The **sender** is the originator of the

FIGURE 1–3 Information-Communication Model

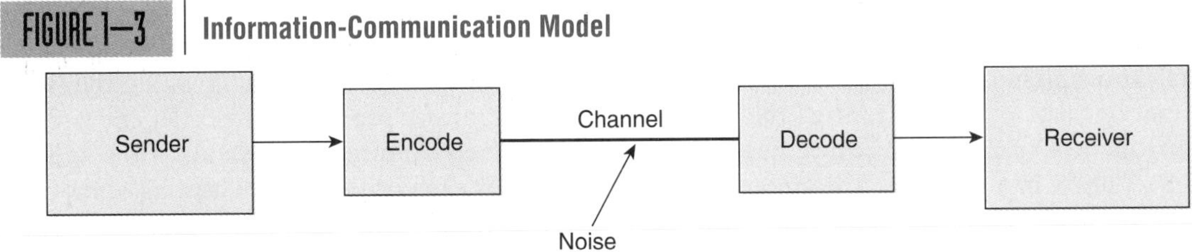

Box 1–1 Definitions of *Information*

in·for·ma·tion
noun
Pronunciation: "in-f&r-'mA-sh&n

1. The communication or reception of knowledge or intelligence
2. a. Knowledge obtained from investigation, study, or instruction
   b. The attribute inherent in and communicated by one of two or more alternative sequences or arrangements of something (as nucleotides in DNA or binary digits in a computer program) that produce specific effects
   c. (1) A signal or character (as in a communication system or computer) representing data (2) Something (as a message, experimental data, or a picture) which justifies change in a construct (as a plan or theory) that represents physical or mental experience or another construct
   d. A quantitative measure of the content of information; specifically: a numerical quantity that measures the uncertainty in the outcome of an experiment to be performed
3. The act of informing against a person
4. A formal accusation of a crime made by a prosecuting officer as distinguished from an indictment presented by a grand jury

From Information. In *Merriam-Webster online: Merriam-Webster's collegiate dictionary.* (2000). Retrieved October 8, 2000, from the World Wide Web: http://www.m-w.com/dictionary.htm.

message. The **encoder** converts the content of the message to a code. The code can be letters, words, music, symbols, or a computer code. For example, the modem on a computer acts as an encoder when it converts a file from a digital form to an analog form so that it can be sent over telephone lines that carry analog sound waves. The telephone line is the **channel.** A channel carries the message. Examples of channels include sound waves, telephone lines, and paper. Each channel has its own physical limitations in terms of the size of the message that can be carried. **Noise** is anything that is not part of the message but occupies space on the channel and is transmitted with the message. Some examples of noise include static on a telephone line and background sounds in a room. The decoder converts the message to a format that can be understood by the **receiver.** When one is listening to a phone call, the telephone is a decoder. It converts the analog signal back into sound waves, which are understood as words by the person listening. The person listening to the words is the receiver.

Shannon, one of the authors of the Shannon and Weaver information-communication theory, was a telephone engineer. He was not concerned with the semantic meaning of the message but rather with the technical problems involved in signal transmission across a communication channel or telephone line. He used the concept of entropy to explain and measure the amount of information in a message. The amount of information in a message is measured by the extent that the message decreases entropy. The unit of measurement is a bit. A bit is represented by a *0* (zero) or a *1* (one). The two sides of a coin can be used to explain this concept. If a coin is thrown into the air, it may land on either of two possible sides: heads up or tails up. This can be coded as 1 for heads up and 0 for tails up. Using this approach, the message concerning which side is up is transmitted with 1 bit. If there were four possible states, additional bits would be needed to transmit the message. For example, if the message could be north, south, east, or west, it might be coded 00 for north, 11 for south, 01 for east, or 10 for west. Computer codes are built on this concept. For example, how many bits are needed to code the letters of the alphabet? What other symbols are used in communication and must be included when developing a code?

Warren Weaver, from the Sloan-Kettering Institute for Cancer Research, provided the interpretation for understanding the semantic meaning of a message (Shannon & Weaver, 1949). He used Shannon's work to explain the interpersonal aspects of communication. For example, if the speaker is a physician who uses medical terms that are not known to the receiver (the patient), there will be a communication problem caused by the method used to encode the message. However, if the patient cannot hear well, he or she may not hear all of the words in the message. In this case the communication problem is caused by the patient's ear, which is having difficulty converting the sound waves into neurological impulses that the brain can decode.

The communication-information model provides an excellent framework for analyzing the effectiveness and efficiency of information transfer and communication. For example, a physician may use a computerized order entry system to enter orders. Several questions illustrate the information transfer process. Is the order entry screen designed to capture and code all of the key elements for each order? Are all aspects of the message coded in a way that can be transmitted and decoded by the receiving computer? Does the message that is received by the receiving department include all of the key elements in the message sent? Does the screen design at the receiver's end make it possible for the message to be decoded or understood by the receiver?

These questions demonstrate three levels of communication that can be used in analyzing communication problems (Hersh, 1996). The first level of communication is the technical level. Do the system's hardware and software function effectively and efficiently? The second level of communication is the semantic level. Does the message convey meaning? Does the receiver understand the message that was sent by the sender? The third level of communication is the effectiveness level. Does the message produce the intended result at the receiver's end? For example, did the physician order one medication but the patient received a different medication with a similar spelling? Some of these questions require a more in-depth look at how health care information is produced, transferred, and used. Bruce Blum's definition provides a framework for this more in-depth analysis.

Blum's Model

Bruce L. Blum developed a definition of information from an analysis of the accomplishments in medical computing. In his analysis Blum identified three types of health care computing applications. He grouped applications according to the objects that they processed: data, information, or knowledge. He defined **data** as uninterpreted elements, such as a person's name, weight, or age. **Information** was defined as a collection of data that has been processed and then displayed as information. An example is the patient's medical record. **Knowledge** results when data and information are identified and the relationships between the data and information are formalized. A knowledge base is more than the sum of the data and information pieces in that knowledge base. A knowledge base includes the interrelationships between the data and information. A textbook can be seen as containing knowledge (Blum, 1986).

In their classic article "The Study of Nursing Informatics," Graves and Corcoran (1989) used the concepts of data, information, and knowledge to explain the study of nursing informatics. Graves and Corcoran identified four types of knowledge: empirical, ethical, personal, and aesthetic. Nelson and Joos (1989) extended this data to include **wisdom.** Figure 1-4 demonstrates the relationships among these four concepts. Wisdom is defined as the appropriate use of knowledge in managing or solving human problems. It is knowing when and how to use knowledge to manage a patient need or problem. Wisdom requires a combination of values, experience, and the four types of knowledge. In Figure 1-4, the concepts of data, information, knowledge, and wisdom overlap. This is demonstrated by the overlapping circles, as well as the overlapping activities included in the circles. As one moves along the continuum, increasing interaction and interrelationships within and between the circles produce increased complexity of the elements within each circle. For example, the concept of wisdom is much more complex than the concept of data.

Using the concepts of data, information, knowledge, and wisdom, it is possible to classify the different levels of computing or automated systems. An **automated information system,** such as a pharmacy's information system, takes in

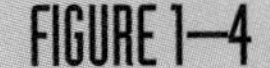

FIGURE 1—4 The Nelson Data-to-Wisdom Continuum

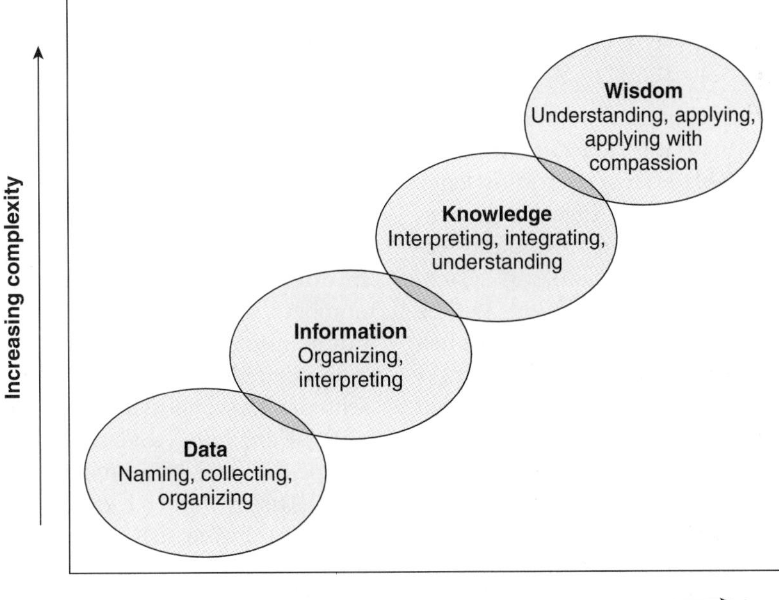

FIGURE 1–5 | **Levels and Types of Automated Systems**

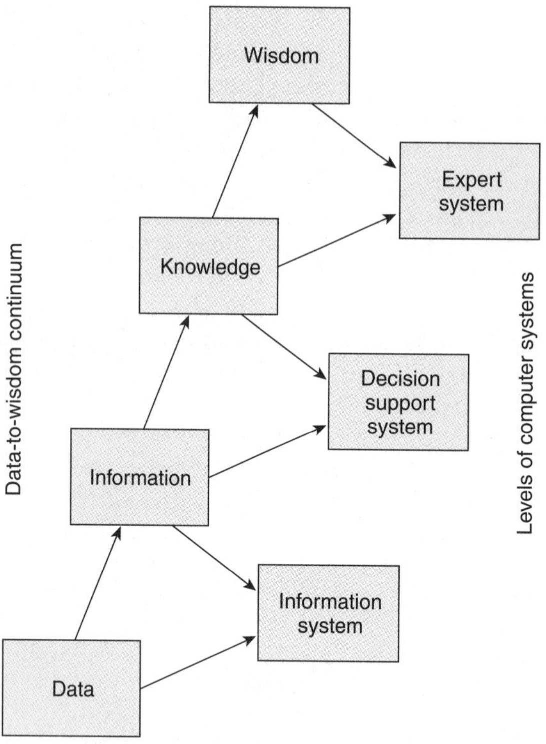

data information, processes the data/information, and puts out new information. An **automated decision support system** uses knowledge and a set of rules for using the knowledge to interpret data and information to formulate recommendations. With a decision support system the user decides if the recommendations will be implemented. A decision support system relies on the wisdom of the user. An **automated expert system** goes one step further. An expert system implements the decision of the computer system without control by the user. The relationships among the concepts of data, information, knowledge, and wisdom, as well as information, decision support, and expert computer systems, are demonstrated in Figure 1-5.

Effective automated systems are dependent on the quality of data, information, and knowledge processed. Table 1-1 lists the attributes: good-quality data, information, and knowledge. These attributes provide a framework for developing evaluation forms that measure the quality of data, information, and knowledge. For example, health care data are presented as either text, numbers, or a combination of text and numbers (alphanumeric). Good-quality health data provide a complete description of the item being presented with accurate measurements. With the use of these attributes, an evaluation form can be developed to judge the quality of a completed patient assessment form or to judge the quality of a health care Web site on the Internet. The same process can be used with the attributes of knowledge. Think about the books or online references that one might access in developing a treatment plan for a patient, or consider a knowledge base

Table 1–1 Attributes of Good Data, Information, and Knowledge

	Attributes
Data	Descriptive
	Measurable
Information	Quantifiable
	Verifiable
	Accessible
	Free from bias
	Comprehensive
	Clear
	Appropriate
	Timely
	Precise
	Accurate
Knowledge	Accurate
	Relevant
	Quality

that is built into a decision support system. What would result if the knowledge were inaccurate or did not relate to the patient's problem, or if suggested approaches were ineffective for treating the patient's problem?

Although this section has focused on computer systems, humans can also be conceptualized as open systems that take in data, information, knowledge, and wisdom. The process is called learning. Learning theory provides a framework for understanding how humans as open systems take in, process, and put out data, information, knowledge, and wisdom.

LEARNING THEORIES

Learning theories attempt to determine how people learn and to identify the factors that influence the learning process. **Learning** is defined as an increase in knowledge, a change in attitude or values, or the development of new skills. Several learning theories have been developed. Each theory reflects a different paradigm or approach to understanding and explaining the learning process. One example that demonstrates the wide range of learning theories is the Theory Into Practice (TIP) database. TIP is a database containing summaries of 50 major theories of learning and instruction (Kearsley, 2000).

Learning theories are not mutually exclusive. They often overlap and are interrelated. This section focuses on four types of learning theories: behavioral; cognitive, or information processing, theories; adult learning; and learning styles. Learning theories are important to the practice of health care informatics for three reasons. First, health care informatics specialists plan and implement educational programs for teaching health care users to use new applications and systems. Second, learning theory is helpful in designing computer screens and developing computer-related procedures that are effective for health care users. Finally, these theories are helpful in understanding and building decision support systems in health care.

Behavioral Theories

The behavioral approach to learning, which was developed around the turn of the twentieth century, focuses on the smallest units of learning. In this theory the basic unit of learning is conceptualized as the stimulus-response (SR) unit. The stimulus is the input to the system or learner. The response is the output, or behavior exhibited by the learner. **Behavioral learning theories** provide two key concepts that can be used in informatics to explain learning. These are pairing and reinforcement. Pairing was first demonstrated by ringing a bell when offering food to a dog. The dog would salivate when the food was presented. Over time the sound of the bell alone would result in the dog's salivating (Booth-Butterfield, 1996). Thus the food and the bell were paired. The process of pairing is one approach to understanding computer phobia. New computer learners frequently make mistakes and become frustrated. Over a short period of time the negative experience can be paired with the computer, so that the presence of the computer itself can stimulate anxiety. Such pairing can be avoided if the learners' initial experience is carefully planned to encourage success, thereby minimizing the impact of mistakes.

The concept of reinforcement can also be used to explain computer phobia. Reinforcement may be positive or negative. Positive reinforcement encourages the learner to continue with correct behaviors. An example of positive reinforcement is telling the learner, "You are doing well" or "That is right." Negative reinforcement makes it possible to identify mistakes and correct them. An example of negative reinforcement is telling the learner, "You will need to spend more time working on this procedure" or "No, that is not the correct way to do this procedure; here is what you need to do." Effective learning involves both negative and positive reinforcement. However, if learners experience mostly negative reinforcement when learning to use a computer, they may begin to associate negative reinforcement with the computer in general rather than with the specific mistakes that should be corrected.

The behavioral approach to learning theory explains complex learning processes by breaking down learning into the smallest units. As a result, behavioral theory is referred to as the reductionist approach to learning. Although the behavioral approach demonstrates the relationship between a stimulus and a response, it does not explain the process of learning. This can be seen with systems theory and Figure 1-1. The behavioral approach includes the input to the system and the output from the system but does not deal with the processes within the system. At mid-century a new group of theories concerned with complex learning, such as problem solving or critical thinking, began to evolve. These theories fit with the systems theory approach and included input, processes, output, and feedback. These are the information processing, or cognitive learning, theories.

Information Processing, or Cognitive Learning, Theories

Information processing theories, or **cognitive learning theories**, divide learning into the following four steps:

1. How the learner takes input into the system
2. How that input is processed
3. What type of learned behaviors are exhibited as output
4. How feedback to the system is used to change or correct behavior

Input of Information

Data are taken into the system through the senses—vision, hearing, smell, taste, touch, and position. Several factors may influence the input process. First, data may be distorted or excluded if there is a sensory organ defect. Second, movement of data across the semipermeable boundary of the system limits how much data can enter at one time. For example, if one is listening to a person who is talking too fast, some of the words will be missed. In addition, the learner will screen out data that are considered irrelevant or meaningless, such as background noise. Data limits are also increased if the learner is under stress. Learners who are anxious about learning to use a computer program will experience higher data limits and thereby less learning.

New information that is presented using several senses at the same time is more likely to be taken in. For example, if a new concept is presented with the use of slides that are being explained by a speaker, the combination of both verbal and visual input makes it more likely that the learner will grasp the concept. As data enter the system, the learner structures and interprets these data, producing meaningful information. Previous learning has a major effect on how the data are structured and interpreted. For example, if a health care provider is comfortable using Windows and is now learning a new software program based on Windows, that learner will be able to quickly structure and interpret the new information using previously developed cognitive structures. If new information cannot be related to previous learning, learners will need to build the interpreting structures as they take in the new information. For example, a person who is reading new information may stop at the end of each sentence to think about the content in that sentence. Learners build interpreting cognitive structures as they import data. Learners who are hearing new information and taking notes at the same time may have difficulty capturing the content that they are trying to record. The more time needed to interpret and structure data, the slower the learners will be able to import data. Assessment of the learners' previous knowledge can help the instructor identify potential problems. Relating new information to previously learned information will help learners develop interpretive structures and in turn learn the information more effectively.

Input Processing

Short-Term Memory New information is interpreted and stored in short-term memory first. Short-term memory consists of the information that is currently being processed by the learner. It is the information that the learner is thinking about at a moment in time. An example is a telephone number that has just been found in a telephone book. The learner will hold the number in memory and actively work to retain the number. This type of memory has several characteristics similar to RAM in a computer. First, short-term memory has a limited capacity, holding about 7, plus or minus 2, bits of information. The size of the bit is determined by how the information is chunked. The number *1952* may be retained as four digits, or if the learner has interpreted this as a year, it may be 1 bit of data. The technique of using organizing structures (such as outlines), giving examples, and explaining how new information relates to previously learned concepts encourages the learner to develop chunks and increases retention.

The second characteristic of short-term memory is that the information is maintained in the temporal order that it was presented. Think of the way a phone number is remembered in order. This is important when presenting new information to a learner. If the information is presented in different temporal orders, it will be more difficult for the learner to retain. For example, an instructor is reviewing a list of commands. At the same time, the learners are given a written handout listing the commands. With computers there may be several approaches that can be used to achieve the same end. If the order that the instructor uses in presenting the commands is different from the order presented in the written materials, the learners can easily become confused. This same confusion occurs if different terminology is used. For example, a phone extension was dictated as "two zero four one." When it was repeated, the speaker said "twenty forty-one." "Twenty forty-one" and "two zero four one" are two ways of saying the same series of digits, but the human mind must do a conversion to create the same mental image of these numbers. The same thing happens when an instructor tells the novice user to "hit the return key," or "hit the enter key."

The third characteristic is that loss of information from short-term memory is inevitable. This occurs by fading or, as new information moves into short-term memory, replacing information in short-term memory. If the replaced information is moved to long-term memory, it can be recalled at a later date. However, when one is learning new information, there may not be time to store the information in long-term memory before it is replaced with more new information. This can often be seen when novice users are learning basic computing skills. First they are presented with a new skill. They understand the skill. They have interpreted the information, and it has meaning. This may be a new command that the learners have completed once or twice by following the directions of the teacher. Next the learners are presented with a second new command or more new information. If the first skill has been interpreted but not stored in long-term memory, the learners may have recognition but not recall. They cannot remember the steps for the first command. However, they will be able to recognize these steps when the instructor repeats them. This process, often seen with novice users learning new systems, is a source of frustration. For example, a novice user has just learned how to do a new procedure such as "cut and paste." The learner is sure he knows how to do this procedure. Next he learns how to change the name of a file after it has been saved. At this point the learner may not be able to recall all of the steps for doing the "cut and paste" procedure. If the instructor now repeats the steps, the learner will recognize each step and be frustrated that that he could not recall the steps on his own. Well-designed handouts and guides play a major role in helping learners deal with this phenomenon.

Long-Term Memory For learning to be maintained over time, the information must be stored in long-term memory. Information is retained in three common formats: episodic order, hierarchical order, or linked. For example, life events are often retained in episodic order. A list of computer commands is also retained in episodic order. Psychomotor episodic learned commands can become automatic. An example of this can be seen in the simple behavior of typing or the more complex behavior of driving a car. Cognitive learning tends to be retained in hierarchical order. For example, penicillin is an antibiotic. An antibiotic is a drug. Finally, information is retained because it is linked or related to other information. For example, the concept of paper is related to a printer. The process by which information is retained in long-term memory can be reinforced by a variety of teaching techniques. Providing students with an outline when presenting cognitive information helps to reinforce the retention of information in hierarchical order. Telling stories or jokes can be used to reinforce links among concepts. Practice exercises that encourage repeated use of computer commands assist with long-term retention of psychomotor episodic learning.

Although long-term memory can retain large amounts of information, two processes can interfere with the storage of information in long-term memory. First, new information or learning may replace old information. For example, health care providers may become very proficient with an automated order-entry system. However, over time they may not remember how to use the manual system for placing orders. This can be a problem if the manual system is the backup plan for computer downtime. Second, previously learned information can interfere with the learning of new information. This can be seen when a new computer system is installed and new procedures are implemented. Experienced users of the old system must remember *not* to use the old procedures that were part of that system. If the instructor for the new system includes clues to remind the experienced users of the change, the process of replacing old learning with new information can be reinforced.

When planning educational programs for health care users, the health care informatics specialist must first plan for intake of the new information via short-term memory and then for transfer of the new information to long-term memory. Several factors assist in moving information from short-term to long-term memory. A list of these factors and examples of each can be seen in Table 1-2. Information that is stored in long-term memory is used in critical thinking, problem solving, decision making, and a number of other mental processes.

Output Behaviors

Learned behaviors are exhibited as output. Three types of output behaviors are usually considered: cognitive, affective, and psychomotor. Cognitive behaviors reflect intellectual skills. They include critical thinking, problem solving, decision making, and a number of other mental processes. These are the skills that are used when designing a procedural manual for users of an automated

Table 1–2 Techniques for Moving Information From Short-Term to Long-Term Memory

Principle	Example
Distribute the learning over time.	It is more effective to schedule four 2-hour classes in 1 week than to schedule one 8-hour class in 1 day.
Plan to retain the information.	Before teaching new content, explain to the learners why the information will be important and when they will need to recall the new information.
Review the materials.	When presenting a list of new ideas, stop after each idea is explained and list each of the ideas that have already been explained.
Overlearn the content.	Once a group of learners has mastered certain concepts, give the group several exercises to reinforce the concepts.
Increase the time spent on task.	This does not mean increase the time scheduled for class; rather, increase the amount of time the learner is actively working on the content to be learned.

health care information system or troubleshooting a computer system that is not transmitting information correctly.

Affective skills relate to values and attitudes. Planning for the learning of appropriate values and attitudes is often overlooked yet can have a major impact on the implementation of an automated health care information system. Automating health care delivery requires change. This can be stressful for health care providers. Often, training programs focus exclusively on how to use the system. There is rarely time to discuss how to integrate the new system into patient care. There is limited discussion of the benefits of change and little support for the development of positive attitudes toward a new system. However, the development of positive values and attitudes can be important to the ongoing maintenance of automated systems in health care. Attitudes play a key role in users' decisions to suggest new and innovative uses for computer systems. Affective knowledge can be key to implementing security systems to protect the confidentiality of patient data. If a high value is placed on the confidentiality of patient data, the development and consistent implementation of security procedures will reflect that value.

Psychomotor skills involve the integration of cognitive and motor skills. These types of skills require time and practice to develop. During the time period when these skills are being developed, productivity is often decreased and users are often frustrated. When new health care information systems are implemented, the institution is usually very interested in measuring the impact of the new system. However, while new users are in the process of developing the psychomotor skills that are part of using the new system, it is ineffective to measure either the impact of the new system or user satisfaction.

Use of Feedback

During implementation, the focus should be on supporting the user's adjustment and troubleshooting problems. Any decision to make significant changes to a new system based on user feedback must be carefully evaluated.

Adult Learning Theories

Adult learning theories focus on the unique learning characteristics of adults. Andragogy is the art and science of helping adults learn (Knowles, 1970). Knowles's model proposes that adults share a number of similar learning characteristics and that these characteristics can be used in planning adult educational programs. Table 1-3 lists a number of these characteristics

Table 1–3 Adult Learning Characteristics and Related Applications

Learning Characteristics	Application
Adults are self-directed.	When planning the implementation of a new system, review with the users what they think they will need to learn about the new system.
Adults have accumulated a number of life experiences and cognitive structures. These are used to interpret new learning.	When teaching a new system, ask the students to provide examples from their experience and use these to explain how the new system will function.
Adults are practical and look for immediate application of learning.	Orientation to a new system should occur no more than 4 weeks before the actual implementation.
Adults are more interested in learning how to solve problems than in retention of facts.	When teaching adults about computer application, use real-life examples that can be expected to occur on the clinical unit.
Adult learners expect to be treated with respect and to have their previous learning acknowledged.	When explaining a new system, ask the students what they already know about the new system.

and provides examples of how these characteristics can be used to plan for teaching adult users.

Learning Styles

Since all learners are not alike, they learn in different ways. They vary in how they take in and process information. There are preferential differences in seeing and hearing new information. Some learners process information by reflecting; others process information by acting. Some learners approach reasoning logically; others are intuitive. Some learners learn by analyzing; others learn by visualizing. Learning theories concerning **learning styles** attempt to explain these differences. Experiential learning theory is one example (Kolb, 1984). The first stage of Kolb's theory involves concrete experience. For example, the learner may learn by viewing a demonstration of a new health care information system.

As learners begin to understand how the system works, they begin to think about how the system would work in their health care setting. This is the second stage, or reflection. In this stage learners reflect or think about the concrete experience. As they continue to think, they begin to form abstract conceptualizations of how the system functions. This is the third stage. Finally, learners are ready to try using the system. This is the fourth stage, when learners use their abstract conceptualization to guide action. In the model these four stages exist on two intersecting continuums. These are as follows:

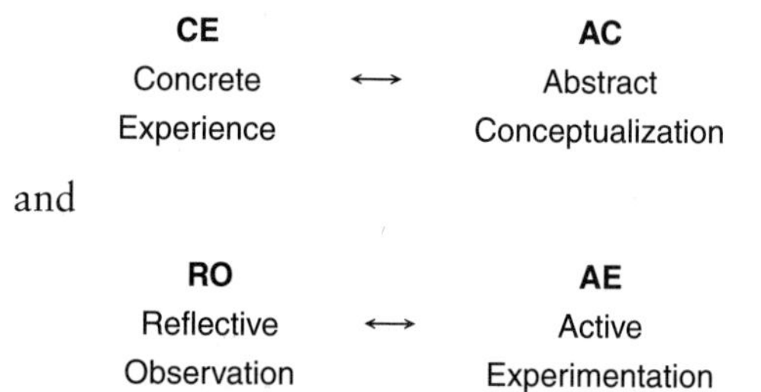

Learners differ in how they use each of these four stages in their individual learning approaches, but all learners ultimately learn by doing. Using this model, Kolb developed a learning assessment tool for identifying individual learning styles. The intersection of the two continua forms four quadrants: diverger, assimilator, converger, and accommodator. These are the four in-

Box 1–2 Learning Principles for Instructional Design

- Meaningfulness assists learning.
- Only so much input can be handled at one time.
- Timing of learning is critical.
- Participation and practice support retention.
- Conceptual learning is enhanced with concrete examples.
- Taking in new material through more than one modality can facilitate learning.
- Learning is enhanced when the teaching method includes the cognitive, affective, and psychomotor domains in concert.
- Learning takes place intentionally and unintentionally.
- Individuals learn at different rates and in different ways.
- Learning is contagious.

dividual learning styles in Kolb's model. The learner plots a score along the CE-AC scale, and the RO-AE scale to identify the quadrant that reflects his or her learning style.

A second widely used measure of individual learning styles is the Myers-Briggs Type Indicator (Myers & McCaulley, 1985). This theory identifies four continua:

Thinking ⟷ Feeling
Sensing ⟷ Intuition
Extroverted ⟷ Introverted
Judging ⟷ Perceptive

A series of questions are used to determine where the learner falls on each continuum. For example, a learner may be thinking, sensing, extroverted, and judging (TSEJ). The combination of where the learner falls on each of the four continua is then used to form a composite picture of the learner's preferred learning style.

A health care informatics specialist plans and implements educational programs for a variety of groups within the health care delivery system. These may include physicians, nurses, unlicensed personnel, administrators, and others. These groups vary widely in learning ability, education, motivation, and experience. However, there is also a great deal of variation among the learners within each group. An understanding of learning styles helps to explain these differences and to plan instructional strategies that are effective for individual learners within a group. Each of the four types of learning theories discussed in this chapter provides insights into effective approaches to teaching. Box 1-2 lists some examples of principles that are derived from these theories.

CHANGE THEORIES

Each of the theories presented in this chapter includes an element of change. As pointed out in the discussion of systems theory, all things constantly change. **Change theory** is the study of change in individuals or social systems, such as organizations. An understanding of change theory makes it possible to effectively plan and implement change in organizations and other social systems. Health care information systems have a major impact on the structure and functions of health care delivery systems. They bring about significant change. The approach used to manage the change process may result in a more effective and efficient health care delivery system, or it may result in increased dissatisfaction and disruption. Health care informatics specialists play a major role in planning for, guiding, and directing these changes. In other words, health care informatics specialists act as change agents.

The change process can be analyzed from two perspectives. The first view is demonstrated by Kurt Lewin's theory, which focuses on how a change agent can guide the change process. This is referred to as planned change. The second view focuses on the process by which people and social systems make changes. Research in this area has demonstrated that people in various cultures follow a similar pattern when incorporating innovation and change. Both views of change provide a framework for understanding how people react to change and for guiding the change process.

Planned Change

The father of change theory is Kurt Lewin. Lewin's theory of planned change divides change into three stages: unfreezing, moving, and refreezing (Schein, 1999). As demonstrated in the discussion of homeostasis, systems expend energy to stay in a steady state of stability. A system will remain stable when the restraining forces preventing change are stronger than the driving forces promoting change. Initiating change begins by increasing the driving forces and limiting the restraining forces, thereby increasing the instability of the system. This is the unfreezing stage. The first stage in the life cycle of an information system involves evaluating the current system and deciding what changes need to be made. The pros and cons for change reflect the driving and restraining forces. If changes are to be made, the restraining forces that maintain a stable system and resist change must be limited. At the same time, the driving forces that encourage change must be increased. For example, pointing out to users the limitations and weaknesses with the current information management system increases the driving forces. Asking for user input early in the process before decisions have been made decreases the restraining forces. Once a decision is made to initiate change, the second stage—moving—begins.

The moving stage is the implementation of the planned change. By definition this is an unstable period for the social system. Anxiety levels are increased. The social system attempts to minimize the impact or degree of change. This resistance to change may occur as missed meetings, failure to attend training classes, and failure to provide staff with information about the new system. If the resistance continues, it can cause the planned change to fail. Health care informatics specialists, as change agents, must anticipate and minimize these resistive efforts. This can be as simple as providing food at meetings or as complex as a planned program of recognition for early adopters. For example, an article in the institution's newsletter describing and praising the pilot units for their leadership will encourage the driving forces for change.

Once the system is in place or the change has been implemented, additional energy is needed to maintain the change. This is the refreezing phase and occurs during the maintenance phase of the information system's life cycle. If managed effectively by the change agent, this phase is characterized by increased stability. In this stage, forces resistant to change are encouraged. Some examples include training programs for new employees, a yearly review of all policies and procedures related to the change, and continued recognition for those who become experts with the new system.

Diffusion of Innovation

Individual Responses to Innovation

The **diffusion of innovation** theory, developed by Everett Rogers, explains how individuals and communities respond to new ideas, practices, or objects (Rogers, 1995). Diffusion of innovation is the process by which an innovation is communicated through certain channels over time among members of a social system. Innovations may be either accepted or rejected. Health care automation, with new ideas and technology, involves ongoing diffusion of innovation. By understanding the diffusion of innovation process and the factors that influence this process, health care informatics specialists can assist individuals and organizations in maximizing the benefits of automation.

Social systems consist of individuals within organizations. Both the individuals and the organization as a whole vary in how they respond to innovations. The individuals can be classified into five groups based on their responses to change.

These groups are innovators, early adopters, early majority, late majority, and laggards. **Innovators** are the first 2.5% of individuals within a system to adapt to an innovation. These individuals tend to be more cosmopolitan. They are comfortable with uncertainty and above average in their understanding of complex technical concepts. These are the individuals who test out a new technology; however, they are not usually respected by other members of the social system. They will not be able to sell others on trying the new technology. This is the role of the **early adopters.**

Early adopters are the next 13.5% of individuals in an organization. Early adopters are more local in focus. They are perceived as discreet in their adoption of new ideas and serve as role models for others in the organization. Change agents should work at identifying these individuals and providing recognition for their efforts. Because of their leadership role within the organization, the support of early adopters is key when introducing new approaches to automation. If the early adopters accept an innovation, the **early majority** will follow their example. This is the next 34% of individuals in an organization. Members of the early majority are willing to adapt to an innovation but not to lead. However acceptance by the early majority means that the innovation is becoming well integrated into the organization.

The **late majority** is the next group to accept an innovation. The late majority makes up 34% of individuals in an organization. Most of the uncertainty that is inherent with a new idea must be removed before this group will adopt an innovation. They adopt the innovation not because of their interest in the innovation but rather as a result of peer pressure. The late majority is followed by the last 16% of individuals in an organization. These are the **laggards.** Laggards focus on the local environment and on the past. They are resistant to change and will change only when there is no other alternative. They are suspicious of change and change agents. Change agents should not spend time encouraging laggards to change but rather should work at establishing policies and procedures that will incorporate the innovation into the required operation of the organization.

Organizational Responses to Innovation

Just as individuals vary in their response to innovations, organizations also vary. There are five internal organizational characteristics that can be used to understand how an organization will respond to an innovation (Trujillo, 2000):

1. Centralization—Organizations that are highly centralized, with power concentrated in the hands of a few individuals, tend to be less accepting of new ideas and therefore less innovative.
2. Complexity—Organizations in which many of the individuals have a high level of knowledge and expertise tend to be more accepting of innovations. However, these types of organizations can have difficulty in reaching a consensus on approaches to implementation.
3. Formalization—Organizations that place a great deal of emphasis on rules and procedures tend to inhibit new ideas and innovation. However, this tendency toward rules and procedures does make it easier to implement an innovation.
4. Interconnectedness—Organizations in which there are strong interpersonal networks linking the individuals within the organization are better prepared to communicate and share innovation. This can be seen, for example, in organizations that use eMail as an integral part of organizational communication.
5. Organizational slack—Organizations with uncommitted resources are better prepared to manage innovation. These resources may be people and/or money.

Although these characteristics help to explain how an organization as a whole will respond to an innovation, they can be analyzed from both an individual and an organizational level. For example, adapting to new software involves a certain degree of complexity. Think about what is involved when an individual must select a new word processing program. Now think about what is involved if an organization decides to select new word processing software as its standard software.

The perceived attributes of the innovation, the nature of organizational communication channels, the innovative-decision process, and the efforts of change agents influence the possibility that an innovation will be adopted and the rate of adoption. There are five attributes that can be used to characterize an innovation:

1. Relative advantage—Is the innovation an improvement over the current approach?
2. Compatibility—Does the innovation fit with existing values, past experiences, and individual needs?
3. Complexity—Is the innovation easy to use and understand?
4. Trialability—Can the innovation be tested or tried before individuals must make a commitment?
5. Observability—Are the results of using the innovation visible to others?

If each of these five questions related to the five innovative attributes can be answered with a "yes," then it is more likely that the innovation will be adopted and that the adoption will occur at a rapid rate. If, on the other hand, an innovation is not gaining acceptance, these characteristics can be used as a framework for evaluating the source of the problem. For example, it may take more time to document a patient assessment with an automated system. As a result, nurses will prefer the manual system because of the relative advantage.

Stages of Acceptance

The decision of individuals and organizations to accept or reject an innovation is not an instantaneous event. The process involves five stages. These stages can be demonstrated when a health care institution considers providing eMail to all professional staff. The first stage of the innovation—the decision stage—is knowledge. In the knowledge stage the individual or organization becomes aware of the existence of the innovation. Mass communication channels are usually most effective at this stage. For example, the institution's newsletter may carry a story about eMail and how staff could use it to support interinstitutional communication with other institutions. If there are no mass communication channels open to the change agent, the knowledge stage may be significantly delayed. Whereas personal-type information moves quickly via informal face-to-face communication channels, cognitive information does not move quickly through these types of channels.

Once individuals become aware of an innovation, they begin to develop opinions or attitudes about the innovation. This is the persuasion stage. During the persuasion stage, interpersonal channels of communication are more important, and early adopters begin to play a key role. In the persuasion stage, attitudes are not fixed but are in the process of being formed. The health care informatics specialist should work closely with the early adopters in developing and communicating positive attitudes to others in the organization.

As these attitudes become more fixed, individuals make decisions to accept or reject the innovation. This is the decision stage. It is at this point that individuals will decide to try the eMail system. For each person this decision can occur at a different point. Early adopters will decide to try the system before the early majority. The individual will test out the system during the implementation stage. In testing out the system, most people begin to discover new features or functions of the system. As they gain a better understanding of how the new eMail system functions, modifications and adjustments are made. For example, eMail is a more informal form of communication. Will individuals be addressed by their first names, or will professional titles be maintained? The health care informatics specialist needs to be sensitive to these modifications. Modifications take on an added significance when formal and informal policies and procedures are developed. The final stage is confirmation. At this point the innovation is no longer an innovation. It has either been rejected or has become the standard procedure. For example, key interinstitutional communication will depend on staff using eMail. Change at this point requires a new innovation.

Using Change Theories

Effective change requires a champion(s) with a clear vision, a culture of trust, an organizational sense of pride, and the intense involvement of the people who must live with the change. The champion must have the institutional resources to support the change process. These resources include leadership skills, personnel (including change agents), money, and time. The change agent uses change theory to understand and manage reactions to change throughout the change process. Reactions to change may be negative, such as resistance, frustration, aggression, surface acceptance, indifference, ignoring, or organized resistance. Or the reaction to change may be positive, such as a sense of pride, supporting and encouraging others, demonstrating how the innovation improves the organization, and overall acceptance. Change agents usually discover both positive and negative reactions during the change process. It is usually more effective to support the positive reactions to change than it is to spend time and effort responding to negative reactions.

CONCLUSION

Health care is an information-intensive service. Automation and the use of technology provide an effective and efficient means to manage the large volumes of data and information with knowledge and wisdom. However, the move from a manual to an automated world is changing every aspect of health care. This degree of change brings excitement, anxiety, resistance, and pride. Health care informatics specialists function at the very core of this change. They play a major role in implementing, managing, and leading health care organizations as they move forward with automation. To play this role, they work directly with the clinical, administrative, and technical personnel in the organization. For health care informatics specialists to provide effective leadership, they must understand the institutions, the people, and the processes within the organizations. The theories presented in this chapter provide a framework for supporting and managing the enormous degree of change experienced by the health care system and the people within the health care system.

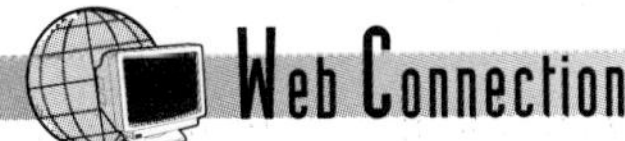

Theories and models are used to explain ways of viewing the world. Concepts come together in relationships to form theories and models. As noted in this chapter, the basis of all of the theories used in health care informatics is system theory. It is suitable then that we use a preeminent system—the World Wide Web—to continue with our learning. Using the World Wide Web as a portal to data and information can facilitate the development of our knowledge. In the Web Connection for this chapter, activities will be offered to reinforce theories, models, concepts, and relationships that are described and illustrated in the chapter. These activities will allow you to make and reinforce the connections that are introduced in the chapter. You will explore the ways in which the concepts of "data," "information," "knowledge," "wisdom," and "change" are used today.

discussion questions

1. List and explain how theoretical knowledge can be used to plan future approaches, as well as to solve current problems, related to informatics.
2. Examine the following icon. Use this icon to explain systems theory (include characteristics of systems and how change impacts systems).
3. Use Shannon and Weaver's model of information to describe communication in a health care informatics class.

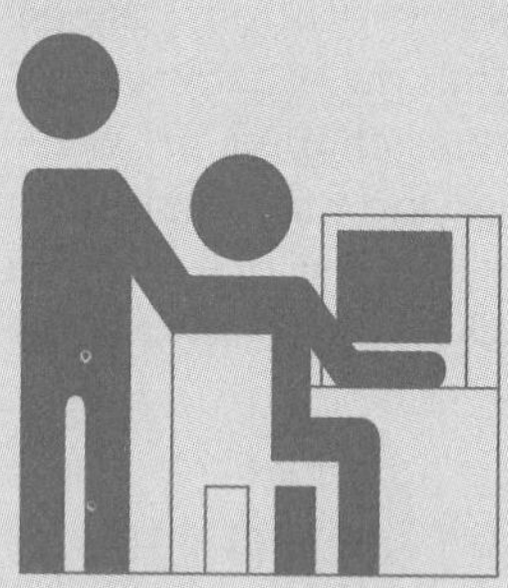

4. Use Blum's model of information to explain how computers are now used and may be used in the future to support health care delivery.
5. Define the concepts of data, information, knowledge, and wisdom. Explain the relationships among these concepts.
6. This chapter includes four types of learning theories. Use each of the types of learning theories to explain how people learn when learning about computers in health care.
7. The response of individuals to innovations has been classified into five groups. List and describe the five groups.
8. List and explain the five internal organizational characteristics that can be used to predict how an organization will respond to a change in automation. Use these five characteristics to predict how the American health care delivery system will respond to health care computing innovations in the next 5 years.

REFERENCES

Blum, B. (1986). *Clinical information systems.* New York: Springer-Verlag.

Booth-Butterfield, S. (1996). Classical conditioning. In *Steve's primer of practical persuasion and influence.* Retrieved July 6, 2000, from the World Wide Web: http://www.as.wvu.edu/~sbb/comm221/primer.htm.

Graves, J., & Corcoran, S. (1989). The study of nursing informatics. *Image: The Journal of Nursing Scholarship,* 21(4), 227-230.

Hawking, S.W. (1988). *A brief history of time.* New York: Bantam Books.

Hersh, W. (1996). *Information retrieval: A health care perspective.* New York: Springer.

Information. In *Merriam-Webster online: Merriam-Webster's collegiate dictionary.* (2000). Retrieved October 8, 2000, from the World Wide Web: http://www.m-w.com/dictionary.htm.

Joos, I., Nelson, R., & Lyness A. (1985). *Man, health and nursing.* Reston, VA: Reston Publishing.

Kearsley, G. (2000). *Explorations in learning and instruction: The theory into practice database.* Retrieved June 19, 2000, from the World Wide Web: http://www.gwu.edu/~tip/index.html.

Knowles, M. (1970). *The modern practice of adult education: Andragogy versus pedagogy.* New York: Associated Press.

Kolb, D. (1984). *Experiential learning: Experience as the source of learning and development.* Englewood Cliffs, NJ: Prentice-Hall.

Myers, I.B., & McCaulley, M.H. (1985). *Manual: A guide to the development and use of the Myers-Briggs Type Indicator.* Palo Alto, CA: Consulting Psychologists Press.

Nelson, R., & Joos, I. (1989). On language in nursing: From data to wisdom. *PLN Visions, Fall,* 6-7.

Rogers, E.M. (1995). *Diffusion of innovation* (4th ed.). New York: The Free Press.

Schein, E. (1999). *Kurt Lewin's change theory in the field and in the classroom: Notes toward a model of managed learning.* Retrieved June 4, 2000, from the World Wide Web http://learning.mit.edu/res/wp/10006.html#toc.

Shannon, C.E. (1948). A mathematical theory of communication. *Bell System Technical Journal,* 27, July, pp. 379-423, and October, pp. 623-656. Retrieved June 2, 2000, from the World Wide Web: http://www.stat.purdue.edu/people/yiannis/info.html.

Shannon, C., & Weaver, W. (1949). *The mathematical theory of communication.* Urbana: University of Illinois.

Trujillo, M.F. (2000). *Diffusion of ICT innovations for sustainable human development—Problem definition.* Retrieved June 27, 2000, from the World Wide Web: http://payson.tulane.edu/research/E-DiffInnova/diff-prob.html.

Von Bertalanffy, L. (1975). General systems theory. In B.D. Ruben & J.Y. Kim (Eds.), *General systems theory and human communication.* Rochelle Park, NJ: Haydan.

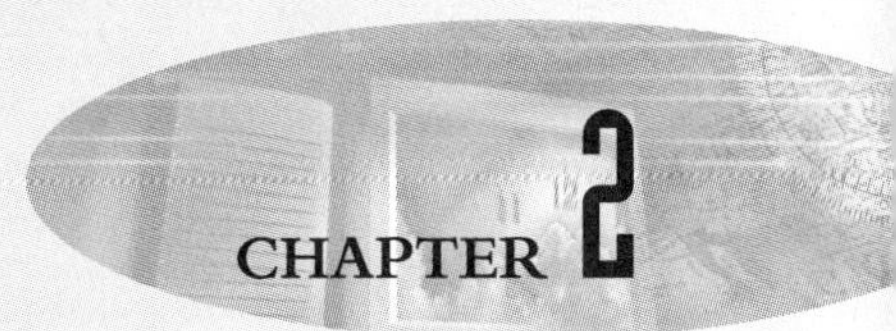

Computer, Information, and Health Care Informatics Literacy

JULIA R. SHAW-KOKOT
KATHLEEN A. MCGRAW
MARGARET EILENE MOORE

Learning Objectives

Upon completion of this chapter, the reader will be able to:

1. ***Define*** *information, computer,* and *health care informatics literacy.*
2. ***Identify*** key literacy terms and components.
3. ***Discuss*** the skills required for information and computer literacy.
4. ***Apply*** computer and information literacy skills to the health care setting.

Outline

Information Literacy
- *Cognitive Information Literacy Skills*
- *Identifying and Defining*
- *Searching and Locating*
- *Evaluating and Retrieving*
- *Organizing, Managing, and Using*

Computer Literacy
- *Hardware*
- *Connectivity*
- *Software*

Evaluating and Improving Literacy
- *Diversity of Skills*
- *Identifying Literacy Objectives and Measuring Existing Knowledge*
- *Offering Training to Increase Knowledge*
- *Evaluating the Results of Training*

Applications of Professional Knowledge
- *Lifelong Learner*
- *Clinician*
- *Educator/Communicator*
- *Researcher*
- *Manager*

Key Terms

access
AMIA
bibliographic managers
bit
Boolean operators
byte
CILM
CINAHL
cognitive skills
computer literacy
controlled vocabulary
data
data sets
delivery methods
Delphi technique
FITness
full text
hardware

Key Terms—cont'd

HealthSTAR
ICPC
IMIA
informatics literacy
information
information competencies
information literacy
information need
input devices
ISI
knowledge
logic
MeSH
needs statement
open source software
operating system
output devices
resources
SNOMED
software
software applications
static information
storage devices
strategies
terms
textwords
truncation
UMLS
vendor
wildcard
WYSIWYG

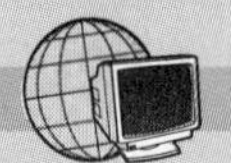

Web Connection

Go to the Web site at http://evolve.elsevier.com/Englebardt/. Here you will find Web links and activities related to computer, information, and health care informatics literacy.

Health **informatics literacy** occurs at the intersection of information literacy, computer literacy, and the application of professional knowledge during the delivery of health care services. Figure 2-1 illustrates this relationship. **Information literacy** is defined as the ability to identify an **information need,** locate pertinent **information,** evaluate the information, and apply it correctly. **Computer literacy** is defined as the ability to acquire and apply a basic understanding of current computer hardware systems and software applications to a problem in a particular work or personal setting. The professional **knowledge** that an individual practitioner draws on to provide health care services results from the combination of education and experience. Ideally, health informatics at the intersection of these three complex sets of skills facilitates the delivery of efficient, cost-effective, high-quality care.

INFORMATION LITERACY

Why is information literacy vital to health care informatics? Information is everywhere, and the literate provider must have the skills to negotiate the information jungle, identify the best resources for the given need, and use the knowledge gained. "In an era when today's 'truths' become tomorrow's outdated concepts, individuals who are unable to gather pertinent information are almost as helpless as those who are unable to read or write" (Breivik & Gee, 1989, p. 23).

No one person or group can keep up with the constant changes in information resources, **access,** and **delivery methods.** Colleagues, books, journals, films, Internet sites, **data sets,** eMail, mailing lists, newsgroups, and computer files are a few of the information **resources** used for problem solving and decision making.

In the past, someone needing to search a database of references would go to a library and talk

FIGURE 2–1 | Health Care Informatics Literacy

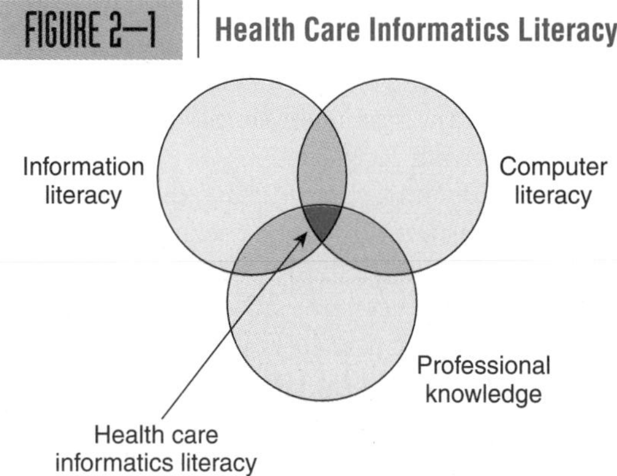

to a librarian. Now those databases and increasing numbers of **full text** journals are available via computer networks wherever the information is needed, and the person looking for information does not need to go to the library.

Many types of information resources can be accessed and retrieved from the office, home, beach, or any other location via desktop, laptop, or handheld computer with an Internet connection. An intermediary can be contacted by phone, eMail, or teleconference, but the searcher in most cases needs to have the skills necessary to independently complete the information-seeking process.

Increasingly, professional associations and groups are grappling with defining and evaluating information literacy. Health care groups, such as the American Nurses Association (ANA), the National League for Nursing (NLN), the American Association of Colleges of Nursing, the Association of American Medical Colleges (AAMC), and the International Medical Informatics Association **(IMIA)**, have defined information literacy competencies.

There are many ways to define core **information competencies** or skills. The information-literate health care provider has developed the necessary information literacy skills and the ability to use these skills to solve problems and make decisions in all practice roles. The AAMC Medical Informatics Advisory Panel has identified five professional roles requiring information competencies: (1) lifelong learner, (2) clinician, (3) educator/communicator, (4) researcher, and (5) manager (Medical school objectives project, 2000). The AAMC's roles are present in all health care professions and can be matched with corresponding Pew Commission Competencies found in the Third Report of the Pew Health Professions Commission (Critical challenges, 1995). Although the information needed for each role may be significantly different, the **cognitive skills** or critical thinking skills necessary to retrieve and use information are the same.

Cognitive Information Literacy Skills

Why stress the cognitive, or critical thinking, rather than the task approach? Tasks change rapidly, and skills must be transferable to new tasks. The underlying knowledge of the process used to identify an information need, locate pertinent information, and evaluate the information must be sound in order to master the transfer. Information that remains the same after publication, **static information,** is frequently used for overviews, background, and historical perspectives. Although books provide a good basic introduction to a clinical problem, the most current and in-depth information will be found in current journal articles or specialized sites on the Internet.

The dynamic nature of information access and transfer is especially evident in health care. For example, a patient is seen in a health care facility and wants to know if his rash could be caused by his medications. The health care provider reviews this patient's record using a computer, checks for drug interactions via a computerized drug information system, and searches a computerized database of journal articles for additional information. She prints out the drug information and discusses the side effects with the patient, quickly scans a couple of full text articles, and orders laboratory tests via the electronic ordering system. The next day she gets an eMail message telling her that the laboratory results are ready, checks the results, notifies the patient via eMail about the findings, and sets up another appointment. The point of this example is that each provider is a member of a group of experts who have combined their skills to produce the materials used to respond to a particular need. But the individual provider is the information seeker who synthesizes, analyzes, and reports the findings.

Over time, the tasks required for information access and retrieval have changed as the information delivery methods have changed. However, the cognitive approach to the information-seeking process has remained the same:

1. The need(s) is identified.
2. The types of information required to meet the need(s) are defined.
3. A search of the information resources is conducted.
4. The information found is evaluated.
5. The items appropriate to the information need are retrieved.
6. The information is organized and disseminated in a useful manner.

Identifying and Defining

Identifying and defining the information need is the foundation for all information literacy skills. A clear understanding of the information need, meaning of the specific information needed and how it will be used, increases the ease and efficiency of searching, locating, evaluating, retrieving, organizing, and managing the resources required to meet the need (Schloss & Smith, 1999).

Developing a Needs Statement

The first information literacy skill is developing a needs statement. Other terms frequently used synonymously with **needs statement** are problem statement, topic statement, and search statement. No matter what term is used, developing the statement before starting the search is the same as planning an itinerary before a trip. It gives direction. There may be detours and serendipitous findings, but the statement should prevent heading in the wrong direction.

The needs statement differs depending on how the information will be used. For example, information is needed about the computerized patient record. This needs statement is much too general; however, it reflects the way that needs statements are often stated. How can this needs statement be refined to meet the specific need? Determine how the information will be used, and come up with a more specific statement to get to the end point. See Box 2-1 for examples of how needs statements can be refined for the different professional roles. The literature on research methods and evidence-based medicine offers tips on refining information needs statements (Brodie, Williams, & Owens, 1994; Richardson et al., 1995; Wood, 1996) The needs statement will continue to be refined throughout the information-seeking process.

Identifying and Defining Terms

Identifying **terms**—words or phrases used to identify information needs—would be easy if the uses of terminology were consistent, but terms frequently have different meanings depending on context, topic area, region, or country. Therefore it is important to remember that terms and spelling may be different for different groups. These variations must be taken into consideration. This concept of multiple meanings is especially true when dealing with abbreviations. One example is the abbreviation *PID,* which can stand for pelvic inflammatory disease in a clinical setting and personal identification in computer terminology. Another example is the term used for sudden death of infants. The term *sudden infant death syndrome* is used in the United States, but in British Commonwealth countries the term *cot death* is used. Another variation is spelling. For example, in the United States the word for the specialty area that deals with the blood and

Box 2–1 Needs Statement Related to Role

- *Lifelong learner:* End use—Develop a basic knowledge of computerized patient records systems. Statement—Identify the vocabulary, concepts, issues, and trends related to computerized patient records systems.
- *Clinician:* End use—Provide a secure computerized patient records system that protects private and confidential information. Statement—Investigate issues, policies, and procedures related to the privacy and confidentiality of computerized patient records.
- *Educator/communicator:* End use—Develop, implement, and evaluate staff training for the computerized medical records system. Statement—Find information on how other facilities have developed, implemented, and evaluated training activities for computerized patient records, and look at concepts and trends in training staff to use these systems.
- *Researcher:* End use—Establish the relationship between computerized patient records systems and decreased patient care errors. Statement—Find studies and data on the effectiveness of computerized patient records systems in preventing patient care errors and comparisons with traditional medical records handling.
- *Manager:* End use—Develop a policy and procedures manual for the facility. Statement—Identify concepts, skills, and resources for inclusion in a policy and procedures manual.

blood-forming organs is *hematology*. The British spelling of the same term is *haematology*. Although many of today's electronic search systems compensate for these variations, others still require exact term matches. Before starting a search, the searchers should think about these variations. Several examples of possible terms for computerized patient records systems are included in Box 2-2.

The best advice is to know the requirements of the search tool. Every print, database, and Internet search tool has a unique structure, a unique language, and unique functions. This becomes even more apparent with resources that provide statistics, images, data sets, or full text documents.

Box 2–2 Alternative Terms for Computerized Patient Records

- Computerized medical records systems
- Medical records systems, computerized (Medical Subjects Headings [MeSH])
- Computer-based patient records
- Electronic patient records
- Digital patient records
- Clinical data repository

Developing Search Strategies

Once the information need has been identified and defined, the next step is to develop search strategies. Search **strategies** are the techniques used in the investigation. Strategies need to be fluid and flexible but structured enough to provide focus for the search. No matter how well the terms and approaches are identified, new terms, resources, formats, and other avenues will appear as the information search progresses. It is important to be able to use the appropriate newly discovered alternatives, but not to get sidetracked from the overall strategy. If the needs statement is the itinerary, the well-planned strategy is the road guide. The following are key concepts to consider.

Textword and Controlled Vocabulary Searching

Textword—natural language—and **controlled vocabulary**—subject heading—are two structures for accessing information. Textword or keyword searching is totally flexible. With this approach, the exact word or phrase searched for is retrieved by the search tool from any area of the information included in the record. This could be a full text article, a Web site, a data set, or any other resource. Therefore it is imperative to use multiple terms. Most Internet search sites use textword searching. The following are problems that arise when using textword searching:

- Lack of precision
- Retrieval of terms that may not be related or in the desired context
- Massive retrieval when the word occurs in multiple entries
- Difficulty narrowing the retrieval down to the items needed

When a database has a controlled vocabulary, indexers assign subject headings to each record on the basis of an established list of criteria. These lists, which usually include synonyms and antonyms, are frequently called *thesauri.* A thesaurus is usually available in print and/or electronic format from the resource producer. Subject headings take much of the guesswork out of what terms to use. The problems that arise when using controlled vocabulary include lack of currency because of the time required for the indexing process and exclusion of new terms until the next updating of the thesaurus.

The best-known example of a controlled vocabulary in health care is Medical Subject Headings (**MeSH**). The MeSH thesaurus is published by the National Library of Medicine (NLM) in print form and is also available electronically from the NLM Web site. See Box 2-3 for an example of MeSH terms and structure. Other schemas are in use or are being developed by health care groups. Some of these schemas include the Unified Medical Language System

Box 2–3 Example of MeSH Structure

- Medical informatics
  - Medical informatics computing
    - Computer literacy
    - Computer systems
      - Computer communication networks
        - Internet
        - Local area networks
    - Computers +
      - Computing methodologies
        - Algorithms
        - Artificial intelligence +
        - Automatic data processing +
        - Computer graphics +
        - Computer simulation
        - Image processing, computer-assisted +
        - Mathematical computing +
        - Signal processing, computer-assisted +
      - Software
        - Data display +
        - Database management systems
        - Grateful Med
        - Hypermedia
        - Programming languages
        - Software design
        - Software validation
        - User-computer interface
        - Video games
        - Word processing

Compiled from the NCBI MeSH Browser, December 2000 (http://www4.ncbi.nlm.nih.gov/htbin-post/Entrez/meshbrowser).
+ Represents additional terms.

(**UMLS**), International Classification of Primary Care (**ICPC**), and Systematized Nomenclature of Human and Veterinary Medicine (**SNOMED**) (Duisterhout et al., 1997). These controlled vocabularies or standard languages are discussed in detail in Chapter 18.

Some resources allow the use of both controlled vocabulary and textword searching. The ability to use both search strategies corrects many of the problems associated with the two searching schemes but requires an understanding of when to use one approach or the other. Reading the help file(s) provided by each search tool is an important way to develop an understanding of the resource and associated searching schemas.

Truncation **Truncation** is the use of symbols to represent letters to search for variations in spelling or forms of a word. By using wildcards, one can retrieve different character combinations for a given word. **Wildcards** are symbols, such as asterisks, that are used to represent the characters in the truncation process. Depending on the database, these symbols can be used anywhere within the word, but the most common place for truncation is at the end of a word. See Box 2-4 for examples of internal truncation to assist in overcoming spelling variations, as well as end-of-the-word truncation to retrieve variant endings. Each resource and/or system has established rules for truncation and wildcard symbols. Again, the system help files will help in identifying wildcard symbols and rules for their use.

Boolean Operators **Boolean operators** represent a form of **logic** used to combine terms in searching. The three most frequently used operators are *and, or,* and *not.* These are used in searching most electronic database systems and the Internet. Use of Boolean operators optimizes retrieval. See Figure 2-2 for a graphical depiction of these operators. Further discussion of Boolean operators can be found in Chapter 3.

And requires both terms or phrases to be included in a search and helps to narrow a search.

Box 2–4 Examples of Truncation

- Internal truncation: h#ematology = hematology or haematology
- End-of-word truncation: comput$ = computer, computers, computing, computerized, etc.
- Common wildcard symbols: *, $, #, and ?

FIGURE 2–2 Boolean Operators

AND Both terms must be present

Diabetes AND Diagnosis

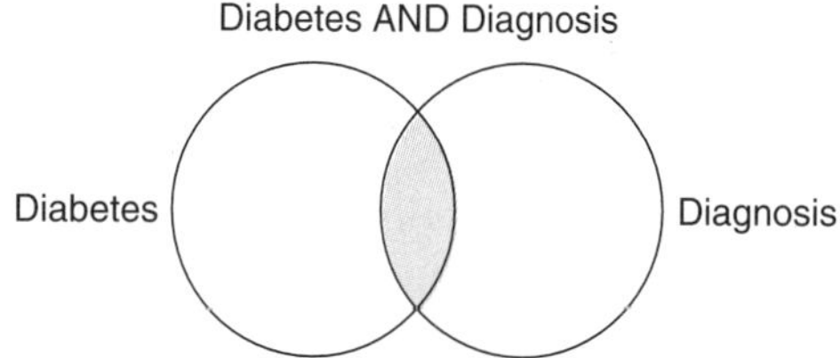

OR Either term is present

Cancer OR Neoplasm

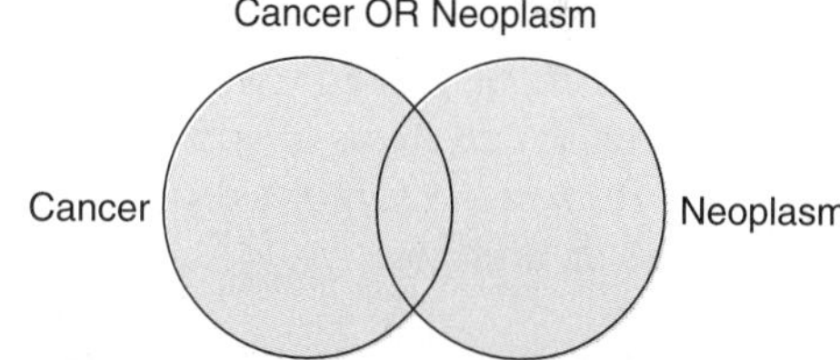

NOT Term does not appear

Prozac NOT Depression

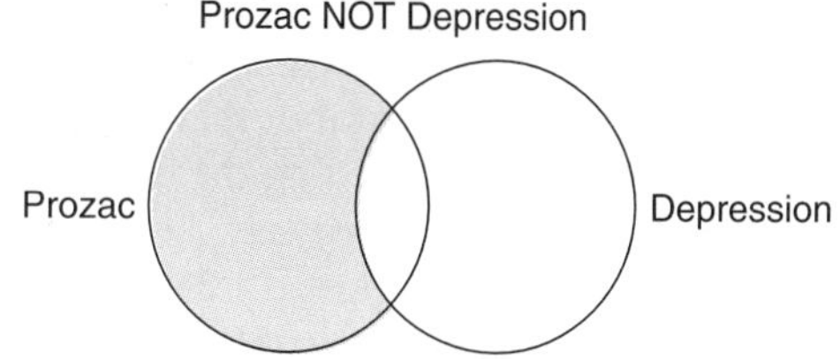

This is especially important when a large number of citations are returned. Many Web-based systems automatically use *and*. The Centers for Disease Control and Prevention's CDC Wonder databases, for example, require selecting a combination of terms to find the **data** required. Once the selections have been made, the computer automatically combines the selections using the *and* operator.

Or requires either of the terms or phrases to be included and helps to broaden a search. This is especially important when searching topics with multiple terms or synonyms. For example, when searching for information about a drug, it is important to search for both the trade and generic names and often the registry number. Although information can be retrieved using any of these terms, the only way to ensure seeing all of the information is to add *or* when searching for the terms together.

Not requires that a term or phrase not be present. This is another way of narrowing a search. Because it is totally exclusive, using the *not* operator is riskier and less dependable than using the *and* operator to narrow a search. For example, when seeking information on electronic communication tools other than eMail, it would be tempting to search for electronic communication tools "*not* eMail." Any resource that had the word eMail would be dropped, and relevant articles could easily be missed. *Not* is appropriately used to eliminate items already reviewed. See Table 2-1 for search examples demonstrating the use of *and, or,* and *not.*

Table 2–1 Use of Boolean Operators in Searching

No.	Search History	Results
And		
1	Informatics	1,453
2	Nursing	36,675
3	1 *and* 2	47
Or		
1	Lorazepam (generic name)	1,612
2	Ativan (generic name)	33
3	846-49-1 (CAS registry number)	1,423
4	1 *or* 2 *or* 3	1,612
Not		
1	Hospital information systems	2,660
2	Laboratories, hospital	1,138
3	1 *and* 2	16
4	Medical records systems, computerized	3,411
5	2 *and* 4	12
6	5 *not* 3	9

Based on numbers from a December 2000 OVID search.

Searching and Locating

The information-seeking skills used to search and locate information include inquisitiveness, persistence, and adaptation, along with knowledge of the resources available. The itinerary is set and the trip marked out, but there will probably be detours before reaching the destination. For example, a search strategy can be developed for finding a free color image of a heart in a specific graphical interchange format (GIF) without copyright restrictions to illustrate a patient education pamphlet. Several sites on the Internet with good color images can be found, and these sites have links to other sites and references to CD-ROM (compact disk read-only memory) clip art programs. There are many variations in the image size, color, and appearance that can be selected, but the identified need in this case emphasizes the format and copyright needs. Looking for images that meet this requirement is more efficient than going through all of the images.

Identifying Resources and Formats

The next step in the searching and locating process is to consider the types of resources that will satisfy the information needs. At this stage it is helpful to cast a wide net and to consider all options. A resource may be a person, a database, a book, a journal, a collection of materials, a patient record, or any other contact or material. Format relates to how the resource is accessed and how the information is presented. For example, contact with a colleague could be face-to-face, by phone, by mail, by eMail, or by other electronic communication.

Increasingly, publicly available resources are accessed via electronic information retrieval. Much of the information collected, such as books, journals, patient information, images, or phone books, is available in electronic format. The move to electronic information retrieval is welcome, but the transformation is a work in progress. Format can be further broken down on the basis of the access method (e.g., accessible on the Internet) or by location (e.g., a library or agency). Format considerations also include the amount of information presented. Brief information, such as a citation, offers only the basic information needed to assist in locating the complete information. Complete information frequently includes full text articles, images, and data files. For example, a chapter in a general text might be found in either printed or electronic format. The electronic format could either include a CD-ROM, a Web-based source, or a handheld device application. Because information formats are still in transition, the search should avoid limiting information selection to one format. Tips on selecting a resource are given in Box 2-5.

Print Resources Even as the move to electronic resources accelerates, much information is still found in print. Many academic institutions, as well as state, local, and hospital libraries, have open access online catalogs for identifying and locating print books and journal titles. Items that are not available locally can often be obtained by interlibrary loan. A good place to identify titles on a health topic or to find out what is in print is the National Library of Medicine's (NLM's) online library catalog, called LOCATORplus. LOCATORplus is not an inclusive list, but it does offer a wide range of resources.

Box 2–5 Resource Selection Tips

- For a quick overview of a topic, try a chapter in a general text, a review article, or a book using an online library catalog by searching for broad subjects or by keywords.
- For in-depth background information, try a text on a specific topic, or search an Internet site for a specific field.
- For the latest research or to look for details not found in texts or books, use an electronic database; an Internet site for a specific field; or a person, agency, or association that specializes in the information needed.

Electronic Resources Electronic resources are the fastest-growing areas of information access and delivery. These resources are convenient, but accessing them is not always an easy task. They often require user IDs and passwords, special configurations such as proxy servers, and/or agreements or association with institutions. Electronic resources can be broken down into at least three general groups: literature databases, journals, and the Internet.

Literature Databases Literature databases are collections of literature related to a specific topic or domain. A growing number of databases, or collections of literature, are available over the Internet. Literature databases are evolving from a bibliographic format (with just the basic information needed to locate a resource) to a full text format offering the complete item. Most databases are subject specific. The information-literate professional should be familiar with many different literature databases. Four major databases provide access to health care–related literature: MEDLINE; **HealthSTAR** (Health

Services, Technology, Administration, and Research); Cumulative Index to Nursing and Allied Health Literature (**CINAHL**), and Institute for Scientific Information (**ISI**) Web of Science.

Two databases—MEDLINE and HealthSTAR—are freely accessed via the NLM or, like CINAHL, are available from local libraries or by subscription from a vendor such as OVID or SilverPlatter. A database **vendor** is a company that presents the data in a format that is consistent with the other resources it distributes and adds enhanced features such as links to full text articles. No matter how the database is provided, the basic information is the same. Individuals can usually negotiate access through a vendor, but access is most often obtained via an institutional or association subscription. A variety of databases useful to health care professionals are available. Some of the most important and common databases in health care include the following:

- MEDLINE is the largest biomedical literature database in the world, covering the literature of medicine, nursing, and dentistry. There are many ways to access the MEDLINE database. Two versions of the MEDLINE database—PubMed and Internet Grateful Med—are available without a password and free of charge from the NLM Web site. Although both are predominantly bibliographic databases, PubMed is beginning to provide links to full text articles.
- HealthSTAR is a significant source of information in the area of health policy and administration. Produced jointly by the American Hospital Association and the NLM, there is some duplication between this database and MEDLINE, but there are many unique HealthStar entries. Both NLM databases use MeSH terms, which allows for easy cross-database searching.
- CINAHL is produced by CINAHL Information Systems and indexes most English-language nursing and allied health publications, as well as publications of the American Nurses Association and the National League for Nursing. CINAHL includes the bibliography of many current articles and some full text articles. This literature database uses CINAHL subject headings. Although these headings are unique to CINAHL, many correspond with MeSH terms. A vendor such as OVID or SilverPlatter distributes CINAHL. As with the NLM databases, the presentation format may be different with each vendor, but the basic information is the same.
- ISI Web of Science is a resource produced and distributed by the Institute for Scientific Information. ISI Web of Science allows searching of topics in both the science and social sciences fields. The real strength of this database is citation searching. The searcher can find articles that have cited a specific author and/or article. Primarily a bibliographic database, there are some links to full text articles. ISI Web of Science uses a textword-searching vocabulary and is only available from the producer.

Journals Some electronic-format journals are electronic copies of print journals (e.g., *Healthcare Informatics*), whereas other electronic journals (e.g., *Online Journal of Issues in Nursing*) are only in electronic format. Electronic publishing is a growing field. Publishers, organizations, associations, and vendors such as OVID are all involved in making electronic articles available. As with databases, there may be multiple ways to access a given electronic journal, and the format and amount of content may be different depending on the vendor or access method. For example, one vendor may offer access to the table of contents, whereas a second vendor may offer full text access to the articles in the journal.

Internet Most people with Internet access begin the search for information on the Web. Information about anything and everything can be found on the Internet and is easily accessed by World Wide Web (WWW) browsers. There are many excellent Web sites, and there are more not-so-good sites. For example, the U.S. government has made an effort to place much of the information generated by specific government agencies on the Internet. In the past, this information has frequently been hard to find and out-of-date, but now Web-based government resources are generally freely accessible and timely. This is especially true for census data. However, there are many sites on the Web that express personal opinions or give false information. Therefore information found on the Web must be carefully evaluated.

The numbers of special information databases on the Internet are growing. Topics covered by these databases include collections of statistics and genetic data and images. CDC Wonder (health statistics), the Genome Sequence DataBase (genetic data), and Findlaw Medical Images are sites that offer specialized information:

- CDC Wonder is produced by the Centers for Disease Control and Prevention (CDC) and includes CDC reports, guidelines, and numeric public health data. Some information is available to the general public; however, other information is available only to registered users. An example of the type of information found in this database is the AIDS Public Use Data Request. This database collects counts of acquired immunodeficiency syndrome (AIDS) cases reported to the CDC by state and local health departments. Case counts can be retrieved by demographics, case definition, date of diagnosis, date of report, human immunodeficiency virus (HIV) exposure group (risk factors), and mortality.
- The Genome Sequence DataBase, produced by the National Center for Genome Resources, is a relational database of publicly available nucleotide sequences and their associated annotations. The data are acquired each night from the International Nucleotide Sequence Database Collaboration. Information includes images and structures.
- Findlaw Medical Images is an example of the growing numbers of commercial sites that "sell" information. Images can be purchased and used as desired. FindLaw Medical Images was developed for legal professionals to use with cases. A medical illustrator prepares each image.

Privacy issues are a growing concern in relation to Web resources. Many sites require setting up a free account so that the information entered and retrieved can be tracked. As a result, the user information can be passed along to others (Dublin, 2000). For example, clinicians can write prescriptions and print customized patient information after registering for some Web sites. The site administrators can then use, or sell, the information collected from the prescriptions or patient information. Based on the information collected, the clinician and the patient may receive promotional information. It is very important to read the privacy policies for Web sites. However, a study by the California Health Care Foundation found that privacy policies and practice are often inconsistent (Privacy, 2000).

Unpublished Information The previous discussions have dealt with published information.

Sometimes the information needed may be too new (or too old), too specialized, or just unavailable in published format. One example of information that falls into this category is statistics. When looking for unpublished information, the best approach is to decide who might collect the information and contact that source. In the case of statistics, for example, local, state, or federal organizations frequently collect statistical information. Identifying and contacting these sources has gotten easier, since many agencies and organizations now have an Internet site that lists phone numbers and eMail addresses.

Evaluating and Retrieving

Evaluating and retrieving the selected information is the critical thinking part of the trip. The savvy traveler will most likely evaluate the resources before retrieving them. Therefore evaluation is a vital part of the process. There is always the initial "this looks good" or "this might work," but the key is to pick the appropriate information that meets the information need.

Evaluating Information

There are many ways to evaluate any resource. The factors to be considered for any format are credibility, bias, accuracy, currency, relevance, significance, intended audience, and usability. These factors build on the attributes of quality information presented in Chapter 1. Box 2-6 gives examples of data that can be used to measure these factors. For example, one approach to evaluating the credibility of a resource is to review the credentials of the author. Using a clearly defined needs statement and evaluation criteria will make identifying relevant resources easier. Chapter 12 presents a specific set of Web site evaluation criteria.

Box 2–6 Evaluation of Information Resources Considerations

- Credibility
  - Credentials
- Arguments
- Documentation
- Bias
  - Agenda
  - Advertisers
  - Conflict of interest
- Accuracy
  - Facts
  - Documentation
- Currency
  - Last update identified
- Relevance to search topic
- Significance to needs
- Intended audience
- Usability

Retrieving Information

Multiple retrieval options are available. Depending on where the information is found, retrieval options include photocopying, eMailing, downloading, saving to a floppy disk or handheld device, and importing directly into a bibliographic manager. eMail has become a primary method of communication and is increasingly being used to transfer information from electronic resources. Saving information to a disk or handheld device also allows for more rapid integration into programs such as spreadsheets, databases, or documents. Information databases, Internet sites, and eMail can be imported directly into bibliographic managers. This ensures a consistent format. All of the above methods decrease the time and errors associated with repeated human data entry. Information-literate professionals will use all these methods.

Organizing, Managing, and Using

Once the resources are retrieved, their organization and management are determined by how they will be used. Sometimes the information is needed quickly and requires no retention of the resources. Most often there is an advantage to storing and organizing resources, items, and/or information retrieved for future reference.

There are many ways to store, manage, and use the resources and/or information retrieved. Resources or information may be placed in databases, files, Web pages, or other storage media. After they are stored, the resources are managed by deleting, updating, or moving, as need dictates. This can be a complex and time-consuming part of the process.

Storage and management can be made easier by the use of bibliographic managers. **Bibliographic managers** are software programs that create reference databases, allow search and retrieval of the data, and integrate with word processing software. Use of bibliographic managers saves time and effort needed to maintain files of resources, to create articles or other documents for publication, and to produce bibliographies. Bibliographic managers also allow for the creation of various databases of subject-specific information that can be used independently, merged, or shared with others. These tools are designed to store citations, full text articles, correspondence, Internet information and sites, patents, and a variety of other information resources. The resources in the database can be searched. Specific selected items can be formatted appropriately as references for articles, bibliographies, or reprint management. Current software versions allow for direct links to universal resource locators (URLs), or addresses, of WWW pages and for direct searching and importing of resources from selected information collections. Because of the rapidly changing information environment, bibliographic formatting software is updated frequently. The enhancements in each new software version increase the functionality and compatibility of the software. Three popular bibliographic managers are EndNote, ProCite, and Reference Manager.

When information is being accessed, copyright and intellectual property rights are important issues that must be considered. Appropriate use of resources requires that copyright and intellectual property rights be respected. Unless information is clearly in the public domain, it is wise to assume that it is copyrighted. Using the Internet adds another layer of complexity, including issues related to international copyright laws (Goudreau, 1999). Spallek and Schleyer's article (1999) on educational implications for copyright includes an excellent list of Web sites dealing with copyright issues. The information-seeking trip is over. After creating a good plan, executing a productive search, selecting the best and most appropriate resources, organizing the resources in a useful manner, and using the knowledge gained to meet the information need, it is time to move on to another search. The information-literate health care provider is able to navigate the process with ease.

COMPUTER LITERACY

Achieving information literacy is dependent on being computer literate, since computer technology is used to access information. However, computer literacy requires more than being able to use computers to find information. The Computer Science and Telecommunications Board (CSTB) of the National Research Council has defined computer literacy for all college graduates as fluency with information technology (FITness). **FITness** is acquired through three kinds of knowledge: foundational concepts concerning how technology works, contemporary skills using computer applications, and the intellectual ability to apply that knowledge and adapt to change through lifelong learning (Lin, 2000). To meet these criteria, the computer-literate health care provider must possess a basic understanding of computer hardware, of the common types of software, and of the different ways in which software applications can be used. In addition to this foundational knowledge about computer technology, computer-literate health care providers know how to use the particular computer systems and applications found in their workplace. They are also aware of and able to evaluate potential or evolving computer applications that may be suitable to their workplace. As computer technology and its applications develop over time, the computer-literate health care provider must be committed to keeping up with change through lifelong learning.

Hardware

The physical parts of a computer—the **hardware**—perform the functions of data processing, storage of data and programs, input of data, and output of processed information.

Central Processing Unit and Memory

The data processing functions of a computer are controlled by the central processing unit (CPU), which has two main parts. The control unit retrieves commands and data, executes commands on data, and stores the results. The arithmetic logic unit (ALU) performs all arithmetic and logic functions. Two types of memory are essential for the functioning of the CPU:

1. Read-only memory (ROM) is manufactured with stored information about the hardware of the computer and cannot be changed.
2. Random access memory (RAM) functions as the working area of a computer that can be written to and read from but does not permanently store data. All of the active programs and data in use at a given time must be loaded in RAM.

Bytes

Memory, storage capacity, and file size are measured in bytes. A **byte** is composed of 8 **bits,** each bit representing either a one or a zero in the binary notation used by digital computers. *Kilo* (1000), *mega* (1 million), and *giga* (1 billion) are prefixes frequently used as multipliers, with the root *byte* indicating the size of an electronic file or the potential capacity of memory or a storage device.

Storage Devices

Data and programs need to be stored when not in use and, at times, transferred from one computer to another. A variety of **storage devices** are available.

Magnetic Storage Personal computers (PCs) contain internal hard disk drives composed of magnetically sensitive metal disks that can hold many gigabytes (GB) of data. Most PCs are also equipped with additional drives to read and/or write data to and from removable disks. A floppy disk drive reads and writes to magnetic diskettes, which are inexpensive and easy to use when transferring data from one computer to another. A high-density 3½-inch diskette stores up to 1.44 megabytes (MB) of data. Several kinds of removable-media drives with high-capacity disks are available for use when larger amounts of data need to be transferred, such as for multimedia presentations. For example, the Iomega Zip disk stores up to 250 MB of data, the Iomega Jaz disk stores up to 2 GB of data, and SyQuest's Quest cartridges store up to 4.7 GB.

Optical Storage CD-ROM disks are optical storage devices that can store up to 640 MB of data. CD-ROM drives read the disks with a laser but do not write to the disk. Compact disk read-write (CDRW) drives both read and write to compact disks. DVDs have been developed for use with data, as well as for video and audio. DVD-ROM (read only), DVD-R (write once) and DVD-RAM (rewritable) can hold many gigabytes of data, depending on the number of sides and layers.

Input Devices

Input devices are the pieces of hardware that capture data in digital format so that they can be manipulated by software applications. Common input devices capture alphanumeric, voice, and image data entry.

Alphanumeric and Function Entry Text, numbers, and function commands are usually entered with a keyboard. The standard 101-key keyboard includes alphanumeric keys, function keys, and cursor movement keys. A mouse directs graphical user interfaces to manipulate programs and data on the screen through pointing, clicking, highlighting, and dragging. Tablets and pen-based technology capture data from handwritten input. Touch screens allow a computer program to be directly manipulated by pressing the screen either with a finger or a stylus. The stylus is one of the techniques used with small, handheld computers to input data.

Voice Entry A microphone coupled with a sound card can capture voice input, convert speech into an electrical signal, and digitize the signal. In a speech recognition unit, the data are analyzed phonetically by speech engine software and mapped into words using a phonetic dictionary. A standard dictionary can be supplemented by adding terms to the system's vocabulary either individually or with specialized dictionaries. Both general medical dictionaries and dictionaries for specific areas of medicine are available. In health care settings this technology is being explored as a replacement for the patient report dictation and transcription processes. Voice input eliminates the time lag between seeing the patient and creating the report, producing an electronic document at a lower cost (Zafar, Overhage, & McDonald, 1999).

Image Entry Scanners capture pictures, print, slides, and radiographs as digital images. Handheld scanners and light pens are special kinds of optical input devices used to capture descriptive data about a particular object stored in a bar code. An example of the use of bar codes in health care is for patient identification and medication dispensing (Walsh, 2000). Digital cameras take both still pictures and video in a format that can be directly loaded into a computer. Digital images can be added to an electronic patient record, eMailed as part of a consultation, or used in a computer presentation (Ratner, Thomas, & Bickers, 1999).

Output Devices

An **output device** creates a visual display, hard copy, or audio record of computer-generated information. Monitors are commonly used output devices that display programs, data, and information on a screen. Screen size and resolution control the monitor display quality. Resolution is measured in the number of pixels per inch. Monitors smaller than 17 inches are usually set at 640 × 480 pixels, 17-inch monitors are set at 800 × 600 pixels, and 20-inch monitors are set at 1024 × 768 or 1280 × 1024 pixels. The higher number means more dots per inch and yields a sharper image. Printers are frequently used output devices that employ dot matrix, ink jet, or laser technology to transfer computer data to hard copy. Plotters are specialized printers used to output graphics such as maps and blueprints. Speakers are often included as part of a computer system to output digitized voice and music audio files.

Connectivity

In many settings, from homes to schools to small businesses to multinational corporations, PCs can be used more effectively and efficiently if they are connected to other machines. Connectivity facilitates resource sharing and communication. Software and output peripherals, such as printers, can be shared; pertinent data and files can be stored in one location and retrieved wherever the information is needed; and communication among individuals and groups can be accomplished using eMail, mailing lists, real-time chat, or videoconferencing.

Wired Networks

Wired networks are groups of computers that are physically connected by cables to enable sharing of software, devices, and files. A network is often defined by the terms *local area network (LAN),* describing connected computers in close proximity, such as within a building, and *wide area network (WAN),* describing widely dispersed connected computers, such as for a national corporation.

Wireless Networks

Wireless networks commonly use spread-spectrum radio transmission to transmit data from a wired LAN through wireless hub access points to an unattached computer. The computer, often a laptop or a handheld computer, must be equipped with a wireless network card. These networks are frequently called WLANs (wireless local area networks) because they cover a local area. Set free from a wired workstation, the health care provider can capture and retrieve patient and treatment information at the point of service anywhere within the coverage area of the access points. A wireless modem can extend information transmission to external clinics and emergency or home health care settings (Walsh, 2000).

Modem and Cable Connections

Modems are devices that connect one computer to another or to a network via telephone lines or cable television lines. *Modem* is an acronym for *modulate/demodulate,* referring to the translation from digital computer data to the analog format of wired telephone technology for transfer and then back. The most common use of modems is by individuals or small businesses connecting to an Internet service provider (ISP). The transmission speed for modems that use standard telephone lines can be as high as 56 kilobits (1000 bits) per second (kbps). Cable modems connect a computer to the Internet using the same lines that deliver cable television service and can download data between 3 and 10 million bits per second (mbps). Digital subscriber lines (DSLs) run on standard phone lines but use special compression techniques that improve download speeds up to 26 mbps. These lines are available only within close distance from a telephone switching office. Both cable and DSL services are purchased by the month at rates similar to the basic rate for telephone or cable television service (Bergeron, 2000).

Internet

The Internet, the world's largest network, is composed of a vast web of diverse computer networks that connect via a set of standardized communication protocols known as transmission control protocol/Internet protocol (TCP/IP). In development since the late 1960s, the Internet became increasingly popular in the 1990s with the development of the WWW. WWW pages include embedded hypertext links presented as highlighted word(s) or image(s) that can be selected to move to another part of the document, or to another document anywhere on the Internet (Whalen, 2000). The WWW has grown into a vast collection of Web pages presenting an ever-changing selection of information and services covering any conceivable interest. An extensive amount of health care information for professionals and consumers is available. The Internet is seen as a potential platform to streamline a variety of health care information transfer procedures ranging from purchasing medical supplies to accessing electronic patient records with embedded links to information sources such as MEDLINE. Increased use of the Internet for health care applications will depend on improvements in bandwidth, response time, data security, reliable availability, and ubiquity of access (Networking health, 2000). Applications related to eHealth are discussed in Chapters 7 and 13.

Software

Computer hardware without software is as useless as a video player without videos. To successfully function as a tool, the computer hardware uses **software,** which is a set of instructions written in a structured programming language that is translated into the binary code of digital computers. Basic computer literacy requires an understanding of the common types of software and the different ways in which software applications can be used.

Operating Systems

An **operating system** is the software program that controls the functioning of the computer by managing tasks, data, and devices. It is the link between the hardware and the software. All software applications installed on a computer must be written to communicate with the specific operating system running on the computer. Common operating systems include the following:

- Microsoft's Windows is the most frequently used operating system for PCs. Windows NT is the network version of this software.
- Apple's Mac operating system established the ease of a graphical user interface but has a much smaller market share than Windows.
- UNIX was developed as a system for use on various hardware platforms that permit multitasking and communication between computers.
- Linux, a product that grew out of UNIX, is an example of **open source software,** a program whose source code can be downloaded at no cost and developed. Developed commercial versions, which come with documentation and support, are usually very low cost, and free versions are available.

Graphical User Interface Functions

With the Mac operating system, Apple computers established the graphical user interface (GUI) as a design that simplified the interaction between users and the software on their computers. A GUI allows the user to interact with software by using a mouse to click on icons and menu items instead of (or in addition to) using function keys or cryptic command terms entered from a keyboard. The GUI can be part of the operating system, as in Windows 2000 and the Macintosh, or it can exist as an additional piece of software between the operating system and the application, as in Motif for UNIX. A GUI establishes a consistent look to programs by using the same icon in the same place for similar functions across software applications. A comparison study of nurses using a GUI interface and a text-based interface revealed that users tend to find a well-designed GUI interface easier to learn and more satisfying to use than a text-based interface. This study also found that nurses have a faster response time and fewer errors with a GUI interface (Staggers & Kobus, 2000).

Software Applications

Software applications are programs developed to perform specific tasks with a particular operating system. Some commonly used software applications are described here.

Word Processing Word processing programs are primarily used to create text documents and provide extensive editing and formatting capabilities. A selection of fonts and colors coupled with the ability to insert graphics allows advanced word processing programs to function as desktop publication software for the production of fliers and newsletters. Mail merge permits the creation of personalized letters generated from text templates. Some word processing programs export text documents in the code necessary for posting on the Web, thus serving as simple Web publishing programs. Commonly used word processing programs are Microsoft Word and Corel WordPerfect.

Spreadsheets Spreadsheet programs are used primarily to manipulate numbers and provide the ability to perform arithmetic and logic operations on a chosen data set. These programs have many specific uses, including budgeting, accounting, and the analysis of data for planning. Spreadsheets open with a ledger of intersecting columns and rows. Numbers, formulas, and labels can be inserted into the cells, and the data in one cell can be referenced from another. A particular sheet or set of sheets can be set up to calculate the figures needed for a particular purpose. Changing the number in one cell will change the calculations of any related cell. This process makes it very easy to perform "what if" analysis of the data. Data output can be presented in a number of different graphical perspectives, such as a bar graph or pie chart. Commonly used spreadsheet programs are Microsoft Excel and Lotus 1-2-3.

Database Management A database management system (DBMS) allows the user to store data in a structured way so that the data can be searched and sorted in response to a specific information need. Data are stored in records made up of fields defined by type, format, and size. A flat file database is one in which every record contains all of the fields and all of the records are stored in one table. A relational database system contains more than one table. Each table contains records with fields describing specific aspects of the entities. The ability to extract necessary information from a database depends on a well-thought-out design of the data structures. Extracted information can be manipulated and formatted using the report function. Scripting and programming languages facilitate the creation of specialized user-friendly data input, query, and report interfaces. Microsoft Access is one of the more commonly used database programs for PCs. Databases are discussed in Chapter 3.

Bibliographic management programs, mentioned earlier in the chapter, are a special type of database application used to capture, store, and organize references to various kinds of publications.

Presentation Presentation programs are used to add graphics to a series of successive slides to be used as visual aids for a lecture or training session. Handouts of a presentation can be created that contain a column of screen shots next to a column for taking notes. These programs include special tools to enhance the visual impact of presentations. Still and animated images can be added, as well as sound. Hyperlinks can be made between slides, to other documents, or to a Web site. A broadcasting feature enables either a live Web broadcast of a person making the presentation or the ability to record the full delivery with audio or with audio and video for posting on the Web. A presentation can be saved as a Web document, although it may lose some of the special features in the process. PowerPoint, another Microsoft program, is the most widely used presentation program.

Graphics Graphics programs are used to create, import, and manipulate digital images. Images can be cropped, resized, and layered. Colors can be changed, the whole image or areas can be lightened or darkened, and special effects can be added. It is possible to zoom in on part of the image and work in fine detail. Text can be created as an image or inserted in any font or color. Adobe PhotoShop is one example of a full-featured and widely used graphics program.

eMail eMail programs facilitate the exchange of electronic messages using computers connected to a network. eMail was first limited to transmission between computers on a specific network, such as within a business, or computers using the same ISP. Although some businesses and organizations still use separate eMail systems, most eMail systems now connect with the Internet. The expanded scope of eMail via the Internet created a worldwide network with the ability to send a message to anyone with an Internet-based eMail account. Many people acquire eMail accounts through work, school, or an ISP. There are also many free eMail services available on the WWW.

eMail applications are used to send text messages that can include file attachments in any electronic format. Graphical eMail programs include images and embedded hyperlinks to Web pages within the message. Subject-oriented mailing lists, often referred to as listservers, broadcast an individual's eMail message to a group of subscribers, creating international virtual communities of shared interests and knowledge. In most professional settings eMail has replaced the office memo. The ability to send and respond to messages between multiple people in multiple locations adds to the speed and efficiency of professional communication in all areas, including health care. Some health care providers use eMail to communicate with patients, although there are legal and ethical concerns with this new format. To address those concerns, the American Medical Informatics Association (**AMIA**) created communication, medicolegal, and administrative guidelines for using eMail with patients (DeVille & Fitzpatrick, 2000).

Web Browser Web browser software offers a user interface, usually graphical, for navigation of the extensive collection of information available via the WWW. Web browsers are also used to navigate intranets—Web sites that can connect to the Internet but can only be accessed by a particular group, such as the employees of a company. The browser interprets the formatting language, hypertext markup language (HTML), and scripting languages, such as JavaScript, on Web pages. Both Web browsers and formatting languages are continually evolving to expand their functionality. Extensible hypertext markup language (XHTML), an advanced version of HTML, is defined within the restrictions of extensible markup language (XML). XML is under development as a new coding language and is designed to define the data structure of the content in a document. XML requires a document-type definition (DTD) that defines the element names, types, occurrences, and relationships for a particular type of document. The National Library of Medicine (NLM) has chosen XML with a DTD as the only format for distributing MEDLINE starting in 2001 (National Library of Medicine, 2000). Two of the most popular PC Web browsers are Microsoft Internet Explorer and Netscape Navigator.

Web Authoring Web authoring programs function as specialized word processor/desktop publishing software offering a "what you see is what you get" (**WYSIWYG**) interface for creating Web pages. However, page creators who know HTML often prefer the increased design control provided by programs that allow direct manipulation of the code. Some programs include Web site management tools to track the linking relationships between all of the pages on a site and to allow editing the same element across many pages. Popular programs include Allaire's HomeSite, Macromedia's Dreamweaver, and Microsoft's FrontPage.

EVALUATING AND IMPROVING LITERACY

Diversity of Skills

Academic programs and businesses frequently evaluate the information literacy and computer literacy of newcomers to the organization. Evaluations done in these settings reveal that people entering similar situations usually have widely different levels of literacy. For example, a self-assessment survey given to first-year medical students at the State University of New York at Stony Brook in 1997 revealed that students had "computer skills ranging from complete novice to that of a systems engineer" (Gibson & Silverberg, 2000, p. 159). A study of the information technology skills of incoming nursing students also found students with different levels of computer knowledge (Sinclair & Gardner, 1999). The diversity of experience of incoming students and employees complicates the attempt to improve literacy for these groups.

Identifying Literacy Objectives and Measuring Existing Knowledge

The first step in evaluating and improving literacy is to clearly identify what people need to know to succeed in a particular setting. The focus should be on articulating levels of cognitive understanding, as well as detailing specific skills that need to be in place. Saranto used the **Delphi technique** to identify and rank the basic information technology skills needed by nurses to describe what should be included in nursing education (Saranto & Leino-Kilpi, 1997).

With defined objectives in mind, an evaluation tool can be created or revised and used to measure what individuals already know. Examples of measurement tools for information and computer literacy can be found in the literature. TekXam, a new examination created by the Virginia Foundation of Independent Colleges (VFIC), has been developed to help liberal arts students demonstrate their knowledge of information and computer resources. One section of this test requires students to find answers to specific questions by using an Internet browser and search engine. Another part of the test requires students to create a multimedia page for the WWW. Currently being evaluated, TekXam was administered at 63 colleges in October 1999 and has the potential to become a standard evaluation tool (Liberal arts grads, 2000). **CILM** (Computer Interface Literacy Measure) is an example of a computer literacy measurement tool that includes both a self-report section and a knowledge application section (Turner, Sweany, & Husman, 2000).

Offering Training to Increase Knowledge

Once current knowledge is evaluated, the next step is to design curricula and training to provide groups and individuals with the means to fill in the gaps between existing knowledge and the required skills. Training can take many forms, such as lecture and demonstration, hands-on exercises, or independent study. It is difficult to meet the needs of a group with diverse levels of skills using the same curriculum. If at all possible, it is best to separate groups by skill level or to allow advanced students to enter a series of courses after the basic content has been taught. One way to approach a group with diverse skills is to present the course as independent study modules. Areas of competence must be clearly defined and resources provided to guide the student in gaining the necessary knowledge and skills. Resources can include readings, online tutorials, exercises, and classes. Learning contracts and assessment exercises can help independent study students track progress and stay motivated (Independent study, 2000).

In education, one approach to improving information and computer literacy is to integrate these competencies within required courses. Students must complete specific assignments to be considered literate. For example, to measure the use of electronic resources for patient care competency, medical students at the University of Rochester Medical Center must review a chart, write a differential (diagnosis), and order tests as part of a hospital information system prototype exercise assignment (Informatics competencies, 1995).

Evaluating the Results of Training

The focus of information and computer literacy training should be on real-life use and lifelong learning. Evaluation should continue after the initial training to measure the outcomes of improved literacy for improving performance in professional roles. Many trainers suggest using Kirkpatrick's four levels of evaluation (Kirkpatrick's four levels, 1996):

1. Reaction—captures the trainee's immediate assessment of the training experience
2. Learning—uses tools such as tests to measure changes in knowledge, skills, and attitudes

3. Behavior—measures actual changes on the job
4. Results—attempts to tie the effect of training to achieving the goals of the institution

Reaction and learning are the most commonly used evaluation strategies. Measuring behavior and results is more complicated and costly. However, because of the investment of time and money in training programs, organizations are concerned with measuring training outcomes. It is recommended that the training programs closely tied to an organization's priorities use evaluations that are focused on behavior and results. These more complicated levels of evaluation are easier to achieve if the expected outcomes are identified and measurement tools are developed as a training program is planned (Geber, 1995).

APPLICATIONS OF PROFESSIONAL KNOWLEDGE

Why do health care professionals combine knowledge of their disciplines with computer and information literacy to support health care through informatics? Computers, software, connectivity, and the vast array of information resources are powerful tools that assist in providing cost-effective, efficient, quality health care services. What are the major areas in which informatics literacy is applied? Ten aims and tasks of health informatics are as follows (Ball, Douglas, & Hoehn, 1997; Haux, 1997):

1. Diagnosis
2. Therapy
3. Simulation training
4. Early recognition and prevention
5. Compensating for physical disabilities
6. Consulting
7. Reporting
8. Health care information systems
9. Computerized patient records
10. Decision support systems

Information and computer literacy progress in each of these areas has been steady in spite of political, educational, attitudinal, environmental, and economic barriers (Moehr, 1997).

How might professionals apply health informatics literacy? The following scenarios illustrate how professionals in each of the five roles identified by the AAMC Informatics Advisory Panel might apply health informatics. (Scenarios are constructed on the basis of statements from the Phase 1 Summary Report of the AAMC Delphi study at http://www.aamc.org/better_health/delphi.htm.)

Lifelong Learner

Jenny White, a community pharmacist, subscribes to a new service offered by the pharmacy school where she received her PharmD degree 15 years ago. When she fills a prescription that has never been filled before, or if her pharmacy's internal system warns her of a potential drug interaction, she is prompted to check relevant online continuing education modules and/or readings. Today two of her regular customers came in to fill prescriptions for a new antidepressant, and they were both worried about potential side effects. When she enters the name of the drug, the pharmacy's computer program gives her access to a topical Web page that lists several good Web sites selected by experts in the field, a section from an electronic pharmacy text, and two articles in recent journals. She starts with the textbook, which is continuously updated on the basis of relevant new research. The program also lets her link directly to the full text of the journal articles. She gets continuing education credit after she passes an online quiz.

Clinician

Barry Dawson is setting up his private dental practice and needs to select and purchase computers and software for scheduling, billing, purchasing, patient records, and access to professional information resources. The state dental association's Web site has evaluations of several integrated dental practice packages that have modules for each of these functions along with dentists' comments regarding their experiences with each system. One dentist describes how the integrated system he uses has made it easier to send patient records to specialists with referrals. For more current information and unusual cases, the search system in the package has a link to the NLM's free Internet-accessible MEDLINE database, where practitioners can find research articles and case reports. The dentist can also check dental practice guidelines that are updated at least once a year on the basis of current research.

This integrated system appeals to Dr. Dawson because of the referral and information access features. He is considering several optional features that would allow him to capture, store, and access dental x-ray films or images taken by an intraoral camera. He would like to be able to transfer these with the patient record. Dr. Dawson already has an arrangement with the closest dental school library that allows him to link directly to the electronic full text of many articles through their Web site and a contract to obtain articles through the NLM's electronic document delivery service. This combination expands his information access methods.

Educator/Communicator

Marge Harris, a certified diabetes nurse educator, is working with a group of young adults with diabetes. Members of the group are having problems controlling their disease. She finds an authoritative, well-organized interactive Web site with images and online texts that explain diabetes, provide self-management tips, and explain long-term consequences of poor control. Ms. Harris knows that all of the group members have PCs and eMail accounts. She gives the group members the URL for the diabetes Web site and sets up an online discussion forum. She also gives them a software package that records, analyzes, and graphs blood glucose test results. Ms. Harris also explains how to send their test results and their daily food-intake and exercise logs to her at the diabetes care center once every week. She monitors the results that become part of their computerized medical record and follows up by eMail or phone with constructive feedback. Over the following weeks, each patient visits the interactive Web site and sends his or her personal diabetes self-management goals to Ms. Harris. They have some lively discussions with other group members. A few comment on how talking with others, setting priorities, and monitoring their condition have helped them meet their goals. Others share new "cool" Web sites with interesting health information. Sometimes both Ms. Harris and a specialist comment on outcomes, answer questions, or correct false assumptions.

Researcher

Dr. Conrad Green is the principal investigator at one of five centers participating in a clinical trial. His staff uses an online form to submit the latest patient data, which are aggregated with data from other patients at his center and across the five centers. Biostatisticians at another center analyze and compare the data according to the study protocol. Dr. Green has a hypothesis that might explain an unexpected finding. Fortunately, the five centers participating in this particular trial agreed 5 years ago to pool their clinical data in a large Internet-accessible database that protects patient privacy. Dr. Green tests his hypothesis against the pooled clinical data and finds the results statistically insignificant. He is able to rule out this hypothesis before the investigators' next teleconference.

Manager

Kevin Madison is the hospital's risk manager and a member of the quality improvement council chaired by the vice president for continuous quality improvement. Mr. Madison has been appointed chair of a quality improvement team charged with investigating a sentinel event. In this case three inpatients committed suicide on the same unit over the last 6 months. He and the team, which includes a staff psychiatrist and a medical social worker, review the incident reports and list possible root causes based on what they know about each case. Mr. Madison tests these hypotheses using the hospital's management information system. Through an interactive Web link to the hospital library, he asks the librarian to help him find relevant literature. The librarian points him to an online chapter from a recent electronic text on suicide that puts the problem in a larger context. Later, she eMails him copies of several recent journal articles describing how other hospitals have approached this problem. Mr. Madison and the quality improvement team review the data and the literature before they develop strategies, actions, and follow-up assessments that will help them evaluate their interventions. They file a report to the quality improvement council that will be reviewed before the next site visit by a review team from the Joint Commission on Accreditation of Healthcare Organizations (JCAHO).

CONCLUSION

The scenarios presented show how a pharmacist, dentist, nurse educator, physician researcher, and hospital manager might apply computer and information literacy in their daily work and professional roles. The scenarios demonstrate how health care professionals use their professional knowledge, their problem-solving skills, and technology to access literature, data, and information to provide high-quality, cost-effective health care. Professionals apply information literacy by defining information needs, locating pertinent information, and evaluating the information. They apply computer literacy by demonstrating a basic understanding of current computer hardware systems and software applications and applying this knowledge to a problem in a particular work setting.

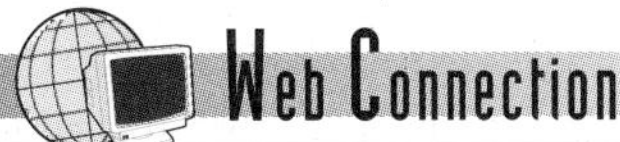

Web Connection

Rapidly becoming a primary source of data and information, the World Wide Web provides an information jungle with hidden dangers like outdated information, incorrect information, and malicious information. Negotiating the information jungle requires developing a plan and demonstrating persistence, flexibility, and adaptability. Knowing the capabilities of other information resources such as institutional and governmental databases, local libraries, patient records, and media such as CD-ROM collections offers ways to extend and enhance Web resources and to validate some of the information. Before this begins, you need to assess your information literacy skills. In the activities for this chapter, you will explore information literacy elements and enter the jungle of information to discover what the World Wide Web has to offer.

discussion questions

1. Describe a scenario demonstrating how you might apply health informatics literacy in your discipline.
2. List several ways that you will continue to develop health informatics literacy now and in the future.
3. What are the four main steps in the information literacy process?
4. You have a stack of photographs that you would like to put into digital format. What hardware do you need to use to perform this task? What kind of software application would you use to manipulate the images?

5. Think about a record-keeping task that you would like to computerize. What kind of software would you select to perform this task?
6. What processes can be used to evaluate information and computer literacy?

REFERENCES

Ball, M.J., Douglas, J.V., & Hoehn, B.J. (1997). New challenges for nursing informatics. In U. Gerdin, M. Tallberg, & P. Wainwright (Eds.), *Nursing informatics: The impact of nursing knowledge on health care informatics* (pp. 38-43). Amsterdam: IOS Press.

Bergeron, B.P. (2000). Need more power in your communications technology? Increasing bandwidth will improve speed and expand options. *Postgraduate Medicine, 197*(2), 35-38.

Breivik, P.S., & Gee, E.G. (1989). *Information literacy: revolution in the library.* New York: American Council on Education & Macmillan.

Brodie, D.A., Williams, J.G., & Owens, R.G. (1994). *Research methods for the health sciences.* Chur, Switzerland: Harwood Academic.

Critical challenges: Revitalizing the health professions for the twenty-first century (3rd ed.). (1995). San Francisco: Pew Health Professions Commission.

DeVille, K., & Fitzpatrick, J. (2000). Ready or not, here it comes: Legal, ethical, and clinical implications of e-mail communications. *Seminars in Pediatric Surgery, 9*(1), 24-33.

Dublin, A.H. (2000). Web-based technology: What every physician practice needs to know. *New Jersey Medicine, 97*(8), 51-55.

Duisterhout, J.S., et al. (1997). Coding and classification. In J.H. van Bemmel & M.A. Musen (Eds.), *Handbook of medical informatics* (pp. 81-98). Heidelberg, Germany: Springer-Verlag.

Geber, B. (1995). Does training make a difference? Prove it! *Training,* 27-33.

Gibson, K. E., & Silverberg, M. (2000). A two-year experience teaching computer literacy to first-year medical students using skill-based cohorts. *Bulletin of the Medical Library Association, 88* (2), 157-164.

Goudreau, K.A. (1999). The copyright quagmire on the Internet. *Computers in Nursing, 17*(2), 82-85.

Haux, R. (1997). Aims and tasks of medical informatics. *International Journal of Medical Informatics, 44*(1), 9-20; discussion, 39-44, 45-52, 61-26.

Independent study for building computer and information retrieval competencies. (2000). Charlottesville, VA: University of Virginia Health Sciences Library. Retrieved September 28, 2000, from the World Wide Web: http://www.med.virginia.edu/hs-library/info_serv/pathfinders/hes/hes.html.

Informatics competencies for medical students at the University of Rochester Medical Center: Planning document, 1995. (1995). Rochester, NY: Edward G. Miner Library. Retrieved September 27, 2000, from the World Wide Web: http://www.urmc.rochester.edu/Miner/Educ/medinfostudents1.html.

Kirkpatrick's four levels. (1996). In C. Nilson (Ed.), *Training and development yearbook 1996/1997* (pp. 5.21-25.22). Englewood Cliffs, NJ: Prentice Hall.

Liberal arts grads seek employability proof. (2000). *Techniques, 75*(2), 10.

Lin, H. (2000). Fluency with information technology. *Government Information Quarterly, 17*(1), 69-76.

Medical school objectives project: Medical informatics objectives. (1999). Washington, DC: Association of American Medical Colleges. Retrieved September 27, 2000, from the World Wide Web: http://www.aamc.org/meded/msop/informat.html.

Moehr, J.R. (1997). Grand challenges in health informatics: An information system perspective on Haux. *International Journal of Medical Informatics, 44* (1), 27-37.

Networking health: Prescriptions for the Internet. (2000). Washington, DC: National Academy Press.

NLM to use XML and DTD for MEDLINE data. (2000). National Library of Medicine. Retrieved December 5, 2000, from the World Wide Web: http://www.nlm.nih.gov/news/medlinedata.html.

Privacy: Report on the privacy policies and practices of health Web sites. (2000). Oakland, CA: California Health care Foundation. Retrieved September 27, 2000, from the World Wide Web: http://admin.chcf.org/documents/ehealth/privacy Webreport.pdf.

PubMed Journal Browser. National Center for Biotechnology Information. Retrieved November 15, 2000, from the World Wide Web: http://www.ncbi.nlm.nih.gov:80/entrez/jrbrowser.cgi.

Ratner, D., Thomas, C.O., & Bickers, D. (1999). Uses of digital photography in dermatology. *Journal of the American Academy of Dermatology, 4*(5 Pt. 1), 749-756.

Richardson, W. S., Wilson, M. C., Nishikawa, J., & Hayward, R. (1995). The well-built clinical question: A key to evidence-based decisions. *ACP Journal Club, 123*(3), A12-A13.

Saranto, K., & Leino-Kilpi, H. (1997). Computer literacy in nursing: developing the information technology syllabus in nursing education. *Journal of Advanced Nursing, 25*(2), 377-385.

Schloss, P.J., & Smith, M.A. (1999). *Conducting research.* Upper Saddle River, NJ: Prentice-Hall.

Sinclair, M., & Gardner, J. (1999). Planning for information technology: Key skills in nurse education. *Journal of Advanced Nursing, 30*(6), 1441-1450.

Spallek, H., & Schleyer, T.K. (1999). Educational implications for copyright in a digital world. *Journal of Dental Education, 63*(9), 673-681.

Staggers, N., & Kobus, D. (2000). Comparing response time, errors, and satisfaction between text-based and graphical user interfaces during nursing order tasks. *Journal of the American Medical Informatics Association, 7*(2), 164-176.

Turner, G.M., Sweany, N.W., & Husman, J. (2000). Development of the computer interface literacy measure. *Journal of Educational Computing Research, 22*(1), 37-54.

Walsh, P.J. (2000). Wireless technology transforms health care delivery and tracking. *MDComputing, 17*(2), 45-48.

Whalen, T.V. (2000). Internet: Past, present and future. *Seminars in Pediatric Surgery, 9*(1), 6-11.

Wood, G.L. (1996). Planning and implementing a research project: Part 1. *Journal of Transplant Coordination, 6*(4), 204-207; quiz, 208-209.

Zafar, A., Overhage, M., & McDonald, C.J. (1999). Continuous speech recognition for clinicians. *Journal of the American Medical Informatics Association, 6*(3), 195-204.

CHAPTER 3

Understanding Databases

LINDA Q. THEDE

Learning Objectives

Upon completion of this chapter, the reader will be able to:

1. ***Identify*** and ***define*** the parts of a database.
2. ***Discuss*** the types of data manipulation that a database permits.
3. ***Plan*** a small relational database.
4. ***Identify*** health care situations in which a relational database is needed.

Outline

Database Models
- *Hierarchical Databases*
- *Network Databases*
- *Relational Databases*
- *Objected-Oriented Database Management System*

Why Use a Database?

Anatomy of Databases
- *Fields*
- *Records*
- *Tables*

Physiology of Databases (Data Views and Data Manipulation)
- *Data Views*
- *Basic Data Manipulation*

Overview of Database Features

Obtaining the Answers to a Simple Question
- *What Information Is Needed?*
- *What Data Are Needed to Answer the Question?*
- *How Will the Data Be Manipulated?*

Relational Databases
- *Getting Information From More Than One Table*
- *Entering Data Into a Relational Database*

Overview of Planning a Relational Database

Planning a Database for a Specific Situation
- *Types of Data and Fields*
- *Accuracy of Data*
- *Queries*
- *Data Entry User Interfaces or Forms*
- *Reports*
- *To the Computer*

Key Terms

algorithm
atomic-level data
Boolean logic
child table
data
data dictionary
data sets
database
database management system (DBMS)
database model
date arithmetic
detail table
embedded form
field
field entry
field name
flat database
foreign key
form
grouping
key fields
look-up table
master table

Key Terms—cont'd

one-to-many
parent table
primary key
primary sort
query
record
relational database
reports
secondary sort
sorting
table (in a database)
tertiary sort
unique identifier
wildcard

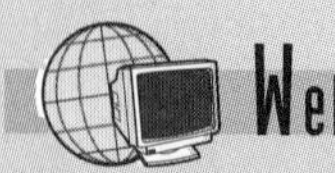

Web Connection

Go to the Web site at http://evolve.elsevier.com/Englebardt/. Here you will find Web links and activities related to understanding databases.

This chapter introduces the reader to databases. It also addresses in detail the anatomy (structure) and physiology (functions) of relational databases. It also explains how a database structure allows **data** to be manipulated to produce information and knowledge. Finally, the chapter addresses the steps involved in planning a relational database to answer clinical questions.

Each individual operates from a personal database (Thede, 1999). When caring for patients, health care providers collect and store data and information in their personal database—memory. When clinical decisions need to be made, these data and information are retrieved and synthesized. Electronic databases work in much the same way, but their data, data structure, and syntheses are visible, unlike the data and processes an individual uses.

A formal **database** is a structured collection of individual data elements. Most health care personnel are already familiar with paper databases. They have used a telephone book, an address book, and a printed patient record. They have probably also used an electronic bibliographic database for finding articles or books. Anyone who has used the paper version of either a bibliographic reference database or a card catalog, as well as an electronic bibliographic database, is aware of the ease and speed that electronic searching has brought to finding references. Health care, however, has been slow to fully use databases. Although clinical documentation may be done electronically, few institutions use only electronic documentation. Of those who do use electronic clinical documentation, there are few that effectively search the clinical data to uncover the hidden knowledge in these databases. This failure is often caused by concepts and data access approaches that are holdovers from the paper database age. For example, through clinical experience a health care provider may develop a theory about the results of a specific treatment. Finding the data needed to test the theory in paper clinical records is a time-consuming and labor-intensive process. Therefore it is seldom done without outside funding for the research. This paper record mindset can be changed if the user becomes aware of how electronic databases can be used to transform data into information, knowledge, and wisdom. For a detailed discussion of the transformations from data, to information, to knowledge and wisdom, see Chapter 1.

DATABASE MODELS

A **database management system** (**DBMS**) is a software program that is used to manage, organize, and retrieve data and information from a database. When databases are being discussed, the terms *DBMS, computer,* and *database* are sometimes used interchangeably. However, there is an important distinction. The DBMS is the software. The computer is the hardware used to run the DBMS. The database is the collection of data.

A **database model** is a model that is used to structure the data in a database. A specific DBMS will use a particular model to store, retrieve, and transform data.* This chapter emphasizes the relational database model. This is the model that is used by the database programs in the PC-based software office suites (e.g., Microsoft Office). It is also the model that is used most often by health care personnel who are not informatics specialists. Other database models that are briefly explained in this chapter include the hierarchical, network, and object-oriented models.

Hierarchical Databases

Hierarchical databases can contain many levels. They can be conceptualized as a family tree wherein each child has one parent. The root is the head of the family. The branches, or second level, are the children who are descended from the root. The third level, the grandchildren, are descended from the second-level parents. Communication among the descendants occurs by passing information up or down to the common parent or child until the desired level is reached.

This model was used to develop many of the older mainframe DBMS programs. However, it has several limitations with large data sets (Sol, 1999a). It works well for **data sets** with one-to-many relationships. For example, each patient in a hospital is assigned to one clinical unit. The unit can be represented as the parent, and each patient can be represented as the child. However there is significant redundancy when the model is used for many-to-many relationships. For example, a patient may have more than one physician, and a physician may have several patients. In addition, any change necessitates a great deal of programming. Hierarchical databases are still used in situations of one-to-one relationships. Several of the DBMSs designed to manage qualitative data use this model.

Network Databases

The network database model was designed to solve the redundancy problem that occurs with the hierarchical model (Sol, 1999b). Although this model is very similar to the hierarchical model, children are permitted to have more than one parent. The records are linked together by pointers that use a key piece of data (e.g., a patient medical record number). Which pieces of data are linked influences the way that the data are accessed (Saba & McCormick, 1995). This type of database, like the hierarchical database, requires professional programmers for implementation and maintenance.

Relational Databases

The relational database model was developed in the 1980s from work done by E.F. Codd at IBM in the late 1960s (Sol, 1999c). The basic structure in this model is a table. The database consists of several tables. A unique field within the tables is used to combine or join the tables. In contrast to users of hierarchical and network databases, users of relational databases need to know only the name of a table in order to locate data.

*The term *database model* may also be used to refer to either a conceptual (user) view of data or the physical structure of the data and objects in a database. In this chapter the term *database model* refers to the type of database (e.g., relational, object oriented).

Object-Oriented Database Management System

Relational databases are popular because of the simplicity of the underlying concepts and query languages (VanBemmel, 1999). They are fine for several aspects of the traditional patient record. However, in a relational DBMS there is a separation between the data storage and the manipulation methods. This separation of data and methods for manipulating those data add to the complexity of the database. This is especially true with large databases.

With the object-oriented model, each object belongs to a class and has a given set of attributes that can be applied to it. Users of operating systems with graphics, such as Windows, are familiar with this model. Right clicking on a selected object yields a menu of options that can be applied to the selected object. The same principles apply to data in an object-oriented DBMS.

Under this scheme, the data and the functions that can operate on these data are stored together. To illustrate, a patient's name would belong to the name category. The options for this category might be that it can be combined with a unit and/or a medical record number, with the results shown on the screen (Montlick, 1999). Some categories can be contained within other objects in a nesting manner. For example, all of the data from a patient's physical examination, although separately available as an object, can be represented in total as one object. Thus objects can be used independently of where they are stored.

One of the advantages of an object-oriented DBMS is that it reduces the amount of programming needed. In addition, an object-oriented DBMS permits the storage of complex data that are not easily accommodated by a relational DBMS (Software Technology Review, 2000). Because of these advantages, many of the more traditional types of databases are incorporating facets of object-oriented database management into their programs. For example, the relational databases present in the office suites use object-oriented programming for their objects, such as fields, tables, and forms.

WHY USE A DATABASE?

Two experienced labor and delivery personnel were discussing whether labor is shorter when the membranes are artificially ruptured (artificial rupture of membranes [AROM]) or when they rupture spontaneously (spontaneous rupture of membranes [SROM]). The practice in their unit varied, which resulted in this discussion. "You know," one said to the other, "We collect a lot of data in the computer. Do you suppose we could get some data and take a look at it?"

"It's worth a try," the other replied. "I certainly would not have attempted this when we were using paper records, but they keep telling us that when information is recorded electronically, it can be used to answer questions."

When the two health care personnel talked to their information services (IS) liaison, she was happy to help them but asked them what data they required. She also suggested that they could import the data and use the database that was part of the office suite package on the computer in their unit. As they talked more with the IS liaison, they found that they needed to understand more about databases before they could determine what data they needed. They also learned that they needed to know how to manipulate the data once they received it.

ANATOMY OF DATABASES

Understanding databases starts with understanding their parts and features. A database consists of fields, records, and tables. Table 3-1 represents the entities that are part of a table: fields and records. Tables are the basic building blocks of a relational database.

Fields

A **field** is a vertical column in a database. It contains data that represent the same charac-

Table 3–1 Anatomy of a Table

	Fields						
	First Name	Middle Initial	Last Name	Street Address	City	State	Zip
Records	Lisa	T	Salmonetti	2 East Side Drive	Missoula	Montana	88514
	Steve	O	Stevens	3 Capital Drive	Columbus	Ohio	45222
	Jane	E	Aarons	25 Forest Drive	Orlando	Florida	52215
	George	V	Brown	232 Lake Drive	Cleveland	Ohio	44256

teristic, or entity, for all of the records. For example, a column labeled "First Name" would include the first name of each individual. Each first name is in the field for that record. Fields in a database contain **atomic-level data,** or the smallest recognizable entity necessary to obtain meaning. The label at the head of a column is called a **field name.** There are usually several fields in a table, each one containing a piece of data relating to the entity. To keep data at the atomic level, three fields are used to collect a name—first name, middle initial, and last name—as seen in Table 3-1. The address is divided into the street address, city, state, and zip code. Keeping data at this lowest level provides flexibility in data use.

Records

In Table 3-1 all of the data in the fields in the horizontal row starting with "Lisa" pertain to that person, whereas the data in the rows starting with "Steve," "Jane," and "George" contain data pertaining to those individuals. These horizontal rows are called **records.** A record contains the different pieces of data belonging to a given entity. In this table the entity is a person, and the fields contain his or her name and mailing address. Thus a record is made up of fields, with each field containing data pertaining to the entity that the record represents.

Tables

A **table** consists of all of the records. Structuring the data in fields and records in a table makes it possible to manipulate and/or select records or fields based on specific data elements in the fields. The process of selecting desired records is called querying, and the feature that permits this is a **query.** To illustrate this, in Table 3-1 the records that contain "Ohio" in the state field could be separated from the rest of table and brought up for view by using a query. The query could also be used to specify that the display contains only the first- and last-name fields for any record that has the entry "Ohio" in the state field. Queries work because when the data are structured in a table, the DBMS knows exactly where to look for the specified piece or pieces of data. It can then easily and quickly determine if the datum in the field matches the search criteria.

PHYSIOLOGY OF DATABASES (DATA VIEWS AND DATA MANIPULATION)

The structure, or anatomy, of a database makes it possible to look at the same data in more than one format and to manipulate the data to provide information. These features provide the physiology of a database. A well-constructed database uses the "one piece of data, many uses" principle. Under this principle, a piece of data is entered only once but is used in many different views. This principle makes monitoring the data and trends in an electronic database far easier than working with the data in paper format. All of the features addressed in this section are available in any of the database programs included in the professional version of the current office suites.*

Data Views

Tables, such as the one in Table 3-1, are the heart of all databases. Views of the data, although they are of the data in a table, are not limited to the table format. The same data can be viewed in a manner that shows only the fields for one record, or only the fields that a person needs to see. This view is called a **form.** Another way to view data is in a report. In a report, records can be grouped on the basis of a similar characteristic, and calculations can be done for an individual record, a group of records, or the entire set of records. The ability to view the data in either a form or report format is present in the database programs in the current popular office suites.

Forms

Forms can contain all or selected data from one record, or they can be designed to show specified data from many records. They can contain fields from more than one table. Forms are designed by the database creator for specific situations. A form may be designed either to guide data entry or to view specific data on a screen, or for both purposes. Figure 3-1 shows a form view of Table 3-1, with the addition of the individuals' home phone, work phone, birth date, identification (ID) number, and hire date. If these data were all in one table, a table view would not display all of the fields at once. Or, if some of the data were in another related table, a table view would not provide this information on one screen. A form view with fields from one or more tables can also be used for either entering or viewing data.

Notice on the form in Figure 3-1 that there are instructions along with easy navigation buttons (e.g., "Find Record") for the person entering data. A form designer can place any information on the form that might be helpful to the data user or person entering data. These types of instructions prevent errors. In many cases the form is the user interface. A form does not have to contain all of the fields in a table. For example, perhaps a user needs to see only the address and work phone number. When designing the form, the designer omits the other fields.

Also when designing a form, the designer places the fields in the order that is most beneficial to the user, not in the order they occur in the underlying table or tables. The data, however, will originate from entries in the table(s). In this way, a form can be used to display data to meet the needs of the various system users, thus fulfilling the "one piece of data, many uses" principle. In a health care information system, for example, name fields showing the patient's name can be displayed on a form that a physician uses to enter orders as well as on a form used to list diet requests for a clinical unit.

Reports

Another view of data is made possible by reports. Generally, one uses a **report** when one wants a paper version of the data. Reports vary from a simple printout of the data in a table format to complex reports based on queries and containing calculations for various groups. Like a form, reports are not limited to just the data in one table, nor is the placement of the data on the report limited to its location in a table.

Reports have the ability to sort the records by multiple criteria. For example, a report can be sorted first by diagnosis; then within each diagnosis, the names of the clients can be alphabetized. In a report this is known as **grouping.** If the database also contains a field with the length of

---

*To have a database program included in an office suite, it is necessary to purchase what is called the "professional" version of the suite. Database application programs can also be purchased separately.

FIGURE 3–1 Form View of Table 3-1

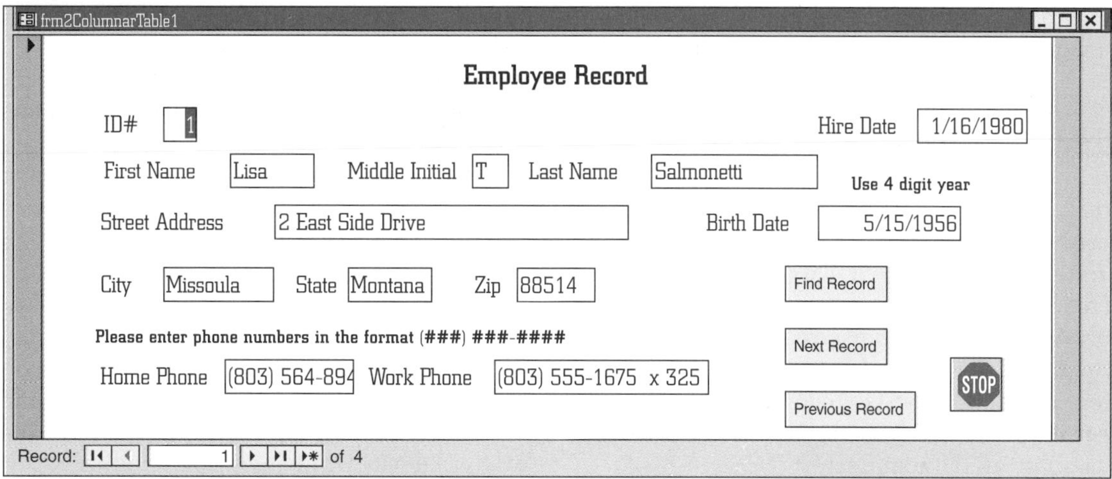

stay for each client, an average length of stay for each diagnosis can be calculated and placed on the report. An average length of stay can also be calculated and reported for all the records in the report.

Basic Data Manipulation

Computers work well for performing functions that require decisions when the decisions follow known and stated rules. For example, when records contain names and addresses, these can be sorted alphabetically by last name. The computer simply follows the rules of alphabetization. These are easily stated as an **algorithm,** or a set of rules to follow that are inclusive of all cases. Anything that can be reduced to an algorithm can usually be performed by a computer with greater speed and accuracy than by a human.

Thus when data are in a table format, in which it is easy for the computer to locate specified pieces of data, such as a last name, the computer can easily re-sort the records so that they are indexed alphabetically by last name. It can just as easily alphabetize by first name or middle initial, or by city. When asked to perform a function, a computer does not stop to think whether performing this feat is of value; it just does it. This is important to remember when working with databases of any sort, including spreadsheets and statistical packages.

Forms and reports are based on the results of data manipulation. There are two overall types of data manipulation in a database: sorting the data and querying the data. Both of these manipulations are dependent on the structure of the data and the entries in the fields. The structure is concerned with the fields and how these fields are combined into tables.

For the results of a sort or query to be accurate, the entries in a field must be identical for the same entity. For example, using Table 3-1, if the computer is queried for all individuals containing "Ohio" in the state field, it is necessary for the search criteria to use "Ohio." If some of the fields contained "OH" in the state field, those records would not be included in the query results. With a DBMS the data field either meets the query criteria, or it does not. There is no gray area. Thus the entries in a field that represent a given item must be identical. If one enters an abbreviation for a state in one record and the full name of the state in another, the computer will regard these as two different states. This need for unequivocal definitions is one of the primary driving forces for using standardized languages.

Another often-overlooked principle underlying database searching is that databases can only provide answers to questions using the data that they contain. For example, Table 3-1 cannot be used to search for the phone numbers of the individuals in Table 3-1. Those data are not included in the table. Not only must the data be present in a table, but also the table must be structured so that the data are retrievable. Therefore planning the structure of a database on paper is an essential first step before designing the database on the computer.

Sorting

Sorting, or reordering records, is relatively easy to understand because of familiarity with this phenomenon in the paper world. When a DBMS is used to sort the records alphabetically by last name, the process is the same whether the database is represented by a table such as Table 3-1, which contains only the four records seen, or a table with 1000 names. Although the process is the same, it would, of course, take longer to sort the larger database. Like querying, sorting occurs without any permanent change in the data or the table itself.

Secondary and Other Sorts Sorting by one field does not always provide the answer that one wants. It may be necessary to sort records by an overall field and then by several fields within that field. To illustrate, if Table 3-1 had 1000 records, it might be necessary to sort the records by state, then by the cities within each state, and then still further by the zip codes within each city. The first sort, by state, would be a **primary sort.** Sorting by the cities within the states would be a **secondary sort.** Ordering the records so that those with the same zip code in each city were next to one another would be a **tertiary sort.** If the alphabetizing of last names within each zip code were required, a quaternary sort would be performed. These levels of sorting are used when grouping records in a report.

This approach can be demonstrated using the example of a health care database that includes data reflecting the occurrence of postoperative infections. First, the records are selected for those patients who had a postoperative infection. A primary sort by organism, a secondary sort by clinical unit, and a tertiary sort by physician are completed. If these results do not provide the needed insight, the same data can be resorted. A primary sort by physician, then a secondary sort by organism, and then a tertiary sort by unit would provide a different view of these data. With a DBMS all of these sorts could be performed in less time than was required to read this paragraph.

Querying

Selecting the records of those patients who had a postoperative infection is a simple query. The criteria that identify the desired records are entered into the query form, and then the query is run. The DBMS produces the records that meet the specified criteria. Queries can also be used to perform calculations on the data in specified fields. Just as sorts can be based on more than one field, a query can also be designed to find records that meet more than one specification or to create calculations.

Boolean Arithmetic Boolean arithmetic, named for the nineteenth-century mathematician George Boole and introduced in Chapter 2, provides the underlying logic for queries, or searches, when a DBMS is used to search a database. In **Boolean logic** all decisions are reduced first to "true" or "false." By combining these true and false decisions, complex decisions are made. This type of decision-making is a form of algebra that works well in computers. In the previous example, Boolean logic is used to locate the records for those patients with postoperative infections.

When the datum in the appropriate field indicates that an infection was present, the criterion for "true" is present. A true response is generated, and the record is shown. If the datum in the appropriate field does not indicate that an infection was present, the criterion for "false" is present. The false response is generated, and the record is not shown. Essentially, Boolean logic breaks down to whether an entry matches the criteria as stated.

And/Or/Not A few of the words that can be used to make a request more specific are *and, or,* and *not.* Boolean logic is used when one wants records that meet multiple criteria. For example, let's say that there is a table of names and addresses that contains 1000 records from all over the United States. One is making a trip and wishes to contact all of the persons in the table who live in Liberty, New York. The database contains records of individuals who live in Liberty, New York; Liberty, Ohio; and Liberty, Missouri. To obtain just the records for Liberty, New York, it would be necessary to enter criteria in two fields: city and state. That is, for a record to be selected, the criteria in both fields must be met; "Liberty" must be the entry in the city field and "New York" must be the entry in the state field. This is an *and* query. An *and* query narrows a search.

Perhaps one also wishes to contact all of the persons in the table who live in Rhode Island and Connecticut. In this case one needs to find the records of the individuals who live in those states. This requires an *or* query; that is, one wants to find records with *either* "Rhode Island" or "Connecticut" in the state field. An *or* query broadens a search.

How to enter the criteria so that the fields in the desired records will match will vary according to the database application program used. The biggest difficulty is that the word *and* is often used to mean *or,* as would occur in the example if the requirement were written "Rhode Island and Connecticut." The criteria that determines whether to use *and* or *or* is whether one wants to broaden (or) or narrow (and) a search.

The use of *not* can further define the criteria. Using the same example, one might want all of the records that have "Rhode Island" or "Connecticut" in the state field, but not any that have "Stamford" in the city field. This is also a way to narrow a search.

Other Symbols Boolean searching is not limited to the use of *and/or/not* in selecting records. There are times when one wants to find records based on partial information in a field. To do this, one uses a **wildcard.** The character that is used for a wildcard may differ from one database application program to another, but the process can be seen in Table 3-2. Other characters may be used instead of the asterisk.

The "greater than" (>) and "less than" (<) signs are useful tools. They may even be used with text, in which case something is "less than" when it is closer to the beginning of the alphabet. Note that in Table 3-2, when the equals sign is used with another symbol, it always follows the symbol. Study Table 3-2 to gain an idea of the Boolean logic symbols that are useful in querying a database.

By creatively combining any or all of these operations, searches can be created that select exactly the records needed. Using combinations of these operations can be complex. When constructing complex searches, it is wise to use a test set of data for which the "answer" is known in order to test the query construction before using it with a large set of records.

Calculated Queries Databases, once in use, have a tendency to become very large. This can create data storage problems on any computer. Because most databases have to compete for space with other applications, one of the precepts in creating a table is to never include a field that can be calculated from other data. For example, if the age of a person is desired, instead of using age as a field, the age can be calculated

Table 3–2 Symbols Used in Boolean Searching

Expression	Definition	Example	Returns
Asterisk (*)	Wildcard	*ight	Records in which the **field entry** ends with *ight*
		i	Records in which the field entry contains the letter *i* anywhere
		12*	Records in which the field entry starts with *12*
>	Greater than	>5	Records in which the field entry is a numerical value of 6 or higher
>=	Greater than or equal to	>=10	Records in which the field entry is a numerical value of 10 or higher
<	Less than	<7	Records in which the field entry is a numerical value of 6 or lower
<=	Less than or equal to	<=7	Records in which the field entry is a numerical value of 7 or lower
<>	Not equal to	<>10	Records in which the field entry is any numerical value except 10
Between	Value lies between two givens	Between >=5 And <=10	Records in which the field entry is a numerical value greater than 4 *and* less than 11 (i.e., 5, 6, 7, 8, 9, and 10)
	For dates	Between 3/1/01 and 3/31/01	Records in which the field entry is a date in March 2001
Not	Does not contain	Not F	Records in which the field entry does *not* contain an *F*
Null	Empty	Null	Records in which the field is empty or blank

These can all be used in combination with one another as well as with *and/or/not.*

using the birth date. This also ensures that the current age will be returned when the database is queried. In addition to **date arithmetic,** queries can perform calculations based on any formula. For example, if there is a need to see the pulse pressure, instead of a field for this datum, the pulse pressure can be calculated from the data in the systolic and diastolic fields. This calculation saves room, as well as data entry time.

OVERVIEW OF DATABASE FEATURES

Relational databases consist of four main objects: table, query, form, and report. The table, with the data organized into fields (vertical columns) and records (horizontal lines), is the heart of any database. A table is where one starts when physically constructing a database. Without it, none of the other objects can be created.

The decisions made about field content and allocation to a table determine how the data can be manipulated. A systolic reading is datum at the atomic level; a combination of systolic and diastolic readings is not. If the required data include blood pressure without a separate field for both the systolic and the diastolic pressure, it will be difficult, if not impossible, to graph these data. Even when the original purpose of a database does not require a separation of data, uses for the data will increase when the database is used. It is easier to start with atomic-level fields than to break the fields into smaller fields later when new uses for the data have been discovered.

The use of one piece of data many times is facilitated by the different views that can be obtained from data, as well as the ability to sort and query the data. Data in a database can be viewed in a table, a form, or a report. Without changing any of the data in the underlying table, the records can be reordered by sorting and retrieved using queries based on a given set of criteria.

OBTAINING THE ANSWERS TO A SIMPLE QUESTION

Once the two health care personnel in the scenario at the beginning of this chapter (who wanted to know whether labor is shorter in patients when the membranes are artificially ruptured [AROM] or when they rupture spontaneously [SROM]) had an understanding of databases, they were ready to plan a database that would answer their questions.

What Information Is Needed?

The first step in planning a database is to specify exactly the information that is desired from the database. Questions cannot be answered if the data are not available. Thus the first step in planning a database is to write down exactly what one wants to know. The health care personnel in the scenario with the question regarding the length of labor would state this question in writing. Putting questions in writing avoids fuzzy thinking and later questions.

What Data Are Needed to Answer the Question?

The individuals in the scenario found that the data they needed to answer their question were (1) the length of labor and (2) the method of membrane rupture. They also decided that they would need a **unique identifier** for each record (a way to identify each record so that it would not be duplicated in the table). They decided that the medical record number would be a good unique identifier. In addition, they decided that they would begin by looking at the data for the last 3 months. Later they might expand their inquiry. Thus they also needed the date of delivery. Accordingly, they asked their IS person for data for (1) the length of labor,* (2) the method of membrane rupture, (3) the date of delivery, and (4) the unique identifier.

How Will the Data Be Manipulated?

In the scenario the IS individual provided the requested data for the preceding 12 months. The health care personnel first selected the records for only the last 3 months by asking to see all of the records between the first day of the first month and the last day of the last month. To gain the information they desired, they could have used a query that would have provided the averages for each group. However, they wanted to print the results, so instead they designed a report that would perform the needed calculations.

To provide an average for each group, it was necessary to group the records by method of membrane rupture. This allowed them to calculate the following:

- The average length of labor for patients in each group
- The average length of labor for patients in both groups
- The number of individuals in each group
- The total number of patients

In addition, they created a report that listed each record. The data that they received from the IS person can be seen in Table 3-3, and the report that they created is provided in Table 3-4.

---

*In the main database the length of labor would be calculated from the time and date of the start of labor to the time and date of delivery.

Table 3–3 Raw Data From Information Services

Medical Record No.	Date of Delivery	Hours of Labor	Method of Membrane Rupture
1	1/20/01	10.5	AROM
3	1/22/01	11.33	SROM
4	1/23/01	12.07	AROM
6	1/23/01	14.67	AROM
11	1/26/01	8.78	SROM
13	1/26/01	8.95	SROM
12	1/27/01	3.9	AROM
14	1/29/01	9.78	AROM
15	1/29/01	11.37	AROM
19	1/29/01	11.03	SROM
23	1/30/01	8.2	SROM
27	2/1/01	11.92	SROM
30	2/2/01	7.88	SROM
31	2/3/01	7.63	SROM
33	2/3/01	21.53	AROM
46	2/13/01	4.3	SROM
47	2/11/01	2.05	SROM
48	2/14/01	10.5	SROM
52	2/15/01	5.75	SROM
53	2/16/01	13	SROM
71	3/1/01	11	AROM
72	3/2/01	9.5	SROM
73	3/2/01	1.5	SROM
74	3/1/01	18.27	AROM
75	3/2/01	7.03	SROM
76	3/3/01	12.82	SROM
77	3/4/01	15.33	SROM
78	3/5/01	12.05	AROM
79	3/5/01	5.55	SROM
80	3/7/01	9.58	SROM

AROM, Artificial rupture of membranes; *SROM,* spontaneous rupture of membranes.

Although it looks like patients with SROM have shorter labors, these data have not been subjected to statistical analysis, so conclusions cannot be drawn about the outcome. It would be a relatively simple maneuver, however, to export the data to a statistical package for analysis. If these results were not statistically significant, these health care personnel might decide to examine data from a longer time period. This would strengthen any conclusions based on the results.

Even with additional data, the decision about whether their results were valid would depend on many things. Some other factors that could influence the results include the number of prior labors each parturient had, the age of the parturient, and even the identity of the physician. It should not be forgotten that this type of data manipulation is a form of research, which is often performed without the "up front" literature review. Conclusions should be considered only with an adequate literature review and follow-up to consider other causes. If a literature search is performed before a database is designed to answer clinical questions, variables that are useful in making decisions can be incorporated into the database. Used properly, databases can help to identify the scientific basis for a health care discipline. They can also demonstrate the value that each discipline adds to health care.

RELATIONAL DATABASES

Relational databases are databases that consist of more than one table. The database application programs in the professional office suites are all relational databases. Any of these relational databases can be used to create a single table, as well as multiple tables with related data.

The question that the health care personnel in the scenario wanted answered could easily be answered with a single table. A database consisting of a single table is called a **flat database.** There are times, however, when a flat database will not provide the needed data in an efficient manner.

Table 3–4 Report (Average Length of Labors by Method of Membrane Rupture)

AROM

Length of labor in hours:

3.90
9.78
10.50
11.00
11.37
12.05
12.07
14.67
18.27
21.53

Number of deliveries for AROM: 10

Average length of labor for AROM: 12.51

SROM

Length of labor in hours:

1.50
2.05
4.30
5.55
5.75
7.03
7.63
7.88
8.20
8.78
9.50
9.58
10.50
11.03
11.33
11.92
12.82
13.00
15.33

Number of deliveries for SROM: 20

Average length of labor for SROM: 8.63

All deliveries

Average length of labor for all 30 deliveries: 9.97

AROM, Artificial rupture of membranes; *SROM,* spontaneous rupture of membranes.

For example, suppose the two health care personnel, after looking at their results for the length of labor, decided that they wanted to look at the Apgar scores* for the newborns. In this agency Apgar scores were done at 1- and 5-minute intervals and every hour until the individual responsible was satisfied that the infant was stable.

If this were attempted in a flat database, the options would be as follows:

- Add fields to the table.
- Place multiple entries in the table.
- Create duplicate records for each Apgar score.

*An Apgar score is a rating of five items that was developed in 1953 by Dr. Virginia Apgar to assess a newborn's condition at birth. The items assessed are heart rate, respiratory effort, reflex irritability, muscle tone, and color.

Table 3-5 shows the result of adding fields to a table. There are several problems with this approach. The database designer has to make an arbitrary decision about the number of fields to add. In this case five fields were added. Not all of the fields, however, have an entry in them. Yet once a record is created in a database, it requires the same amount of storage space whether the fields have data in them or not. Thus space is wasted. In large databases this can rapidly take up storage space. There are several other problems with this approach. There will be times when more than five fields are needed. In addition, trying to print a report that groups the Apgar scores by time will be impossible.

In Table 3-6, multiple entries were put into one field. This creates several problems. One, it does not permit sorting by one entity. Nor will this solution permit one to easily create a report

Table 3–5 Multiple Fields

Medical Record No.	Delivery Date	Hours of Labor	Method of Membrane Rupture	Apgar 1 Min	Apgar 5 Min	Apgar 60 Min	Apgar 120 Min	Apgar 180 Min
1	1/20/01	10.5	AROM	8	9	10	6	
3	1/22/01	11.3	SROM	8	10	10		
4	1/23/01	12.07	AROM	9	10	10		

AROM, Artificial rupture of membranes; *SROM,* spontaneous rupture of membranes.

Table 3–6 Many Entries in One Field

Medical Record No.	Delivery Date	Hours of Labor	Method of Membrane Rupture	Apgars
1	1/20/01	10.5	AROM	6, 8, 9, 10
3	1/22/01	11.3	SROM	8, 10, 10
4	1/23/01	12.07	AROM	9, 10, 10

AROM, Artificial rupture of membranes; *SROM,* spontaneous rupture of membranes.

that distinguishes the time of the Apgar score. Another difficulty is that one does not know how large an area to designate for this field. Database designers have to indicate the length of a field so that the database will know how much room to provide for the data.

Creating duplicate records, as seen in Table 3-7, in addition to being labor intensive, hence expensive, opens the door to errors. Each time that data are entered, it is possible for errors to occur and for data that are not identical to the original entry to be used. Duplicate entries also increase the size of the database. Hence these solutions are unsatisfactory because they do not allow the data to be manipulated adequately or they jeopardize the accuracy of the data.

The best solution is to create another table that is related to the first one. This relationship is constructed by creating an identical field in both tables. The field that would be selected for both tables is the medical record number field from Table 3-3. The medical record number field in Table 3-3 is called a unique identifier. With a unique identifier no other record in that table can have the same datum in that field. For example, if the number "4502" is entered in the medical record number field for one patient, the database will not allow another entry of "4502" in the medical record number field of another record. The unique identifier allows the data from records in one table to be combined with the data from records in another table. Creating two or more tables that are related by unique identifiers creates a relational database. These unique identifiers are called **key fields.**

Table 3-8 displays the new table that would be developed in the scenario to contain the Apgar scores. Note that under this scheme there can be as many or as few Apgar recordings as are needed. Relationships such as these, in which there is more than one record in Table 3-8 that matches a record in Table 3-3, are known as **one-to-many.** The table in which there is only one record that matches is the **master table** (sometimes called the **parent table**), and the table that has many records that match is the **detail table** (sometimes called the **child table**). Thus Table 3-3 is the master table, and Table 3-8 is the detail table.

Table 3–7 **Duplicate Records**

Medical Record No.	Delivery Date	Hours of Labor	Method of Membrane Rupture	Time of Apgar in Minutes	Apgar
1	1/20/01	10.5	AROM	1	6
1	1/20/01	10.5	AROM	5	8
1	1/20/01	10.5	AROM	60	9
1	1/20/01	10.5	AROM	120	10
3	1/22/01	11.3	SROM	1	8
3	1/22/01	11.3	SROM	5	10
3	1/22/01	11.3	SROM	60	10
4	1/22/01	12.07	AROM	1	9
4	1/22/01	12.07	AROM	5	10
4	1/22/01	12.07	AROM	60	10

AROM, Artificial rupture of membranes; *SROM,* spontaneous rupture of membranes.

Table 3–8 Apgar Detail Table

Medical Record No.	Time in Minutes	Apgar
1	1	8
1	5	9
1	60	10
1	120	6
3	1	8
3	5	10
3	60	10
4	1	9
4	5	10
4	60	10

Getting Information From More Than One Table

Take a look at Tables 3-3 and Table 3-8. What is the delivery date for the infant whose Apgar scores in Table 3-8 are represented by medical record number 1? And what was the method of membrane rupture for this delivery? The delivery date was 1/20/01, and the method of rupture was artificial (AROM). That conclusion was reached by matching the number in the medical record number field of Table 3-8 with the number in the medical record number field in Table 3-3. This is a simple algorithm that the computer can be programmed to follow. The computer also performs this feat much more rapidly and with greater accuracy than humans.

With the data in Table 3-3 combined with the data in Table 3-8, the result looks like the data in Table 3-7 with duplicate entries. This result is achieved, however, by using what is already in the database, not by entering data twice or storing duplicate data. This is another example of how data can be manipulated to present different views without disturbing the underlying data structure and without the difficulties that would occur if the flat table design seen in Table 3-7 were used.

Entering Data Into a Relational Database

At this point, a logical question to ask would be how one could ensure that the medical record number field for the records in Table 3-3 would be identical to the medical record number field in Table 3-8, given that human beings are prone to errors. In a relational database, forms can be created that display fields from both the master table and the detail table. Figure 3-2 demonstrates such a form. It contains fields from Tables 3-3 and 3-8. With the use of this form, known as an **embedded form,** the information from the primary key field (the medical record number field in Table 3-3) in the master table is automatically copied to the foreign key field (the medical record number field in Table 3-8) in the detail table.

OVERVIEW OF PLANNING A RELATIONAL DATABASE

As was seen when the labor and delivery personnel in the scenario planned their database, the first step in creating a database is to determine the questions that the database will answer. The data that are needed are determined from these questions. The needed data elements are used to identify fields. Decisions are then made about what fields belong in which tables. Once the tables are planned, the unique identifier for each record is determined. A decision is then made concerning which table will be the master table and which tables will be the detail tables.

With relationships identified, one can identify primary keys and foreign keys. A **primary key** is the key field or fields in a master table. A **foreign key** is the exact match of the primary key in the detail table. Foreign keys are not unique identifiers and thus can be duplicated in the detail table but not in the master table. A detail table should have another field that is a unique identifier for itself that is *not* the foreign key.

FIGURE 3–2 | An Embedded Form

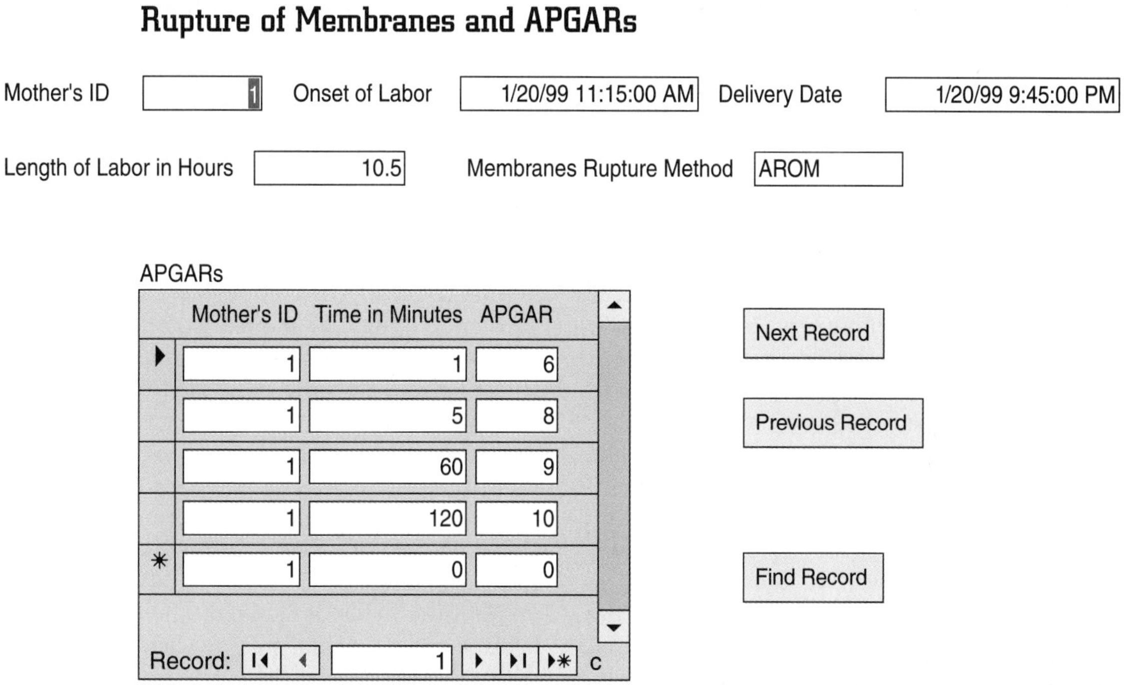

Rupture of Membranes and APGARs

Mother's ID [1] Onset of Labor [1/20/99 11:15:00 AM] Delivery Date [1/20/99 9:45:00 PM]

Length of Labor in Hours [10.5] Membranes Rupture Method [AROM]

APGARs

	Mother's ID	Time in Minutes	APGAR
▶	1	1	6
	1	5	8
	1	60	9
	1	120	10
*	1	0	0

Record: |◀ ◀ 1 ▶ ▶| ▶* c

Next Record

Previous Record

Find Record

To determine if the answers to the desired questions can be obtained using the planned table structure, it may be helpful to plan the queries that will be needed. It is not unusual at this point to have to add or reassign fields and create additional tables or change relationships. Because forms and reports can be based on queries, planning for queries will often need to be revisited when these are designed.

The next step is to consider how the data will be entered. This information will be used to create data entry forms. It should be noted that ease of data entry results in forms with fewer data errors. In a relational database, forms can be created that allow data entry into more than one table. During the process of designing the needed data entry forms on paper, it may be necessary to alter the table and relationships again, in which case one would again check to be certain that the desired questions can still be answered.

Deciding how the data will be viewed is done next. During this phase the screen or paper forms are designed. Screen and paper data views should be designed on paper before they are created. Once the screen and paper views are designed, the tables and related fields should be examined to determine if the relationships that have been created will allow the data to be displayed in the desired manner. Necessary changes are made, and the design of the database is again reviewed to determine if the modified design will be functional.

As can be seen, the design of a database is an iterative process. Besides checking to be certain that the planned design will function, it is an excellent idea to share with other potential users the current efforts. This is the time to identify further needs. It is far easier to make changes before physically creating the database on the computer. Investing time in creating forms and reports before finishing the process of planning the database is usually inefficient. In addition, it is helpful to test some assumptions by creating test tables with data.

PLANNING A DATABASE FOR A SPECIFIC SITUATION

Let's suppose that a unit manager wants a list of employees' addresses, home phone numbers, and dates of hire. In addition, this manager needs to track various types of recertifications that occur at 6-, 12-, and 24-month intervals. Many certifications are based on the classification of each employee. The unit manager wants to be able to send a notice to each employee a month in advance of the recertification date. He would like to have a list of recertification dates for all employees grouped by each month. Finally, he would like a report for each department responsible for the recertification that contains the names of employees who will be requiring the recertification. To meet these needs, the required data for each employee in the database are name, address, and phone number; classification name of the recertification that was completed; and date of the last recertification.

The unit manager reduces these data to atomic level and places each field name on a separate row in a table. See Table 3-9 for the table that this unit manager creates to identify each field. Initially, the unit manager uses only the leftmost column; the others will be used later in the planning process. At this point, the key fields are not yet identified; thus the fields marked with an asterisk are not yet in the table. Also, the need for a field for the date of next recertification has not yet been identified. Note that the field names have no spaces in them, but the words are demarcated with capital letters.* Although most modern databases allow spaces in field names, they create problems when doing some manipulations. Because databases tend to expand as they are used, the best idea is to start with field names without spaces. Using names that accurately reflect the data in the field makes it easier to understand the database.

The next column in Table 3-9 asks for the source of the data. This information is useful in making decisions about data entry. The unit manager knows that the basic demographic information about the employees is available from administration and requests permission to import it. Ideally, of course, there would be an automatic update or import from the administration data to the manager's database. This would ensure that the data used by this manager were always up-to-date. Errors creep into databases when more than one source of the same data are used. This leaves only two fields for which the unit manager will need to enter data: the type of recertification and the date it was completed.

With the fields designated, one can allocate fields to tables. In studying these fields, it can easily be determined that there are two main topics represented: demographic data and recertification data. The fields that represent unique information about each employee are assigned to one table. Because they represent employees, the descriptive title "Employee" is assigned to this table. The fields "TypeOfCertification" and "DateCompleted" represent the topic certification and therefore become another table titled appropriately "Certification."

At this point, one looks at each table and either designates a field that is present as a key field or adds a field that can act as the unique identifier. In this example the unit manager decides that "EmployeeID" will be the primary key in the Employee table. In the Certification table at present there is not a field that will serve this feature; thus one is added—"CertificationID." This field has no actual relationship to the data that the table will contain but is assigned as a unique identifier. Each is designated with an asterisk.

*Some database designers use the underscore (_) to connect words in field names.

Table 3–9 Fields for the Planned Database

Field Name	Source of Data	Table	How Entered	Type of Table	Type of Field	Length of Field
*EmployeeID	Administration	Employee	Import	Master to certification	Text	6
FirstName	Administration	Employee	Import		Text	15
MiddleInitial	Administration	Employee	Import		Text	1
LastName	Administration	Employee	Import		Text	20
StreetAddress	Administration	Employee	Import		Text	50
City	Administration	Employee	Import		Text	25
State	Administration	Employee	Import		Text	2
Zip	Administration	Employee	Import		Text	10
HomePhoneNumber	Administration	Employee	Import		Text	14
DateOfHire	Administration	Employee	Import		Date	
Classification	Administration	Employee	Import		Text	10
*CertificationID (a primary key for the Certification table)	In computer	Certifications	Automatically	Detail to employee	Auto-number	
TypeOfCertification	From certificate given me by employee	Certifications	Self		Look-up	15
DateCompleted	From certificate given me by employee	Certifications	Self		Date	
**EmployeeID	In Administration table	Certifications	Automatically		Text	6
DateNextCertification	From certificate given me by employee	Certifications	Self		Date	

*Primary key.
**Foreign key.

The unit manager now refers back to the desired information and determines the necessary table relationships. It will be necessary to link a name with a certification to produce the desired information; thus a link between these two tables will be needed. It is obvious that each record in the Employee table will represent only one employee, although there may be several records in the Certification table for each employee. This then becomes a one-to-many relationship, with the Employee table serving as the master table (one record) and the Certification table serving as the detail table (many records for each record in the Employee table).

With the relationship identified, it can be seen that for the Certification table to be linked to the Employee table, a linking field will be necessary. The logical field that provides accurate identification of the data in the Certification table is the employee ID; thus it is added to that table. In this relationship the Employee table is the master table and the Certification table is the detail table. Thus "EmployeeID" becomes the primary key in the Employee table and the foreign key in the Certification table.

A solution that prevents these problems yet still provides the needed information is seen in Table 3-10. With this design, a report could be created that was printed every month and grouped by the type of recertification (e.g., cardiopulmonary resuscitation [CPR], fire safety). With the design in Table 3-11, one would need to create a separate report for each category. The report would list the names of the individuals who needed to fulfill a given requirement and the date by which this must be done. Although the table itself contains the date from the previous certification, using date arithmetic, it would be possible to have the report print the date when each item was due instead of the date on which it was completed the previous year. Because each year a new entry could be made, this structure would preserve a history that could be used to find any employees who were habitually late in recertifications.

Table 3–10 Best Structure for Certification Table

ID No.	TypeOfCertification	DateCompleted

Types of Data and Fields

For a DBMS to effectively manipulate the data in a field, it is necessary to designate the type of data that is stored in the field. There are many different types of data; major data types are text, date, and numeric. One other type of field is called an object linking and embedding (OLE) field. This type of field can contain graphics. Most other data types are modifications of these. For example, a text field may be further designated as a look-up field. Table 3-12 lists some of the available data and field types.

An often-used type of numeric field is the auto-number field. When an auto-number field type is designated, the computer automatically creates a new number for each record. This number will not be duplicated even if the original record assigned that number is deleted. The auto-number field is useful as a unique identifier when another field does not lend itself to the

Table 3–11 Beginner's Conceptualization of Detail Table

ID No.	CPR Date	Fire Safety Date	Name of Certification	Certification Date

task. The unit manager in the example could use this type of field for the certification ID.

The design of a database requires that fields be assigned a specified length. The only exception to this rule is a memo field. The size of the memo field is determined by the software. A memo field is used for entries that are lengthy and that will not be used in data manipulation. An example would be a comments field. When one designs a database the lengths of all fields that are assigned, except for memo fields, are provided. The size of a memo field is determined by the software. Decisions about the length of fields should be made to include the most unusual case. For this example, the length of the fields for the demographic information would have been set by the administration table. The certification field length should accommodate the longest certification available and perhaps a few more characters. Spaces are included in counting characters for field length.

Table 3–12 Some Database Field Types

Type of Field	Use
Text/alphanumeric	All fields that will not be calculated; must designate a length for these fields; limit 255 characters
Numeric	Use only for numeric fields on which calculations will be performed; should not include alphanumeric fields that consist of numbers only (e.g., phone numbers, zip codes, employee numbers); there are many different subtypes of numeric fields (e.g., currency, byte, integer)
Time/date	Fields that will contain dates and/or times
Memo	A field that contains text of more than 255 characters
Look-up	Fields in which one can specify a list of data from which entries can be made
Auto-number	A field that automatically creates a new number for each record that will not be duplicated even if the original record assigned that number is deleted; useful for keys when another field does not lend itself to this task of being a unique identifier
OLE	Short for object linking and embedding; used to provide links to graphics or other objects

Once the information about columns in Table 3-9 is completed, the information can be used to construct a **data dictionary.** A data dictionary is a table that provides information about the database. It is a table of tables that contains a list of all of the tables in the database, as well as the fields in the tables and a description of the fields. The only addition needed is a description of the contents in a field. Although the field names themselves are descriptive of the field contents, the data dictionary provides additional detail. It is also wise, after finishing the planning process, to create another table that lists any queries, forms, and reports and provides information about the fields they reference and the tables they represent. Planning a database is facilitated by the use of a word processor, or paper process, to create the tables used for planning. When actually creating the database, these tables are created as part of the database to ensure that they will be readily available to anyone who needs them.

Data dictionaries are useful as a quick reference or for anyone who needs to update the database design. For example, the unit manager might decide that it is necessary to have information about the length of time between recertifications for each type of certification. Using the data dictionary would make it much easier to add a table that includes this information. The larger the database, the more imperative keeping a quickly referenced data dictionary becomes.

Accuracy of Data

As the earlier example using the state of Ohio demonstrated, in order for a database to effectively provide information, all of the characters used to indicate a given data element must be identical. Using the employee example, "cardiopulmonary resuscitation" and "CPR" could not both be used in the certification field to indicate CPR. To protect against different terms being used for the same data element, look-up tables can be included in the database. The **look-up table** contains the specific terminology to be used for each condition. When data are entered in that field, a box drops down from which the appropriate term can be selected. The database will limit the entries in that field to only what is on that list. The field can also be designated to allow free text entry.

Another way to increase data accuracy is to stipulate the lowest and highest numbers that can be entered in a numeric field. It is also possible to create a default entry. A default entry is data that are automatically placed in a field unless overwritten by the person entering data.

None of these techniques ensures complete accuracy, but they prevent many errors while making data entry easier. As a rule of thumb, look-up tables should be used for as many fields as possible. On the database in the example, a look-up field would be appropriate for the field labeled "TypeOfCertification."

Designing look-up tables begins by identifying the terms to be used in the table. This usually requires working with those responsible for entering the data. There must be agreement about what terms will be included, and each term must be unambiguously defined.

Queries

Queries are the power of a database. As stated earlier, planning queries provides a further check on whether all of the needed data are included and structured appropriately. They can also be used as a basis for developing forms or reports. Database software differs on whether the information produced in a query is a replica of the table or the actual table; thus whether a query can be used as a basis for a form for data entry depends on the software.

In the example the unit manager began by creating a query of the employees' phone numbers and addresses. The manager looked at the fields in the Employee table to be certain that the needed information was available. Using paper, a name was assigned to the query, a purpose written, and the fields needed listed. After planning this query and starting the next step, planning a report, the unit manager realized that the report could be done without first producing a query. The unit manager then changed the query to a report, an easy step in the planning process and one that saved a step in the creating process. In general, if a report needs information from only one table and only summarizes calculations (e.g., sum, average), the report can be created without first creating a query.

To retrieve the data for the three additional reports needed—one for the employee, one for the manager's reference, and one for the department responsible for the recertification—it was necessary to create a query. The query required both tables. The query would retrieve the ID number, first name, middle initial, last name, and type of recertification needed on the basis of the date of the last recertification. Here the unit manager realized that because there was a different time length between the various types of recertifications, it would be easier to select the records by the date of the next recertification and thus added that field to the Certification table. With this new field it now became possible to select the records using the field for the date of the next recertification. To illustrate, when the unit manager created a report for those employees due for recertification in May 2002, the criterion was "Between May 1, 2002, and May 31, 2002." The unit manager created the plan seen in Table 3-13 for the needed query. The unit manager used this to match the query against the

Table 3–13 Query Plan

Name of query: Certifications needed
Description: Provides a list of those needing recertification for the next month

Table	Fields	Criteria and/or Comments
Employee	FirstName	
	MiddleInitial	
	LastName	
	EmployeeID	
Certification	TypeOfCertification	
	DateNextCertification	Between the beginning and end of the next month

information already in the plan to determine if the planning so far was adequate.*

Data Entry User Interfaces or Forms

In the example, with the addition of a field for the date of the next recertification, the unit manager determined that all of the necessary fields were present. The unit manager was now ready to design forms for data entry. Because this manager had arranged to import the data in the employee table, a form to enter these data was not needed. The only data that the unit manager needed to enter pertained to certifications in the Certification table. The unit manager decided that it would be helpful to have the employee's name, ID number, and date of hire visible when data were entered. Using a table similar to the one in Table 3-13, the unit manager listed the fields needed in the form, as well as the table where the entered data would be stored. A picture of the proposed form was then sketched. The form contained the needed fields from the master table and the detail table. Data were automatically copied into the employee ID field from the master table, and the computer automatically assigned a number to the certification ID field. The design resembled Figure 3-2, but with the appropriate tables and fields.

Whether one is designing a small database for individual use or a large hospital information system, creating a user interface that makes data entry easy can be the key to the success of the project. The form in Figure 3-1 is a user interface for Table 3-1. On this form the database designer used labels for each field. The designer also added instructions to make it easier for the person entering the data. In addition, the designer provided easily accessible buttons to simplify some of the routine tasks related to entering data. When designing these types of forms, it is important to think about the related human factors. Chapter 15 focuses on this topic. Conferring with the individuals who will enter the data before finalizing a design can improve the form and help create a sense of ownership.

---

*To save data entry, a table for the length of time between each recertification would be created. This would be used to calculate the date for the next recertification. This query would then be used to request the specific records in which recertification was due in the next month. To keep this example simple, this step is not being done here.

Field placement on a database form is *not* determined by the field's location in the table. A field can be placed anywhere on the form. If the user must enter data from a paper form, the database form should be designed to follow the printed form exactly. Also, the form should be organized so that those items that need to be seen together are on one form and present a logical view.

The ergonomics of a user interface is very important to the success or failure of information systems (Thede, 1999). When data entry screens are not designed to mirror how the individual works, errors and frustration are invited. In the process of designing screens, the importance of listening to those who will be using and entering data cannot be overemphasized. Users will not accept a system that is difficult to use or counterintuitive. If they are forced to use it, problems such as incorrect or incomplete data will result.

Reports

Forms are designed for onscreen viewing, whereas reports are designed for printed presentations. Like forms, reports can be based on one or more tables or on a query. The same table format (i.e., Table 3-13) used in planning a query is used to plan a report. In the example the unit manager lists the fields needed for each report and the table or query from which each will be retrieved. If it is desired that the records in a report be alphabetical, a comment is added stating which field will be used to alphabetize the records. Comments will also be added if grouping of records by a given field is wanted. A sketch of the planned report is then made.

The unit manager has already created reports that will produce a list of names and addresses and one that will produce just the names and phone numbers. This was done while planning queries. The query for the three recertification reports was designed earlier. For the department responsible for the recertification, it is necessary to print a report with the names of employees who need the certification offered by the department. This report requires that the records be grouped by type of certification. The report that is created for the employees will include the type(s) of recertification required by the following month. This report will have to be grouped by employee. The unit manager also plans a report listing the recertifications needed listed alphabetically by employee last name with a space between each employee's name. This report will be grouped by employee last name. Each of these reports can be based on the query described earlier. Using this information, the unit manager designs on paper how each of these reports should look and adds the notes regarding the grouping that will be needed when the actual report is constructed. In the paper sketch, a differentiation is made between data that will be retrieved and data that will be added to make the report clear to the recipient. Using a highlighter for the data to be retrieved will achieve this.

The paper planning process is iterative. As each step is completed, one should check to see that previous steps do not need to be modified. The importance of planning a database on paper before attempting to construct one on the computer cannot be overemphasized. The later in the creation process that a database must be changed, the more expensive and time consuming the changes will be. An outline of the steps in planning a database can be seen in Box 3-1.

To the Computer

With a paper plan completed, one is ready to use the computer and the DBMS. The first items to be designed are the tables. Before progressing to forms and reports, it is helpful to enter a few records, create a query, and see if the appropriate data are available. This step is a final check on the written plan. It is not a substitute for careful planning before the computer is approached. The earlier that errors are found when creating a database, the easier it will be to correct them.

Box 3–1 Outline of Steps in Planning a Database

1. List questions to be asked.
2. Determine fields needed to provide the answers and list them.
3. Study the fields to see what topics they represent.
4. Allocate the fields to tables based on the topic.
5. Identify primary key fields.
6. Determine the relationships between the tables.
7. Add foreign key fields where needed.
8. Designate the types of fields and allocate space for fields that will contain text.
9. Designate terminology for any look-up fields.
   a. Confer with users.
   b. Write a description of the terms.
   c. Get agreement from users for definitions and terms.
10. Plan the queries needed and ascertain if the structure supports the queries. Replan where necessary.
11. Plan the forms for data entry and ascertain if the structure supports the forms.
    a. Add notes for constructing the form.
    b. Make a sketch of the proposed form.
    c. Confer with those will enter the data.
    d. Replan where necessary.
12. Plan the reports and ascertain if the structure supports the forms.
    a. Add notes for constructing the report.
    b. Make a sketch of the reports.
    c. Confer with those who will enter the data.
    d. Replan where necessary.
13. Design views for the data—both screen (forms) and paper (reports)—and ascertain if the structure supports the queries. Replan where necessary.
14. Study the entire plan to be certain that it is valid.

CONCLUSION

A database is a very powerful tool. The increased access to data provided by a DBMS significantly increases the ability of health care providers to make practice-based decisions. To effectively use these data in a database system, the user must understand database structures and the types of data manipulation possible. Databases can be used by health care professionals in administrative positions for many items that they need to track on a routine basis. Careful planning of these databases will decrease considerably the time involved in constructing and maintaining them.

Databases also have a place in helping health care professionals discover clinical information. Some nurses are now using existing clinical data to support clinical and management decisions (Minarik, 1999). One example is the use of laboratory reports and nursing acuity scores to identify inpatients at risk for skin breakdown. In this capacity, however, it is not a tool to be used lightly. Recall the two individuals who were trying to determine if labor was shorter when the membranes were ruptured artificially or spontaneously. Even if the data turned out to be statistically significant, they needed to consider other factors before coming to any conclusions.

In health care problems there is often debate about which type of care is most beneficial. A database could help to answer many of these questions. For example, there are many different treatment approaches used to treat chronic wounds. But which approach results in the best outcome in the shortest period of time? In a long-term care facility, pressure ulcers are often a problem. Which type of mattress produces the least number of pressure ulcers? The results of these databases, however, are better designed and more reliable if an appropriate literature review is the first step in the database design.

In short, the power of a database rests with the vision of the individual health care provider. When one understands how a database functions and is curious about the "why's" of health care procedures and treatments, many opportunities for gaining the knowledge and wisdom for improving patient care will present themselves.

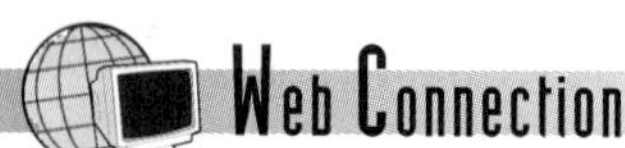

Web Connection

Health care professionals are becoming increasingly dependent on databases to support their work because of the vast array of information available to them through databases. Besides developing databases to support their work, health care professionals need to become knowledgeable about evaluating existing databases. Through the Web activities for this chapter you are given the opportunity to explore some popular databases, paying particular attention to the elements of the database that are useful in helping collect needed data or information. The purpose of exploring databases is to provide you with the ability to identify the elements of good database design as it has been described in this chapter, as well as to develop skill in performing searches within different databases.

discussion questions

1. Name three health care questions that could be approached using a database. Explain your answer.
2. Identify three questions that might be asked of health care data contained in a patient's health care record. What specific data elements would be needed to answer these questions?
3. Identify a specific health or health care delivery problem and plan a database for the management of that problem.

REFERENCES

Minarik, P. (1999). Using hospital databases. *American Journal of Nursing, 99*(2), 54.

Montlick, T. (1999). *What is object-oriented software?* Retrieved April 2, 2000, from the World Wide Web: http://www.soft-design.com/softinfo/objects.html.

Saba, V., and McCormick, K.A. (1995). *Essentials of computers for nurses.* New York: McGraw-Hill.

Software Technology Review. (2000). Retrieved June 3, 2000, from the World Wide Web: http://www.sei.cmu.edu/str/descriptions/oodatabase.html.

Sol S. (1999a). *The hierarchical database model.* eXtropia. Retrieved April 3, 2000, from the World Wide Web*: http://www.extropia.com/tutorials.html/sql/hierarchical_databases.html.

Sol S. (1999b). *The network database model.* eXtropia. Retrieved April 3, 2000, from the World Wide Web*: http://www.extropia.com/tutorials.html/sql/network_databases.html.

Sol S. (1999c). *The relational database model.* eXtropia. Retrieved September 4, 2000, from the World Wide Web*: http://www.extropia.com/tutorials.html/sql/relational_databases.html.

Thede, L.Q. (1999). *Computers in nursing: Bridges to the future.* Philadelphia: J.B. Lippincott.

VanBemmel, J.H. (Ed.). (1999). *Handbook of medical informatics.* Retrieved September 4, 2000, from the World Wide Web: http://www.mihandbook.stanford.edu/handbook/home.htm.

*The URL given is the actual URL, but to access these references, you must first go to http://www.extropia.com/, click on "tutorials," scroll down to "Introduction to Databases for Web Developers" and select from that menu. The eXotropia company develops full-featured, well-tested, install-out-of-the-box Web applications for Web designers.

CHAPTER 4

Supporting Administrative Decision Making

MICHAEL H. KENNEDY

Learning Objectives

Upon completion of this chapter, the reader will be able to:

1. ***Describe*** an administrative decision support system.
2. ***Distinguish*** between administrative and clinical decision support systems.
3. ***Discuss*** administrative decision support system components.
4. ***Identify*** contemporary decision support system applications by administrative health care venue.
5. ***Discuss*** emerging developments in administrative decision support systems.

Outline

Key Terms

agency relationship
clinical data repository
criterion of rationality
criterion of realism
data definition language
data dictionary
data manipulation language (DML)
data marts
data warehouse
database
database management system (DBMS)
decision analysis
decision support system (DSS)
demand management
economic order quantity (EOQ) model
electronic data interchange (EDI)
expected value (EV) criterion
field
file
forecasting

Key Terms—cont'd

geographical information system (GIS)
graph theory
group decision support systems
homegrown product
inventory models
linear programming
maximally effective care
maximax criterion
maximin criterion
maximum likelihood criterion
minimax regret criterion
model library
model manager
network problems
optimally effective care
query language
queuing theory
record
report writer
simulation
spreadsheet
user interface

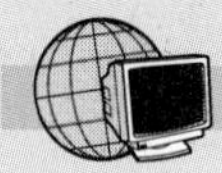

Web Connection

Go to the Web site at http://evolve.elsevier.com/Englebardt/. Here you will find Web links and activities related to supporting administrative decision making.

There are two primary types of decision support systems (DSSs) in health care: administrative and clinical. This chapter distinguishes between the two types and focuses on administrative DSSs. The administrative DSS is formally defined, and typical decision support applications and software packages are discussed. The algorithms and decision models embedded in many administrative DSSs are reviewed, as are the strengths and weaknesses of the rudimentary decision support tool kit offered by spreadsheets and databases. The chapter concludes with a discussion of emerging developments.

OVERVIEW OF ADMINISTRATIVE DECISION MAKING AND DECISION SUPPORT

Historically, the perspectives assumed and processes employed by health care personnel making decisions have differed depending on whether they were fulfilling administrative or clinical roles. The **agency relationship** assumed that the clinician made decisions to ensure the welfare of the individual patient and, by extension, family members and others who cared about the patient (McLean, 1997). In that context the clinician's primary focus was directed toward ensuring health care interventions on behalf of the individual patient that continued as long as positive benefits were achieved. Concerns about resource consumption and costs were largely secondary. Donabedian (1995) has described this approach as **maximally effective care.** The health care institution benefited from this approach as positive individual patient outcomes aggregated to produce a collective reputation for quality.

Health care personnel operating in administrative roles have generally embodied a systems perspective. Under this approach, decisions were made to conserve finite institutional resources by supporting useful additions to health care until the differences between the benefits received and the costs to deliver that care were maximized. Donabedian (1995) has described this approach as **optimally effective care.** Optimality identifies the point beyond which the benefits received for one additional dollar of health care begin to decrease. For example, at the point of optimally effective care the patient may receive a benefit worth $5 for every dollar spent. The additional provision of health care beyond the optimal point may result in $4 of benefit for every dollar spent. Effective and efficient health care delivery processes resulting from fiscal stewardship translated into patient care that exceeded an acceptable-quality threshold while offering the potential for improving access to care.

That was then; this is now. Grossman (1994) has reviewed the changing marketplace incentives caused by the transition from cost-plus reimbursement to prospective payment. Under the previous system, providers were paid to dispense units of health care and were reimbursed for the costs of providing services. Increasing service volume increased revenue. Less attention was paid to producing the best outcomes as efficiently as possible. Under the new system, revenues are prospectively determined. The best result accrues when an agreed-on threshold of quality is achieved or exceeded at lowest cost. Measurement of outcomes becomes crucial to ensure that the process of care delivery produces the expected result and to counter the incentive to withhold necessary medical services. Focusing on outcomes involves a tremendous volume of highly fragmented data and information. The complexities that this fosters demand solutions provided by information technology. Although it is difficult to extract information for clinical decision making, the challenge administrators face is "to track and organize a welter of data to distinguish between necessary and inappropriate services, to identify opportunities for greater efficiency, and to project the cost implications of substituting one form of treatment for another" (Grossman, 1994, p. 24). Sophisticated information and networking technologies help administrators make decisions about the consumption of resources and selection of processes to support the delivery of health care.

Kvedar (2000) has also examined the "unparalleled change" that health care in the United States is undergoing. Projected increased demands for health care run counter to growing third-party payer reluctance to foot the bill for noninflationary costs. Health care providers are increasingly challenged to find a business model that accommodates both patient demand and payer constraints. Information technology has provided core solutions to similar problems faced by both financial services and airline industries (Kvedar, 2000). Many of the transactions supported by bank tellers and airline ticket agents can be completed by the customer with the support of the decision support functions of an automated teller or ticket agent. Health care has been slow to make a similar investment. The typical health care information expenditures are 2% to 3% of the organization's operating budget compared with 7% to 9% for retail and financial organizations.

Administrative Decisions Typically Faced by Health Care Leaders

Health care leaders are faced with the need to make a variety of nonclinical decisions designed to support and facilitate the delivery of reasonably priced, high-quality health care in an environment constrained by resource limitations. This environment is further complicated by the following:

- Evolving decision paradigms that modify decision objectives and constraints
- Rapid technological change that increases the opportunity for successful health care interventions
- Patients and payers who are better informed of these opportunities and increasingly reluctant to assume the burden of increasing costs

Objective decision making that is timely and informed by data provides the basis for effective competition and even survival in the medical marketplace.

The quantity and complexity of decisions faced by the health care executive demand standardized decision processes (Fralic & Denby, 2000). The creation of credible and effective DSSs has become a core executive competency. DSSs must help the executive to respond to the following five themes that shape the current health delivery paradigm:

1. The mandate by patients, payers, and compliance agencies to precisely measure and quantify services provided and their costs and quality
2. The need to respond to financial pressure stemming from the increasing demand for and intensity of services provided, which is balanced against a growing payer revolt against the associated price of care
3. The pressures to recruit, retain, pay, and effectively deploy the health care workforce
4. The management of workload variability either caused by fluctuations in demand for care and intensity of services or resulting from directional strategies employed by the health care institution
5. The efforts to reduce variation in practice reflected by protocol-based health care

In responding to these five themes, health care DSSs must meet the following criteria (Fralic & Denby, 2000):

- Timeliness—Data must be input, alternatives generated, and recommendations rendered within a relevant time frame.
- Objectivity—Decisions must be made in response to identified criteria, and the decision process must be explicit.
- Integration—Decisions must be made within the context of the entire organization.
- Scope–Information collected must be bounded by the demands of the decision under consideration.
- Priority—DSSs must help prioritize among the range of decisions facing the health care executive.

Decision Venues

Several taxonomies have been used to present the major decision-making categories. According to Fralic and Denby (2000), decisions can be categorized as clinical, financial, operational, strategic, or some mix of these categories. Decisions can be differentiated on the basis of the frequency with which they must be made—whether they must be made on an ongoing and daily, periodic, or one-time basis. Improving DSSs requires an understanding of each of the decision categories and how they interrelate. A vision of what decisions require better information and how that information can be collected should also be communicated. Finally, the appropriate decision support infrastructure must be constructed and staff members trained on the system. Effective DSSs are needed to free health care executives from routine, day-to-day operational decisions. The role of the health care leader is to set the strategic direction of the health care organization, not to "put out fires."

DSSs are ideally used to support the semistructured and unstructured decisions that health care leaders often face (Turban, 1993). This support also requires an adequate information technology infrastructure.

To be effective, DSSs depend on accurate information that is quickly retrievable across the entire enterprise. Both the DSS and sources of organizational information must be tied to the organization's business rules, and applications such as cost accounting, product line analysis, episodic grouping, revenue modeling, and provider profiling must be deployable to information users throughout the organization (Nunnelly, 1997).

Griffith and King (2000) have identified eight categories of decision processes. Six are distinctly administrative—governance/strategic management, financial planning, planning and marketing, information services, human resources, and plant services. Two are distinctly clinical—clinical quality and clinical organization.

A problem exists when the health care leader is unaware of the results of literally decades of research in the associated fields of management science that could provide insights, methods, and tools for solving administrative problems. Blumenfield (1997) has addressed the problems clinicians face as a result of data overload, inaccessible reference sources at the point of decision, and inability to pose the correct question. To be effective, point-of-care decision support must be offered within the appropriate clinical context through convenient, real-time reference to a clinical knowledge base. The knowledge base can be filtered to anticipate and answer questions that should be asked by the clinician. For example, an order for a specific drug may prompt a warning regarding potential interactions (Blumenfield, 1997).

In a similar fashion, executives addressing nonclinical problems need point-of-decision support within the appropriate management venue through convenient, real-time access to information about the health care organization and available methods or tools. As with clinical systems, administrative DSSs should anticipate or suggest to administrators appropriate questions to ask. However, ensuring confidence in the recommendations of the DSS requires an understanding of algorithms and decision models.

The discussion that follows provides an overview of algorithms and decision models that are useful to administrative decision making. Then an examination of two tools that are not fully evolved DSSs is presented. These are spreadsheets and databases. Discussions regarding advances in the science of decision making often focus on the input and output only. The decision processes captured by the decision models and algorithms are relegated to a "black box" without revealing how the data are processed. Data processing is accepted as a magical occurrence. The discussion that follows is intended to open this "black box."

Opening the Black Box: Algorithms and Decision Models

Levin et al. (1992) have noted that management science/operations research helps managers make better decisions by employing a quantitative approach. The authors have cataloged the contributions of many disciplines, including physics, engineering, mathematics, probability, and statistics. Since World War II the field of quantitative research and its contributions to management science have continued to expand. An overview of the history of operations research is reflected in Table 4-1 (Rubbo, 1992).

Quantitative specialists can assist and support organizational leaders in the process of decision making. Levin et al. (1992) found that the manager and the quantitative specialist typically have different roles in problem recognition, formulation, and solution. The astute manager discerns a problem from organizational symptoms. Together, the manager and the quantitative specialist model the problem by identifying the variables involved and quantifying the relationships among them. The quantitative specialist investigates approaches and tools for solving the problem, makes assumptions, and produces alternative solutions. Together, the manager and the quantitative specialist determine the impact of each solution on the organization and determine which solution is best, given the environmental constraints. Final responsibility for choosing the solution to be implemented rests with the manager as the decision authority. Managers and quantitative specialists have applied operations research/ management science (OR/MS) algorithms and

Table 4–1 Significant Events in the History of Operations Research/Management Science

Date	Significant Events
1942	J. Tate recruits P.M. Morse to form the "Baker's Dozen"
1945	RAND founded
1947	G.B. Dantzig debuts the simplex algorithm; J. von Neumann introduces duality for linear programming (LP); J. Laderman solves the Diet Problem via calculator
1951	"Karuch-Kuhn-Tucker" conditions introduced for nonlinear programming
1953	T.M. Whitin introduces stochastic inventory models
1954	Petroleum blending problem solved by LP; W. Orchard-Hays develops commercial LP software at RAND
1957	Smith's rule published regarding shortest processing time optimality; J.R. Jackson establishes Jackson Queueing Networks
1958	R.E. Gomory publishes cutting plane solution for integer programs; program evaluation and review technique (PERT) and critical path management (CPM) project management methods established by Booz, Allen, and Hamilton and by J.E. Kelly and M. Walker, respectively
1961	S. Johnson publishes Johnson's rule for two-machine scheduling; IBM produces commercial version of GPSS by G. Gordon; J.D.C. Little produces his queuing formula ($L = \lambda W$)
1964	Simscript simulation program produced
1967 to 1968	Foundation scheduling (Conway, Maxwell, & Miller, 1967) and operations research textbooks (Hillier & Lieberman, 1967; Wagner, 1968) published
1975 to 1977	Personal computers made available to average consumer with Altair and Apple II
1979	L.G. Khachian's ellipsoidal algorithm translated and publicized
1982	Simulated annealing based on idea by N. Metropolis
1984	N. Karmarkar's algorithm published based on ellipsoidal LP algorithm

Data from Rubbo, E.G. (1992). ORSA turns 40: OR pioneers tell of four decades of achievement, anecdotes. *OR/MS Today, April*, 50-52.

techniques to accounting, finance, marketing, production and operations management, organizational development, and human resources management. Given the importance of these areas to contemporary health care management, OR/MS continues to have a significant role in the efficient and effective operation of health care organizations.

Unfortunately, the value of quantitative methods in the effective management of health care and other organizations is often overlooked or misunderstood, particularly as the quantitative techniques and algorithms become embedded in the tools facilitated by modern information technology. Once committed to software, the solution approaches become part of a "black box" that the naive or uninformed manager fails to understand.

Opening the "black box" involves the examination of the algorithms and decision models employed to solve problems. Representative quantitative techniques include forecasting, decision analysis, inventory models, linear programming, graph theory and network problems, queuing theory and waiting line problems, and simulation.

Table 4–2 Deciding Among Feasible Hospital-Based Ambulatory Care Construction Alternatives: Payoff Table

	Feasible Hospital-Based Ambulatory Care Construction Alternatives		
States of Nature (Demand)	**Status Quo**	**Renovation**	**Construction**
Low	$0	−$100,000	−$300,000
Moderate	$100,000	$200,000	$300,000
High	$200,000	$400,000	$600,000

Forecasting **Forecasting** takes advantage of experience. Basically, knowledge about what happened in the past should improve the ability to estimate what will happen in the future. For example, documentation of the pattern of arrivals to the emergency department during the previous year will identify trends, as well as seasonal and random variation. These can be used to project future emergency department arrivals. A variety of mathematical techniques can be employed to develop a projection of future demand. Time series data collected at regular intervals (daily, weekly, and yearly) can be used by a variety of extrapolation methods. Causal methods explore the relationship between the variable of interest (e.g., number of arrivals to the emergency department) and other variables (e.g., patient demographics, insurance status, proximity to the facility). Judgmental forecasting solicits consumer feedback or expert opinion (Levin et al., 1992).

Decision Analysis **Decision analysis** is concerned with making the best decision possible on the basis of the information available. Chapter 4 of the text by Levin et al. (1992) serves as the basis for the discussion of decision analysis that follows. When a decision is to be made, three steps are often followed. First, feasible alternatives are considered. For example, a hospital may be considering alternatives to meet the projected demand for ambulatory services. Some possible alternatives are to retain the status quo, renovate available space within the hospital, or initiate new construction. Second, possible states of nature are identified. These decision states are mutually exclusive future events affecting the decision. In the ambulatory services example the states of nature concern the level of demand for ambulatory services. The future demand state for ambulatory services might be low, moderate, or high. Finally, a payoff table is constructed, listing the consequences for each alternative selected in conjunction with each decision state. A 3 × 3 payoff table (Table 4-2) lists the consequences for the nine possibilities related to this example.

Important administrative decisions in health care are generally made in one of two environments: conditions of uncertainty or conditions of risk. When the decision maker operates under conditions of uncertainty, insufficient knowledge exists to assign probabilities to the various demand states. Under conditions of uncertainty for the problem described, an informed decision maker would not be able to assess the probabilities associated with each of the demand states for ambulatory care. In this situation the decision maker would make a decision by selecting from one of four criteria.

The **maximax criterion** is an optimistic criterion that assumes the maximum payoff for each alternative, and the decision maker chooses the alternative representing "best of the best" payoffs. For Table 4-2, the maximum payoffs for status quo, renovation, and construction are \$200,000, \$400,000, and \$600,000, respectively, and the alternative chosen would be construction.

The **maximin criterion** is a pessimistic criterion that assumes the minimum payoff for each alternative, and the decision maker chooses the alternative representing the "best of the worst" payoffs. For Table 4-2 the minimum payoffs for status quo, renovation, and construction are \$0, −\$100,000, and −\$300,000, respectively, and the alternative chosen would be status quo.

The **minimax regret criterion** takes a different tack by first assessing the opportunity costs (regret) associated with each decision (demand) state. The maximum regret for each decision alternative is highlighted, and the "minimum of these maximums" is chosen. Table 4-3 reflects the regret table associated with this problem and the selection of renovation as the preferred alternative.

The **criterion of realism** is a weighted average computed for each decision alternative with the use of a coefficient α bounded by 0 and 1, called an "index of optimism." A sample computation of a measure of realism for the status quo alternative follows, with the index of optimism set at $\alpha = 0.6$:

Measure of realism (Status quo) =
$$[(\alpha) \times (\text{Maximum payoff for status quo})] +$$
$$[(1 - \alpha) \times (\text{Minimum payoff for status quo})] =$$
$$[(0.6) \times (\$200{,}000)] + [(0.4) \times (\$0)] =$$
$$\$120{,}000$$

A measure of realism is also computed for the alternatives of renovation (\$200,000) and construction (\$240,000). The decision maker selects the construction alternative, producing the highest-valued weighted average of \$240,000.

When the decision maker operates under conditions of risk, probabilities are associated with each decision state. Under conditions of risk for the problem of ambulatory services, a decision maker would decide among one of three building alternatives. The **expected value (EV) criterion** computes a weighted average for each decision alternative. The weighted average is composed of the payoff for the alternative associated with a particular decision state multiplied by the prob-

Table 4–3 Deciding Among Feasible Hospital-Based Ambulatory Care Construction Alternatives Under Conditions of Uncertainty: Table of Regret

	Feasible Hospital-Based Ambulatory Care Construction Alternatives		
States of Nature (Demand)	**Status Quo**	**Renovation**	**Construction**
Low	\$0	\$100,000	**\$300,000**
Moderate	\$200,000	\$100,000	\$0
High	**\$400,000**	**\$200,000 (select)**	\$0

abilities associated with the decision state. This method is simply illustrated for the status quo alternative of the problem introduced previously:

EV (Status quo) = [Pr (Low demand) × (Monetary payoff for selecting status quo given low demand)] + [Pr (Moderate demand) × (Monetary payoff for selecting status quo given moderate demand)] + [Pr (High demand) × (Monetary payoff for selecting status quo given high demand)]

Assuming Pr (low demand) = 0.20, Pr (moderate demand) = 0.50, and Pr (high demand) = 0.30, the computations for the status quo problems become:

EV (Status quo) = [(0.20) × ($0)] + [(0.50) × ($100,000)] + [(0.30) × ($200,000)] = $110,000

Similarly, the EV (renovation) and the EV (construction) are computed to produce results of $200,000 and $270,000, respectively. Construction would be selected as the alternative with the highest computed value.

The **maximum likelihood criterion** selects the decision state with the highest probability and selects the alternative with the highest payoff for that decision state. In the example provided so far, the moderate demand state has the highest probability (0.50), and construction provides the highest payoff ($300,000) within that demand state.

The **criterion of rationality** assumes that all decision states are equally likely—in this case Pr (all decision states) = 0.33, with construction selected as the alternative producing the highest expected value of $198,000.

Inventory Models Inventory presents a conundrum for health care organizations. Inventories of medical materials are maintained by health care facilities to support scheduled procedures and examinations and to respond to emergencies as they occur. Failure to maintain an adequate inventory results in several costs, including lost opportunities to garner revenue by providing care, special costs associated with expeditious procurement requests, and costs associated with harm to the patient—even possible loss of life—caused by unavailable materials. On the other side of the ledger, storage costs accrue as warehouse space is consumed, materials or pharmaceuticals expire from age, labor is devoted to maintaining the inventory, and other opportunities lie fallow as funds are spent on inventory purchases. Inventory decisions represent a balancing act—how to balance the costs of maintaining inventory against the costs of running short.

Ravindran, Phillips, and Solberg (1987) have documented the successive stages of inventory theory development begun during the 1920s. Two parallel paths evolved. The first path was concerned with optimal management of one item of inventory. Simple deterministic **inventory models**, such as the **economic order quantity (EOQ) model**, were developed, followed by the development of probabilistic models begun in the 1950s. According to Ecker and Kupferschmid (1988), a variety of solution techniques have been applied to include a variety of optimization models (constrained and unconstrained), integer programming, and dynamic programming.

The second inventory theory path noted by Ravindran, Phillips, and Solberg (1987) dealt with the management of many lines of inventory at the same time—a process concerned with effective record keeping and processing of inventory requests. This process, called inventory control, has more recently been facilitated by the automation of effective paper-based systems. In the early 1970s material requirements planning or, alternatively, manufacturing resource planning (MRP) revolutionized the management of production line inventories. By the early 1980s the concept of a virtually inventory-free workplace gained popularity. This concept was supported by just-in-time (JIT) deliveries from a select number of primary vendors. JIT deliveries refer to the practice of shipping a product only in direct response to a confirmed order. The goal is to decrease inventories and thereby decrease holding costs. This trend in inventory control has coincided roughly with the quality movement in health care.

Linear Programming **Linear programming** is generally used to determine the best consumption of resources in order to meet some objective. This solution method can be adapted to apply to a broad range of problems. In health care, linear programs can be used to schedule staff and facilities, design the optimal production of medical services or goods, establish the most efficient routes for transporting patients, solve production problems, and determine the most efficient use of space.

The general form for a linear program follows:

Maximize (or minimize)	A linear objective function of two or more variables
Subject to	Linear equality or inequality constraints
	Nonnegativity constraint

The linear constraints form a convex solution space that can be expressed in a tabular form known as a tableau. George Dantzig devised the simplex algorithm in 1947 to solve linear programs based on an extension of wartime research that he and his colleagues conducted for the U.S. Air Force. His solution method for executing row operations within the tableau (known as pivots) is performed iteratively until optimal form is achieved or the problem is determined to be unbounded or without solution (Ecker & Kupferschmid, 1988).

Variants of linear programs include models for network flows that include transportation, transshipment, and assignment problems for which special tableaus facilitate a solution approach that is different from the simplex algorithm. Solutions may be constrained to integer values, or they may be constrained even further to binary values (0 or 1). Both kinds of problems can be solved using the "branch and bound" algorithm (Ecker & Kupferschmid, 1988). Goal programming is designed to address multiple criteria for a solution (Ravindran, Phillips, & Solberg, 1987).

Other classes of algorithms or solution methods designed to achieve optimal solutions include nonlinear programming, dynamic programming, and stochastic programming (Wagner, 1975).

Graph Theory and Network Problems **Graph theory** was born with Leonhard Euler's formulation and solution of the Königsberg bridge problem in 1736, wherein seven bridges connected two islands to each other and the rest of the city. Euler addressed a problem regarding whether it was possible to begin at home and return home by using a route in which every bridge was crossed exactly once. Graphs and networks can be used to represent these types of problems. Graphs are represented by points (vertices) and the lines (edges) that join them. When the edges of the graph have one or more numbers associated with each edge, representing physical distances, times, costs, etc., the graph becomes a network. Graphs and networks can represent many problems in health care associated with the flow or movement of patients and staff, vehicles, cash, and communications. Let's assume that apothecaries were located on each island and the far riverbank. Each was supplied from the same single source on the near riverbank. The supplier stocked all of the apothecaries on a single run and was concerned about finding the shortest supply route. This is known as a "traveling salesman problem" that can be concisely modeled using a network (Figure 4-1). With computers and the advent of linear programming, graph and **network problems** have increasingly become the focus of solution by optimization (Evans & Minieka, 1992).

FIGURE 4–1 | Network Representation of Apothecary Resupply

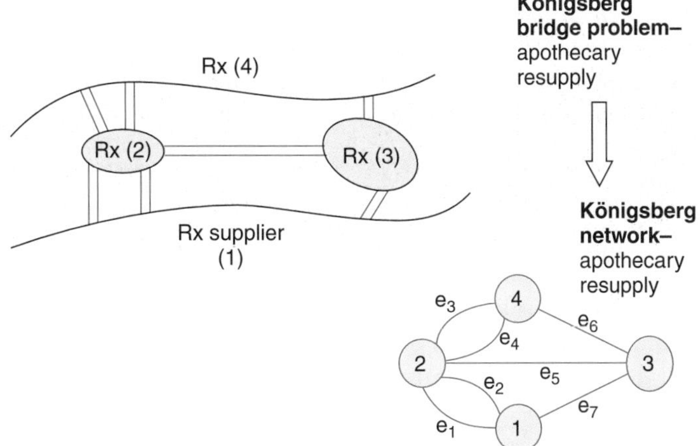

Modified application of the Königsberg bridge problem–apothecary resupply. *(Modified from Figure 1.2 of Evans and Minieka [1992, p. 2] by courtesy of Marcel Dekker, Inc.)*

An important subset of network problems relates to project management. A Program Evaluation Review Technique (PERT) network is used in PERT analysis to determine the start and stop times of activities, the critical activities that must be completed on time to prevent delay to the remainder of the project, and the completion time for the entire project. Critical path management (CPM) is an associated technique that integrates activity costs (Levin et al., 1992).

Queuing Theory and Waiting Line Problems

Waiting for care is symptomatic of the health care experience at many facilities. According to Ecker and Kupferschmid (1988), any system wherein a line (or queue) builds as people wait for service can be described by how customers arrive (the input process), how they are selected to receive services (the queuing discipline), and how services are performed (the service mechanism). Levin et al. (1992) have addressed three parts of queuing systems: (1) the calling population—characterized by size, arrival characteristics, and behavior; (2) the waiting line—finite or infinite length; and (3) the service facility—characterized by the number of channels and servers, the queuing discipline (e.g., first come, first served), and the distribution of service times. For queuing systems meeting certain assumptions, formulas exist to compute the mean number of patients in the waiting line and in the system, the mean time that patients spend in the waiting line and in the health care facility, and the probability that the server in the health care facility is busy. These formulas allow health care facilities to adjust the characteristics of waiting line systems (e.g., number of servers, waiting room capacity, and server performance characteristics) to produce optimal performance. Two limitations to the **queuing theory** exist: (1) sometimes the system of interest does not match one of the queuing systems for which formulas have been derived, and (2) queuing formulas are only accurate once the queuing system reaches steady state; for example, a clinic opening at 8:00 AM may not reach equilibrium until mid-morning.

Simulation

Simulation "is the imitation of a dynamic system using a computer model in order to evaluate and improve system performance"

(Harrell, Ghosh, & Bowden, 2000, p. 5). Discrete event simulation may be used in complex health care systems not meeting the assumptions required by the queuing formulas or for solutions to problems occurring as a system is in transition before reaching equilibrium. At their most basic, health care systems can be modeled using arrival patterns of patients who subsequently receive service. The pattern of arrivals, usually posed as interarrival times, can be "fit" to a theoretical mathematical distribution, as can the service time durations, to produce a theoretical model of the health care system under study. The computer simulates the passage of patients through the system by generating random variants in accordance with the arrival and service time distributions. A schedule of arrival and service events is derived, and the relationship of discrete events to time is recognized. The discrete simulation model runs as the computer advances as scheduled through the list of clock times.

In practice, the simulation model is run in thousands of iterations. However, the following hypothetical schedule of three patient arrivals and services is sufficient to illustrate how a queue forms and how the server spends times (both busy and idle) during the execution of the schedule. Assume that the arrival-generating function produces the following interarrival times: 1, 3, 3; and that the service time–generating function produces the following values: 4, 1, 3. The interarrival times convert to the following clock schedule: 1, 4, 7. Service occurs when arrivals present to the server for service, unless the server is still occupied serving the previous arrival. The first patient arrives at time 1 and is served until time 5. The second patient arrives at time 4 but spends 1 time unit in the queue because the server is not available until time 5. The server is freed of the first patient at time 5 and serves the second patient until time 6. The third patient arrives at time 7, and as a consequence, the server who was freed of the second patient at time 6 has spent 1 time unit idle. The third patient is served at time 7 and released from service at time 10.

Two things happen as the simulation schedule executes. First, the generating functions representing the arrival and service time distributions produce random values that when aggregated after numerous iterations, do indeed form the characteristic distributions. Second, execution of the scheduled events produces results representative of the health care system being modeled. The simulation software records information similar to that produced by the queuing formulas—the mean number of patients in the waiting line and in the health care facility, the mean time that patients spend in the waiting line and in the health care facility, and the probability that the server in the health care facility is busy. In practice, the simulation model representing the status quo can also represent alternatives under consideration. For example, the number of servers could be changed. The performance of the status quo and the alternative models are then examined to determine the effects of possible changes. Modern simulation software packages incorporate animation to aid in model construction and representation of the problem.

The Rudimentary Tool Kit

Many of the decision algorithms or models that have been discussed are incorporated in spreadsheet and database applications. Beginners or those who have superficial knowledge of spreadsheets and databases may be unaware of their untapped potential to support the decision process.

Spreadsheets: Strengths and Weaknesses

The modern **spreadsheet** provides the adept health care administrator with a capable quantitative modeling and decision support tool. Imbedded financial, mathematical, and statistical functions enable ad hoc modeling that is remarkable in scope and complexity. Many spreadsheet applications are also capable of optimization modeling that includes support of linear and nonlinear optimization. Finally, database functions facilitate the manipulation of data input within the spreadsheet.

Irvin and Brown (1999) have provided an example of the use of a self-scheduling spreadsheet application in an emergency department to replace a flawed manual system. The manual system created difficulties because staff members were not aware of unit requirements for the time period being scheduled as they posted their schedule requests. Often, self-scheduling did not provide adequate staff for all shifts. The head nurse manually tallied staffing numbers for nine overlapping shifts and then rescheduled staff to ensure adequate coverage or to correct errors related to the self-computation of hours to be worked. Delays in posting the approved schedule contributed to staff dissatisfaction.

In the revised self-scheduling procedure an Excel spreadsheet was used by the head nurse to common-code a 6-week master schedule with each cell representing a 4-hour block of time. Staff members requested time off that was subsequently posted on the spreadsheet by the department secretary. The schedule was then fine-tuned to even up unit coverage, a process often involving "trades" between staff members, followed by the subsequent approval of revisions by the head nurse. A key contribution of the spreadsheet was the identification and computation of the number of staff members filling each 4-hour period of the schedule.

This example illustrates spreadsheet capabilities and limitations. The spreadsheet that was developed in the example effectively presented both the master schedule and the final product. This contributed to improved interpersonal scheduling dynamics. The head nurse saved 51% of the time previously used to schedule manually, largely because the spreadsheet automatically computed the number of staff scheduled. A limitation of this spreadsheet is that the knowledge base employed by the head nurse to build the master schedule was not captured by the spreadsheet. The quality of the master schedule depends on the ability of the head nurse to remember and effectively accommodate considerations such as staff preferences and scheduling constraints (e.g., a nurse should not be scheduled to work a third shift that is followed by a first shift).

The spreadsheet presents several advantages as a decision support tool. It provides computational power enabled by embedded formulas and functions, as well as optimization capabilities available through the data analysis tools. Spreadsheets also have the advantage of availability. They are bundled as a component of every major software office suite, usually with a word processor, presentation manager, and perhaps a database application. Spreadsheets are also familiar programs to many professionals. Many colleges and universities and an increasing number of high schools provide an orientation to spreadsheets as part of their course offerings.

There are several disadvantages to using a spreadsheet as a decision support tool. Most health care executives who are familiar with spreadsheets use them for arithmetic operations and the graphical presentation of data. They are unfamiliar with more advanced spreadsheet applications. Accurate modeling of health care problems requires the ability to express the objectives of the organization and its constraints in mathematical or logical terms. In the example provided by Irvin and Brown (1999), the knowledge base required to build the master schedule was not built into the spreadsheet. Although the problem to be modeled was clearly understood by the head nurse in this example, this is not always the case. Sometimes the processes and information needed as problem input are not clearly understood. Finally, not all health care executives may have the time to accumulate and then model the disparate pieces of the puzzle and then personally construct a semiautomated spreadsheet solution.

Databases

A **database management system (DBMS)** basically uses the computer to collect and manage data (Date, 1986). The **database** provides the electronic filing cabinet for storing data in a computerized hierarchy of field, record, and file.

A **field** represents a distinct category of collected data, such as personal identification (name), demographic (gender), billing (amount due), or clinical (diagnosis-related group) information. A **record** is essentially equivalent to the file folder stored within a traditional filing cabinet. It represents data items stored within a number of fields for a distinct entity, such as an individual patient. A collection of records is a **file.** Detailed information about databases can be found in Chapter 3. A brief overview of the use of databases for decision support is covered here.

The **data definition language** provides a link between the user and the physical view of the database; the **data dictionary** provides a detailed description of the data elements in the database. In a relational database a common "key field" is used to join records contained in two or more files. For example, a unique patient identifier could be used as a common field to join the clinical and insurance files for a single patient. A **data manipulation language (DML)** allows nonprogrammers to perform a variety of operations on the data contained in the database. A **query language** is a variant of the DML that can be used to directly interact with the database and pose conditions for retrieval via natural language queries, query by example, or structured query language (Austin & Boxerman, 1998).

Two additional constructs build on the foundations of the DBMS. The **clinical data repository** accumulates clinical and operational data from many systems for real-time retrieval and queries to assist clinicians in managing patient care. The **data warehouse** works retrospectively to report trends, offer comparisons, and provide strategic analyses to manage the health care of populations and groups. The data warehouse also includes financial and operational data that are used in administrative decision making. **Data marts** provide a decentralized approach to data distribution (Nunnelly, 1997; Waldo, 1998). Dominant vendors of commercial database software suggest that database technology provides significant and positive decision support.

What's Missing?

Given the computational models already discussed, as well as tools such as spreadsheets and databases, what void exists that needs to be filled by a more maturely developed DSS? Decision support in health care can be argued to range across a continuum, rather than existing narrowly. Decisions in health care may engage the total effort of the human decision maker with relatively little extraneous support from an external knowledge base. Alternatively, expert systems may be created to capture the content and process of reasoning to solve problems when accessed by persons with little expertise. At this far end of the continuum, some believe that expert systems should provide solutions comparable to those of human experts, replace numeric and algorithmic procedures with symbolic and heuristic reasoning, separate knowledge from inference procedures, and offer insight into the decision process (Buchanan, in Delaney et al., 1999).

Spreadsheets and databases rightfully belong within the decision support continuum. Spreadsheets magnify the computational expertise of the human decision maker and provide a nice framework for the management and representation of the problem to be modeled. Databases excel at organizing and managing information and are capable of presenting information in a variety of formats. Both spreadsheets and databases depend on a certain level of sophistication by the user in formulating the problem and managing the models needed for the solution. The following section demonstrates how classically defined DSSs offer more than spreadsheets and databases.

WHAT IS AN ADMINISTRATIVE DECISION SUPPORT SYSTEM?

Definition

Turban (1993) has provided the following working definition of a **decision support system (DSS):** "At a minimum we can say: A DSS is an interactive, flexible and adaptable computer-based information system (CBIS), specially developed for supporting decision making related to the solution of a particular management problem. It utilizes data, it provides easy user interface (UI), and it allows for the decision maker's own insights." Turban extends the definition even further by recognizing that the sophisticated DSS "also utilizes models (either standard and/or custom-made), is built by an iterative process (frequently by end-users), supports all the phases of the decision making, and includes a knowledge base" (p. 87).

Components of a Decision Support System

DSSs include the following components:

- **User interface**—facilitates communication between the executive and the DSS
- **Model manager**—accesses the collection of available models
- **Model library**—includes a variety of statistical, graphical, financial, and "what if" models
- Databases—provide clinical and financial data needed for decisions
- Database management system—accesses the available databases to provide data directly to the model manager or to the user
- **Report writer**—formats and produces the written output (Austin & Boxerman, 1998).

Austin and Boxerman (1998) have mapped the types of DSSs with Alter's categorization of information system uses (Alter, 1976). Table 4-4 is a modification of their presentation.

Answering the Question (What Is an Administrative Decision Support System?)

In health care, deriving the answer to the question "What is an administrative decision support system?" is not a trivial exercise. Clinical DSSs (CDSSs) seem relatively easier to identify and isolate. Haug, Gardner, and Evans (1999) identified four categories of clinical decision support facilitated by computer: (1) programs assisting the provider in making diagnoses, (2) programs providing alerts to providers (e.g., warnings of

Table 4–4 Mapping Decision Support Systems to Uses of Information Systems

Types of Decision Support Systems	Alter's Uses of Decision Support Systems
Simple database management system with query capability	Retrieve requested data items
Generic statistical package spreadsheet package with statistical module	Perform ad hoc data analysis of a modern data file
Decision support system with a report generator; executive information system	Aggregate data in a standard report
Decision support system with "what if" capability	Estimate consequences of a proposed decision
Decision support system with optimization modeling capability	Propose decisions to management
Expert system; decision support system with artificial intelligence	Make decisions according to predetermined algorithms

Modified with permission from Figure 13.4, *Information Systems for Health Services Administration, 5th Edition,* by Charles J. Austin and Stuart B. Boxerman (Chicago: Health Administration Press, 1998).

drug interactions), (3) programs providing guidance as orders are issued to alter care, and (4) applications supporting quality assurance activities. (A complete discussion of CDSSs is found in Chapter 5.) Administrative DSSs are defined in part by what they are not. They are not CDSSs. If health care administration consists of those processes providing the infrastructure for care and supporting the delivery of care, then administrative DSSs empower health care leaders to make nonclinical decisions within these venues.

Commercial DSSs are offered to provide assistance in the following areas:

- Strategic planning and marketing
- Process improvement
- Finance
- Human resources management
- Materials management
- Management of competition and markets
- Management of the demand for services
- Physician practice management
- Scheduling of personnel and facilities

SURVEY OF ADMINISTRATIVE DECISION SUPPORT APPLICATIONS AND SOFTWARE

The need for administrative decision support has stimulated the development of several different software packages. This section provides several examples of decision support software and demonstrates the features and functions offered by such software. Perhaps the most basic of the contributions of administrative DSSs is the management of information overload. Often an administrative DSS supports the decision maker by cleaning up distracting "information clutter." For example, according to Rick Seigrist, President of HealthShare Technology, financial and clinical information required by government and regulatory agencies is only rarely used to full advantage. HealthShare Technology provides services and software to clean up the clutter of information from a variety of sources and present it in a user-friendly format. For example, HealthShare One provides a database to capture adjusted information regarding severity of illness in relation to costs, charges, case mix, payer mix, length of stay, and market share for specified groups of inpatients and hospitals. HealthShare Two uses the payer's or provider's internal data to support decisions. For example, the software provides comparative information for all patients served by the health care facility for any category of patients or physicians. A patented reporting technology is used that couples an executive summary, including visual analysis and recommendations for change, with data mining capabilities to perform much more complex analyses (Walker, 1999).

For a complete list of software applications and a list of commercially available health care data warehouses related to the digital transfer of information via **electronic data interchange (EDI)**, refer to the *1999 Healthcare Sourcebook and IT Buyer's Guide* (Fantle & DiLima, 1999). EDI allows linked computers to conduct business transactions such as ordering and invoicing over telecommunications networks.

Strategic Planning and Marketing

Strategic decision making is enhanced by the use of group DSSs. These computer-based interactive systems facilitate the solution of unstructured problems by a group of decision makers. The software supports consensus building, usually by facilitating brainstorming, narrowing of alternatives, and voting by group members. For example, the chapter author participated in a Department of Defense initiative in the mid-1990s, called the Joint Service Executive Skills Training Program. This program attempted to explore the executive competencies needed by facility commanders in the military health service system to lead effectively and then attempted to identify or develop curricula and training programs to teach those competencies. Ventana Group Systems software was used to facilitate agreement among subject matter experts regarding the skills, knowledge, and abilities associated with the identified competencies.

Business Resource Software, Inc., also provides software to directly support the strategic planning process. This company provides two products: Business Insight and Quick Insight. Business Insight (Business Resource Software, n.d.a) is an expert system software product that does the following:

- Evaluates marketing strategy against a knowledge base of expert system rules
- Criticizes the strategy using the same model as a Harvard MBA consultant
- Identifies strengths and corrects weaknesses
- Pinpoints the factors that can threaten success

Quick Insight (Business Resource Software, n.d.b) was developed from Business Insight to include a set of expert system rules to quickly and accurately analyze the market potential for products or service.

Organizations may choose to employ a DSS as a marketing tool to help their customers select from among its products. One example of an organization using a DSS this way is a long-distance telephone provider that routinely provides feedback to customers based on their patterns of use and then suggests more cost-effective long-distance plans.

One health care example is BLUeCHOICE offered by Highmark Blue Cross Blue Shield. BLUeCHOICE is an Internet-based, paperless health insurance program providing a choice of 16 different health plans (Highmark, 2000). A unique decision support feature of this Web site is an algorithm that asks beneficiaries to rate the attributes that are important to them, such as low co-pay, preventive benefits, or choice of provider. Plan recommendations are made online after consideration of beneficiary input.

Process Improvement

Process improvement represents another opportunity for decision support. The following example demonstrates how this might work. The Maine Medical Services Bureau coupled a data warehouse with a DSS to query Medicaid data in real time. Thirty-three million records representing 5 years' worth of data have been loaded into the system. The system's background processing capability permits queries by multiple users. Detail screens are provided to let users query the data in reference to providers, claims, clients, and prior authorization issues and includes a screen for customized queries. A three-tiered design permits access to the Medicaid business rules and the integration of both provider and patient records. This system allows the state of Maine to use information about both patients and providers to analyze outcomes of care to improve process delivery. This DSS primarily depends on the capabilities promoted by a data warehouse with query capability, but with the business rules also available, cases of fraud can be uncovered. For example, more than a million dollars' worth of duplicate pharmaceutical billings was uncovered in a single morning (Gilhooly, 1997).

Finance

Financial applications were among the earliest automated administrative applications. Payroll and accounting functions supported by the mainframe began to emerge in the 1960s (Austin & Boxerman, 1998). Specific applications packages for managing accounts receivable and payable, budgeting, and cost reporting emerged, as did entire financial management information systems. These financial applications evolved as the hardware changed from mainframe, to smaller minicomputers, to PCs, and finally to electronic data networks. Today, the enterprise data warehouse supports decision support functions such as budgeting (including case-based budgeting), cost accounting, revenue management (including managed care contract modeling) and profitability analysis (Waldo, 1998).

Financial management, decision support, and outcomes applications are among those that must be successfully incorporated into the information technology infrastructure of an integrated delivery system (IDS). According to Mousin, Remmlinger, and Weil (1999), "To achieve economies of scale, an IDS can adopt a central business office strategy, which involves consolidating patient management and patient accounting, general accounting, materials management and managed care contract administration" (p. 48). However, most administrative DSSs are inpatient focused, require manual manipulation of data, and function only within single enterprises.

Financial suites typically include modules for cash ledger, general ledger, activity-based costing, activity management, project accounting, accounts receivable, accounts payable, asset management, employee expense, budgeting, average daily balance, allocations, currency, and asset management (Lawson, 2000).

Financial stewardship is another aspect of financial management that is facilitated by decision support applications. Health care institutions must competently manage both the excess of revenue over costs and the cash on hand. According to Cleverley (1997), hospitals have larger sums of funds available for investment than other comparably sized institutions; one example is a facility that maintained almost 30% of its total assets in short-term cash, marketable securities, and other investments. Health care organizations also have a need for investment management for capital replacement, self-insurance, management of gifts and endowments, funding of defined benefits for employees (such as pension plans), and servicing of debt. The use of decision support software for portfolio management software will become increasingly common in the future

Human Resources Management

Human resources management software fulfills a variety of functions that include recruitment and retention, personnel administration, management of payroll against budget, training, and performance evaluation. The software serves as repositories for documents and records, thereby facilitating data-driven decision making. Some software includes embedded human resources expertise regarding federal and state regulatory requirements related to recruitment, personnel administration, or position management. The software matches regulatory requirements against human resources records to ensure compliance. In addition, changes in employee status can be flagged to alert the manager to the need to modify compensation or benefits administration. Several vendors offer comprehensive, enterprise-wide software solutions for human resources management (Fantle & DiLima, 1999).

Management of compensation and benefits has become an increasingly complex task facilitated by decision support. One of the responsibilities of the human resources manager is to develop a competitive compensation package of salary and benefits while controlling costs. This is particularly important in a labor-intensive industry like health care, where labor costs are a significant percentage of the overall costs of delivering care. Gupta and Scott (1996) have created a DSS for employers to control insurance costs by examining alternative premium structures and reimbursement schedules in conjunction with the previous medical history of the beneficiary and the beneficiary's family. A form of breakeven analysis is employed; if the value of projected medical expenses (co-pay and deductibles) is less than the premiums paid for an insurance option under consideration, then another option should be chosen.

Once a benefit package is established, managing it is a challenge because of employee and organizational changes that typically occur. Loofbourrow (2000, p. 37) has suggested the use of a human resources knowledge base to "provide the business logic, rules, and content to create a knowledge resource that can be delivered online, so that a desktop PC can provide personalized information to employees." Properly designed, the knowledge base can assimilate input (such as the birth of a child), guide transactions (such as the election of maternity leave and selection of health insurance options), and provide feedback regarding the impact of choices. A variant of this approach can be used to update benefits verification for physician practices. A human resources knowledge base could facilitate the development and integration of other applications and assist with compliance reporting to meet government and accreditation agency requirements (Loofbourrow, 2000). To that end, Human Resource Management System (HRMS) data will be increasingly leveraged for other purposes. Decision support software is also of value in managing issues related to credentialing and compliance (Marzulli, 2000).

Training management modules are among those applications being introduced to core HRMS products. Vendors at the Softworld Resource and Payroll Expo (Gunsauley, 1999b) introduced modules that integrate training program administration with career development and succession planning. Health care institutions could integrate these modules to manage competency training and documentation as required by the Joint Commission on Accreditation of Healthcare Organizations (JCAHO) and other accrediting organizations. Other benefits offered by HRMS software is the integration of training management with other services such as counseling, performance management, recruiting, compensation, skills tracking, and succession planning.

eBusiness will transform traditional personnel practices from personnel recruitment to retirement. Using the Internet, "health care organizations can, and should, automate and re-engineer job candidate registration, recruitment, and selection processes. . . . In today's dynamic business environment, successful health care organizations are steadily beginning to realize and understand the power of the Internet. For health care organizations to achieve and surpass their expected outcomes, they must fully embrace not only the vision, but also the reality of a comprehensive e-business management system" (Marzulli, 2000, p. 20).

Materials Management

As noted earlier, the development of materials management software is based on two distinct concerns: (1) how to optimally manage single lines of inventory and (2) how to simultaneously manage many lines of inventory.

The market provides several examples of materials management software. Dade Behring, Inc., a prominent manufacturer and supplier of medical equipment, used modern approaches to warehouse management to improve on an already outstanding paper-based system that had achieved 96% inventory accuracy and a shipping error rate of less than 1%. With the use of a "smart warehouse" consisting of warehouse management software, bar coding, and radio frequency (RF) technology, performance improved to 99% inventory accuracy and a shipping error rate of less than 0.05%. Enhancements supporting and automating inventory decisions include automatic order processing, inventory placement within the warehouse based on demand frequency, efficient routing of workers, and the use of a separate algorithm for each product to support storage decisions (Making, 1998).

Philips Medical Systems uses SAP software to provide enterprise-level visibility of inventory to manage its service/parts supply chain; the inventory includes 65,000 active part numbers, and 26% of the inventory is used in any given month. Consumers of the company's three lines of diagnostic imaging equipment demand immediate availability of each of the parts. The operating environment places a premium on same-day delivery of parts and service. Philips previously had made several strategic decisions to restructure its service/parts supply chain. The company had (1) transferred manufacturing to Europe by the early 1990s, (2) relocated its centralized operations base to Memphis, Tennessee (near Federal Express), and (3) distributed inventory among six stocking hubs to facilitate same-day service. The visibility of inventory afforded by using SAP software facilitated the transition to demand-based forecasting (Andel, 1999). Tools for real-time planning and decision support, for advanced forecasting and demand planning, and for supply network and production planning are included in SAP's supply chain management applications. These tools enable detailed scheduling and offer global availability for matching product supply with customer demand.

Montefiore Medical Center in New York has also had success employing SAP technology. Implementation has eliminated paper order forms, flattened supply chain administration, reduced the personnel overhead, and reduced order turnaround time significantly (Agins, 1998). In addition, this software supports selection decisions by automatically selecting the lowest-priced vendor in the contract file.

According to Perry (1998), conventional wisdom has changed with respect to purchasing materials management information systems. The evolving wisdom advises the purchaser to change focus from buying the best possible materials management system to buying a system that incorporates both function and organization-wide communication applications. Organizations should buy a system that combines proven value with the ability to link to other systems. The ability to accept a variety of input devices and channels, including the bar code reader, electronic data interchange, and Web capability, is important. Vendors and purchasers should share responsibility for installation, training of end users, and successful implementation.

Fortunately, a rapid return on investment is possible from materials management software. According to Straub (1997a), information collected from an integrated materials management system provides information about product usage, mixes, and costs that facilitates the effective negotiations of supply contracts with the potential for producing significant cost savings.

Management of Competition and Markets

Many managed care organizations are at the forefront of effective management of the marketplace and the competition for market share, but in reality, all health care organizations are similarly engaged. According to Rothenberg (1995), a health care organization should consider purchasing managed care software when actively seeking managed care contracts. Money will be saved as the software replaces the labor-intensive efforts of manual data collection. Such software supports decision making by calculating contract profitability and by managing the complexity of benefit and provider compensation structures. Key software capabilities include automatic payment of providers in accordance with contract specifications, enrollment, authorization of services, claims processing, and adjudication. Increasingly, the ability to accomplish each of these tasks electronically has become an essential system capability.

Managed care organizations face the challenge of supporting a delivery system that serves a broader community whose social characteristics, demographics, and pattern of health care use must be identified. The managed care information system must identify patient and community health status, provider capability, and changes in health status (Grazier, 1998). Effective managed care approaches require that the information technology include the use of data warehouse and DSSs to manage risk and customer satisfaction, the use of data analysis to cost-effectively manage preventive care and health care interventions, and the ability to measure the effect of interventions. Finally, the Internet will allow managed care organizations to cost-effectively exchange information with providers, payers, and patients (Schaich, 1998). Schaich concludes that current legacy systems must be converted or replaced to adapt to the new managed care paradigm. Specialized niche software packages offer support for claims auditing, case management, demand management, provider contract administration, and provider profiling. Decision support add-ons typically enhance ad hoc analysis, reporting, and graphical presentation of results regarding operational and financial performance (Waymack, 1999).

Rock (1999, p. 39) has identified Synertech, Inc., as "one of the few companies to license information system software to managed care organizations and, at the same time, use its own software and staff to administer a wide range of managed care services." As with many decision support products, the main advantage of the software appears to be the leveraging of easy information access to facilitate decision making. Inherent capabilities include an easily updated database structure, the ability to link with third-party products, the optional Synertech Data Warehouse to facilitate informed decision making, and Synerview, a Windows-based graphical user interface that produces real-time data views.

As another example, the New York State Department of Mental Health developed a DSS to track behavioral health care provider productivity. The system is designed to convert data into information by adhering to the following principles: (1) extensive screen design to produce a screen-oriented system, (2) top-down orientation so that the user can proceed from summaries to increasing levels of detail, (3) use of exception reporting and trend analysis using graphical information to flag problems, and (4) compact design. The provider database captures 30 activity-based variables and performs case-mix analysis. The final output tracks productivity, and root causes can be traced to make improvements (Mohan, Muse, & McInerney, 1998).

Computers and the Internet also provide the key to managing the public's perception of managed care. Computers can be used to provide patient data to decision makers that may be difficult to retrieve manually and to serve as input for treatment protocols. Clinically tested, evidence-based "best practices" that are automated into treatment protocols make rational decision support evident. The Internet can subsequently be used to share clinical successes with providers, consumers, and accrediting agencies concerned about positive patient outcomes (St. Clair, 2000).

Managed care plans are evaluated against three criteria: cost, quality, and accessibility. Software such as GeoNetworks (produced by GeoAccess) uses the longitudinal and latitudinal coordinates provided by a **geographical information system (GIS)** to measure the distance between patients and providers. This allows consumers to identify the nearest provider. Another software product, Directories Online, is used to make information about network health care providers available over the Internet. This software supports the most basic types of decisions for the patient ("Where can I go for care?) and the managed care provider ("How shall we recruit and distribute providers to optimize access for our enrollees?") (McCue, 1998). Blue Cross/Blue Shield of Georgia uses cartography software to woo third-party payers to purchase coverage by mapping employee addresses with overlays of provider locations. Mapping software is also capable of importing data important to marketing, such as patient demographics and the services provided to patients (Villalon, 1999). In this way the software provides marketing value when contracting with third-party payers and during employee enrollment.

Predictive software offers decision support when coupled with claims processing, benefits verification, or plan administration. Rules-based decision support can be integrated to flag high-cost providers, patients who are seen frequently, or fraudulent billing. Automatic implementation of coverage constraints or negotiated discounts is also possible. An example of this kind of software is VeriComp, produced by HNC Software Solutions (Thomas, 1998).

Management of the Demand for Services

Queuing methods are used to solve a variety of demand-for-services problems in health care. Some demand-for-services problems are episodic, and therefore ad hoc approaches using queuing formulas or stochastic simulation are appropriate. Based on the demand for services, these approaches can be used to determine facility capacity or the number of servers, or to define how other resources should be committed to the delivery of care.

Demand management takes a different approach. Rather than addressing the question "How do we provide services to patients as they arrive?" questions such as "Must patients be treated at the time and place where they initially present for service, or can services be provided less intensively or by a less costly provider?" are posed. Consideration of these questions is important because "appropriate utilization fosters appropriate care at reasonable costs" (Jacobs, 1997, p. 41). DSSs may be used to respond to the demand for service by referring the patient to the appropriate source of care or facilitating self-selection.

Patient call systems can manage demand simply by routing the caller to the appropriate number: "press 1 for . . . , press 2 for . . . ." The decisions supported are the patient's, and the support offered is a timely reference to information or to the appropriate provider. Although this is a rudimentary example, an institution using staff to address random misdirected requests for information could use this more efficient alternative with the caller having the option to escape the system to talk to a human operator.

More complex demand management systems that perform triage services deserve special attention. Telephone-based health care demand management generally has taken two forms: either "nurse advice" or "patient risk assessment" (Bell, 1996). Nurse advice serves to inform the consumer about the promotion of changes in health behaviors. Nurses performing a patient risk assessment use protocols or care algorithms to provide guidance regarding self-care or the best means to access medical services. According to Bell, the transition from nurse advice to telephone risk assessment has been facilitated by computer-assisted medical DSSs that help nurses triage patients into various risk categories and then provide referral to the most appropriate level within the health care system. "The old-fashioned approach of deploying a smart nurse with a few reference texts is no longer acceptable and very risky. Today's environment requires a computer-based clinical decision-support system with software that provides standardized algorithms, protocols, and a documentation function" (Rhinehart, 1998, p. 20).

An example of a telephone-based health care demand management system is a system by Intracorp. Call center nurses using this system have access to an online database of clinically validated, symptom-based medical guidelines. Approximately 54% of callers seeking emergency department care and 22% of callers seeking physician care are rerouted to less costly alternatives. Most of the calls Intracorp receives are symptom based. Approximately one third of the calls are health information requests, and the remainder are related to health plan coverage and benefits (Gunsauley, 1999a).

According to Jacobs (1997), contradictory environmental factors simultaneously encourage both overutilization (as a result of provider and patient expectations that are a legacy of an indemnity insurance system paid by third parties and buffered by tax breaks) and underutilization (fostered by managed care financial and administrative controls that may inappropriately create incentives to underutilize resources). Clinical decision support tools combine practice guidelines and appropriateness criteria to mitigate against overutilization and underutilization.

Practice guidelines can incorporate cost control decisions by choosing the lower-cost treatment among alternatives providing acceptable outcomes. Financial pressures on physicians are lessened if appropriate care decisions are based on informed clinical guidance that is a result of agreed-on best practices. CDSSs and their uses are discussed in detail in Chapter 5.

Physician Practice Management

Traditional practice management systems have addressed scheduling, billing, and collections of accounts receivable (Hagland, 1998). To be successful, physician practices must incorporate comprehensive systems that address the electronic medical record, clinical data, order entry, as well as link with outside agencies concerned with accreditation, compliance, and outcomes measurement. In addition, these systems should provide decision support for the physician at the point of service.

An increasingly important aspect of practice management is checking for benefit eligibility. Ignorance of plan benefits can result in significant financial losses for a medical practice. Money is lost in several ways: (1) from performance of uninsured services, (2) from time wasted filing claims that are subsequently rejected, (3) from inappropriate referrals, and (4) from damaged relationships with patients. Automation is the key to effective management of hundreds of different patient benefit packages. **Homegrown products** represented by spreadsheets or databases offer a partial solution. However the main difficulty with these products results from the need to keep the products up-to-date. Increasingly, DSSs are being designed by vendors to advise practices of the presenting patients' eligibility for care. Electronic data interchange supports updates provided by multiple carriers (Larkin, 1999). Although the decision support offered is similar to that offered by a relational database, the technology is evolving to support verification using swipe cards and voice-response systems (Terry, 1999).

Scheduling of Personnel and Facilities

The difficult and time-consuming task of scheduling personnel and facilities in health care organizations can be made easier by computer-aided decision support. In the operations research and management science literature, the nurse scheduling process is synonymous with three-shift, multiple-skill-level scheduling. Multiple-skill-level scheduling is the scheduling of personnel with several different levels of skill. For example, scheduling a nurse aide 1, a nurse aide 2, a licensed practical nurse, a staff nurse 1, and a staff nurse 2 would be multiple-skill-level scheduling. Computer programs that can assist managers with scheduling personnel for around-the-clock coverage, weekend and holiday staffing, vacations, calloffs, and personal requests for time off fall within the definition of a DSS. Managers pay a great deal of attention to scheduling because of the impact on budget, morale, and workload coverage. Several useful criteria for evaluating the quality of decision support offered by scheduling software are fairness, flexibility, and optimality. These are defined from the perspectives of both cost and staff satisfaction (Schaffer, 1994).

According to Schaffer (1994), the generation of a timely, optimal schedule is often not possible given all the constraints involved. Heuristics such as everyone working alternate weekends are often employed. Schaffer's review of software scheduling suggests two typical solutions: (1) the "automated manual system" that essentially stores and presents the solution achieved previously by the human scheduler and (2) the amusingly titled "automated fascist system" whose solution methodology restricts the human scheduler to the constraints of the software package. Schaffer's conclusion is that a true rule-based technology that permits scheduler definition of thousands of scheduling rules offers the best potential for user satisfaction. The spreadsheet self-scheduler described earlier by Irvin and Brown (1999) falls into the "automated manual system" category. Many of the scheduling models based on optimization belong in the "automated facist" category of schedulers.

The typical scheduling problem is difficult and complex. For example, inpatient nurse scheduling involves two processes: (1) staffing (determination of the number of nurses and other personnel needed on each shift based on patient acuity) and (2) scheduling (assignment of personnel to each shift by skill level in response to identified needs). Since 60% to 80% of the hospital budget may be devoted to personnel costs, scheduling is a function with significant impact on the bottom line (McConnell, 2000).

Box 4-1 provides the results of a search of online health care databases for articles addressing the nurse scheduling problem over a period of 15 years. A mix of optimization, heuristic, and mixed models represents solution approaches to the nurse scheduling problem. An example of a scheduling model based on optimization techniques and another based on decision rules follow.

The first example is demonstrated by the software package HOROPLAN (Darmoni et al., 1995). HOROPLAN uses constraint-based programming to produce a noncyclical schedule after consideration of available resources and defined constraints. The software uses Charme, a constraint-based programming language, to employ nine scheduling steps:

1. Allocate nurses from the department pool.
2. Determine the personnel needed to provide a defined level of service.
3. Identify scheduled absences, such as training and paid holidays.
4. List up to five nurse wishes.
5. Fill the night shift.
6. Assign weekends and nights off.
7. Check illegal scheduling patterns.
8. Integrate nurse experience.
9. Check global consistency.

Constraint-based programming reduces the solution space by defining sets of values for the variables that meet the constraints and then attempts to generate the best solution.

The second example of scheduling software is the Physician Scheduler (Physician scheduling software, 1998), produced by MSI Software. This software, designed by physicians, permits physicians to employ their own rule-based scheduling parameters. The software is credited with eliminating problems caused by human error, such as double booking, understaffing or overstaffing, improper workload distribution, and the resulting conflicts. A rule-based DSS permits the user to define various rules, such as ensuring equitable call coverage among a group of specialists while maintaining assignment preferences or blocking the physician who works night call from working the next morning. The system is described as being capable of defining virtually any rule while being flexible enough to accommodate last-minute changes. The associated Web site claims

Box 4-1 Solution Models for the Nurse Scheduling Problem

A quick search of the online health care databases reveals the mix of optimization, heuristic, and mixed models addressing different facets of the nurse scheduling problem over the past 15 years. These models include zero-one linear goal programming (Huarng, 1999), constraint programming and real users' heuristics (Weil et al., 1998), zero-one linear goal programming combined with an expert system program (Chen & Yeung, 1993), linear programming (Harmeier, 1991), simulated annealing combined with a rounding algorithm (Isken & Hancock, 1991), and use of Prolog (Okada & Okada, 1988). Podgorelec and Kokol (1997) have even reported a genetic algorithm-based system for patient scheduling in a highly constrained environment.

that the Physician Scheduler reduces scheduling time by 70% and can be used to equalize or weight physician workloads, incorporates time off and vacations in advance, and tracks and analyzes workload distribution. An intriguing (but unanswered) question is whether this rule-derived schedule produces an optimal solution.

Contemporary personnel scheduling software packages are capable of accomplishing a variety of functions. It is possible to compare staffing scenarios to determine the staffing level that provides the best quality of care at the least cost. In addition, specific scheduling needs can be managed via queries about staff competency or credentials. Rule-based scheduling systems can prompt the patient or provider about actions that are needed before the next appointment or to order medical materials for a scheduled procedure. Increasingly, administrators and clinicians can expect "one-call" systems to schedule a variety of procedures in multiple departments (Cupito, 1998).

Facility scheduling represents a second important branch of scheduling. Operating room scheduling is an important subset of facility scheduling. Effective management of the operating room scheduling template represents an often unrecognized opportunity to enhance revenues. Computerization can help accomplish both the scheduling and the inventory control tasks necessary to manage the operating room environment. According to Bird (1997), in addition to ensuring effective scheduling, the computer system's criteria list should include database functions, compatibility with other facility information systems, and the capabilities to accomplish procedure-based costing, inventory management, interoperative charting and charging, and reporting. Critical components for inventory control include electronic data interchange and bar coding. Decision capabilities supported by contemporary operating room scheduling modules include case selection from a waiting list, automated scheduling search, open scheduling, block scheduling, and online conflict verification. Dexter and Lubarsky (1998) have noted efforts to improve surgical scheduling by predicting case times and the existence of algorithms employing scheduling rules to improve the assignment of cases to the operating room. Perhaps the greatest difficulty comes in successfully accommodating the multiple, conflicting objectives existing in operating rooms with other goals of the health care organization.

Decision support scheduling applications have been successfully applied to cleaning procedures in medical facilities that are complicated by around-the-clock operations, varied service hours, a complex physical plant, and strict environmental and regulatory requirements. Modern decision aides couple computer-aided design (CAD) data (such as layout and square footage) with database and scheduling systems. Hours can be assigned for team cleaning after breaking cleaning tasks into time and labor units and assigning time standards for each room on the basis of prior experience. Scheduling algorithms are used to determine optimal schedules (Wilford, 1998).

EMERGING DEVELOPMENTS IN ADMINISTRATIVE DECISION SUPPORT

Garets and Hanna (1998) have accurately reflected the change in health care from a focus on sick care to a focus on wellness, emphasizing the role that rule-based systems play in managing wellness. According to these authors, decision technology is emerging as an important strategic asset, creating a need for the health care industry to increase funding for information technology.

Health care organizations will continue to strive for improvements in operational effectiveness without causing a decrement in quality care in the twenty-first century. Performance measures will be rigorously tracked to ensure optimal clinical outcomes at the least possible cost. Successful health care organizations will be positioned to leverage technology, particularly decision technologies, for the provision of increased quality at reduced costs. An emerging development in administrative decision support includes the increased use of information technology by administrators. This trend is promoted by the increased need for operational performance indicators. In addition, cost pressures on health care facilities will force information vendors to provide less expensive solutions. This concurrent decrease in the information technology price tag will also increase utilization. Health care organizations that "incorporate a pre-packaged, flexible analytic solution to address these performance indicators will have a significant competitive advantage" (Marzulli, 2000, p. 20). According to Marzulli (2000, p. 20), the organization should receive "standard" performance indicators over the organization's intranet, such as the "cash flow to net patient revenue, days in patients accounts receivable, inpatient payer mix, trend analysis over time, and the HMO discharge percentage." Health care leaders will be increasingly responsible for accurately documenting the return on investment of decision support activities. Payer mix (capitation versus fee for service or per diem) must be discerned to accurately compute cost savings (Rosenstein, 1999). Furthermore, return on investment (ROI) modules could be easily integrated into and routinely used by financial DSSs.

Organizations depend increasingly on technology to improve information input and throughput. Workflow tools for improving clinical and administrative processes will become commonplace. Increasingly, electronic data interchange, the Internet, and eMail are being used to lower the costs of collecting information to support decision making in health care. Workflow tools are designed to automate paper flow; capabilities include automatic distribution of documents for simultaneous consideration, reduction of file redundancy, and capture of information in an electronic format (Latamore, 1999). Workflow tools have evolved over a 10-year period from basic office automation tools to process management products capable of managing high transaction volumes with security and recovery capabilities. Workflow flexibility is enhanced by the rule-based management of business processes (Garets & Hanna, 1998). Order entry systems facilitated by voice recognition or bar code readers, the evolving computerized patient record, "smart cards," and imaging technology are further advances in this area (Ziegler, 1996).

Simpson (1999) has suggested that hybrid software solutions that merge patient care, financial, and operational modules to meet the challenges of understanding costs and allocating resources throughout the organization will also become increasingly common. Data mining is increasingly being used to understand connections between processes and outcomes in clinical, financial, and administrative information sources. Simpson has noted several impediments to improving quality of care via decision support. The impediments identified by Simpson, as well as environmental influences serving to limit the impact of these impediments, are listed in Box 4-2.

Decision technology will increasingly reduce the chaos inherent in a fragmented information environment. An interesting analogy can be made between today's health networks and American railroads of the early nineteenth century. Congress established the track width for the Union Pacific Railroad, which set in motion a uniform rail system. In a similar manner, the Internet and conventions such as the technical standards established by Health Level Seven (HL7) encourage uniform information pipelines in health care (Ziegler, 1996). According to Marzulli (2000), interconnectivity promoted by new standards such as XML, ActiveX, or Enterprise Java Beans, coupled with an infrastructure evolving to support application integration, is the key to the development of new business models.

Many DSSs representing niche solutions or narrow applications within an individual health care facility will increasingly be applied throughout the entire enterprise. Scheduling applications serve as a primary example. Straub (1997b) has cited a variety of health care leaders who believe

Box 4—2 Improving Quality of Care via Decision Support: Point/Counterpoint

Simpson (1999) has noted several impediments (listed below as Point) to improving quality of care via decision support. Environmental influences serving to limit these impediments are offered as counterpoints by the chapter author.

Point: Operational rules and guidelines vary within and by facility; this makes rule-based programming difficult.
Counterpoint: Laws, regulations, and accrediting agencies are increasingly guiding the actions taken by health care facilities.

Point: Facilities lack a standard clinical vocabulary.
Counterpoint: Data warehousing in part translates information into a standard format.

Point: Clinicians are reluctant to adopt tools and technology.
Counterpoint: Administrators commonly believe this fallacy while ignoring other administrators who choose to remain technologically incompetent. In fact, clinicians use enormous amounts of technology every day. The key to acceptance of technology by any user is to make the purpose and value of the technology evident. Developing input mechanisms that are complementary to the normal work pattern also helps.

Point: Outcomes are expensive to measure.
Counterpoint: Implementing processes that produce undesired outcomes represents an expense much greater than the mere measurement of those outcomes. In the face of mandates to measure outcomes, the argument against doing so is also obsolete.

that enterprise scheduling will be a key component of the health information technology infrastructure. New products are being designed to meet the needs of evolving health care networks and enterprise systems. Four propositions support the thesis that informed, shared decision making represents the future of health care (Rockefeller, 1999):

1. The human mind needs assistance to manage the contemporary biomedical knowledge base.
2. Optimal medicine is executed in partnership between an optimally informed patient and an optimally informed provider.
3. Modern decision support tools are essential to effective health care decision making.
4. Information technologies will "rehumanize medicine."

CONCLUSION

DSSs are not immune to the environmental influences that impact the entire industry. The changes that are expected to occur in the health care system imply an increasing need for administrative DSSs. These include (1) the continuing integration of health care delivery organizations, (2) collaboration among health care payers and providers to improve community health status, (3) better-informed patients demanding high-quality care, (4) pressure from third-party payers and patients to control costs and demonstrate the value of the services delivered, and (5) efforts to implement continuous quality improvement initiatives similar to those found in other fields (Dolan, n.d.).

Benefits of decision support that are facilitated by the effective capture, consolidation, processing, and manipulation of data include (1) effective use of historical trends to reengineer the process of health care delivery; (2) creation of "what if" models to assess the risk of various scenarios during managed care contracting; (3) measurement of cost, quality, and resource consumption performance indicators; and (4) support of "data-driven reengineering" through benchmarking, comparative uses of data, and economic profiling of providers (Waldo, 1998).

In this chapter the question has been asked, "What is an administrative decision support system?" Examples of DSSs have been successfully implemented at the level of the spreadsheet and the database. The contributions of this mode of decision support should not be discounted. However, as health care systems continue to evolve in response to the challenges of the marketplace, administrative DSSs must incorporate modern data warehousing, electronic data interchange, a sophisticated knowledge base, and solutions models.

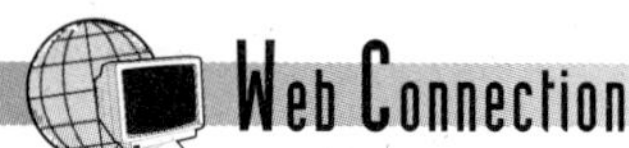

Web Connection

Administrative decision making is getting a new face as developers look to extend software capabilities beyond basic spreadsheet and database manipulations. The Web activities for this chapter are designed to encourage exploration of the current products available, the application of decision-making models, and the evolution of applications. Complex forecasting algorithms and simulations in decision support are replacing simple what if applications that use spreadsheet add-ins. You will gain an overview of both traditional and innovative approaches to decision support software as well as opportunities to examine the processes that have been in the "black box" of decision support until recently. To facilitate your understanding, several of the exercises will explore the world of decision support using demonstration products.

discussion questions

1. Distinguish between a clinical decision support system and an administrative decision support system.
2. What decision support system components are missing from both spreadsheets and databases? Discuss applications that include the missing components.
3. Identify five criteria that health care decision support systems should meet in response to the changing health care paradigm.
4. Name and discuss the decision venues to which administrative decision support systems are successfully applied.
5. Simpson has listed the following impediments to improving quality of care via decision support systems. Discuss a counterargument to Simpson's position; show why decision support systems will proliferate throughout health care in the near future.
   - Operational rules and guidelines vary within and by facility; this makes rule-based programming difficult.
   - Facilities lack a standard clinical vocabulary.
   - Clinicians are reluctant to adopt tools and technology.
   - Outcomes are expensive to measure.

REFERENCES

Agins, C.A. (1998). SAP goes to the hospital. *Across the Board, 5*(36), 36. Retrieved May 31, 2000, from ProQuest online database: http://www.sru.edu/depts/library/ElecJour.htm.

Alter, S.L. (1976). How effective managers use information systems. *Harvard Business Review, 54*, 97-104.

Andel, T. (1999). I need it now! *Transportation and Distribution, 40*(8), SCF13-SCF16. Retrieved May 18, 2000, from ProQuest online database: http://www.sru.edu/depts/library/ElecJour.htm.

Austin, C.J., & Boxerman, S.B. (1998). *Information systems for health services administration* (5th ed.). Chicago: Health Administration Press.

Bell, W.H. (1996). Telephone-based demand management: What you need to know now. *Health Care Strategic Management, 14*(2), 6. Retrieved May 18, 2000, from ProQuest online database: http://www.sru.edu/depts/library/ElecJour.htm.

Bird, L.J. (1997). Computerization in the OR. *AORN Journal, 66*(2), 312-317. Retrieved May 18, 2000, from INFOTRAC online database: http://www.sru.edu/depts/library/ElecJour.htm.

Blumenfield, B. (1997). Integrating knowledge bases at the point of care. *Health Management Technology, 18*(7), 44-46. Retrieved May 31, 2000, from ProQuest online database: http://www.sru.edu/depts/library/ElecJour.htm.

Business Resource Software, Inc. (n.d.a). *Business Insight download.* Retrieved October 29, 2000, from the World Wide Web: http://www.brs-inc.com/binsight.html.

Business Resource Software, Inc. (n.d.b) *Quick Insight download.* Retrieved October 29, 2000, from the World Wide Web: http://www.brs-inc.com/qinsight.html.

Chen, J.G., & Yeung, T.W. (1993). Hybrid expert-system approach to nurse scheduling. *Computers in Nursing, 11*(4), 183-190. Retrieved June 15, 2000, from EBSCOhost database: http://www.sru.edu/depts/library/ElecJour.htm.

Cleverley, W.O. (1997). *Essentials of health care finance* (4th ed.). Gaithersburg, MD: Aspen.

Conway, R.W., Maxwell, W.L., & Miller, L.W. (1967). *Theory of scheduling.* Reading, MA: Addison-Wesley.

Cupito, M.C. (1998). Balancing people, places, and times. *Health Management Technology, 19*(7), 26-34. Retrieved May 31, 2000, from ProQuest online database: http://www.sru.edu/depts/library/ElecJour.htm.

Darmoni, S.J., Fajner, A., Mahe, N., Leforestier, A., Vondracek, M., Stelian, O., & Baldenweck, M. (1995). HOROPLAN: Computer-assisted nurse scheduling using constraint-based programming. *Journal of the Society for Health Systems, 5*(1), 42-54. Retrieved from the World Wide Web: http://www.chu-rouen.fr/dsii/publi/plao.html.

Date, C.J. (1986). *An introduction to database systems* (Vol. 1, 4th ed.). Reading, MA: Addison-Wesley.

Delaney, B.C., et al. (1999). Can computerized decision support systems deliver improved quality in primary care? (Interview by A. Berger). *British Medical Journal, 319* (7220), 1281. Retrieved May 8, 2000, from EBSCOhost database: http://www.sru.edu/depts/library/ElecJour.htm.

Dexter, F., & Lubarsky, D.A. (1998). Managing with information: Using surgical services information services to increase operating room utilization. *ASA Professional Information.* Retrieved June 16, 1998, from the World Wide Web: http://www.asahq.org/NEWSLETTERS/1998/10_98/Managing_1098.html.

Dolan, T.C. (n.d.). *Your career as a healthcare executive.* Retrieved October 29, 2000, from the World Wide Web: http://www.ache.org/carsvcs/ycareer.html.

Donabedian, A. (1995). The quality of care: How can it be assessed? In N. Graham (Ed.), *Quality in health care: Theory, application, and evolution* (pp. 32-46). Gaithersburg, MD: Aspen.

Ecker, J.G., & Kupferschmid, M. (1988). *Introduction to operations research.* New York: John Wiley & Sons.

Evans, J.R., & Minieka, E. (1992). *Optimization techniques for networks and graphs* (2nd ed.). New York: Marcel Dekker.

Fantle, L.A., & DiLima, S.N. (1999). *1999 healthcare software sourcebook and IT buyer's guide.* Gaithersburg, MD: Aspen.

Fralic, M.F., & Denby, C.R. (2000). Retooling the nurse executive for the 21st century practice: Decision support systems. *Nursing Administration Quarterly, 24*(2), 19-28. Retrieved June 10, 2000, from INFOTRAC online database: http://www.sru.edu/depts/library/ElecJour.htm.

Garets, D., & Hanna, D. (1998). Emerging managed care technologies. *Health Management Technology, 19*(11), 28-32. Retrieved May 31, 2000, from ProQuest online database: http://www.sru.edu/depts/library/ElecJour.htm.

Gilhooly, K. (1997). Decision support with down east twist. *Software Magazine, 17*(14), 17-18. Retrieved May 26, 2000, from EBSCOhost database: http://www.sru.edu/depts/library/ElecJour.htm.

Grazier, K.L. (1998). Managed care information systems. *Journal of Healthcare Management, 43*(4), 303-305. Retrieved May 31, 2000, from ProQuest online database: http://www.sru.edu/depts/library/ElecJour.htm.

Griffith, J.R., & King, J.G. (2000). Championship management for healthcare organizations. *Journal of Healthcare Management, 45*(1), 17-31. Retrieved May 30, 2000, from ProQuest online database: http://www.sru.edu/depts/library/ElecJour.htm.

Grossman, J.H. (1994). Plugged-in medicine. *Technology Review, 97*(1), 22-29. Retrieved June 12, 2000, from ProQuest online database: http://www.sru.edu/depts/library/Elec Jour.htm.

Gunsauley, C. (1999a). Telephonic demand management shows savings potential. *Employee Benefit News, 13*(7), 15-16. Retrieved May 28, 2000, from EBSCOhost database: http://www.sru.edu/depts/library/ElecJour.htm.

Gunsauley, C. (1999b). Vendors push to leverage HRMS data. *Employee Benefit News, 13*(12), 1-3. Retrieved May 30, 2000, from EBSCOhost database: http://www.sru.edu/depts/library/ElecJour.htm.

Gupta, O.K., & Scott, C.L. III. (1996). A decision support system for selecting an employee health care insurance plan. *Mid-Atlantic Journal of Business, 32*(1), 47. Retrieved June 14, 2000, from INFOTRAC online database: http://www.sru.edu/depts/library/ElecJour.htm.

Hagland, M. (1998). Practice made perfect. *Health Management Technology, 19*(10), 12, 14. Retrieved May 31, 2000, from ProQuest online database: http://www.sru.edu/depts/library/ElecJour.htm.

Harmeier, P.E. (1991). Linear programming for optimization of nurse scheduling. *Computers in Nursing, 9*(4), 149-151. Retrieved May 29, 2000, from EBSCOhost database: http://www.sru.edu/depts/library/ElecJour.htm.

Harrell, C., Ghosh, B.K., Bowden, R. (2000). *Simulation using Promodel* (3rd ed.). Boston: McGraw-Hill.

Haug, P.J., Gardner, R.M., & Evans, R.S. (1999). Hospital-based decision support. In E.S. Berner (Ed.), *Clinical decision support systems: Theory and practice.* (pp. 77-103). New York: Springer.

Highmark Blue Cross Blue Shield unveils the nation's first-ever Internet-based "paperless" health insurance program. BLUeCHOICE offers businesses and consumers flexibility, online access and choice. (2000). Retrieved May 27, 2000, from the World Wide Web: http://www.highmark.com/whatsnew/nrbluechoice-a.html.

Hillier, F.S., & Lieberman, G.J. (1967). *Introduction to operations research.* San Francisco, CA: Holden-Day.

Huarng, F. (1999). A primary shift rotation nurse scheduling using zero-one linear goal programming. *Computers in Nursing, 17*(3), 135-144. Retrieved June 15, 2000, from EBSCOhost database: http://www.sru.edu/depts/library/ElecJour.htm.

Irvin, S.A. & Brown, H.N. (1999). Self-scheduling with Microsoft Excel. *Nursing Economics, 17*(4), 201-206. Retrieved June 15, 2000, from INFOTRAC online database: http://www.sru.edu/depts/library/ElecJour.htm.

Isken, M.W., & Hancock, W.M. (1991). A heuristic approach to nurse scheduling in hospital units with non-stationary, urgent demand, and a fixed staff size. *Journal for the Society of Health Systems, 2*(2), 24-41. Retrieved May 30, 2000, from EBSCOhost database: http://www.sru.edu/depts/library/ElecJour.htm.

Jacobs, C.M. (1997). Managing demand using clinical decision support tools. *Healthcare Financial Management, 51*(7), 41-42. Retrieved May 31, 2000, from ProQuest online database: http://www.sru.edu/depts/library/ElecJour.htm.

Kvedar, J.C. (2000). Decision support is changing healthcare. *Archives of Dermatology, 136*(2), 249. Retrieved June 10, 2000, from INFOTRAC online database: http://www.sru.edu/depts/library/ElecJour.htm.

Larkin, H. (1999). Stay up to date on patients' health benefits. *Medical Economics, 76*(8), 93-106. Retrieved May 31, 2000, from ProQuest online database: http://www.sru.edu/depts/library/ElecJour.htm.

Latamore, G.B. (1999). Workflow tools cut costs for high quality care. *Health Management Technology, 20*(4), 32-33. Retrieved May 31, 2000, from ProQuest online database: http://www.sru.edu/depts/library/ElecJour.htm.

Lawson is top healthcare financials vendor in KLAS study. (2000.). Retrieved June 14, 2000, from the World Wide Web: http://www.lawson.com/news/pressreleases/2000/2/klas.html.

Levin, R.I., et al. (1992). *Quantitative approaches to management* (8th ed.). New York: McGraw-Hill.

Loofbourrow, T. (2000). HR knowledge base: Making call centers and self-service really work. *Compensation and Benefits Management, 16*(2), 37-41. Retrieved May 31, 2000, from ProQuest online database: http://www.sru.edu/depts/library/ElecJour.htm.

Making a good warehouse better. (1998). *Material Handling Engineering, 53*(11), SCF4-SCF8. Retrieved May 31, 2000, from ProQuest online database: http://www.sru.edu/depts/library/ElecJour.htm.

Marzulli, T. (2000). Achieving a healthy e-business solution. *Health Management Technology, 21*(1), 18-20. Retrieved May 31, 2000, from ProQuest online database: http://www.sru.edu/depts/library/ElecJour.htm.

McConnell E.A. (2000). Staffing and scheduling at your fingertips. *Nursing Management, 31*(3), 52-53. Retrieved May 31, 2000, from ProQuest online database: http://www.sru.edu/depts/library/ElecJour.htm.

McCue, M. (1998). Delivering results without the hype. *Managed Healthcare, 8*(11), 24-26. Retrieved May 31, 2000, from ProQuest online database: http://www.sru.edu/depts/library/ElecJour.htm.

McLean, R.A. (1997). *Financial management in health care organizations.* Albany, New York: Delmar.

Mohan, L., Muse, L., & McInerney, C. (1998). Management smarter: A decision support system for mental health providers. *Journal of Behavioral Health Services and Research, 25*(4), 446-455. Retrieved May 31, 2000, from ProQuest online database: http://www.sru.edu/depts/library/ElecJour.htm.

Mousin, G., Remmlinger, E., & Weil, J.P. (1999). IT integration options for integrated delivery systems. *Healthcare Financial Management, 53*(2), 46-50. Retrieved May 30, 2000, from ProQuest online database: http://www.sru.edu/depts/library/ElecJour.htm.

Nunnelly, J. (1997). Managing with decision support tools. *Health Management Technology, 18*(5), 82. Retrieved February 26, 2000, from EBSCOhost database: http://www.sru.edu/depts/library/ElecJour.htm.

Okada, M., & Okada, M. (1988). Prolog-based system for nurse staff scheduling implemented on a personal computer. *Journal of Computers in Biomedical Research, 21*(1), 53-63. Retrieved May 29, 2000, from EBSCOhost database: http://www.sru.edu/depts/library/ElecJour.htm.

Perry, P.A. (1998). Software shopping. *Materials Management in Healthcare, 7*(5), 24-27. Retrieved June 14, 2000, from EBSCOhost database: http://www.sru.edu/depts/library/ElecJour.htm.

Physician scheduling software. (1998). *Materials Management in Healthcare, 7*(6), 58. Retrieved May 28, 2000, from EBSCOhost database: http://www.sru.edu/depts/library/ElecJour.htm.

Podgorelec, V., & Kokol, P. (1997). Genetic algorithm based system for patient scheduling in highly constrained situations. *Journal of Medical Systems, 21*(6), 417-427. Retrieved May 30, 2000, from EBSCOhost database: http://www.sru.edu/depts/library/ElecJour.htm.

Ravindran, A., Phillips, D.T., & Solberg, J.J. (1987). *Operations research: Principles and practice* (2nd ed.). New York: John Wiley & Sons.

Rhinehart, E. (1998). Demand management moves into the tech era. *Managed Healthcare, 8*(12), 20. Retrieved May 18, 2000, from ProQuest online database: http://www.sru.edu/depts/library/ElecJour.htm.

Rock, S. (1999). Serving your customer, serving yourself. *Managed Healthcare, 9*(2), 39-42. Retrieved May 31, 2000, from ProQuest online database: http://www.sru.edu/depts/library/ElecJour.htm.

Rockefeller, R. (1999). Informed shared decision-making: Is this the future of healthcare? *Health Forum Journal, 42*(3), 54-56. Retrieved May 18, 2000, from ProQuest online database: http://www.sru.edu/depts/library/ElecJour.htm.

Rosenstein, A.H. (1999). Inpatient clinical decision-support systems: Determining the ROI. *Healthcare Financial Management, 53*(12), 51-55. Retrieved June 16, 2000, from INFOTRAC online database: http://www.sru.edu/depts/library/ElecJour.htm.

Rothenberg, F. (1995). Choosing the right software. *Ophthalmology Times, 20*(41), 42-43. Retrieved May 30, 2000, from EBSCOhost database: http://www.sru.edu/depts/library/ElecJour.htm.

Rubbo, E.G. (1992). ORSA turns 40: OR pioneers tell of four decades of achievement, anecdotes. *OR/MS Today, April,* 50-52.

Schaffer, S.C. (1994). Automation: It can help solve staff scheduling—maybe. *Nursing Homes Long Term Care Management, 43*(1), 44-46. Retrieved May 28, 2000, from EBSCOhost database: http://www.sru.edu/depts/library/ElecJour.htm.

Schaich, R.L. (1998). IT implications of the next generation of managed care. *Health Management Technology, 19*(1), 34-36. Retrieved May 31, 2000, from ProQuest online database: http://www.sru.edu/depts/library/ElecJour.htm.

Simpson, R.L. (1999). IT takes lead role in outcomes measurement. *Nursing Management, 30*(8), 12-13. Retrieved February 26, 2000, from ProQuest online database: http://www.sru.edu/depts/library/ElecJour.htm.

St. Clair, D. (2000). The truth about managed care decisions. *Health Management Technology, 21*(2), 30-31. Retrieved May 31, 2000, from ProQuest online database: http://www.sru.edu/depts/library/ElecJour.htm.

Straub, K. (1997a). Chaos theory. *Health Management Technology, 18*(7), 32-35. Retrieved November 5, 2000, from ProQuest online database: http://www.sru.edu/depts/library/ElecJour.htm.

Straub, K. (1997b). Right on schedule? Demand for enterprise-wide scheduling solutions grows. *Health Management Technology, 18*(7), 32-35. Retrieved June 14, 2000, from EBSCOhost data-base: http://www.sru.edu/depts/library/ElecJour.htm.

Terry, K. (1999). Wrestling with the managed care octopus: Cut your losses by verifying patient's coverage. *Medical Economics, 76*(5), 54-71. Retrieved May 31, 2000, from ProQuest online database: http://www.sru.edu/depts/library/ElecJour.htm.

Thomas, T. (1998). Predictive software helps trim costs. *National Underwriter, 102*(48), 16-17. Retrieved May 31, 2000, from ProQuest online database: http://www.sru.edu/depts/library/ElecJour.htm.

Turban, E. (1993). *Decision support and expert systems: Management support systems* (3rd ed.). New York: Macmillan.

Villalon, M. (1999). GIS and the Internet: Tools that add value to your health plan. *Health Management Technology, 20*(9), 16-18. Retrieved May 31, 2000, from ProQuest online database: http://www.sru.edu/depts/library/ElecJour.htm.

Wagner, H.M. (1968). *Principles of operations research*. Englewood Cliffs, NJ: Prentice-Hall.

Wagner, H.M. (1975). *Principles of operations research* (2nd ed.). Englewood Cliffs, NJ: Prentice-Hall.

Waldo, B.H. (1998). Decision support and data warehousing tools boost competitive advantage. *Nursing Economics, 16*(2), 91-93. Retrieved February 26, 2000, from INFOTRAC online database: http://www.sru.edu/depts/library/ElecJour.htm.

Walker, T. (1999). Cleaning up the information clutter. *Managed Healthcare, 9*(3), 42-48. Retrieved May 31, 2000, from ProQuest online database: http://www.sru.edu/depts/library/ElecJour.htm.

Waymack, P. (1999). The managed care technology toolkit. *Health Management Technology, 20*(3), 26-27. Retrieved May 31, 2000, from ProQuest online database: http://www.sru.edu/depts/library/ElecJour.htm.

Weil, G., et al. (1998). The nurse scheduling problem: A combinatorial problem, solved by the combination of constraint programming and real users heuristics. *Medinfo, 9*(1), 508-512. Retrieved June 15, 2000, from EBSCOhost database: http://www.sru.edu/depts/library/ElecJour.htm.

Wilford, M. (1998). Software aids in managing cleaning logistics. *Hospital Materials Management, 23*(8), 12-13. Retrieved May 31, 2000, from ProQuest online database: http://www.sru.edu/depts/library/ElecJour.htm.

Ziegler, J. (1996). Health care's search for an information injection. *Business and Health, 14*(4), 33. Retrieved May 18, 2000, from ProQuest online database: http://www.sru.edu/depts/library/ElecJour.htm.

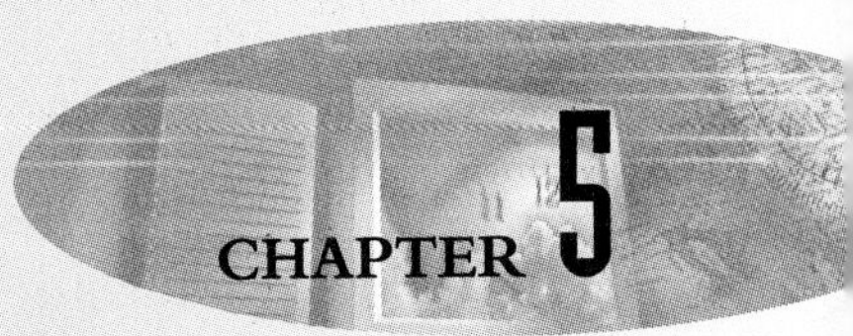

CHAPTER 5

Supporting Clinical Decision Making

PATRICIA A. ABBOTT
MARIANELA E. ZYTKOWSKI

Learning Objectives

Upon completion of this chapter, the reader will be able to:

1. ***Define*** a clinical decision support system.
2. ***Verbalize*** an understanding of how knowledge discovery in large data sets can be used for clinical decision support system knowledge base development.
3. ***Describe*** the challenges inherent in clinical knowledge representation for a clinical decision support system.
4. ***List*** areas of application for a clinical decision support system.
5. ***List*** several challenges to the development and acceptance of a clinical decision support system.

Outline

Key Terms

Arden Syntax
clinical decision support system (CDSS)
data mining
data warehouses
decision making
decision support system (DSS)
guideline interchange format (GLIF)
Health Level Seven (HL7)
inferencing
intelligent agent architecture
knowledge
knowledge discovery in large data sets (KDD)
knowledge-based systems
machine learning techniques
oracle
reasoning

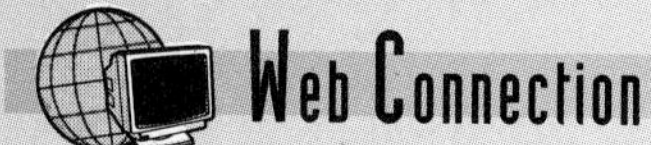

Go to the Web site at http://evolve.elsevier.com/Englebardt/. Here you will find Web links and activities related to supporting clinical decision making.

The 1999 report by the Institute of Medicine (IOM) entitled "To Err Is Human—Building a Safer Health System" states that 44,000 to 98,000 preventable medical errors occur annually, resulting in an estimated cost of $29 billion per year. Specifically mentioned in the IOM report is the need for decision support aids such as automated guidelines, intelligent decision support systems, and alerts that can be used to help prevent medical errors and improve the quality of decisions made in the clinical realm.

Improvements in the processes of care (and consequently the outcomes and costs of care) are dependent on optimal clinical **decision making.** Decisions made in the clinical arena can be enhanced by systems that facilitate, enhance, or expand the clinician's ability to work with data and information. A **clinical decision support system (CDSS)** is an automated **decision support system (DSS)** that mimics human decision making and can facilitate the clinical diagnostic process, promote the use of best practices, assist with the development and adherence of guidelines, facilitate processes for improvement of care, and prevent errors. However, to integrate these systems into the clinical environment, the process of human decision making must be understood and modeled sufficiently. In addition, expert knowledge must be captured, manipulated, and presented in ways acceptable to clinicians. Furthermore, the discovery and representation of **knowledge** that drives decision making require innovative techniques for management and use.

This chapter provides a background on decision support, discusses transition into the use of decision support systems in clinical care, and concludes by presenting new approaches to the development of a CDSS. In particular, attention to innovative pattern recognition and discovery methods such as knowledge discovery in large data sets (KDD) is suggested as a foundation for CDSS model development.

DECISION MAKING IN CLINICAL CARE

In the course of normal clinical activity, health care workers are presented with and manipulate many pieces of data and information. In this presentation and manipulation, decision making occurs—often under conditions of stress, cognitive overload, uncertainty, and increasing levels of scrutiny. These conditions can lead to clinical decisions that are faulty and produce less than optimal outcomes.

The challenges of problem solving and decision making in health care have led to the investigation and development of **knowledge-based systems** that enhance the human ability to analyze, problem solve, treat, diagnose, and estimate prognoses of health-related conditions (Peng & Reggia, 1990). Decisions made in the clinical realm can be enhanced by systems that facilitate, enhance, or expand the clinician's ability to work with data and information. This type of system, the CDSS, is not new to health care. In reality, CDSS applications were first evidenced in the 1970s, yet they have still not achieved widespread acceptance or use in health care. There are many reasons cited for this failure in acceptance:

- Narrowness of scope of the applications
- Mistrust of the clinical decisions made by the system
- Inability to incorporate new discoveries into the rule bases
- Nonportability of the CDSS to other computer systems
- Lack of integration with existing systems

However, the power behind the CDSS is not to be denied, and work continues to harness the capacity of these systems.

The health care environment has changed dramatically over the past two decades. Managed care organizations (MCOs), health maintenance organizations (HMOs), regulatory agencies, the public, and the government are closely monitoring health care. The pressure to "do more with less" has become a way of life. The 1999 IOM report regarding medical errors and the follow-up report, "Crossing the Quality Chasm: A New Health System for the 21st Century (2001)," have added to the frenetic activities aimed at improving the processes and actions surrounding the provision of health care. Improving the processes of care is dependent on developing automated systems that support optimal decision making.

The challenge facing information technologists is how to incorporate the science of decision making into systems that are accurate, descriptive, adaptive, unobtrusive, and usable as a normal part of clinical activity. These ambitious goals are dependent not only on the application level of systems development, which is reflected in what the clinician sees, but also on the conceptual model underlying the creation of the system. It is in this last statement that the questions surrounding the modeling of a CDSS are illuminated. How are the foundations that power DSSs in health care created? How can we capture and represent the knowledge and expertise of humans in a form that is suitable for automated systems? According to Seymour Cray, inventor of the Cray supercomputers, "Adding two and two together is no longer the issue: it's pattern recognition, pattern generation, and interpretation" (McCormack, 1993). A CDSS mimics the human decision-making process. Humans observe aspects of health (pattern recognition), cluster these patterns to identify new patterns (pattern generation), and then plan a course of action based on diagnosis/need (pattern interpretation). This process illustrates a new model that can be used for the development of CDSSs in health care. Adding automated methods of looking for patterns and trends in the data to problem-solving tool kits can be used to augment clinical decision making. Alternative approaches to modeling and supporting the human decision-making process can be aided by new methods (such as those developed by Cray) that foray into nontraditional methods of classification and prediction. This may be particularly appropriate in health care, where the "importance of prediction may begin to exceed that of explanation" (Abbott, 2000, p. 147). Although there are many different approaches to the development of a CDSS, the intent of this chapter is to suggest the use of knowledge discovery and prediction techniques as ways to improve clinical decision making.

BACKGROUND OF DECISION MAKING AND KNOWLEDGE REPRESENTATION

According to Graves and Corcoran (1989), the phenomenon of study in nursing informatics is not the computer technology but rather the data, information, and knowledge of nursing. These authors have described the development of systems that "assist with the management and processing of data, information and knowledge to support the practice of nursing and the delivery of nursing care" (p. 227). To understand the foundation of systems that facilitate decision making in care delivery, a discussion of the background of decision making and how it relates to the data-information-knowledge model posed by Graves and Corcoran is necessary.

Decision Making

A decision is defined as a course of action taken when making a choice between alternatives. The classic view of decision making focuses on the "analysis" between such alternatives. A more comprehensive view of human decision making categorizes it as a knowledge-based activity. The knowledge-based view defines a decision as a "piece of knowledge indicating the nature of an action commitment" (Holsapple & Whinston, 1996, p. 37). In other words, each time a decision is made, a piece of knowledge is generated. Since a decision is a manipulation of a piece of knowledge, making a decision can be likened to creating a new piece of knowledge—hence the term *knowledge based.* One may argue that repetitive, static decision making does not represent the creation of new knowledge. However in observational research, it is said that simply observing a phenomenon makes it different. This point supports the argument that all decision making is knowledge based.

Decision making occurs within a context, or setting. These contexts highly influence any sort of discussion about systems that support decision making. Decisions that work in one context may be totally irrelevant in another. The organizational design, area of application, decision maker, maturity of the setting, and importance of the decision all have an impact on the decision-making process and consequently are important to the development of any systems that facilitate decision making. These issues identify the challenges to developing DSSs that are appropriate to context.

Also critical to this generalized background discussion of decision making is the concept of "decision type." A decision type crosses a spectrum from structured to unstructured. Structured decisions are generally classified as routine decisions that are made day in and day out on the basis of well-established guidelines and static rules. The parameters surrounding structured decision making are known, predictable, and expected. Unstructured decisions, at the other end of the spectrum, are classified as highly unique and often made in emergent situations or in situations where the alternatives are not known or are unclear. A third category of decision type can be classified as semistructured. These situations are those where some of the background information is known and some is unique. This particular decision type is common to health care, where courses of action for general conditions are reasonably well understood, yet the nature of humans makes individual responses and presentations somewhat unstable.

The elements of decision context and decision type are offered to create a foundation for understanding the development of a DSS. This is not to say that these elements are the only considerations behind the design of these systems. In fact, there are entire texts devoted to decision making and support systems. Readers are referred to the work of Holsapple and Whinston (1996) for additional detail. For the purposes of general understanding of CDSSs, knowledge of decision context and decision type is critical.

Knowledge

As mentioned earlier, decision making is often viewed as a knowledge-based and knowledge-intensive activity. New knowledge is created when a decision is made; old knowledge is often altered or discarded after a new decision is made. Frequently, in the course of making a decision, improvement is generated just by the consideration of various courses of action. New ways of doing things may result from such cognitive considerations, leading to improvement of existing processes. Therefore the generation of new knowledge can be viewed and valued as a production or manufacturing process.

A DSS can use both non–knowledge-based and knowledge-based approaches in the production process. In non–knowledge-based approaches, a DSS is simply manipulating data, sometimes transforming it into information for use in certain situations. An example of such a transformation in health care is the graphical representation of physiologic data (flowcharts). The data are manipulated and presented in such a way that they can be readily interpreted and decisions made. This is in contrast to a true knowledge-based DSS, wherein contextual knowledge is contained within the system and the full implications of the Graves and Corcoran model (data-information-knowledge) are evident. The incorporation of knowledge allows the machine to "think" like the user and bases output on logic that has been preprogrammed into the knowledge base of the system. This is where the challenge to the system lies. "Preprogramming" denotes a formalized approach to representing knowledge. It also makes one realize that representing knowledge for a computer to use is a never-ending activity because knowledge is constantly changing. The representation of knowledge is further compounded by the following issues:

- Human decision making is not fully understood; therefore it is not possible to perfectly model the human decision-making process.
- Health care is an ever-changing body of knowledge.
- Biology is not static, requiring adaptive approaches to knowledge base development and maintenance.
- Uncertainty and incomplete knowledge thwart the development of a DSS.
- Development of standards for CDSSs and clinical data representation is in its infancy.

Each of these elements points to the multiple facets that challenge researchers and developers of these systems and leads to a discussion of knowledge and knowledge representation. Is the conundrum of knowledge capture and representation akin to capturing moonbeams in a jar?

Defining Knowledge

What exactly is knowledge? Entire careers have been spent trying to describe and define knowledge. For the purposes of this chapter, a DSS requires a collection of knowledge that is captured and structured in a way that is interpretable by the computer. Knowledge has been formally defined by Vehkavaara (1998) as "a true well-justified belief or proposition. Knowledge is achieved, at least in standard empiricist dogma, by some learning process, either through perception or through the adoption of such a tradition that contains previously gathered knowledge." Holsapple (1983) has described three types of knowledge: descriptive knowledge, procedural knowledge, and reasoning. Each one must be represented in a fashion that a DSS can manipulate.

Descriptive knowledge is simply a description of something. It can be a description of past, present, future, or "what if" situations. Descriptive knowledge is gained by learning and observation. Procedural knowledge focuses on how to do something, usually a step-by-step procedure, and is also gained by observation, learning, and experience. **Reasoning** is knowledge that assists one in drawing conclusions; for example, as certain symptoms cluster together, reasoning is used to assign a diagnosis. Reasoning is also learned, but it is truly a product of experience and exposure. According to vanBemmel, Musen, and Miller (1997), this type of knowledge (reasoning) is highly intuitive, meaning that it is based on "gut" feelings and is a product of "information chunking." In information chunking, humans develop the ability to recognize patterns over time as a product of experience and exposure to certain situations. The way that humans chunk information is almost untraceable, making it difficult to model in a DSS.

These three types of knowledge cover the "know what" (descriptive), "know how" (procedural), and "know why" (reasoning). By combining these three types of knowledge, a decision maker can make a decision. This is also called "drawing inferences." **Inferencing** is the process

FIGURE 5–1 | **Decision Support System Architecture**

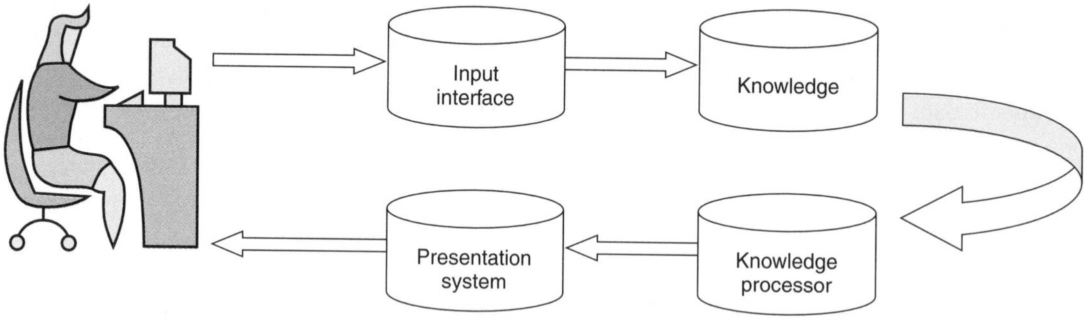

of drawing a conclusion from the evidence that has been presented. It can be based on rules or probabilities. A DSS that has been programmed with descriptive, procedural, and reasoning knowledge, as well as the rules or probabilities necessary to make inferences, consists of a knowledge base and an inference engine.

Representing Knowledge

Representing knowledge for use in a DSS is very challenging. As noted earlier, a DSS requires that knowledge be represented in a fashion that can be stored and manipulated by a computer. For knowledge to be represented, it must be structured in a usable format. A "usable format" implies that there is a pattern of symbols that represents the captured knowledge. A DSS has knowledge-processing ability so that the symbolic representation of the knowledge can be manipulated (Figure 5-1). The relationship between knowledge representation and knowledge processing can be considered as follows: a "DSS cannot process knowledge that it cannot represent. Conversely, a DSS cannot know what is represented by some pattern of symbols that it is unable to represent" (Holsapple & Whinston, 1996, p. 104).

The issues surrounding knowledge representation are very complex, compounded not only by the underlying intricacy of the domain but also by the current dynamic state of the standards movement in health care. In moving from a DSS to the more domain-specific CDSS, Broverman (1999) has asserted that there are three areas of focus related to standards in a CDSS:

1. Consensus on clinical data models
2. Standardized interfaces between the CDSS and underlying systems
3. Consistent representation of guidelines/clinical logic

Active research is being done in an effort to arrive at a consensus concerning standardized reference and information models for clinical data representation. For a CDSS to reach maximum potential, a consistent representation of health care data is mandatory. Two particular knowledge/guideline representation formats that will assist in standardizing the interface between a CDSS and other systems are **Arden Syntax** and **guideline interchange format (GLIF).** Arden Syntax for knowledge representation has been described by Broverman (1999) as "a balloted and internally deployed standard that was created with the goal of allowing users to create and share pieces of medical knowledge in a format that can be implemented by computer systems" (p. 26). The GLIF is an extension of the Arden Syntax that improves the ability of the syntax to represent protocols for care and complex multicomponent guidelines in a temporal fashion.

Standardization of guideline representation is occurring in **Health Level Seven** (HL7), in the American Society for Testing and Materials (ASTM), and in academic institutions.

Active work to incorporate and further develop these representation formats is occurring in the HL7 CDSS technical committee (TC), at the CORBAmed Healthcare Data Interpretation Facility, and at several universities. The HL7 CDSS TC has derived an outline of the components required for a CDSS. The outline includes standardized reference terminology and an information model (RTM/RIM), a standardized query language that taps into the RIM/RTM, and a standardized clinical language. These are large tasks, but work is well underway in each component. Developments at the Second Annual Nursing Vocabulary Summit (June 2000) at Vanderbilt University demonstrated the movement toward convergence of clinical vocabularies and further development/testing of the RTM/RIM. Although a great deal of work in both representation and exchange standards is needed to complete the standardization of components required for a CDSS, it is believed that completion is inevitable. A detailed discussion of standards used in health care informatics is presented in Chapters 17 and 18.

DECISION MAKING IN CLINICAL SETTINGS

The foundations of DSSs for the clinical realm are built on the basics of human decision making and knowledge representation. Understanding how decision types and context influence the process, as well as the manner in which the "what," the "how," and the "why," contribute to the drawing of inferences, is important, especially as the DSS is applied in the clinical domain.

As stated previously, the use of DSSs in the clinical domain began in the 1970s. An excellent review of previous CDSS use has been provided by Miller and Geissbuhler (1998). Ozbolt (1988) has provided a review of earlier CDSS use in nursing. Since the initial CDSS applications, an understanding of how clinicians make decisions has expanded dramatically. In concert, the rapid expansion of information technology, as well as the changing nature of health care delivery, has initiated increased attention on the use of these systems. According to Perreault and Metzger (1999):

> *CDSS, appropriately implemented, can improve the quality of care, reduce costs, and improve patient satisfaction. More and more institutions—academic health centers, community-based organizations, and physician group practices alike—are actively pursuing the goal of implementing patient-care systems that include CDSS, backing their plans with significant investments of capital and staff resources (p. 5).*

Defining a Clinical Decision Support System

Brennan in 1985 defined a CDSS as a tool that can be used to provide "nurses with strategies to analyze, evaluate, develop, and select effective solutions to complex problems in complex environments" (p. 319). A CDSS is any computer program designed to help health care professionals make clinical decisions (Shortliffe, Buchanan, & Feigenbaum, 1979). Early forerunners of these systems focused on diagnostic assistance for clinicians, as evidenced in the definition offered by Miller in 1990 that "a CDSS can be defined as a computer-based algorithm that assists a clinician with one or more component steps of the diagnostic process" (p. 582). Each of these definitions is true. However, on closer examination, Brennen's definition is more visionary. It steps away from a narrow prescription of application to a more holistic view of the diverse complexities that face clinicians. A more modern definition is offered by Perreault and Metzger (1999): "In its ideal sense, CDS [clinical decision support] is a set of knowledge-based tools that are fully integrated with both the clinician workflow components of a CPR [computerized patient record] and a repository of complete and accurate clinical data" (p. 6).

It is becoming more apparent that diagnosis and "clinically" based issues are only two of many facets to be considered for a CDSS. Eight competing demands for CDSS application in the clinical realm include the following (Perreault & Metzger, 1999):

1. Improving patient care
2. Reducing costs
3. Disseminating expert knowledge
4. Managing clinical complexity
5. Monitoring clinical details
6. Managing administrative complexity
7. Educating students and residents
8. Supporting clinical research

Innovative ways for dealing with the knowledge base for a CDSS are required when considering these comprehensive needs. The caveat, however, is one made by Miller and Geissbuhler (1998)—that a CDSS cannot be formulated that can answer every question posed. Instead, the "problem to be solved originates in the mind of the clinician-user" (p. 7). Expecting a CDSS to blindly process every piece of information presented and come up with a definitive diagnosis or plan of action was an original conceptualization of the CDSS and is referred to as the **oracle** model. The *Encyclopedia of Greek Mythology* defines an oracle as "the answer given by a god to a question asked by a mortal supplicant," giving one the idea of a single source of definitive knowledge, which we now know to be impossible. The Greek oracle model was therefore abandoned, and movement toward user interaction with the CDSS was accepted. However, even the notion of traditional user interaction is being called into question. According to Miller and Geissbuhler (1998), "Current CDDSS [sic] models assume that the user will interact with the CDDSS in an iterative fashion, selectively entering patient information and using the CDDSS output to assist with the problems encountered in the diagnostic process" (p. 7). However a second question of equal significance is the issue of "selectively entering" patient information. In other words, the user determines which data will be entered.

In the environment of terabytes of data, traditional approaches, which are based on people dealing directly with the data, require alterations. One alteration is the use of intelligent agents. The term intelligent agent is used to refer to software that can autonomously accomplish a task for a person or other entity. The software has some sort of "trigger" built into it, and once executed, the agent can carry out its function without further intervention. **Intelligent agent architecture** (a model of an intelligent information processing system) and the ability to mine **data warehouses** create a confluence of opportunities for CDSS development. Instead of "selectively entering patient data" when a problem arises, a modern CDSS may be able to extract information from the underlying enterprise information system. These systems may be able to use existing rules, probabilities, and guidelines to provide guidance and support for health care professionals. One cannot expect a system to provide assistance for ill-defined or undefined problems; a CDSS can never totally replace human judgment (Miller & Geissbuhler, 1998). A CDSS can no longer be viewed as an oracle; it cannot know all and see all. The influences of technology and policy will result in a much more powerful and comprehensive approach to CDSS development wherein advanced systems will be able to *support* (not replace) clinical decision making. The power of the CDSS will be evidenced and leveraged.

OPPORTUNITIES FOR NEW APPROACHES

Improvements in information systems, coupled with the mushrooming amount of data being collected, stored, and shared in large health care databases, are changing the fundamental paradigms of information capture, management, and data use. The size of many data sets has already surpassed the ability of humans to work directly with data.

One can look to the size of the data sets that have emerged from the Human Genome project to get an indication of the future size of data warehouses. Genes are made of DNA, and each strand of DNA contains 23 pairs of chromosomes. Each chromosome, in turn, carries thousands of genes arranged like knots on a rope. All totaled, the human genome is made up of 3 billion base pairs of chromosomes (U.S. Department of Energy, Human Genome Program, 1996). If printed out, the entire human genome would fill a 1000-page telephone book. Without advanced methods for analysis of large data sets, searching for certain combinations of gene sequences that denote certain diseases would be like looking for the proverbial needle in a haystack. Although not related to health care, another excellent example of mushrooming data sets is found in the Earth Observing System that NASA launched in 2000. This satellite network gathers 46 megabytes of data per second, requiring massive storage capacity *and* requiring new approaches to analysis.

"Data cemeteries," a term coined by McCormick in 1981, describes the preexisting state of many health care data collections. Data and information were (and in some cases still are) often found in isolated silos with little connectivity or integration. This isolation of data is counterproductive to the development of a reliable and accurate CDSS. The concept of data cemeteries contrasts with current and planned applications where data are shared on an enterprise-wide basis. According to Szolovits and Pauker (1993):

> *Comprehensive on-line clinical databases are really just now becoming a reality, and even today often do not include what is, for clinical decision aids, the most critical component: problem lists, histories and physical examinations, progress notes, the coded results of non-numeric diagnostic tests (e.g., radiology), and diagnostic categories. Early systems were, until very recently, limited to simple trend detection and extrapolation because the only data available to them were numerical records routinely produced in labs. We expect that new kinds of systems, such as decision aids that don't respond to specific requests for assistance but simply monitor the provision of good care, will only be effective if they can provide timely advice to the clinician who is integrating information, designing strategies, and making choices (p. 17).*

The emergence of comprehensive online clinical databases creates many opportunities for CDSS development and enhancement. The augmentation of existing claims-based/administrative data sets with rich multidimensional clinical data opens new avenues for retrospective analysis of patterns and trends. These can be used in CDSS development to guide future decisions, identify areas for process improvement, and refine existing patterns of care. Using data where the outcomes are already known (retrospective data) enables the construction of prediction models that can then be applied prospectively. Furthermore, the coupling of clinical data with administrative data can be referred to as bringing "business to the bedside," facilitating real-time continuous quality improvement. The potential for a positive impact on processes and outcomes of care is considerable. The ability to analyze large collections of data from populations to individuals crosses the spectrum of need for diverse users of health care data. Ultimately, the goal of developing a CDSS is to improve clinical decision making. This goal requires that the data, information, and knowledge on which clinical decisions are made is available, understandable, and usable.

The challenges facing information technologists are as follows:

- To harness and then unlock the multidimensional data caught in these large data sets
- To detect the trends or look for predictors of untoward outcomes
- To incorporate such findings into systems that support decision makers

The webs of causality in health care are exceedingly complex, requiring new approaches to knowledge discovery and application. The use of knowledge discovery in large data sets is one particularly promising method that may be used to unlock the value of data residing in large health care data warehouses.

USING KNOWLEDGE DISCOVERY IN LARGE DATA SETS FOR CLINICAL DECISION SUPPORT SYSTEM DEVELOPMENT

Fayyad, Piatetsky-Shapiro, and Smyth (1996) have defined **knowledge discovery in large data sets (KDD)** as the "non-trivial process of identifying valid, novel, potentially useful, and ultimately understandable patterns in data" (p. 6). In applying this generalized definition to the domain of health care, Abbott (2000) has defined KDD as "the melding of human expertise with statistical and **machine learning techniques** to identify features, patterns, and underlying rules in large collections of health care data" (p. 141). The goal of KDD is to search for consistent patterns and relationships among data points based on analysis of a large set of data and to turn those discovered relationships into a "model." The model is then applied to other test cases to determine if the model will "hold" on new cases (also called model verification). The model can then be incorporated into systems that can support decision making. KDD is sometimes used interchangeably with the term **data mining,** although they are different. Data mining is only one step in the process of KDD (Figure 5-2). However, as a step in the KDD process, the semantic argument can be made that to effectively discover the nuggets of information in large, disparate data sets, the data sets must be quarried for valuable pieces of information. This quarrying process takes place through the application of data mining algorithms. Examples of specific data mining algorithms are presented in Chapter 4.

The concept of KDD is not new, having been used in business and financial environments for more than a decade. Although KDD has been used in claims fraud detection (the financial/reg-

FIGURE 5–2 | **KDD Process**

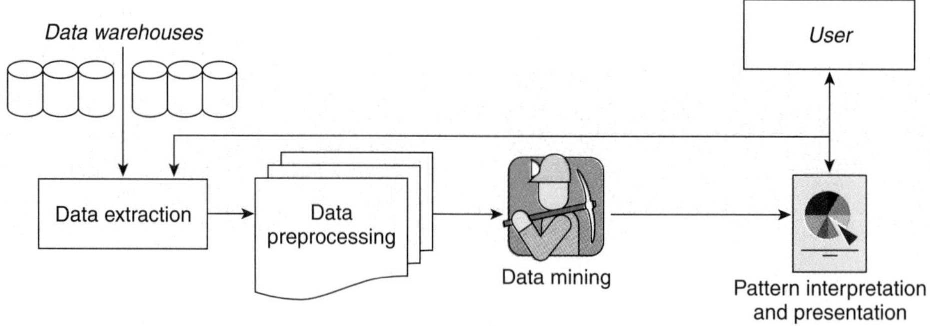

Data extraction: Searching for and choosing data

Data preprocessing: Choosing variables, dealing with noise and multidimensionality

Data mining: Analyzing data using association, clustering, modeling, classification, etc.

Pattern interpretation and presentation: Interpreting, evaluating, and presenting patterns

(From Abbott, P. [2000]. Knowledge discovery in large data sets: A primer for data mining applications in health care. In M. Ball et al. [Eds.], Nursing informatics: Where caring and technology meet *[3rd ed.]. New York: Springer-Verlag.)*

ulatory side of health care), there has been limited use in the clinical side of health care. This is rapidly changing as a result of a dawning awareness of the value of information—particularly in relation to the addition of clinical data to administrative sets, scalable technology, a movement of database ownership from information systems shops to the business/clinical side of operations, and the massive size of expanding health care data sets. Each of these issues has contributed to increased examination of the techniques and application of KDD. Unlocking the patterns, trends, and information that are trapped in these warehouses is critically important to the creation of a CDSS.

Understanding KDD begins by contrasting it with traditional approaches of data analysis. In the traditional approach (also called "verification based"), the hypothesis is given a priori (in advance). For example, in analyzing a large data set from a long-term care facility to determine the predictors of admission to an acute care facility, one may hypothesize a priori that fractures, severe congestive heart failure, and sepsis are the major predictors of admission. The analysis of the data set is undertaken. The three predictors that were hypothesized a priori may emerge as the top contributors to the outcome of admission. However, there is also a possibility that these three will not emerge as major predictors. Instead, new and nonhypothesized predictors might emerge. In a traditional approach, the nonhypothesized variables (outliers) that emerge invalidate the original hypothesis.

By contrast, in the "discovery-based" approach, such as KDD, the outliers are considered the gold mine. In essence, the quest is to find what is not known. Variables that emerge (or are "discovered") from the KDD process are of particular interest. This is not to say, however, that one can blindly use KDD. Using KDD techniques to analyze health care data without health care expert involvement is called data dredging and threatens the reliability of results. An example is when a business analyst or statistician singularly mines health care data with no idea of the clinical relevance of findings. However, when KDD is applied properly, using appropriate expert opinions, it can reveal unknown or nonhypothesized relationships or patterns in the underlying data.

These unknown factors or relationships have strong bearing on the development of the knowledge base that powers a CDSS. The model developed from these relationships can be applied prospectively in clinically based systems, thereby alerting health care workers to impending problems or unexpected variances. Knowing what factors contribute to certain outcomes, being able to predict the occurrence of the factors, and then being able to deliver the information (as part of a CDSS) to providers at the decision-making point is the goal.

The process of KDD consists of five basic steps:

1. Identify and understand the problem.
2. Obtain/access the target data set.
3. Preprocess the data (which includes handling missing or "dirty" data).
4. Apply the data mining algorithm.
5. Interpret the findings.

Each step builds on the preceding one, and the process is iterative. The whole process moves from a large and diffuse collection of data to the end product of knowledge discovery and model development. A detailed description of the KDD process can be found in the work by Abbott (2000), in which large data sets from the Health Care Financing Administration (now the Centers for Medicare & Medicaid Services [CMS]) were mined to determine predictors of hospitalization in long-term care (LTC) resident populations.

KDD should not be construed as a panacea for all woes related to the creation of a CDSS. There are many approaches being used in the CDSS domain. However, the techniques of KDD hold tremendous promise for the development of knowledge bases required to support decision making in the clinical realm. Allowing the data to "speak" without the constraints of traditional approaches will validate what is already known and, in addition, help to discover what is unknown. The harnessing of known and unknown knowledge for use in developing CDSSs will improve the quality and utility of systems that facilitate human decision making.

REQUIREMENTS FOR FUTURE DEVELOPMENT OF CLINICAL DECISION SUPPORT SYSTEMS

This chapter presents many of the challenges that face information technologists in the development, implementation, and maintenance of a CDSS. The issues surrounding the understanding of how humans make decisions, considerations of why these systems have failed in the past, the challenges of knowledge representation and standards adoption, and the pressing issues facing health care delivery contribute to the complexity of clinical decision making. Solving these problems will require massive commitment of financial and intellectual resources. Areas that must be addressed include the following:

- Robust technical infrastructure and integration—The inability to share and exchange data, information, and knowledge is a bottleneck to CDSS development.
- Standards/knowledge representations—The lack of standardized representation for both logic and clinical and health data impedes comprehensive CDSS development.
- Understanding of scope—Diffuse development of ill-defined or poorly conceptualized applications can lead to a CDSS that mimics the oracle approach.
- Support and commitment—Health care knowledge is constantly expanding. A CDSS requires constant maintenance and updating. A high level of commitment with intense buy-in from all stakeholders is needed.
- Understanding of human nature—Not only is it important to understand how humans make decisions important, but also it is important to understand how humans adapt to change.

Implementation of a CDSS requires attention to change management, consideration of process engineering, and an understanding of how humans adapt to innovation. These systems can be perceived as threatening to clinicians for a variety of reasons.

CONCLUSION

This chapter provides a comprehensive examination of human decision making, knowledge representation, decision support concepts, and the domain of clinical decision making. The environment of health care is rapidly changing. Knowledge bases are increasing in size. Health care delivery paradigms are changing. These changes have produced the need to improve the decision-making processes in health care. CDSSs have not been overly successful in the past. However, the increased adoption of integrated computerized patient record systems combined with the growing acceptance of guidelines or protocols of care and new discovery-based approaches to information management are opening new avenues of possibility. The use of discovery-based techniques in large warehouses of clinically oriented data will enable organizations to detect patterns and trends, identify and support best practices, and reengineer the processes of care.

The way in which health care data are used in the development of knowledge-based systems requires new approaches. Clinical data warehouses are rapidly becoming larger than humans can deal with directly. This requires new techniques for identifying the knowledge that is contained within data warehouses. The adoption and utilization of methods that focus on discovery and prediction are suggested as an approach to CDSS knowledge base development.

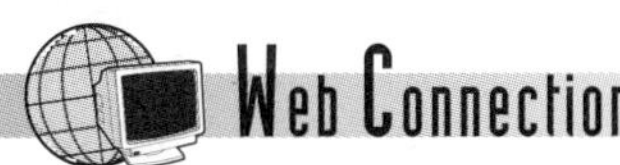

Web Connection

Clinical decision support systems range from those prompting the clinician with reminders to consider best practice aspects of care to more complex applications that simulate outcomes based on patient data and predetermined rules. In the Web activities for this chapter, you will explore a variety of clinical decision support systems and techniques. Through these activities you will learn to develop a decision model using a modeling tool and to form a personal perspective on the state of clinical decision support based on the available literature.

discussion questions

1. Three types of knowledge are discussed in this chapter (descriptive knowledge, procedural knowledge, and reasoning). Create a clinical scenario using the three types of knowledge. Identify the hallmarks of all three.
2. The local university hospital has developed a CDSS that assists emergency department clinicians in determining whether a patient's complaint of chest pain is cardiac related or of epigastric origin. The developers used in-house guidelines and local vocabulary. Cite two reasons why this CDSS would not be transportable to another hospital. How could the interoperability issue be solved?
3. How does the KDD approach differ from traditional approaches to data analysis?
4. A clinician who is unfamiliar with how a CDSS works does not understand why the system is unable to analyze all elements of the patient's record and come up with a diagnosis and plan of care for the patient. How would you explain the inability of the system to perform in this fashion?

REFERENCES

Abbott, P. (2000). Knowledge discovery in large datasets: A primer for data mining applications in health care. In M. Ball et al. (Eds.), *Nursing informatics: Where caring and technology meet* (3rd ed.). New York: Springer-Verlag.

Brennan, P. (1985). Decision support for nursing practice: The challenge and the promise. In K. Hannah, E. Guillemin, & D. Conklin (Eds.), *Nursing uses of computer and information science* (pp. 315-319). Amsterdam: Elsevier.

Broverman, C. (1999). Standards for clinical decision support systems. *Journal of Healthcare Information Management, 13*(2), 23-32.

Committee on Quality of Health Care in America, Institute of Medicine. (2000). To err is human: Building a safer health care system. Washington, DC: National Academy Press.

Committee on Quality of Health Care in America, Institute of Medicine. (2001). Crossing the quality chasm: A new health system for the 21st century. Washington DC: National Academy Press.

Encyclopedia of Greek mythology. Available: http://www.cultures.com/greek_resources/greek_encyclopedia/.

Fayyad, U., Piatetsky-Shapiro, & Smyth. (1996). *Advances in knowledge discovery and data mining.* Cambridge, MA: MIT Press.

Graves, J., & Corcoran, S. (1989). The study of nursing informatics. *Image: The Journal of Nursing Scholarship, 21,* 227-231.

Holsapple, C. (1983). The knowledge system for generalized problem processor. *Krannet Institute Paper, no. 827.* West Lafayette, IN: Purdue University.

Holsapple, C., & Whinston, A. (1996). *Decision support systems: A knowledge-based approach.* St. Paul, MN: West Publishing.

McCormack, R. (1993). One hour with Seymour Cray. *High Performance Computing and Communications, 46,* 7.

McCormick, K. (1981). Nursing research using computerized data bases. In H. Heffernan (Ed.), *Proceedings of the fifth annual symposium on computer applications in medical care.* Silver Spring, MD: IEEE Computer Society Press.

Miller, R. (1990). Why the standard view is standard: People not machines understand patients' problems. *Journal of Medicine and Philosophy, 15,* 581-591.

Miller, R., & Geissbuhler, A. (1998). Clinical diagnostic decision support systems—An overview. In E. Berner (Ed.), *Clinical decision support systems: Theory and practice.* New York: Springer.

Ozbolt, J. (1998). Knowledge-based systems for supporting clinical nursing decisions. In M. Ball et al. (Eds.), *Nursing informatics: Where caring and technology meet.* New York: Springer-Verlag.

Peng, Y., & Reggia, J. (1990). *Abductive inference models for diagnostic problem solving.* New York: Springer-Verlag.

Perreault, L., & Metzger, J. (1999). A pragmatic framework for understanding clinical decision support. *Journal of Healthcare Information Management, 13*(2), 5-22.

Shortliffe, E., Buchanan, B., & Feigenbaum, E. (1979). Knowledge engineering for medical decision-making: A review of computer-based decision aids. *Proceedings of the Institute of Electrical and Electronic Engineers, 67,* 1207-1224.

Szolovits, P., & Pauker, S. (1993). A coherent philosophy for development or a straightjacket for research (Editorial commentary). *Methods of Information in Medicine 32,* 16-17.

U.S. Department of Energy, Human Genome Program (1996). *To know ourselves.* Washington, DC: Author. Available: http://www.ornl.gov/hgmis/publicat/tko/03_introducing.html.

vanBemmel, J., Musen, M., & Miller, R. (1997). Methods for decision support. In J. vanBemmel & M. Musen (Eds.), *Handbook of medical informatics.* The Netherlands: Springer-Verlag.

Vehkavaara, T. (1998). Extended concept of knowledge for evolutionary epistemology and for biosemiotics: Hierarchies of storage and subject of knowledge. In G.L. Farre & T. Oksala (Eds.), *Emergence, complexity, hierarchy, organization* (pp. 207-216). Selected and edited papers from ECHO III. *Acta Polytechnica Scandinavica: Mathematics Computing, and Management in Engineering, Series No. 91.* Espoo, Finland.

PART TWO

Health Care Information Systems

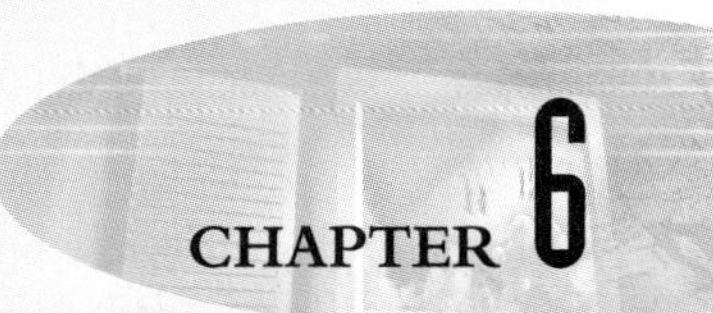

The Purpose, Structure, and Functions of Health Care Information Departments

CHARLES OLESON

Learning Objectives

Upon completion of this chapter, the reader will be able to:

1. ***Describe*** the staff roles within an information systems department.
2. ***Explain*** the scope of responsibility of an information systems department.
3. ***Identify*** factors that interact to influence the success of an information systems department.

Outline

Structure of Health Care Information Departments
- *Departments/Sections/Responsibilities*
- *Roles*
- *Technology Infrastructure*
- *Business Environment*

Key Terms

adds, moves, and changes
critical care monitoring applications
Health Insurance Portability and Accountability Act (HIPAA)
interface engine
production job
system backup

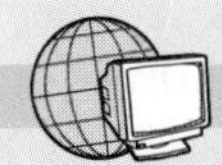

Web Connection

Go to the Web site at http://evolve.elsevier.com/Englebardt/. Here you will find Web links and activities related to the purpose, structure, and functions of health care information departments.

This chapter describes the purpose, structure, and functions of information systems (IS) departments within health care organizations. Although there are significant variations across organizations with respect to how information services are provided, common needs and requirements are addressed. Typical approaches to providing these services are described. The chapter begins with a description of the areas of responsibility within an IS department. The next section describes typical role types within IS departments. The information technology (IT) infrastructure within a health care organization is described from the point of view of the support requirements for an IS department. The business considerations to be addressed in the course of providing information services within a health care organization are discussed. The chapter concludes with a description of a day in the life of a chief information officer (CIO).

STRUCTURE OF HEALTH CARE INFORMATION DEPARTMENTS

Departments/Sections/Responsibilities

The typical departments or sections within the larger IS department are operations, telecommunications, clinical applications, administrative applications, personal computer and help desk support, systems administration, and network support. Small organizations may combine functions or identify individuals who will carry out more than one function. Figure 6-1 illustrates typical department organization and reporting relationships within an IS department. The roles identified in this chart are described in the next section of this chapter. Occasionally other departmental areas are included under the umbrella of information systems. Examples of such areas are medical records and quality management. These departmental areas are discussed and described in Chapter 7.

Operations

The operations department is responsible for the operation and maintenance of the IS hardware, the execution of routine software applications, and the management of the output produced by these systems. Typically an operations section is staffed on a 24-hours-per-day, 7 days-per-week (24/7) basis.

Typical activities of operators include interacting with computer screens to start **production jobs,** monitoring system status, and carrying out system backups. Much of an operator's responsibility is involved with paper processing. These responsibilities include output management, such as separating print jobs and packaging output for delivery to the designated recipients. Examples of such output include laboratory reports, billing reports, and financial reports of various types used within the organization. Other specialized printing responsibilities include printing patient bills and printing payroll checks. These types of jobs often require the use of specific forms that must be loaded into printers and then removed at the end of the print job.

Machine maintenance is another area of significant responsibility for operators. Since printing reports involves a mechanical process related to moving paper across the print area, routine maintenance is required to maintain adequate print quality. Maintenance involves the replacement of ink cartridges and the replacement of guides and moving parts such as rollers and brushes. As a result of the development of remote laser printing capabilities within most health care organizations, operations sections have also often been given responsibility for maintenance of remote printers.

System backup is a daily routine for most operations staffs. Maintaining patient data and billing information is critical to the ongoing operations of health care organizations; therefore precautions must be taken to ensure that data will not be lost in the event of a computer failure. Backup is most often accomplished by copying data from the organization's information systems onto magnetic tapes. The tapes are then usually stored in an off-site location so that they will not be damaged in the event of a disaster such as a fire or flood.

FIGURE 6–1 | Information Systems Organization Chart

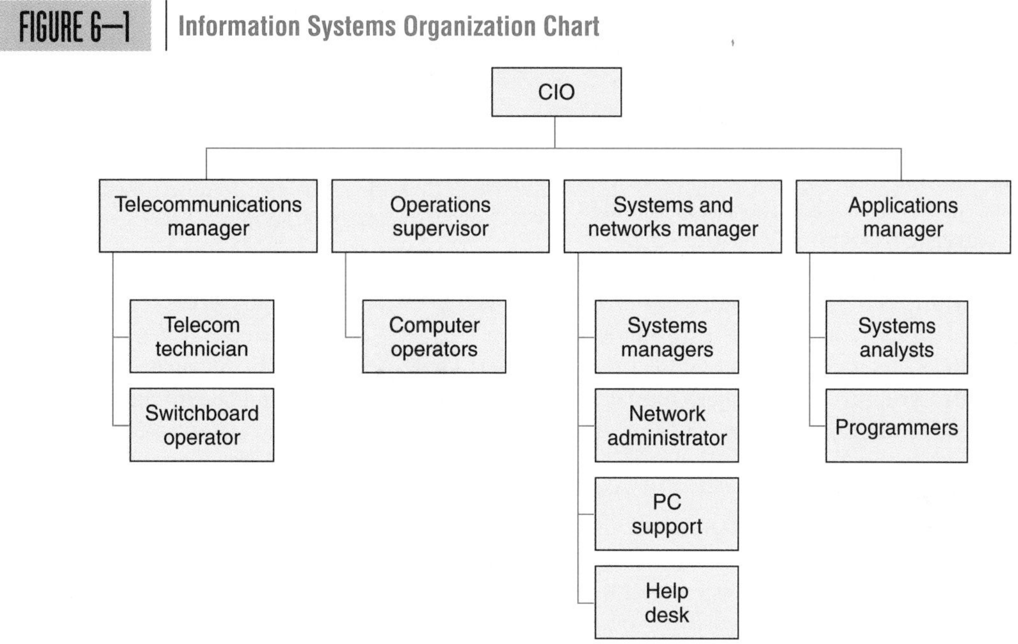

Telecommunications

The telecommunications department provides support for the telephone systems within a health care organization. Support for a main switchboard that handles both internal and external calls, as well as specialized functions such as paging physicians and responding to emergency events such as alarms for fire and emergency (stat) medical events, is part of telephone systems support.

Other responsibilities within the telecommunications department relate to in-house **adds, moves, and changes** requested by users of telephone systems. Rewiring to install additional telephone wall plates and jacks is often involved.

Managerial functions within the telecommunications department require monitoring and verification of billing statements, monitoring of switchboard performance to ensure that acceptable response times are being provided for callers, and planning for system enhancements. Examples of opportunities for system enhancement are the conversion from analog telephone sets to digital sets and the use of fiberoptic wiring and switching devices to support voice and data communications.

Systems Development/Project Management

Traditionally, the systems development section of a health care IS department was responsible for producing computer software to support organizational functions. This production role has shifted in recent years as fewer software systems are produced in-house. The build-versus-buy decision for hospital applications has increasingly favored the buy option. Reasons for this include the cost of maintaining systems, an ongoing need for system changes and enhancements with associated costs, and the economics related to developing a system that is used by many organizations versus a system that is used by only one. The most common in-house–developed applications are small databases and Internet Web sites.

In the wake of the shift from in-house–developed systems to vendor-provided applications, the need for project management support has emerged. In fact, project management assignments have replaced system development assignments for many IS department employees. Project management assignments for IS departments typically are associated with the selection and installation of a new computer system. Such projects are often quite complicated in that they require modification of established business practices, as well as of the underlying technology infrastructure. The project management process is detailed in Chapter 8.

Application Support

Application support is one of the more challenging areas for a health care IS department. Typically, each large software application used within the organization has an associated IS support staff. For large, integrated health care applications, separate modules may require separate support staffs. For instance, an integrated health care information system may support billing, accounting, materials management, laboratory, radiology, and pharmacy. Such a breadth of functionality usually requires individuals with different application knowledge sets to provide the required support.

The application support function is intellectually challenging because it typically requires both IT expertise and application domain expertise. Although the application users have greater domain expertise than the IS application support staff, the support staff must have enough domain expertise to be able to understand both the requirements of the users and the domain functionality provided by the application. Health care informatics specialists with knowledge of both fields are especially valuable in meeting this challenge.

Functionality One area of responsibility for the application support staff is to be a resource for users with respect to application functionality. The support staff must be able to do the following:

- Explain what the application will do.
- Explain the rationale behind the implementation of the function.
- Provide training for new users.
- Answer specific questions from experienced and novice users.

Many questions in this area are of the "if, then" variety. For instance, "If a lab test is ordered using a short-form registration, will the patient's address be recognized by the system at a later time?" The application support staff often investigates such questions using a test system that is maintained separately from the production application for testing purposes.

Troubleshooting A second area of routine activity for the application support staff involves the investigation of problems associated with an application's function. Typically, these activities are initiated by a call from the application users or from the operations department indicating that the application is not performing in the expected manner. Given the dynamic nature of computer systems, system configurations can easily get changed and produce unanticipated effects. In addition, applications sometimes contain errors ("bugs") that show up only under certain circumstances. When these occur, the responsibility of the application support staff is to document the problem, report it to the application vendor, follow up to make sure that the error is corrected, and if possible, provide a temporary solution (work-around) for the problem until it is corrected.

Enhancements Most health care software applications are enhanced on a routine basis by the software application vendor. Health care organizations typically gain access to these enhancements through maintenance agreements for the software that include commitments for ongoing improvement of the application. A typical release cycle for new versions of applications is every 9 to 12 months. Each new release includes enhancements to the previous version of the application. The application support staff has the responsibility to work with application users to determine whether the organization can benefit from use of the enhancements in its routine use of the application. Incorporation of the enhancements may impact business processes and may require significant transition planning and analysis to achieve effective utilization of the enhancement.

Support

IS support is typically provided by a help desk group and a personal computer (PC) support section within the health care IS department.

Help Desk The help desk group provides a first response for solving problems that arise with the use of information systems. An exception to this rule is related to problems with specific application systems for which users have a contact to call within a separate application support staff area. One routine type of call placed to a help desk involves users' loss of or the expiration of passwords that provide access to the computer systems. Organizations have different policies and procedures for use by their help desks to verify the caller's legitimacy and to reinstate access to the computer systems.

The help desk may also be called with reports of network outages or other system failures. In these cases the primary role is as a liaison with the responsible IS staff members to advise them of the problem, to monitor the problem status, and to provide information to users until the problem is resolved.

In recent years, software packages have been developed to support help desk functioning. These packages track the types of calls and provide access to solutions and procedures that address frequently occurring types of problems.

PC Support In contrast to help desk staff members, who are located at a specific call station, PC support staff members spend most of their time working at the user's worksite. These visits are needed to solve problems related to the user's use of the PC, to install new software onto the PC, or to reconfigure existing software to support new uses.

Another function of the PC support staff is related to PC acquisition. The PC support group is usually responsible for tracking the evolution of PC technology and for making recommendations concerning standards for PC hardware and software acquisition within the organization. Once PCs have been ordered and delivered, PC support staff members typically configure the PCs with the software and network capabilities specific to the organization and install the PCs at user worksites.

PC support often requires adjudication and compromise as a result of conflicting objectives of the user community and the PC support group. The user community typically desires unrestricted scope with respect to the hardware and software that is available for their use. In contrast, the PC support group benefits from standardization of hardware and software. Such standardization allows the group to become optimally familiar with the systems and with the types of associated problems. In addition, staff training needs can be limited to supported software packages. The negative side of standardization is that in many instances, users have legitimate needs for software capabilities outside of those authorized. In addition, standardization can lead to complacency in that new, paradigm-changing applications may be ignored because they are not within the "standards."

The resolution of this conflict varies from organization to organization, but in general, as organizational software and hardware decisions become less standardized, the user takes on more responsibility for support of the PC. PC support teams are limited in the extent to which they are able to support nonstandard applications.

Network

Depending on the size of a health care organization, the network section may be a separate group or a subsection within the systems management section. In either case, there may be some overlap between the responsibilities of the network group and the systems management group. The network group is primarily responsible for the wiring that connects computers, the devices connected to the wires, and the management of data traffic across the wires.

Local Area Network A local area network (LAN) is a network within a building that can be managed entirely within the organization. In other words, all of the wiring and communications equipment needed to support the LAN is typically owned and managed by the network group within the organization.

Wide Area Network A wide area network (WAN) generally links a number of LANs owned by the organization so that users can communicate with each other and with the organization's information systems that are accessible over the WAN. In most cases an organization will contract with outside telecommunications vendors for the provision of the network infrastructure (wires and communications devices) that is necessary to accomplish these linkages.

Systems Administration

The systems administration section is responsible for management of the operating systems for all of the health care organization's computers. The operating system of a computer controls all of the computer's basic functions, such as file management, printing, network communication, tape management, and input functions. Most health care organizations support a number of different types of computers. Different computers may employ different operating systems. Typically, systems administration staffs have expertise predominantly with respect to a single operating system. As a result, staffing to maintain backup coverage for each operating system can be a challenge for IS management, especially in smaller organizations.

Security IS security traditionally is the responsibility of systems administration. With the adoption of the **Health Insurance Portability and Accountability Act (HIPAA),** increased standards for information privacy and confidentiality are required. As a result, a preference for a separate and independent IS security capability is being adopted by many health care organizations. See Chapter 20 for a complete discussion of security and protection of patient information and Chapter 19 for additional information on HIPAA.

Upgrades Operating systems are routinely upgraded with new versions in much the same way that application software is periodically upgraded with new releases. In the case of operating system upgrades, a great deal of planning and testing is often needed before migration to the new version can be carried out. In addition, operating system upgrades can require as much as 8 to 10 hours to complete. During this time, the system is unavailable for routine use. To mitigate the impact of these outages, upgrades are often scheduled for hours of low utilization, such as the middle of the night on a weekend. There is always a certain degree of risk associated with upgrades. The upgrade and the system may not function as expected once the upgrade has been carried out. In these cases the outage can be much longer than expected and, as a result, cause much more of a problem.

System Resource Management Oversight with respect to the usage of system resources is another responsibility of the systems administration staff. The key resources of interest are generally computing power and data storage capacity. Increases in the level of computing usage by system users can result in degradation of the system response time to unacceptable levels. To avoid this deterioration, ongoing monitoring of the level of system usage is required. When increased-usage data suggest that the system's capacity cannot keep up with demands, it is time to upgrade the computer system. The configuration, ordering, and installation of a new computer system can be a time-consuming process. Therefore adequate planning is needed in order to have the new system operational before the old system is unable to provide acceptable response time.

With respect to system storage, multiple application systems are often run from a single mainframe computer. Since these applications share system resources, adequate allocation and safeguard policies need to be put in place to ensure that one application does not consume all available data storage capacity and thereby prevent other applications from storing data. In addition, many uses of data storage are temporary or discretionary, such as when systems are tested. Given the discretionary nature of the use of data storage resources, it is important that system administration staff members routinely monitor the system for changes in the expected level of use by each application. A key part of this responsibility is working with the institution's administrative staff to determine both short- and long-term needs for data and information.

Roles

Chief Information Officer

The primary leadership role within a health care IS department has a variety of titles. The most commonly used titles are chief information officer (CIO), vice president of information systems, and director of information systems. Similarly, the leader of the IS department may report to a variety of persons within the organization. The most common of these are the chief financial officer (CFO), the chief operating officer (COO), and the chief executive officer (CEO). The reporting relationship to the CFO is derived from the early uses of computers in health care when the primary use was for financial purposes. Since information systems are now used in all areas of a health care organization, the head of the IS department is likely to report to either the COO or the CEO.

Typical qualifications for a CIO are a master's degree in a health care informatics discipline, information science, computer science, or business and 10 or more years of experience with administrative and management responsibilities in a health care computing environment.

The CIO's responsibilities and daily activities vary depending on organizational size, organizational culture, and personal style. Some CIOs demonstrate hands-on involvement in the activities of the department; others prefer to engage in discussions outside of the department with the goal of identifying user needs and discovering opportunities based on emerging technology developments.

Generally, the CIO has the final approval responsibility for technology purchases and acquisitions. Hiring decisions for the department may reside with the CIO, but in larger IS departments the primary hiring recommendation is made by the responsible manager and approved by the CIO. The CIO typically has overall budgetary responsibility for the department and is held accountable for budgetary performance.

A key area of responsibility for the CIO is the development of the organization's IS strategy. This function is often undertaken with the assistance of a steering committee made up of key representative administrators and users of information systems within the organization. Alignment of the IS strategy with the overall organizational strategy and the development of support and approval (as well as funding) for the IS strategic plan are critical to an effective IS department. Chapter 8 includes additional information on strategic planning.

Director

Director positions usually provide leadership for one or more sections within an IS department. Examples of common areas of responsibility for director-level positions are telecommunications, networking, systems management for application systems, and operations.

Directors generally report to the CIO and have managers reporting to them. Typically, director-level positions require a master's degree in a related field and 5 to 7 years of related administrative/managerial experience. Director-level positions are most commonly found in larger health care organizations. Recent trends to reduce the number of levels and thereby reduce overhead in organizations have created pressures to eliminate middle management (director-level) positions in many health care organizations.

A director's day includes substantial time spent in meetings. Some meetings are with internal clients to discuss their needs and desires regarding the selection and enhancement of an information system. Other meetings are with vendors and other external information resources about potential services and IS solutions.

Manager

A manager usually has responsibility for one or more of the sections within an IS department. Managers usually have staff members reporting to them. They may report to department directors in large organizations or to the CIO in small organizations. Qualifications for managerial positions usually include a bachelor's degree in a related field and 5 or more years of experience relative to the area of responsibility in the IS environment.

On a day-to-day level, a manager's time is usually divided between time spent with staff members dealing with specific issues and time spent with users and user groups from the areas for which the manager is responsible. For instance, if a manager has responsibility for the laboratory system, it can be expected that the manager will spend a significant amount of time with users of the laboratory system to deal with problems, to plan for more effective use of the system, and to identify needs for additional functionality or upgrades to the system.

The operating budget for a section is often developed at the manager level. Responsibility for the capital budget is usually at the director or CIO level. Hiring responsibility usually resides with the manager.

Supervisor

A supervisor in the operations section of an IS department reports to a manager. Supervisors perform hands-on functions with the staff members whom they supervise. An analogous position in a manufacturing setting is that of foreman.

The primary job qualification for a supervisory position is years of experience performing the functions associated with the jobs of the staff employees being supervised. Another important qualifying characteristic for supervisor is the ability to provide direction and leadership to staff members. Supervisors may or may not have responsibility for performing job evaluations. However, a supervisor does not make hiring decisions. As with persons in most leadership positions, supervisors have a strong influence on the morale and effective job performance of their staff.

Operator

Operators perform their jobs within the operations section of an IS department. The typical qualification for an entry-level operator is a 2-year degree from a computer technical school. This position usually involves shift work and often requires weekend shifts. Many organizations have developed variable shift patterns to provide 24/7 staff coverage.

Telecommunications Technicians

The responsibilities of telecommunications technicians are related primarily to providing support for the adds, moves, and changes of telecommunications equipment that are required in the normal course of events in a health care organization. Smaller organizations may use outside contractors to support these functions if the level of such activity is not enough to support a full-time employee.

Telecommunications technicians have had training in the wiring methods required to support telephone wiring. Expertise includes familiarity with patch panels and the programming of telecommunications switches to support moving a telephone number from one phone jack location to another. Other functions relate to configuring the telecommunications switch to support service requirements, including turning on and off such features as voice mail, dial-out capability, and call forwarding.

Telecommunications technicians may perform telecommunications wiring tasks, or outside contractors specializing in telecommunications may install the wiring required for larger projects.

Telecommunications Operators

Telecommunications operators manage the switchboard for health care organizations. Previous experience or training in the operation of a switchboard is required for employment in these positions. Telephone coverage is required 24 hours a day, 7 days a week; therefore 24/7 staffing patterns are needed. Effective operator performance is essential to the smooth flow of critically important information. The operator interfaces with patients' families, friends, and physicians and other health care providers on a routine basis and in so doing creates a lasting impression of the organization. Paging physicians is a routine responsibility. The management of emergency situations such as fire alarms and crisis events requires substantial ability to perform efficiently under severe pressure. A portion of the telecommunication operator's tasks are now managed with automated phone systems.

Systems Analyst

The systems analyst role is normally associated with the application support or development/project management sections of an IS department. Systems analysts are expected to bridge the technology gap between IS knowledge about a specific application and domain-specific knowledge that applies to the business function that the application supports.

Systems analyst qualifications include a bachelor's degree in a related field and usually 1 to 3 years of experience in the particular application area to which they are assigned. As with many of the other roles within IS departments, there may be as many as three separate levels of systems analyst job grades that reflect increasing responsibility and reimbursement levels.

Systems analysts typically spend a large percentage of their workday fielding telephone calls and investigating problems reported by their application users. Another typical activity of a systems analyst is to generate reports based on ad hoc requests for specific information not provided as part of the application's standard set of reports. This is often an entry-level position for a health care informatics specialist.

Programmer

Programmers traditionally have worked in the development section of an IS department. As less software development is being done within health care organizations, the number of programmers employed has declined. Programmers are more often employed by the vendors of health care software applications.

Qualifications for programming jobs include a bachelor's degree in computer science or software engineering or a bachelor's degree in another subject with substantial course work or experience in programming. Programmers tend to have less interpersonal contact with system users than systems analysts and managers. They usually spend the majority of their time specifying, implementing, and testing computer programs.

Consultant

Computer consultants generally are not employed by a health care organization's IS department. Rather, the services of consultants are usually acquired on a contract basis for a specific time duration to perform a specific service. IS consulting projects may involve the selection and installation of application systems with which staff members of the health care organization have little knowledge or expertise. An example of the use of a consultant might be for the development of an Internet Web site or for assistance with the installation and initial use of business intelligence software to support executive decision support capabilities.

Technology Infrastructure

The infrastructure for information systems consists of the hardware and operating systems software that enable all of the computations performed within an organization. The primary components of this infrastructure are the computers, the data communications network, and the computer peripherals that are used within the organization.

Computers

Computers perform the computational tasks required to process the information required by health care organizations. The size, cost, and computing capacity for computers vary widely. Since the early 1980s the ability and need for computers to communicate with each other has increased dramatically. Before 1980 it was not unusual for an IS department to be primarily concerned with the operation of a single computer. In today's environment, even within small health care organizations, the IS department is usually responsible for the operation of hundreds of computers.

The primary factors producing this transition are the development of microcomputers and of computer networking technology. The microcomputer has enabled the pervasive use of low-cost personal computer workstations within most health care organizations. These workstations were first used in stand-alone mode to support such tasks as word processing and spreadsheet calculation functions. The emergence of computer networking has allowed the personal computer workstations to be linked to the central shared computers that run a hospital's primary administrative and clinical software applications.

Mainframe Computers Mainframe computers are the computers at the high end of the cost and capacity spectrum. Typically, the cost for a mainframe computer ranges from $300,000 to several million dollars. Usually a mainframe computer is used to run a large health care organization's core software applications. Because of the cost of such systems and increases in the capacity of lower-cost systems, there has been a trend over the past 15 years for health care organizations to transfer most of their new computing applications to less expensive mid-range and minicomputers.

Another disadvantage of mainframe computers is their reliance on proprietary operating systems. Generally, proprietary operating systems are more expensive and require more specialized staff training and expertise than the operating systems for mid-range computers and minicomputers.

Mid-range Computers Mid-range computers cover the price range from $50,000 to $300,000. These computers are typically used by large health care organizations to support specialized software applications such as laboratory or radiology systems. Medium and smaller organizations often are able to run their core software applications on these systems because of lower demand for computational capacity driven by smaller numbers of computer-using employees and smaller database requirements.

Mid-range computers may use operating systems that are proprietary to a single vendor, such as IBM's AS400, or they may use operating systems that are available from a number of vendors. Unix is the predominant operating system of this type.

Another factor that distinguishes whether an organization is more likely to use mainframe, mid-range, or smaller computer servers is the age of the application that is in use. Older applications (sometimes called legacy systems) tend to require mainframe computing support, whereas newer applications are usually developed for more economical mid-range and smaller computers.

Servers Low-cost server systems were heavily deployed during the 1990s. These systems typically cost from $10,000 to $50,000 and use either the Unix or Microsoft Windows NT operating systems. Such systems are capable of supporting specialized applications for both large and small health care organizations. Computer networking technology allows such systems to interact with each other. Networking allows for a great deal of flexibility for IS departments to manage the need for computing capacity. When a new application is to be installed in an organization, a decision to support the application on a dedicated, low-cost application server is often the preferred path. The use of dedicated servers for individual applications simplifies capacity management problems. Similarly, when applications share the same server, they can create technical problems for one other. This is not an issue if the applications are on their own computer.

Workstation Computer workstations are used throughout health care organizations to support staff members for both local and remote computing functions. Examples of local computing on a workstation are word processing and spreadsheet functions. Remote computing involves using the workstation to access application servers that run centralized applications such as patient accounting, registration, scheduling, and payroll. Another example of remote computing is to use the workstation to access information via the Internet.

Portable Computers Portable computers are increasingly used to enable clinical staff to document patient information electronically at the point of care. A typical configuration involves installing a notebook computer on a movable stand. Wireless networking may be used as the communication method to support access from the portable computers to application servers.

Handheld Devices The use of handheld computing devices to access health care data is emerging as a preferred mode of interaction for many clinicians. Personal digital assistants (PDAs) such as the Palm Handhelds, Handspring Visor, and HP Journada promise low cost and reasonably high functionality. The integration of wireless and cellular telephone capabilities in these devices suggests scenarios whereby clinicians can have access to information regarding their patients at virtually any time and in any place. These devices are discussed in Chapter 7.

Networks

IS departments in health care organizations have primary responsibility for the design, implementation, and maintenance of the computer networks used within their organizations. As is true in other areas of IT, computer networking has been an area of explosive growth; expectations for improved computer networking support continue to increase.

The most obvious example of this growth in computer networking is the Internet. Health care IS users now expect access to the Internet to support routine job functions. But the issues for IS departments in providing this access are not trivial. These issues include concerns related to information security and confidentiality, to employees' misuse of the Internet, to adequate expertise within the IS department staff, and to providing adequate network bandwidth for acceptable response time. Internet applications are discussed in Chapter 11.

Data communications networks are composed of transmission cable and network devices that control the flow of information across the cable. Types of cable commonly used include fiberoptic cable and shielded and unshielded copper wire. Coaxial cable may also be used in some organizations, but it is being phased out of use because of the reduced cost and easier application of copper wire.

Types of network devices that an IS department is likely to deploy to support its network include network hubs, routers, and switches. Network hubs are used to link devices that are intended to participate in the LAN. Any computer in the LAN can access all communications through a network hub. Messages on the network are addressed to designated target computers. Routers and switches have the capability to link multiple LANs to create a WAN. Part of the function of these devices is to pass messages from one LAN to another. In the process they perform a filtering function so that only those messages designated for computers on the other LANs are sent forward.

The primary network activities of IS departments are to configure the network and devices so that communication on the network is enabled, to monitor network utilization to ensure adequate speed of messages across the network, and to troubleshoot problems that arise with network function. Specialized devices such as network "sniffers" and other specialized monitoring software are used for these purposes.

Peripherals

Computer peripherals are input and output devices used by computer systems. Examples of types of peripherals are printers, magnetic tape devices, computer terminals, scanners, and projectors. The operations section within the IS departments of most health care organizations provide most of the required support for computer peripherals. Some exceptions are scanners and projectors, which are usually installed and maintained by the PC support section The primary activity related to computer terminals is to replace them when they fail with a supply of spares that is maintained for this purpose.

The peripheral device on which the operations section expends the greatest level of effort is the printer. In addition to loading paper and managing printed output, operators frequently are called on to replace toner cartridges and troubleshoot problems related to the generation of printed output by users. Other functions related to printing include monitoring the output queues associated with printers to ensure that all reports are printed in a timely manner.

Various types of printers are found within a health care organization. Laser printers usually serve local printing needs at various sites throughout an organization. Label printers may be installed remotely to support certain clinical department needs, such as the labeling of blood samples for the laboratory. These printers may also be capable of printing bar codes.

Impact-type printers are likely to be installed in the operations area of an IS department. The advantage provided by impact printers is that they can be used to produce printed output on multipart forms. Such multipart forms are frequently used to prepare billing statements and other financial documents.

Although printers may be linked directly to individual computers, there is often a strong preference for printers to reside on data networks so that all computers can direct output to them. Most IS departments have the majority of their printers accessible via computer networks.

Business Environment

The possibilities inherent in IT can be seductive for organizations by seeming to promise benefits that may be difficult to realize. Organizational decisions have been made to purchase and install expensive IS projects that have turned out to be failures. Reasons for failure include immature technology, lack of alignment of objectives of the IS project with overall organizational strategic objectives, inadequate planning and transition management, underestimation of resources required to complete the project, and overestimation of the benefits that are expected from the project. For these reasons, business considerations should be primary drivers of the decisions made in health care IS departments.

Clients

A key contributor to the success of an IS department is the relationship that the department has with its clients. IS clients are made up, by and large, of users of the computer systems that are supported by the IS department.

The primary users of information systems within a health care organization are the internal staff. The quality of an organization's information systems has a direct impact on patients, but they are not generally users of the systems. Similarly, health care providers may be thought of as clients of IS departments in that they make use of the clinical information that is stored in the organization's computers. Organizations vary in the degree to which health care providers within the organization directly use the software applications of the organization.

Administrative departments such as registration, materials management, general accounting, and patient accounting, as well as clinical departments such as laboratory, radiology, pharmacy, cardiology, nursing, and critical care medicine, make extensive use of information systems. In many organizations a tension exists regarding where the expertise regarding particular applications should reside. User departments typically wish to rely on the IS department for the support of their department-specific applications. In contrast, IS staff members may claim that they lack the domain expertise required for mastery of department-specific applications. Most IS staff members believe that mastery of specialty applications is the responsibility of the user department staff. One of the most satisfactory solutions to this tension is the employment of health care informatics specialists, who bridge the technical and clinical worlds.

IS staff members often perform organizational improvement roles for their clients by identifying opportunities for process improvement and then proposing ways that IT can be effectively used to support process improvements. In this way they also function as change agents by first bringing new opportunities to the awareness of their clients, demonstrating the potential benefits of the new processes, and then carrying forward the implementation of the required changes. Supporting organizational improvement in this way requires analytical aptitude, as well as IT and business domain expertise.

Types of Expectations: Cultures

Because of the breadth and depth of impact that information systems have on a health care organization, a variety of performance expectations often accrue to the staff and to the leadership of IS departments.

Technical Expectations First, IS departments are expected to be masters of technology. This expectation is not easily realized. IT is an incredibly complex field. Not only are the various domains such as networking, operating systems, and programming separate and diversified, but also individual software applications require specific, detailed levels of knowledge in order to provide effective support. In spite of these challenges, IS leadership must be able to assemble "big picture" strategies and the means to continue to keep up with ever-evolving technology.

Professional Expectations The staff members of IS departments are expected to be professionals who function as consultants, project managers, and providers of services. Levels of accountability are standardized, and in the area of network administration, certification processes are in place.

Administrative/Entrepreneurial Roles Members of IS leadership are expected to fulfill administrative and entrepreneurial roles within their organizations. The CIO is viewed as an administrative officer of the organization and, as such, is expected to provide organizational leadership in such areas as strategic planning, monitoring, and analysis of financial and business issues, as well as public relations and marketing.

IS department personnel fill entrepreneurial roles by identifying opportunities for the department to perform revenue-generating services.

One example is developing the ability to act as an Internet service provider for physicians' practices or providing billing services for physicians' practices. Another example is the development of software packages that have potential commercial value. A final example is providing outsourcing services to health care organizations that may not have sufficient resources to implement IT projects on their own. All of these potential revenue-generating opportunities provide ways to contribute to the overall well-being of the parent organization.

Scientific Pursuits Scientific pursuits within a health care IS department occur mainly in academic health care organizations. In these settings, funded research projects are commonplace. Investigators in research projects often rely on individuals or groups within the IS department for support of and participation in the IT components of the projects. These projects may involve database management activities, statistical analysis program development, or access paths to clinical and administrative data from the organization's health care information system. Research project involvement creates additional expectations and workloads that must be juggled and addressed in concert with all of the other departmental performance obligations.

Types of Organization

The characteristics of IS departments in health care organizations may vary considerably according to the specific type of organization that is being supported.

Community Hospital Community hospital IS departments are motivated to find middle-of-the road solutions to delivering IS capabilities to their organizations. Resources within this context are limited, and the ability to recruit staff members may be difficult. Community hospitals typically support their IS requirements using mid-range or smaller computer systems. Health care software vendors with integrated support for multiple functions are often viewed favorably, since the single-vendor approach simplifies support requirements.

Teaching Hospital IS departments within teaching hospitals are often urged to pursue solutions at the cutting edge of technology. Many teaching hospitals are also research organizations, and the research orientation contributes to the organizational culture. Many medical IS advances have come out of systems development projects at teaching hospitals. Examples include the development of the HL7 standard for medical information interchange (this standard is described in Chapter 17), the development of digital radiology imaging and archival solutions, as well as the development of **critical care monitoring applications.**

Of particular note in teaching hospital settings is the need for IS integration capabilities. A best-of-breed approach to systems acquisition is often used at teaching hospitals. Inevitably, the need for interaction between independent systems is identified. For instance, a radiology system should have access to patient demographic data from the registration system so that the identifying information need not be reentered.

For information to be shared across systems, a systems integration interface engine is needed to reliably pass messages between the systems. The role of the **interface engine** is to ensure that messages between two or more systems are communicated effectively. For instance, in the example just mentioned, the radiology system may be unavailable because of a system problem or because of scheduled system maintenance. The registration system continues to manage the admission, discharge, and transfer of patients during the radiology system outage. For the radiology system to be appropriately updated when it is functioning again, the interface engine stores the messages from the registration system. When radiology comes back online, the interface engine forwards these messages to the radiology system.

The implementation and management of such integration capabilities require a specialized level of expertise. Therefore integration services are often contracted to consulting organizations that have specific expertise.

Health Care System An integrated delivery system (ISD) poses challenges of another type for an IS department. Typically, ISDs have been formed from the merger of several formerly independent community hospitals, clinics, physician practices, nursing homes, and home health agencies. Each of these formerly independent organizations might have had IS capabilities of its own.

The most likely situation is that individual institutions have distinct IS capabilities that vary a great deal with respect to hardware, software, and networking technologies. Decisions to standardize across the system on a particular set of IT solutions can be both costly and difficult. Many software applications are tightly coupled to the business processes that they support. Changing these processes can be very disruptive to organizations that have already been stressed by merger and acquisition activities. In addition, the separate IS departments also undergo stress and power struggles when merged together.

Other Settings: Clinics, Nursing Homes, Physicians' Offices, and Home Health Care Clinics, nursing homes, physicians' offices, and home health care organizations usually do not have adequate resources to support an extensive IS department. Therefore IS support in these settings is often provided via contracted arrangements with system vendors who provide the system hardware and software, training, and support for the system.

CONCLUSION

A DAY IN THE LIFE OF A CIO

The workday for a CIO can be quite varied and differs from organization to organization; however, the interactions described in the following scenario can be expected to occur with high frequency:

- Beginning of the day—Put on your pager, drive to work, turn on the PC, get a cup of coffee, check and respond to any voice mail and eMail that has accumulated, check regular mail, and discard items of little interest. Repeat checking of voice mail and eMail throughout the day as time allows.
- Routine scheduled meetings—Meet with staff members or a project team to review details and issues associated with a current project. For example, meet with network staff members to discuss a project to enhance network capacity to support transmission of computerized radiology images across the network. Attend weekly administrative team meetings to review and discuss issues of current interest.
- Administrative tasks—Sign time sheets, conduct a performance review for a direct-report staff member, produce status reports, and review and forward items being circulated for administrative review.
- Vendor interaction—Interact with vendors via phone or in person to discuss planned purchases of new systems or upgrades to existing systems. Vendors provide a positive impact with respect to providing education and explanation to IS staff members regarding technology functionality and applicability. At the point of purchase of new hardware or software, participate in negotiations along with the purchasing department to ensure that the organization receives a beneficial contract.
- Problem management—Deal with technical issues. When technical issues arise, it often falls to the CIO to explain the nature of the problem and

the course of action that will be taken to correct the problem. This usually involves a fairly extensive problem investigation so that good information regarding the problem can be communicated to the organization.

- Peer networking—Interact with peers on the administrative staff to establish open lines of communication and to share "news and views" regarding the health care organization. This type of informal communication is critical to the successful performance of a CIO, since it provides information at a level of detail and in a form that is not otherwise easily available. This is the CIO's connection to the organization's informal "grapevine" (i.e., information that is not part of the formally communicated organizational news stream).
- External environment monitoring—The CIO keeps in touch with what is happening in the external environment for information systems by attending meetings and conferences where topics of interest are presented. These can range from 2-hour sessions at a local meeting site to 5-day conferences thousands of miles away. The meetings are important because they provide a means for the CIO to keep current on solutions that may be available for use by the health care organization in the future.
- Wrap-up of the day—Review articles of interest in journals and trade magazines that have recently been received. Respond to the last eMail and voicemail of the day. Process any unfinished paperwork. Prepare a task list for the next day.

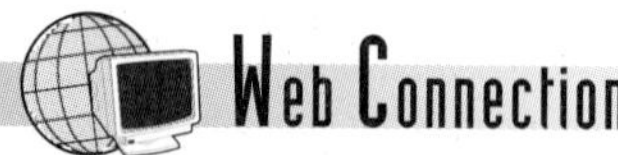

The role of health care information departments has become critical to successful operation of integrated health care networks and other forms of health care service provision. To understand how information departments are integrated into the business of health care, the Web activities for this chapter examine departmental structures, roles, and responsibilities and evaluate market conditions that influence today's chief information officers (CIOs). These activities will demonstrate the colorful world of advertising that entices CIOs to purchase particular products, consultative services, and outsourcing resources.

discussion questions

1. Imagine that you are the CEO of a 150-bed community hospital. Describe the organizational structure that you would use to support the IS needs of your hospital. Give your rationale for each position.
2. Consider the conflicting IS needs among departments in an academic medical center. Describe two potential conflicts, and propose appropriate ways to deal with the conflicts.
3. Computer hardware and software continue to evolve at a rapid rate. As head of the IS department within a health care organization, what problems would this create for you? How would you deal with these problems?

CHAPTER 7

Applications for Health Care Information Systems

MARGARET M. HASSETT

Learning Objectives

Upon completion of this chapter, the reader will be able to:

1. ***Discuss*** the components of a health care information system.
2. ***Discuss*** five application classifications for health care information systems.
3. ***Identify*** at least three constraints in the use of health care information systems.

Outline

Systems Overview
What Is a Health Care Information System?
Data Handling
Types of System Applications
Institution-wide Applications
Specialty Support Systems
Documentation Systems
Administrative Systems
Operations Support Systems
Information System Configuration

Key Terms

admission, discharge, and transfer (ADT)
aggregate
best of breed
clinical data repository
data archive
data purging
database
client server
core vendor
electronic medical record (EMR)
end user
health care information system (HIS)
information services department (ISD)
infrastructure
input
integration
interface
network
output
point of care (POC)
point of service (POS)
queries
radio frequency (RF)
stand-alone system
system architecture
trending data
voice recognition

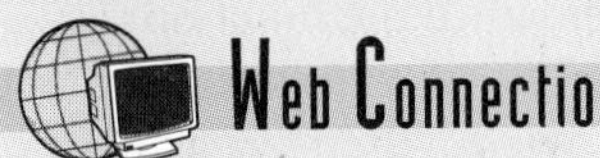

Web Connection

Go to the Web site at http://evolve.elsevier.com/Englebardt/. Here you will find Web links and activities related to applications for health care information systems.

The integration of information systems into clinical practice workflow is challenging information technology (IT) professionals to provide systems, services, and leadership to their end users in new and different ways. An **end user** is the person who will use the components of a system. As technology rapidly evolves and applications are adapted to meet professional requirements, health care is being presented with a vast array of system solutions by a growing number of IT vendors. **Information services departments (ISDs)** are responsible for developing initiatives that provide technical information and vision to support the collection and management of information to meet the expectations of health care enterprises. Four perspectives are considered in the development and implementation of a hospital or **health care information system (HIS)** (Celli, 1999):

1. Clinical—speed, reliability, and best practices support
2. Enterprise—best practices, patient satisfaction, and ability to generate revenues
3. Technical—**infrastructure** to support a myriad of applications and to integrate system applications for collection, management, and storage of data that are accurate, complete, and comparable
4. Client or customers—access to data and information, including contracts, schedules, and medical histories in the HIS

SYSTEMS OVERVIEW

An information system is an assemblage of computer technologies that first captures data. **Input** occurs via three paths:

1. Users enter data using devices such as keyboards, touchscreens, and personal digital assistants (PDAs).
2. Data are transferred from interfaced systems.
3. Automatic data transfer occurs from other systems and reporting programs.

The information system then processes or **aggregates** the data into information and provides the user with reports, graphs, printouts, or screen displays (system **output**).

An information system can be constructed or configured to maximize the collection and communication of data and information among users in a variety of ways. System configuration is dependent on the organization's existing information systems and applications (Saba, Pocklington, & Miller, 1998).

The mainframe configuration supports multiuser computers that are designed to meet some or all of the computing needs of a large health care organization. Information is stored, sorted, and reported from the mainframe to printers or dumb terminals on the patient care units. All applications and data are maintained on the mainframe rather than on individual personal computers (PCs).

Microcomputers are the PCs that many people have at home or at work. These computers are either stand-alone machines or are networked to other personal computers. A **stand-alone system** is one in which the computer is not connected to other computers via a network. The direct sharing of data or applications between stand-alone computers is not possible. In other words, the user is able to store and retrieve data and information; however, the data and information are limited to what the user enters into the computer. Applications such as word processing or spreadsheets are often installed individually on each PC and maintained on a one-to-one basis.

Networked microcomputers (PCs) or handheld devices greatly enhance the functionality of information sharing. With a **network,** data and files can be shared by providers regardless of their location and can be sorted to represent the specific information needed to support an effective patient encounter. An example of information sharing to support the patient care process is demonstrated using a laboratory order and results scenario:

1. The physician on the clinical unit inputs a set of orders for specific blood work into the clinical information system. For example, the physician may order a complete blood count and liver function tests.
2. These sets of orders are broken down into individual orders, which are sent over the network to the laboratory information system. The laboratory system communicates the requests to the laboratory personnel and the phlebotomists.
3. The blood is drawn and analyzed using the laboratory information system. The resulting data from laboratory tests are sent back to clinicians across the network.
4. The laboratory results on the network are viewed by the following:
   - Nursing staff before medication administration
   - Pharmacy for assembling medications and intravenous solutions
   - Physician to determine continued treatment

Networking and linking also allow an institution to share applications such as word processing or databases in what is called a networked environment. Additional licensing is usually required by the software vendor because most applications are not written to support multiple users or they restrict the number of concurrent users. Networked configurations are popular in clinical environments, but increased numbers of concurrent users can cause slow network performance. Networking also requires attention to important security issues.

The level of data sharing in an organization is determined not only by the technology but also by institutional security and access policies. Passwords and log-in IDs are created to identify which data should be available to which users. For example, physical therapists might have access to their list of patients but may be limited to specific inpatient areas or to the outpatient census. A supervisory dietitian, however, may have access to all newly admitted patients so that the new patients can be assigned dietary consults. Another example of how the system limits data access is with laboratory results and demographic information. Most clinicians are permitted read-only access to test results or demographic information. This means that they can view test results or demographic data but cannot enter new laboratory results or change the current demographic data. Laboratory technicians, on the other hand, may have both read and write access for laboratory data. They can view the laboratory results, as well as enter new results. However, these same laboratory technicians may have read-only access to demographic data. Registration personnel can enter and edit demographic information but do not have either read or write access to laboratory results. Data access is controlled through user ID and system rules. Additional information regarding system security can be found in Chapter 20.

PCs can also be configured to function as workstations. Workstations are PCs that communicate with a file server or a central computer via a network. The benefits of workstation configurations are standardization of the system, as well as shared applications and data.

A **point-of-service (POS)** device is a computer or information system that is located where information is required or where the data are collected. For example, a laptop PC may be used by the admitting department to admit patients who are located throughout a facility. The laptop is taken to the patient's location, data are entered, and the health care organization's network is accessed via distributed plug-in sites or radio frequency. Another POS device is a PDA such as a Palm Handheld. PDAs allow users to receive and send information from multiple locations in a manner similar to the way that cell phones are used. The major limitations of PDAs are the small screen size, requiring data to be truncated or structured into drop-down lists and the limited storage capacity.

Radio frequency (RF) usage is becoming common in patient care environments. This technology allows clinicians to work with mobile systems. These are usually portable computers that link to the network's infrastructure via radio waves. The wiring of older buildings to support radio frequency technology is expensive, and there may be interference with data transfers. Therefore although the technology may provide users with more portability, the information and data transfers may be slower to process than when using a system that is hardwired directly to the network.

A **client server** is system architecture that splits an application into a front-end client application and a back-end server component as the basis for distributed applications. The term *client* in this context refers to the computer. The front-end application running on a workstation collects information from the user and prepares it for the server. The server receives results from a client application, processes them, and distributes the information to the appropriate client. The client then presents the information to the user.

WHAT IS A HEALTH CARE INFORMATION SYSTEM?

An HIS encompasses a wide array of applications and information systems that are linked or interfaced. An HIS supports the provision of care to patients and the business aspects of the health care organization by communicating information. The assembly of information systems and the architecture by which they are integrated is unique for each organization.

Health care organizations have managed and communicated information since the days of Florence Nightingale. Early manual systems evolved to automated stand-alone systems. Current systems are well integrated. Two or more components that are merged together into one system are often referred to as an integrated system. The development of integrated systems is more pronounced today as information and its efficient communication have become vital to the survival of health care organizations in today's economy and regulatory world. The systems have expanded beyond small fiscal systems with manual form supports to multiapplication systems that are interfaced to share data and networked to support multiple institutions in one health care organization. This expansion is evidenced by the integration of IT into almost every practice's workflow (Saba & McCormick, 1996).

Organizational strategic goals and business plans determine the composition of the applications, hardware, and network structure that make up an individual HIS. The type of data and information that are collected or reported in an efficient manner are determined by the specific composition of the HIS and its integration with other systems or networks. Readily available and current information enables administrators in departments and those in executive positions in organizations to make informed decisions that enhance the development and direction of the services to be provided (Dick & Steen, 1991).

A single piece of data (such as a patient's ID number) can be used many times by a variety of practitioners in a multitude of locations through the integration of the various components of an HIS. The development and planning of an HIS are dependent on the following:

- Strategic goals of the institution that drive the selection and prioritization of systems
- Practice needs of the care providers that shape the content and functionality of systems
- Business needs of the organization that shape the scope of an IS department's strategic plan.

DATA HANDLING

The generation, collection, management, and reporting of data are the primary functions of each information system within the an HIS. Each function is addressed by the organization's integrated information systems. For example, to meet the billing and regulatory requirements for an outpatient visit, the following data are captured and communicated:

- Patient demographics
- Medical record and account number
- Time and location of the appointment
- Name of the primary care provider
- Services provided
- Charges with associated documentation on an encounter form

To accomplish these functions, an HIS includes components that support patient registration, scheduling, charge capture, clinical documentation, and billing. In some cases, manual forms track patients through portions of their visit and then data are subjected to batch data entry at a later time to complete a **database.**

Primary access to databases, either to enter data or to view reported data, is a crucial component of the success and endurance of any application. This access is dependent on the system architecture. The computer systems throughout an HIS are linked together via a structure of networks, interfaces, or input devices. This structure enables the communication and sharing of data. System architecture is the design of an HIS including the hardware, software, methods of connecting the parts of the total system and protocols used. The **system architecture** ensures efficient and effective access to data by enabling rapid screen flips or field filling, consistent and timely network communication, and decreased downtime. In addition to the speed and reliability of the system, the placement and availability of PCs have an impact on data access. Finally, security requirements and policies regarding "user's need to view" limit some access to data. Organizational policies and procedures are reviewed and revised if the needs for data change.

Collection of data is another consideration that may affect the look and feel of an HIS. Data may be entered into a system through the use of a keyboard and mouse. However, imagine the impact on portability if the data entry can be accomplished using **point-of-care (POC)** PCs or laptops connected to the hospital network via wireless RF. These variations on the keyboard input of data enable practitioners to capture data at its source in a timely and more accurate way.

Another data input option is **voice recognition.** Voice recognition systems are used in some radiology and emergency department systems. These are systems whereby the user inputs data by speaking to the computer. Another approach, direct download of data from physiological systems such as cardiac monitoring devices and ventilators, enhances data input by eliminating the human "copying" factor. As Web technology continues to develop and provide solutions in health care arenas, additional opportunities will present themselves for secure data capture directly from a variety of sources. The structure of information systems and their integration into the clinicians' or end users' workflow help to determine the type of data collected while eliminating the use of paper notes. No longer do clinicians need to transcribe documentation from scratch notes made during a variety of encounters on whatever handy form of writing medium is available (McDermott, 1994).

Equally important in information management is the fact that information and data entered into a system can be presented in a variety of formats (e.g., documents, reports, data tables, bills, and graphs). The ability of a system to generate meaningful information for the user is directly related to the quality of the data collected and the integrity of the aggregated data or information. Measures used to improve data consistency and quality include the following:

- Data selected from drop-down lists containing structured notations or terms

- Blocked or required fields that limit or mandate information in a specific format
- System checks, such as time factors for medication administration
- Out-of-range error alert that requires the user conform unusual or unrealistic data such as a body weight of 450 pounds or an age of 150 years
- Audits to determine system use and security compliance

Storage of data and system access to data enhance the functionality of a system. The availability of data to support **queries** on a system, such as past laboratory results or clinical history, is very desirable in an HIS. However, large quantities of data have a direct impact on system performance. Large amounts of data stored and queried by a system present design challenges. As databases are constructed, attention must be paid to the following issues (Zielstorff, Hudgings, & Grobe, 1994):

- Names of data fields
- Relationship of data fields
- **Data archive** (how long should data be kept)
- **Data purging** (what should be deleted, and when)

Queries of large data sets require system functionality that supports data sorting, aggregation, and report production. Reports can be as simple as the last patient visit or as complicated as the **trending data** for the last 300 patients treated in an ambulatory center by a designated provider. Trending data are reports and/or graphs that display data collected from a variety of sources over time. The information displayed can enable projections to be made based on data reports. Both examples require sorting through a significant amount of registration and provider data. The length of time that the data are kept has an impact on the number of patient admissions, number of providers, and number of sites to be sorted.

Many of these issues are foundational to the development of the **electronic health record (EHR)**. The vision of many health care providers is to have an EHR that supports the capture, storage, and reporting of data across the continuum of care (Ball et al., 1995).

TYPES OF SYSTEM APPLICATIONS

Several different types of system applications are used by patient care facilities to build their HIS. These applications communicate information that is needed to maintain good patient care and to support business needs. Individual applications are usually transparent to the end user of a clinical workstation. The display of needed information is dependent on applications functioning adequately and interfacing with other applications (Hassett, 1999).

The applications that support the hospital's business needs and patient care provision can be categorized into systems that have a primary function to support the following:

- Institution-wide needs
- Specialty and ancillary support
- Clinical documentation
- Administrative needs
- Operational support

Institution-wide Applications

Information systems or applications that are accessible throughout the institution support the exchange or collection of data that are required across departmental lines. These applications enable the provision of basic services, such as the collection of patient demographics and charges, tracking orders and results, and communication such as eMail. Usually they allow a consistent approach to or standard view of a service that is offered in variable environments. Examples of these kinds of systems include admission, discharge, and transfer systems; financial systems; and order entry and results reporting systems.

Admission, discharge, and transfer (ADT) applications are the backbone of most HISs. ADT systems collect, store, and track patient information from admission to discharge. Such data elements as demographics, insurance information, medical record number, care provider, and next of kin are tracked and facilitate functions such as bed control and records of patient census. All patient care and treatment interactions are tracked or linked to this basic information.

Financial systems are another distinct application in the HIS. Fiscal reporting includes patient services billing, accounts receivable (AR), accounts payable (AP), and general ledger (GL). An **interface,** or an exchange of information between systems, supports data sharing and avoids redundant data entry. An order entry system, for example, retrieves patient demographic information from the ADT system and feeds the service or test information to the fiscal system, where a cost is attached and a bill created.

Order entry applications, which are in place in many health care institutions, are regularly used by clinicians. The order entry system provides for several automated solutions for order entry, communication of orders to ancillary departments, service or test inventory for departments, and billing tracking. Clinical tests and services are typically ordered by selecting a patient in the system and then selecting the ordered test. A number of ancillary departments can be represented in an order entry system. Services and tests can be electronically ordered at the POS of the patient (Drazen et al., 1995).

Information that is captured in an order entry system includes specific service or charge IDs maintained in a database, notations related to each of the services, and order preferences by provider. Reports can be generated to answer a number of business questions about usage, quality issues related to test results, and the volume of providers using services.

Results reporting systems greatly enhance patient care and ancillary departmental operations. Results reporting applications allow for the automated reporting of individual test results, such as x-ray studies and laboratory tests. Reports are displayed as text reports, graphical charts, or actual visual views of radiology procedures such as x-ray studies and magnetic resonance imaging (MRI) scans. Available displays are dependent on the applications and systems that are part of the HIS, as well as on the architecture of the HIS network and the kind of data and information transfer that are supported. For example, the visual display of x-ray studies requires a more robust network than the display of a graph of a laboratory test report.

Specialty Support Systems

Ancillary applications allow for the structured integration or sharing of information among the ADT, order entry, results reporting, and financial management systems. In addition, ancillary practice-specific data are captured and reported to support the unique coding practices, ordering needs, or reporting format required by a department. Examples of such applications are specialty systems that support the radiology, laboratory, dietary, anesthesia, and physical therapy departments. Test processing, reporting, and documentation are individualized by supporting daily operational needs, such as schedule and supply tracking. Quality control testing in the laboratory environment, assessment write-up, and equipment billing in a physical therapy department and film tracking in a radiology system are examples of specific information support provided by an ancillary system.

Several ancillary support systems with their unique functions are compared in Table 7-1. The systems include some features that are the same, such as interfacing with the ADT system for patient information or the financial system for billing, and some that are unique to each application.

Specialty systems are continually being developed to meet the specific needs of specialty groups. Unmet information needs of a specific

Table 7–1 Comparison of Specialty Systems Functionality

System	Major Functionality	Specific Functionality
Radiology	Supports the operations of a radiology department, including film tracking	Tracks files or x-ray studies Schedules x-ray studies Tracks patients and radiology transport Supports a database of services that are provided by the department and billed against
Laboratory	Supports a laboratory department, including machinery that processes laboratory specimens	Tracks and performs quality testing on laboratory equipment Tracks orders, specimen receipts, reorders, processing, and results Maintains database to support normal result ranges, specific test numbers, and suppliers
Pharmacy	Supports the operations of a pharmacy department; can be evaluated to support either inpatient or outpatient services	Provides quality control for total parenteral nutrition (TPN) mixtures Communicates orders Controls stock and reorders Counts and tracks narcotics Records and tracks drug reactions

specialty group are usually the driving force for a vendor to develop such systems. These systems collect and manage patient data elements specific to the practice of the specialty group. Selected test results are recorded and placed in a report designed to meet the specialty practice needs. For example, a system has been developed to meet the needs of a practitioner who specializes in the gastrointestinal system by collecting specific patient history information related to gastrointestinal symptoms and history. An endoscopy is performed, and the images from the test are automatically attached to a report generated from the accumulated information. Although the use of this system will directly support the specific practitioner's needs, there can be issues concerning how the data in the specialty systems are communicated and used in other systems. The reverse can also be true. Other information systems may not be able to share data with the specialty system. For example, the specialty system may not be able to import ATD data from the HIS. This inability of the specialty system to integrate data with other information systems in the HIS may limit its overall usefulness.

Individual practitioners may see a specialty system as the answer to their information needs. However, one of the biggest challenges with most specialty systems is the integration of information between systems. Patient information should ideally be provided automatically from the ADT system, results should be provided to the practitioners via the results reporting system, and the bills should be generated by the financial system. However, some specialty systems are unable to provide for that exchange of information. Therefore personnel in the specialty area enter patient information, reports are generated for the financial area, and hard copy reports are distributed. This increases both the workload and the potential for error.

Documentation Systems

Documentation applications are available in a variety of formats. To provide full benefit, a documentation system needs to be part of the clinical workflow and communicate real-time information so that the need to "go find the chart" is eliminated. For example, at change of shift several practitioners should be able to use the same patient record at one time. Data collection should be designed in such a way as to support clinical workflow rather than distracting from it. Screens can be designed to support assessment documentation by listing body systems, or practitioners can be "cued" by the system to complete or verify vital information, such as allergies, with a "pop-up" box.

Systems that have been developed to capture physiological data (such as vital signs, monitor information, or pulmonary wedge pressures) directly from physiological monitoring equipment and feed the data into fields in a clinical documentation system greatly enhance functionality.

Interfaced systems require increased troubleshooting and support from IS support personnel. A support issue with integrated systems involves understanding how the system is functioning. For example, a system's interfaces may be programmed so that a heart rate captured in one system can be used to populate a field on a progress note screen in a separate application used for clinical documentation. This communication of data from the physiological monitoring system to the clinical documentation system is invisible to the end user. When there is a problem with the capture of the heart rate, the support of IS personnel and their understanding of the system's functionality is critical to the smooth operation of both systems. As systems become more and more integrated, this relationship with IS personnel in the day-to-day clinical work will be increasingly important.

Communication and documentation that allow each discipline participating in the patient's treatment plan to see the whole picture and know the precise current patient status enable quality, cost-efficient care. This concept is demonstrated in the following example comparing clients with the same nursing diagnosis: A multidisciplinary group has reached agreement on a treatment plan. The treatment plan is used to develop care maps that encompass a variety of care issues related to a number of specialties such as laboratory tests, medications, physical therapy orders, and discharge plans. The automation of these plans ensures better communication for orders and results, patient progress, and practitioner evaluation among all care team members.

The length of stay (LOS) for the identified diagnosis is defined as the precise number of days to allow for specific predetermined interventions to achieve specific outcomes. Care providers' documentation can compare patients' progress in achieving the desired outcomes by noting the documentation of results or patient responses in a progressive and interrelated format such as a critical path. This documentation also allows for comparison of clinical data regarding interventions, outcomes, and multidisciplinary approaches.

Administrative Systems

Administrative systems support functions required to manage service lines or specific departments, such as patient care services, food services, and materials management. The primary function of these systems is to document administrative activities and facilitate directed decision support for the identified service. Administrative systems require a significant amount of organizational support and planning.

For example, case management systems specifically support primary care case managers by using ADT information to locate patients, provide patient demographics, list diagnoses, and identify primary care provider and contact information. Clinical documentation systems can be used to determine risk and establish the interventions required according to a case management plan. In addition, the systems support case management workflow by enabling scheduling of patients and services, as well as providing reminders and flags for case managers (Drazen & Metzger, 1999).

Acuity applications provide for the classification of patients or services in an attempt to quantify activities and the resources needed to provide care. These systems may be integrated with the ADT, documentation, staffing, and scheduling systems to support resource planning, such as scheduling of staff and medical supplies.

Scheduling applications support the scheduling of patients, procedures, supplies, and staff. These applications can be used to schedule patients, staff, or services for a specific department, such as radiology, or across several departments, such as all services in an ambulatory clinic. Scheduling systems offer added benefits if they are integrated with other administrative systems. For example, the patient scheduling system is enhanced when it shares data with a materials management system for supplies or stock related to scheduled procedures, the ADT system for patient demographics, and the financial system for cost-accounting purposes.

Staff scheduling, on the other hand, is enhanced when information is shared with the hospital personnel or human resources department and fiscal systems to enable timely and accurate tracking of personal and scheduling data, such as the following:

- Hire date for benefits and merits administration
- Number of hours and shift worked for payroll information
- Shift or schedule preferences for scheduling of staff
- Emergency contact for notification

Decision support systems provide data in a manner that supports decision making. The data that reside in the HIS are formatted in different reports and communicated as trends or real-time events. These reports support informed decisions regarding patient care, budget, outcomes planning, strategic goals achievement, determination of care or population trends, and financial directions. The decision support system interfaces with all other existing systems for its data. Logical and relationship statements can be incorporated into the systems to generate the integrated documentation and order entry systems. Additional information on decision support systems is provided in both Chapters 4 and 5.

Operations Support Systems

Operations support systems address the direct day-to-day operations of an institution. Some operations support systems address office applications and communication systems that are used throughout an institution. Enhancement of daily operations can be attained by standardizing and networking office applications such as word processing, spreadsheet, database, presentation, and others. Standardization greatly enhances the ability of the IS department to support users. Standardization of office applications accomplishes the following:

- Decreases user confusion and questions
- Allows for consistent training and user support
- Permits a standardized approach to upgrades and required system changes

Standardization of the communication systems addresses all forms of communication used in the organization, such as phone, paging, eMail, and Web pages. The ISD usually makes decisions regarding these systems. The communication systems allow for the timely exchange of information within the organization, as well as with other individuals and groups outside the organization. The increased information flow has already demonstrated a significant impact on clinical practice.

Human resources or personnel systems enable facilities to track and store information about personnel management: prospective hires, new hires, active employees, and past employees. Such systems enable more efficient tracking and posting of open positions, salary schedules, pending job opportunities for approval, and hiring trends.

Materials management systems are expansive and high-profile systems in the environment of just-in-time inventory control. Medical and office supplies that are used on a regular basis are tracked and ordered as needed. An accurate inventory allows an institution to provide efficient services while tracking the financial impact of the care effectively.

INFORMATION SYSTEM CONFIGURATION

The integration of IT into the clinical and business environment of any organization is accomplished in one of four ways. Each method has its own benefits and limitations. The four methods are as follows:

1. Choose a single vendor for the majority of applications.
2. Establish a **core vendor system,** and require other applications and systems to integrate or interface with the core vendor. A core vendor is the primary vendor supplying the information system that serves as the basis for any other systems that are integrated within an organization. This vendor provides the backbone architecture for the HIS. Other applications are either purchased from the core vendor or able to interface/integrate with the core vendor.
3. Select multiple systems that represent an approach that is considered "best of breed" for each department or specialty area represented, and network these together.
4. Develop a hybrid structure using any combination of the above three approaches.

An organizational selection process determines the system integration method to be implemented. This process includes close work with both administrators and end users. The goal must be to clearly understand what the informational needs are and will be in the future. Close scrutiny and evaluation by the IS team helps to identify the type of IT an organization's infrastructure, end users, and health care network will support. Specifically, an IS assessment determines the selected technology or specific system or application that can be supported by the current IS department. In addition, the assessment identifies technology enhancements and staff training that must occur to enable success with the chosen system. Finally, budget constraints also contribute to the final system selection. The budget amounts have an impact not only on system purchases but also on required hardware, training, consultant support, reconstruction, wiring, etc. The bottom dollar amount that can be provided to make this selection must be established early in the process (Middleton, 1998).

Single-vendor solutions provide applications within a suite of products that enable an organization to support the full array of departmental needs using only one vendor. This can include capabilities related to medical records, order management, ADT functions, patient accounting, and general accounting. Departmental supports are realized in areas such as pharmacy, nursing, patient accounting, laboratory, and radiology. Benefits realized by institutions with this kind of system integration have a standard approach and similar functionality for users, limited interfaces, and transactions with the same vendor.

The core-vendor method supports a core of data functions such as medical records, order management, patient accounting, and patient management. Other applications, such as pharmacy, radiology, laboratory, ambulatory care, and operating room applications, can be provided by different vendors. Any system that is brought into the organization is evaluated on the basis of how it will interface with the existing core system, as well as how it will provide for the selected departmental need. The IT infrastructure and end user support for this kind of system integration is more extensive than with the single-vendor method.

The best-of-breed approach is the most complicated of the three in its network and integration architecture. The **best of breed** seamlessly integrates data and information from a variety of applications and systems to support the use of other applications and to increase each system's robustness with data entered in other systems and reported in each connected system. That is to say, there would be separate system supporting the data collection, communication, and reporting of the core functions of the organization, as well as the accounting functions and individual clinical functions.

Integration of these systems requires that each computer system speaks to each other and exchanges data to provide information to the user. A good example is the exchange of data between a patient management system and a laboratory system and then the patient accounting system. The patient management system shares a patient's demographics, medical record number, etc., with the laboratory system. The laboratory system attaches the demographics and medical record number to laboratory results generated from its system. By attaching the information, the system can track and report results. Then test identification numbers and charges are communicated to the accounting system with the attached demographics and medical record number to support billing (Hannah, Ball, & Edwards, 1994).

This communication among systems demonstrates the interfacing of one system with another to enhance the functionality of all. Effective system interfacing requires that the "source" or "master" for all data be identified. For example, a patient management system is the primary source for patient demographics and as such is the master of edits and changes for these data. However, a laboratory system is the source and master system for laboratory test results. This delineation must be established and maintained to ensure data integrity. Dealing with questions concerning data integrity requires one correct data source.

Data **integration** is accomplished by interfacing a number of information systems as in the preceding example. Another common method is the development of a single database to house data from a variety of systems. One example of this concept is known as the electronic medical record (EMR), which is commonly accomplished by establishing a **clinical data repository.** Essentially, the single database captures information from numerous systems and aggregates the data over time for single use (Ball et al., 2000). The EMR is explained further in Chapter 10.

CONCLUSION

The automation of patient data allows more than one person to find, access, or enter data elements at the same time. In addition, information is provided to the user in what is called "real time," or while the data are current. An example of a patient flow that supports the integration of all of the systems mentioned in this chapter is a patient admitted to an inpatient care unit for pneumonia (ADT). Admission blood tests and a chest x-ray film are ordered (order entry system, laboratory system, radiology system). Medications are also ordered and administered on the various shifts (pharmacy system, staffing system). Assessments are documented on each shift, with improvement in the patient's condition noted, thereby prompting final discharge plans to go into place (care management systems, clinical documentation systems). On discharge, instructions are generated with follow-up instructions and information about whom to contact if there are any questions related to the hospital stay. Finally, a bill is forwarded to the patient for review after the insurance billing is complete (financial systems).

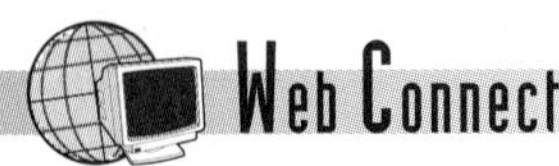

Web Connection

Health care information systems bring together aspects of the individual systems you have read about in previous chapters. As a result of your study of those systems and applications, you understand what makes a well-integrated system. The Web activities for this chapter focus on how the information and communication technology industries have integrated those systems. Through these exercises, you will be able to summarize your assessment of functional systems and some of the barriers to comprehensive information systems.

discussion questions

1. Trace the data flow for a patient's care during one health care visit. Determine how each of the following systems supports the care of the patient:
   - ADT system
   - Order entry
   - Results reporting
   - Clinical documentation
   - Financial system
2. Evaluate one point-of-care event, such as discharge planning, an outpatient MRI scan, or preoperative screening. What data are required to provide safe and complete care and treatment? Where would the data be collected, and who would need to see it? Can you identify information systems that can facilitate this one point-of-care event?
3. Discuss how an HIS supports the information sharing of the following:
   - Order entry system
   - Results reporting
   - Admission, transfer, and discharge
   - Financial system
   - Decision support
4. A patient is scheduled for a knee replacement and receives the following care:
   - Preoperative home visit from a physical therapist
   - Preoperative blood studies, chest x-ray film, and electrocardiogram done in the outpatient area
   - Surgery in the operating room
   - Discharge planning with one home nurse visit, three physical therapy home visits, and outpatient physical therapy follow-up

   What systems can support or enhance the care of this patient by enhancing the information flow?

REFERENCES

Ball, M.J., et al. (Eds.). (1995). *Health care information management system* (2nd ed.). New York: Springer-Verlag.

Ball, M.J., et al. (Eds.). (2000). *Nursing informatics: where caring and technology meet* (3rd ed.). New York: Springer-Verlag.

Celli, M. (1999). Clinical systems applications. *Journal of Healthcare Information Management, 13*(3), 1-3.

Dick, R.S., & Steen, E.B. (1991). *The computer-based record: An essential technology for health care*. Washington DC: National Academy Press.

Drazen, E., & Metzger, J. (1999). *Strategies for integrated health care*. San Francisco: Jossey-Bass.

Drazen, E., et al. (1995). *Patient care information systems.* New York: Springer-Verlag.

Hannah, K.J., Ball, M.J., & Edwards, M.J.A. (Eds.). (1994). *Introduction to nursing informatics.* New York: Springer-Verlag.

Hassett, M. (1999). Information systems. In L. Thede (Ed.), *Computers in nursing: Bridges to the future.* New York: J.B. Lippincott.

McDermott, S. (1994). Interfacing and linking nursing information systems to optimize patient care. In S.J. Grobe & E.S.P. Pluyter-Wenting (Eds.), *Nursing informatics: An international overview for nursing in a technological era* (pp. 197-201). New York: Elsevier.

Middleton, B. (1998). *Introduction to clinical systems.* Health Care Information Management Systems Society annual meeting handout. Chicago: Health Care Information Management Systems Society.

Saba, V.K., & McCormick, K.A. (1996). *Essentials of computers for nurses* (2nd ed.). New York: McGraw-Hill.

Saba, V.K, Pocklington, D.B, & Miller, K. (1998). *Nursing and computers: An anthology, 1987-1996.* New York: Springer-Verlag.

Zielstorff, R.D., Hudgings, C.I., & Grobe, S.J. (1994). *Next-generation nursing information systems.* Washington, DC: American Nurses Publishing.

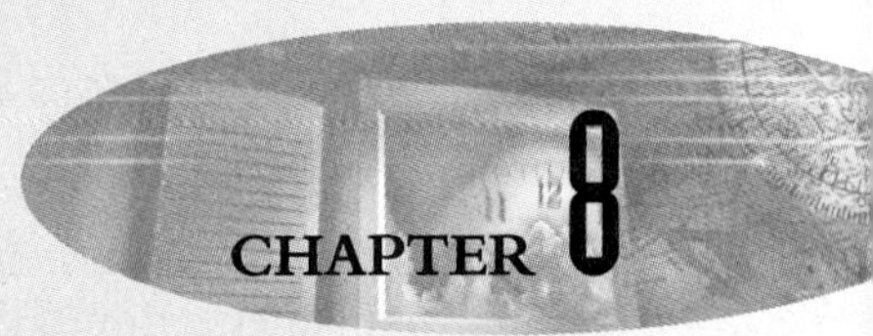

Strategic and Tactical Planning for Health Care Information Systems

MARINA DOUGLAS

Learning Objectives

Upon completion of this chapter, the reader will be able to:

1. ***Discuss*** the key assessment areas required for the development of a health care institution's information systems department strategic plan.
2. ***List*** the main subject headings included in a strategic plan.
3. ***Discuss*** three key differences between strategic and tactical planning.
4. ***Present*** an overview of the five major phases of project management.

Outline

Key Terms

commercial, off-the-shelf (COTS) software
confidentiality
information systems (IS)
information technology (IT)
IS application portfolio
niche software
privacy
project plan
strategic planning
SWOT methodology
tactical planning
technology generation
work breakdown structure (WBS)

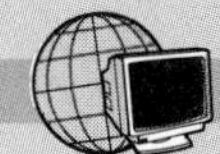

Web Connection

Go to the Web site at http://evolve.elsevier.com/Englebardt/. Here you will find Web links and activities related to strategic and tactical planning for health care information systems.

Planning activities are essential for all successful implementation projects, from a large-scale, multimillion-dollar system to a smaller scale application project. These activities are ongoing at all management levels in organizations. Although planning takes both time and effort, good planning, coupled with the strong execution of plans, has repeatedly demonstrated significantly better outcomes for all **information technology** (IT) projects. Organizations willing to bypass thorough planning in favor of the "let's just get started" mentality soon find projects exceeding budget, unfulfilled user requirements, and frustrated project team members.

This chapter focuses on the planning needs of an **information systems** (IS) department within a hospital-based health care organization. The chapter examines two major planning areas: strategic planning and tactical planning. Much has been written on these subjects. Many of the "best practices" and "lessons learned" come from the experiences of government projects and the construction industry. The body of knowledge for planning, project management, and execution has grown significantly, with educational degrees and certification programs now available.

RATIONALE

Motivating Events

The positive aspects of planning are numerous. Two of the most significant incentives are hard-dollar savings and increased user confidence in the IT department and in the organization as a whole. With strong planning, strategic marketing efforts are made easier. Aggregate patient demographic data, service utilization by patient clusters, and financial performance of service offerings provide the tools to tailor service offerings. Planning for the specific data needs is required to gain the maximum potential value from IT for the organization.

In the current fast-paced financial environment, IT provides the foundation for quick response to both internal organizational trends and external market forces. The ability to aggregate clinical and financial data provides a basis for profit planning. Information on current funds and/or securing funding for future projects, as well as the potential for phased financing of projects, is a powerful and necessary organizational tool.

Planning, while often justified in dollars and cents, also positively impacts the human resources of an organization. An article by LaRouge and Davis (1999) cites the strong increase in productivity of teams when the number of projects, often "priority projects," assigned to a single person is limited. Additional works indicate a stronger sense of satisfaction and team esprit de corps when management exercises appropriate planning of resources (LaRouge & Davis, 1999; Lidlow, 1999).

Lack of Planning: Negative Aspects

Unfortunately, the track record for strong planning within IT environments has not been overwhelming. More than 10% of all IT projects are undertaken with no formal planning (Lewis, 1997). Another 52% of projects will cost 189% of their original estimate by the time they are completed. This figure does not include lost opportunity costs. A staggering 31% of projects will be canceled before completion, accounting for $81 billion in losses (Standish Group, 1995). The two major reasons for canceling a project are (1) poor planning, particularly with respect to resources (human and monetary), and (2) encountering unanticipated requirements (Simpson & Ramsaroop, 1999).

Benefits

The benefits of strong IT planning within an organization are numerous. The cost justifications for IT include many intangible benefits, as well as hard-dollar savings. The business of health care begins with the provision of care. With accurate, easily attainable patient information, the quality of medical decisions and the provision of care are inherently easier for direct caregivers. When clinical information systems and clinical decision support systems are integrated, the results are improved patient care delivery with a decrease in the cost of care (Tierney, Miller, & McDonald, 1990). Avoidance of a single malpractice suit is a significant cost saving for any organization.

Appropriate planning can double the productivity of project teams (LaRouge & Davis, 1999). Current statistics indicate that only 42% of the originally planned features and functions of an information system are implemented when the system is initially activated. Appropriate planning assists in bringing a higher percentage of functionality to the end users sooner. According to Lewis (1997), "A project delivered within budget, but 6 months late, can expect to miss out on one third of the potential profit over its lifetime."

PLANNING

The two primary levels of planning are **strategic planning** and **tactical planning.** Strategic planning is generally the responsibility of senior management—both of the organization, as well as of the IS department. It answers the question "Where/what do we, as an organization or department, want to be in X number of years?" Strategic planning provides the high-level direction needed to reach organizational goals. Tactical planning provides the detail planning for reaching these goals. In this chapter the specific planning requirements for IT project management are included as tactical-level planning. This chapter focuses on both levels of planning within a health care organization's IS department.

Strategic Planning

Management has the responsibility to establish and communicate the strategic direction for the health care organization as a whole as well as for each institutional department. In the past, strategic planning encompassed a 5- to 7-year planning horizon. The 5-year time frame reflected, in part, the current technology generation. **Technology generation** is the length of time needed for a technology innovation to move from a concept to the generally available technology being used within an industry. The 1990s brought a rapid reduction in technology generations. A period of 12 to 18 months is now recognized as the accepted time frame for new technology generation. With a significant decrease in the length of a technology generation, the strategic IT planning horizon is often reduced to 3 years. Development of the strategic plan takes into account the organization's, or the department's, strengths, weaknesses, and opportunities, as well as threats, and the organization's strategic business plan.

To be effective, the IT strategic planning goals must be in concert with the strategic goals and objectives of the organization. In addition, the plan identifies and prioritizes the organization's information requirements. It identifies the IT infrastructure and develops a budget for the resource allocations needed to accomplish the plan (Austin & Boxerman, 1997). The process for developing a strategic plan for the IS department begins with an analysis of the strategic business goals and initiatives of the organization and a review of the organization's mission statement. As a critical piece of the overall infrastructure of the organization, a strategic IS plan must be in alignment with and support the overall business goals and the mission of the organization. Information provides a major source of power for management in meeting organizational goals.

For example, a health system comprising five acute care facilities within a 45-mile radius established a strategic goal of being recognized as the premiere health care system in the area for cardiac care. The supporting IS department's strategic goals included the selection and implementation of a central data repository for all electrocardiograms that would be administered to patients in that health care system. The repository would provide health care professionals access to electrocardiograms from any of the five acute care facilities. With this approach, patients requiring cardiac care within the health care system would be assured that their electrocardiograms were immediately available to their health care providers regardless of their physical location within the health care system. An added advantage would be that the repository would attract physicians to practice within the health care system.

Steps in Strategic Planning

The development of a strategic plan is the responsibility of senior management. This is a multistep process usually requiring a period of 4 to 6 months. The plan traditionally encompasses the following four steps:

1. Development of a mission statement
2. Assessment of the organization's or department's current state
3. Determination of the desired future position
4. Development of the actual strategic plan

The assessment and the planning steps require the scrutiny of six key IT areas. These areas are hardware, software, networks, operations, skill sets, and budget.

Step 1: Develop a Mission Statement President John F. Kennedy delivered a classic mission statement to the American people in 1961. According to President Kennedy, the mission for America was "to place a man on the moon and return him safely to the Earth by the end of the decade." The statement clearly articulated, with a measurable outcome in a defined time frame, the strategic goal for the National Aeronautics and Space Administration (NASA) and the American people. The mission statement provides an organization with a frame of reference. It is a guidepost for the work effort of the organization. Day-to-day decisions are evaluated against the mission statement. In the 1960s the president's mission statement was the yardstick by which day-to-day decisions within NASA were measured.

The mission statement of the organization is the foundation for the development of the department's mission. Box 8-1 presents examples of two health care systems' mission statements. Note that these two mission statements define the purpose of the organization, as well as articulate the beliefs and values underlying the mission.

Step 2: Assess the Current State The development of the mission statement is followed by an assessment of the current state of the organization or department. In the early 1960s, a methodology was introduced to assist businesses in assessing their position in the marketplace (Pearce & Robinson, 1988). This methodology includes reviewing the organization's or department's *s*trengths, *w*eaknesses, *o*pportunities, and *t*hreats and is referred to as the **SWOT methodology.** The SWOT methodology helps to review each component area from both an internal and an external perspective. For purposes of the IS strategic plan development, each of the following areas must be reviewed for its strengths, weaknesses, opportunities, and threats: hardware, software, networks, operations, employee skill sets, and budget.

Hardware Hardware considerations encompass the physical age, as well as the technological age, of the equipment. Leasing, maintenance, and service contracts for each piece of hardware are reviewed. Repair costs and operational logs are included in the review process.

Software Software considerations include major clinical and financial application software, communications and connectivity software, and operating systems software. This includes the software managed by the IS department, as well as that managed by other departments and units within the organization. The IS department must actively

Box 8–1 Examples of Two Health System Mission Statements

Mission statement 1

Purpose

We serve the community by improving the quality of life through better health.

Values

Working together in service to God, our values are:

- Integrity
- Quality
- Serving the customer
- Caring for and developing our people
- Using the community's resources wisely

Mission statement 2

Purpose

We will promote health, ease suffering, heal, and teach.

Values

We believe in the dignity of all individuals. We hold a reverence for life. We will ensure access for all. We view participation and teamwork as necessary for excellence. We recognize diversity and creativity as sources of strength.

Philosophy

We will continually learn, seek, and improve. We will listen to and act upon the needs of the patients. We will meet expectations with the right resources, at the right time. We will relentlessly pursue quality.

Vision

We will be the premier health delivery family for the region.

seek out information concerning the different applications used by various departments within the organization including the use of niche software. **Niche software** is software developed to meet the specific information needs within a department. In large organizations it is not unusual for the IS department to first learn of an individual department's purchase and use of niche software during the strategic IS planning assessment.

In clinical areas, niche software is often associated with specialized treatment areas and medical diagnostic equipment, such as pulmonary function software or nursing acuity systems. In addition, clinicians may use programs developed by members of their staff to fill a specific departmental need. For example, a rehabilitation department may maintain a database of patients and their types of prosthetic devices. Although these small systems are generally not integrated with the main registration, patient billing, or order entry systems, added benefits for the individual departments may be realized if integration can be included as an objective for the IS department.

Financial software review takes into account not only those major applications used to bill and collect patient accounts (the general financial areas of accounts payable, payroll, and specific software for materials management) but niche software as well. Niche software is often used to send financial data to state and federal reporting agencies. Individual insurance companies and health maintenance organizations (HMOs) may use niche software to check patient eligibility status for enrollment and treatment. Software linkages between materials management and their major suppliers may use specialized software; however, this trend is declining in favor of Internet connections.

Networks Review of network architecture will include current-use volumes of intranet and Internet transactions. Telehealth, teleradiology, and teleconferencing usage must be reviewed. In some institutions, communications functions (telephone, pagers, and faxes) are also administered by information systems.

Operations Support desk/help desk functions are reviewed. Customer satisfaction metrics, often called service-level agreements, are reviewed. Service-level agreements may include the length of time between notification to resolution of an IS problem, the number of problems reported grouped by type of problem, and the frequency of unplanned system downtime. Conducting interviews with targeted end users relative to their experiences and perception of IS support is helpful for understanding the needs of the organization.

Policies are reviewed as part of the SWOT assessment. With issues of privacy and confidentiality of patient data in the news headlines and the subject of many debates by private industry, individual citizens, and the federal government, security policies and practices must be closely reviewed. Areas of concern include policies related to end user access of the system, the distribution and use of individual sign-ons, and viewing of patient records by employees when viewing such records are not part of their employment responsibilities. Policies relative to company eMail systems used for personal messaging must also be reviewed. Access to the Intranet is extremely valuable for researching available treatment and disease literature; policies should reflect appropriate use of the Internet for patient care.

The Health Insurance Portability and Accountability Act (HIPAA) of 1996 outlines specific requirements for maintaining a secure environment for electronic storage and transmission of patient data. **Confidentiality** describes a health care professional's duty to protect the secrecy of information about a patient's condition, regardless of its source. **Privacy** is a right of patients to determine what information about their health state they choose to share with their health care team. Policy reviews should be conducted to ensure support of these key tenets.

Procedures within the IS department are reviewed during the current-state evaluation. Assessing these procedures includes evaluating how the IS policies and procedures interface with the policies and procedures of other institutional departments. Several examples demonstrate this issue. Providing IS support and help desk coverage 24 hours per day, 7 days per week (24/7 coverage) requires careful planning. The needs of the departments are anticipated and integrated with the resources of the IS department. Another example involves departmental use of computer resources. Reports detailing the organization's month-end financial summary often use a large amount of the computer's central processing capabilities. Running the reports during times of less system activity and patient care demands may prevent an overall slowing of the system's response time. A final example is the procedure for activating and deactivating user access codes to the hospital information system. These procedures must be reviewed in conjunction with human resources policies related to initiation and termination of employment. The IS department requires advanced notification in order to establish and maintain an accurate list of current employees. This is particularly important when an individual's employment is being terminated as a disciplinary action. The number one security threat to the integrity of an institution's information system is a disgruntled employee (Jones, 1999). Additional information on security issues is discussed in Chapter 20.

Skill Sets A review of the skill sets for each of the employees within an IS department is key to the strategic planning process. Single-source knowledge for any area within information systems is risky. For example, when only one member of the IS staff has knowledge of the interface engine used by the laboratory system, the organization is at high risk should the person be unavailable when the interface system develops a problem. For many in the IT field, the ability to learn new skills is important to continued job satisfaction, and cross-training on multiple systems is often welcomed.

Budget Reviewing budget data is imperative in the development of any plan. Planning for IT growth, as well as business growth, is incorporated into the budget. In the strategic planning process, it is extremely important to understand funding capabilities and sources. Securing appropriate funding for the entire project before beginning the project is crucial. Budgetary planning based on past performance budgeting has been successfully used in the past.

An IS budget includes costs for licensing, maintenance fees, and upgrade fees for software, hardware, and communications. Anticipated costs for personnel training and education, incidentals, fringe benefits, and salaries are reviewed, and calculations for increases in the cost-of-living and consumer price index are evaluated. In some instances the allocations for physical space within the building and an appropriation for utilities used are included in the budget.

Step 3: Define the Desired Future State The third step in the development of a strategic plan is the identification of the desired future state for the organization or department. During this step the "where" and "what" questions of strategic planning are formalized. The answers are based on the strategic business goals of the organization and the IT department, as well as the SWOT assessment. Of paramount concern is the alignment of the IS department's strategic plan with the strategic business plan of the organization. Failure to account for the organization's strategic business plan will result in major internal conflicts between the IS department, the end users, and senior management. In such cases the IS department is perceived to be providing the organization with marginal support. This is due, in part, to IS resources being deployed to IS projects with little support being provided to projects in the strategic planning initiatives. The process of determining the desired future state should include a review of the SWOT assessments in relation to the strategic business goals and the organization's mission.

In some instances the desired state includes new purchases or replacement of hardware, software, or networks; in other instances it includes the upgrading of application releases or hardware to remain in compliance with contractual obligations for maintaining vendor support.

Hardware Hardware considerations include the ongoing upgrade of equipment to support new technologies. In large institutions with hundreds of workstations, personal computers (PCs), or dumb terminals deployed in clinical areas, capital expenditure budgets may include replacement of 25% of the total number of PCs. The older/slower PCs deployed are targeted for replacement. In some situations, leasing equipment is more cost-effective than purchasing new equipment. Members of the institution's finance group will be helpful for determining the appropriate strategy. The shortened time frame for a technology generation must be taken into account when evaluating these options.

Software Strategic goals for the organization may be supported by upgrading current software to a newer version or release level. When goals and objectives are not supported by current software, new software applications may be required. The evaluation, acquisition, and implementation of new applications can be costly, both in terms of dollars and personnel time. Understanding the current state of systems is fundamental to making an informed choice.

Networks As with hardware, advances in the field of networking are occurring at a rapid rate. Local area networks (LANs) and wide area networks (WANs) are being augmented or replaced with the use of the Internet and intranets. The next-generation Internet (NGI) is in the early stages of deployment. It is prudent to include experts in the area of networks and communications in the strategic planning process. Videoconferencing, telemedicine, and teleradiology are fast becoming part of mainstream medical practice.

Operations Helping to define and service the information needs of the organization is part of the mission of most IS departments. As new technologies and functionality are introduced, service levels to the end user must be established. Dumb terminals, as the basic workstations, are being replaced by desktop PCs. Developing and meeting standards for established service levels to the end user is a cornerstone of IT departments. A caregiver working on an off-shift (evenings or nights) and unable to access automated patient data because of nonavailability of a PC or clinical application is unacceptable. Response time for resolution of in-house problems, as well as vendor-specific issues, should be established. Service agreement stipulations within vendor maintenance contracts must be incorporated into the department's service-level standards. An alternative to maintaining a centralized IS staff is to outsource the services to a contractor. For some organizations, outsourcing is a financially viable alternative. For other organizations, outsourcing is not a financially viable alternative.

A number of factors are involved in the outsourcing decision. These include salary and fringe benefit costs, the rate and reason for personnel turnover within the IS department, the skill mix and technical resource availability to support the strategic and ongoing IT goals and objectives, and finally, the pricing structure proposed by the outsourcing organization. A support area often considered for outsourcing is technical support for maintaining desktop PCs and desktop applications. In some larger institutions, upwards of 3000 to 4000 PCs may require centralized support. The organization's health care application-knowledgeable staff may spend significant time supporting the end users for PC and desktop applications. This support time can be at the expense of the strategic initiatives for the specialized health care applications. The outsourcing organization has access to specific technical resources and staff for supporting PCs and desktop application. This approach can provide IS staff members with a work environment where they can specialize in their technical area, an attractive feature for technical professionals looking for advancement in their field. For some IS departments a combination of continuing a limited central IS staff and outsourcing portions of the IS operations, such as desktop support, might be appropriate.

Skills Sets Personnel are an extremely valuable asset to an organization. Planning is required to anticipate the staffing needs and skill mix as an organization grows. If a strategic goal of the organization is to increase name recognition within the community, increased presence of the organization on the Internet will likely be a part of the strategy. Having the technical personnel with the skills to support interactive Web page development and network connectivity will be required. This may require training for the staff. To gain early benefits from the technology, the training should be provided before the technology arrives at the site.

Cross-training is essential to providing departmental depth while maintaining affordable numbers of staff. The opportunity for continued learning is considered a major component of job satisfaction and longevity with an institution. Training and education considerations are particularly important within this group of personnel.

Budget The percentage of the IS budget in relation to the overall operating budget of an organization is an indicator of the importance that the organization places on IT. In the banking world, 10% to 12% of the operating budget is spent on IT. Current figures for health care place the average percentage for IT expenditure at 3%. As new technologies and systems are available to health care organizations and become integrated into the day-to-day workflow, this percentage will increase.

Step 4: Writing the Strategic Plan Once the assessment and the definition of the desired future state have been completed, the strategic plan is written. There are generally eight specific sections to a strategic plan (Austin & Boxerman, 1997). These are outlined in Table 8-1.

Section 1: Executive Summary The executive summary is a 1- to 3-page distillation of the key components of the plan. It is an overview for the target audience of senior executives and places the important aspects of the plan in summary format.

Section 2: Institutional Strategic Goals and Objectives As mentioned earlier, the IS department's strategic planning goals must be in alignment with and strongly support the organization's strategic goals and objectives. In the example used earlier in this chapter, a Midwest health care system has established a strategic goal to be recognized as the premiere provider of cardiac care in their metropolitan region. The IS department's strategic plan supports the organizational efforts toward this goal, such as the implementation of the electrocardiogram central data repository and niche systems involved in cardiac surgery, as well as the smooth operation of the cardiac catheter laboratory system.

Table 8–1 Format for a Written Strategic Plan

Section	Title
Section 1	Executive summary
Section 2	Institutional strategic goals and objectives
Section 3	Information systems department strategic goals and objectives
Section 4	Information systems application portfolio
Section 5	System architecture and infrastructure
Section 6	Software development plans
Section 7	Operational plan
Section 8	Budget

Section 3: Information Systems Department Strategic Goals and Objectives The goals and objectives of IS management are clearly stated. These are stated in measurable terms, with defined dates for accomplishing each. The criteria for measuring the success of each goal and objective are defined. These critical success factors are important for two reasons: (1) they establish the unit of measure for success, and (2) they provide a guidepost for maintaining strategic direction within the department. When unanticipated events occur, knowledge of the criteria for the success of the strategic plan supports informed decision making related to these events. In addition, IS project priorities can be defined more easily.

Section 4: Information Systems Application Portfolio Similar to the concept in investment strategies, an **IS application portfolio** indicates the suite of software applications planned, proposed, or implemented in an organization. In a young organization where IT support is just beginning, the applications available may be newly implemented or in the process of being implemented. There is a higher degree of risk associated with an environment of all new applications. Less risk is generally associated with applications 2 to 3 years following implementation; known operational routines and end user processes decrease the IT risk. The ongoing development of the organization, and therefore the introduction of new applications, provides for a portfolio where some applications are associated with low risk, some are associated with medium risk, and some are associated with high risk.

In this section of the strategic plan, the application portfolio and planned activities are defined. A typical health care organization's portfolio includes application software for the clinical, financial, administrative, and decision support areas. Decision support software exists for many aspects of the organization. The clinical decision software is the newest and most complex decision support addition to the portfolio. Applications used to support the management of the operating systems, communications, and security are included in the portfolio. The portfolio outlines the addition of new software higher-risk projects, as well as projects for upgrading existing applications to new versions—medium- to lower-risk projects.

Section 5: System Architecture and Infrastructure The overall system architecture is established. This includes the infrastructure of networks and communications; the level of access, distribution, and security of information; the network architecture; and the location of data within the infrastructure.

Section 6: Software Development Plans Some level of software development generally does take place within an institution. The intricacies of today's health care information applications, the integration requirements, and the cost of development often preclude IS departments from major in-house development. Small projects can be undertaken to augment **commercial, off-the-shelf (COTS) software.** In some instances a third-party development group is contracted to accomplish the development. These development plans are outlined in this section.

Section 7: Operational Plan Information collected from the operational and skill set assessment and future-state planning is used as the basis for defining the overall operational plan. The operational plan includes the schedule for performing system back-ups, database back-ups, and application back-ups; maintenance procedures; as well as the scheduling of report generation. The operational plan includes the management of software changes, "bug" fixes, and upgrades to the production or live environment. Well-established and well-executed change management procedures are a necessity for smooth operations. Availability of the required skill sets and staffing to accomplish these tasks are necessary.

Section 8: Budget The budget is based on the defined monetary and personnel resource requirements. A capital budget and an operating budget are outlined. The capital budget includes purchases for hardware, software, networks, and communications equipment to accomplish the goals of the plan. The operating budget includes the cost of maintaining the IS department. It includes, for example, personnel and supply costs.

The strategic plan is reviewed by many groups within the organization before it is finalized. These groups usually include members of the senior management team, selected members of the IS steering committee, a member of the finance group, and selected members of the user community. The finalized version of the strategic plan is submitted to the appropriate governing bodies within the organization. Within the IS department, appropriate portions of the plan are reviewed and discussed with department personnel. Sensitive information regarding salary and actual budget figures is sometimes filtered for presentation within the department. As members of the department become familiar with and work toward accomplishment of the outlined goals and objectives, the strategic plan becomes an integral part of the department. The measurable goals and objectives defined in the strategic plan become milestone events and a means for determining the department's progress in supporting the plan. An approved strategic plan is essential to the development of a departmental tactical plan.

Tactical Planning/Project Management

Once the "where" and "what" questions have been outlined in the strategic plan, the IS department can begin to plan for the "how" of carrying out the strategic plan. This is the development of the tactical plan. Tactical planning sets out the details for accomplishing the goals and objectives. The tactical plan defines the following:

- The broad scope of each objective
- The order in which objectives are to be initiated
- The major milestones for each objective
- The project manager and team members for each objective

Feasibility Study

For major, high-risk IT initiatives, a feasibility study is often done before an organization will commit resources to the project. The purpose of the feasibility study is to assess whether the proposed IT initiative is in fact an appropriate avenue for achieving a specific objective or a set of objectives.

The final outcome of a feasibility study is the decision to proceed or not to proceed with the IT project. In some instances other approaches may support the strategic initiatives more completely. For example, a 200-bed urban community hospital has set a strategic goal to increase the revenue generated by their women's and children's center by a total of 15% within 3 years. The tactical plan includes an objective to streamline the registration process for prenatal and laboring mothers. Implementation of a new automated labor and delivery system is proposed. The feasibility study seeks to determine if the impact of the new automated labor and delivery system's registration function will decrease the length of time needed to register the patients. During the feasibility study, the current prenatal and laboring patient registration processes are reviewed. The results indicate that the new system will require three additional screens of information to be collected for each expectant mother and that peak registration times in the perinatal area are covered by only one clerk. In this example, accomplishing the goal of streamlining the perinatal registration procedure may be better served by business process reengineering and potentially increasing registration staff availability during peak registration times.

Project Management

Once the strategic and tactical plans are established and a feasibility study is completed (if required), a project plan is developed. The **project plan** provides the granular details for accomplishing the objective. The project plan, sometimes called a work plan, breaks down the individual tactical objective into tasks and subtasks, assigns task initiation and completion dates, assesses task dependencies, and determines resource requirements. Milestone event schedules within the project plan must coincide with the tactical plan's milestones and can be used to track the project's progress. The work breakdown structure (WBS) of a project is developed from the milestone events, tasks, and subtasks. With the aid of automated project management tools, cost models, and "what if" software functions, scenarios can be established. This provides valuable information for planning and decision making during the initiation and execution phases of project management.

There are two paradigms in project management. The classic conventional planning paradigm establishes a detailed plan with explicit time frames and cost structure. Team members are assigned and given specific tasks to accomplish. All aspects of the finely detailed planning are completed before the work effort is begun. Team meetings during the course of the project may occur on a weekly basis, with a monthly status report to management. The measurement of a successful project is the completion of the project on time and within budget.

The new paradigm uses systematic and integrative planning, with timely decisions made to adjust the plan as needed under conditions of uncertainty. The phases of the project may in fact overlap, and although planning occurs, the details may not be finely delineated before the work effort is begun. Communications between the team and management and among the team members is intensive (Laufer, 1997). The measurement of success for the new paradigm is the completion of a project that meets critical performance, cost, and schedule targets in uncertain environments, under accelerated time frames, and with scarce resources (Laufer, 1997).

The management of projects can become quite intricate. The Project Management Institute in Newtown Square, Pennsylvania, has compiled years of project managers' experiences and currently offers various levels of certification in project management. This organization offers extensive information on project management methods, tools, and certification.

Box 8–2 Top Ten Reasons for Cancellation of a Project

1. Incomplete requirements
2. Lack of user involvement
3. Lack of resources
4. Unrealistic expectations
5. Lack of executive support
6. Changing requirements
7. Lack of planning
8. Technology no longer needed
9. Lack of coordinated management
10. Technology illiteracy

Five Phases of Project Management Whether subscribing to the classic or the new paradigm approach, the planning methodology is defined by five phases:

1. Initiation
2. Planning
3. Execution
4. Control and management
5. Closing the project

Initiation The project initiation phase begins by setting a vision or mission statement for the project. The statement clearly communicates the intent and time frame of the project. Establishing the project team and the project plan are also accomplished in the initiation phase. Selection of the team members is critical to the success of the project. Of the ten top reasons given by chief information officers as reasons for canceling a project (Box 8-2), nine are directly related to interpersonal skills and communications (Standish Group, 1998). The importance of selecting the right personnel for the project cannot be underestimated.

Fredrick Mumma (1998) has described eight team roles required for a successful project team: the roles of leader, moderator, creator, innovator, manager, organizer, evaluator, and finisher. The success of the team rests in large measure on the ability of the team to effectively complete the work of each of these roles during the life cycle of a project. Members may serve in more than one role. Teams lacking a member to assume the responsibilities of a particular role will have a difficult time achieving a successful completion of their project. For those seriously considering a career in project management, further investigation of Mumma's theory is highly recommended. The work of the "creator" role, for example, is to generate original ideas, to view tasks from different perspectives, and to produce several alternative approaches (Mumma, 1998). A team lacking a member to assume the responsibilities of the creator role will have a difficult time thinking of alternative approaches to accomplishing tasks. Approaches to, and potentially the task outcomes themselves, may appear surprisingly similar to the current modes of operations. In some instances "the way it has always been done" may be the best way; however, if there is no one in the creator role to stimulate new perspectives, the team risks seeing "the way it's always been done" as the only approach.

Planning The second aspect of the planning phase is the development of a project plan. The project plan may also be referred to as the work plan. The development of a project plan begins with a clear understanding of the objective and its relationship to the strategic goals of the organization and department. The scope of the project is established during the planning phase. It is extremely valuable to have the project team involved in the project plan development. This provides the team members with an understanding of the problem before the plan is conceived and executed, which significantly increases the potential for the project's success. The team members augment the manager's knowledge. This is helpful in establishing plan details and assists in gaining buy-in from the project team. The project team develops the critical success factors for the objective and incorporates them into the project plan. A thorough understanding of the mission, goal, and scope of the project is fundamental to maintaining the course during the project implementation.

The project plan is developed by dividing the project into manageable tasks. Referred to as the **work breakdown structure (WBS)**, this breakdown of the tasks is the basis for the project plan structure. In the WBS a task is divided into subtasks. The typical WBS has three to six levels of subtasks. Defining the subtasks involves identifying the duration of the task, the estimated amount of time needed to complete the task, start dates and end dates, the resource(s) needed to complete each task, the dependencies of associated tasks, and key milestones.

To illustrate, imagine that the IS department wants to implement online radiology results reporting. One of the subtasks is to survey direct caregivers in the hospital regarding their perception of a newly implemented radiology results reporting display. The duration of time to complete a user survey is estimated to be 3 weeks. The duration accounts for the development and dissemination of the survey, a period of time for the users to respond to the survey, and a period of time to compile the responses. The number of hours estimated for IS resources to complete the task is 25 hours. The task requires 10 hours of a clinical analyst to develop the survey questions and survey format and 10 hours of the analyst's time to disseminate, compile, and analyze the responses. A technical resource will be used for an estimated 5 hours to assist in automating the survey and compiling the responses. Milestones for the project are the development of the survey, the distribution of the survey, and the return of an acceptable sample size for analysis. The granularity of the subtasks is dictated by the ability to estimate the completion of the task with a degree of accuracy in terms of hours. The time line for completion is linear in nature; subtasks occur sequentially. Figure 8-1 demonstrates a simple WBS for this project on the left side of the box and the corresponding Gantt (bar) chart on the right.

The online radiology results reporting example just described is actually a part of a clinical information system (CIS) implementation. In the example the activation of online radiology results follows the activation of laboratory order entry and results reporting by 4 weeks. During the planning phase the CIS project team members thought that a period of time was needed for the staff to become familiar with the automated laboratory processes before activation of the next major department—radiology. Pharmacy order entry and online medication administration records are scheduled to be activated 2 weeks after the radiology activation. Utilization of resources allows members of the laboratory team to be available to assist in the final preparation for both the radiology and the pharmacy activations. In relation to the larger CIS project, the tasks are in fact overlapping; resources are used for multiple tasks, and the timing of the activation of the radiology and pharmacy components is dependent on the reaction of the users to the laboratory activation. The use of an automated project management tool assists in developing a time line for the project and in managing

FIGURE 8–1 Example of a Work Breakdown Structure for a Radiology Results Display Satisfaction Survey

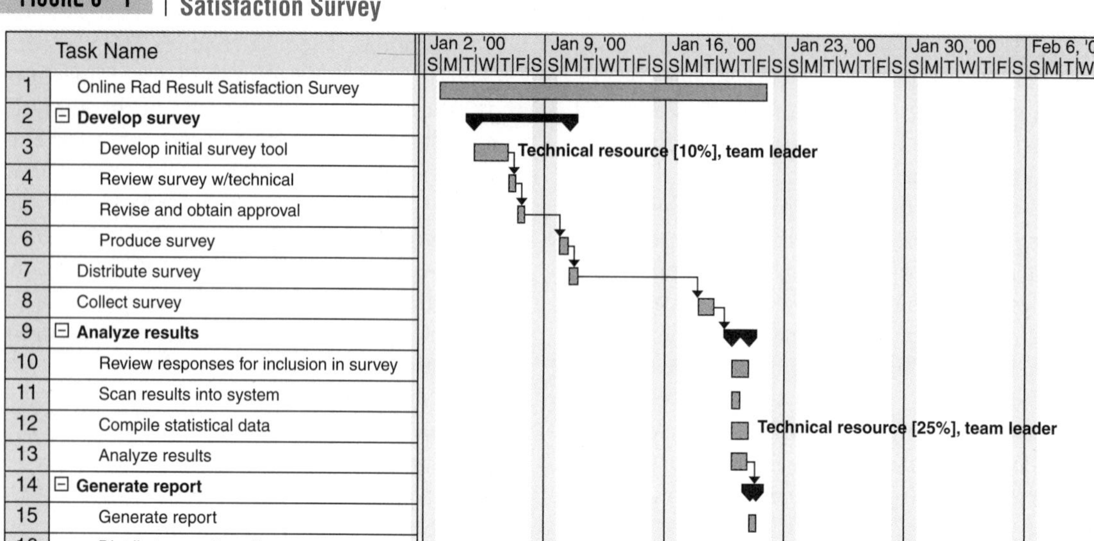

the availability of resources to ensure resource availability.

Within the hospital environment, key events must be factored into project planning. Scheduled surveys from licensing bodies or regulatory agencies (e.g., Joint Commission on Accreditation of Healthcare Organizations [JCAHO], Department of Health and Human Services [DHHS]), Christmas holidays, known periods of high census, and popular vacation times are known to have a severe impact on a project plan and must receive realistic consideration. When creating a new project, project managers often begin by developing the WBS inclusive of start and completion dates. Using automated project management tools, the time line for the project naturally develops. The WBS can also be developed without task start and completion dates; a planned project end date is established, and the automated tool calculates the task start and completion dates on the basis of task durations and task dependencies. The latter methodology is used often in the IT vendor community where a standard methodology has been developed, tested, and refined over many implementations.

Execution Execution of the plan is the third phase of project management. It requires attention to detail by all project team members. The project manager must engineer the environment to foster motivated team members and maintain momentum for completion of the project. The adage "plan the work; work the plan" becomes the mantra. Good communication practices, both verbal and written, are required to keep other team members informed and motivated. Team meetings, both formal and informal, are crucial. Organizational skills are needed to manage complex projects where multiple teams perform multiple tasks with the same objective. Maintaining senior management support during the working phase is imperative to the work of the execution phase. Resources, financial and personnel, become critically important during the execution phase. Rarely is the precise plan that was established during the planning phase executed in its original form. Completion dates slip, resources become unavailable, and acts of nature (e.g., snow storms, hurricanes, and flu epidemics) disrupt work schedules. Recognition of this reality contributed greatly to the new paradigm in project management described earlier. Successful teams celebrate their accomplishments and the attainment of milestones along the way.

Controlling and Monitoring Controlling and monitoring is the fourth phase in project management. This phase overlaps the execution phase and the closing-the-project phase. Although controlling and monitoring are generally the responsibility of the project manager, team leaders and team members have the responsibility to monitor and control their assignment. Projects are most successful when authority for decision making is granted at the lowest possible level. Those project decisions that benefit one department or area at the expense of other departments are detrimental to both the overall project and the organization. Participative management, allowing team members to schedule their work within the scope of the project plan, provides team members with a sense of autonomy; the level of autonomy is ultimately kept in balance with the needs of the overall project by the project manager. Good team members have the ability to see the integration of their portion of the project as a part of the whole.

Monitoring a project requires a plan against which one applies knowledge concerning the status of the project tasks. The types and numbers of monitoring points assigned to a project must be selected carefully. Project time should be directed toward accomplishing the objectives as opposed to spending inordinate amounts time reporting on the project's progress. To control a project, the current project status is compared with the plan. Decisions are then made and implemented in response to deviations occurring in the plan. Often project managers apply many monitoring points but fail to act decisively when plan deviations occur. They do well at monitoring but lack any control.

Automated project management tools monitor the progress of the project through estimates of completion of task—often referred to as the "percent complete" for a particular task. Some project managers require the team leaders and team members to enter the percent complete of their assigned tasks into the automated project plan on a weekly basis. The software program calculates the project's progress and reports on the variances and impact on the project. Another methodology for monitoring the progress of a project is the earned value assessment (EVA). Used frequently in government software projects, the EVA adds an additional level of complexity to the percent complete assessment by requiring additional data points regarding the current status (Flemming & Kopleman, 1998, 1999).

Project status reports are done on a routine basis and at various levels of reporting. Project team members may complete a status report for their team leaders. Their team leaders, in turn, provide a status report to the project manager, who reports to a leadership or steering committee. In the early stages of a project, status reports may be done on a biweekly or monthly basis. As milestone dates or significant testing periods approach, status reports may be requested on a weekly or more frequent basis. Project and team meeting minutes are most effective when they are distributed within 2 to 3 days of the meeting time. In large IT implementation projects, where personnel are diverted from usual duties, the distribution of project meeting minutes are effective when distributed to not only the team members, but to each team member's individual supervisor as well (one over distribution).

Two useful tools of project management are the development and maintenance of an issues list and a project manager's diary. Use of an issues list allows the tracking of all issues affecting the project. The issues may be of any nature—administrative concerns for training schedules, bugs found in the software, current process workflows requiring business process improvement to take advantage of software functionality are but a few. The issues list should be centrally maintained through the use of a database or spreadsheet and accessible so that all team members have quick access to the issues and can easily add issues. A partial list of data fields in an issues list is given in Box 8-3.

The database or spreadsheet best serves the team when reports can be easily created from the list. Reports showing open issues or resolved issues, issues organized by individual application or by responsible party, issues organized by the date initiated or date resolved, the current status of the issues, and the priority of the issues are most helpful. It is critical for the issue-tracking tool to also document the actual resolution of an issue. Often an issue is brought up multiple times by different teams or is revisited by the original team multiple times. The documented resolution provides a reference point for other teams as well. Weekly status meetings may include discussion of any new or unresolved critical issue for the team. During the implementation of one hospital-wide information system, over 700 issues were logged during the course of the implementation. The addition of issues seemed to be exponential during the early phases of the project. As the testing phases of the implementation approached, the list began to reflect the "controlling" work of the team members. At the time of integrated testing, 53 open or in-progress issues were on the list. By the time of the initial activation of the system, only six low-priority issues remained. The team became reenergized as the rate of issue resolution became faster than the rate of new additions to the list.

Use of a project diary to record major project events and decisions has been invaluable to project managers and team leaders. An individual diary kept by the project manager and/or by the team leaders provides the manager/leader with a history of events surrounding the major decisions. On occasion, a team member may challenge an issue resolution or may want to reopen the issue. In some instances this may be appropriate in light of new knowledge or newly available functionality. In instances where the team member has not come to terms with the team's decision on the issue, the diary entries related to the event can clarify why a particular decision or resolution was reached. This helps prevent team energies from being wasted by revisiting closed issues.

Box 8–3 Suggested Data Fields in an Issues List

Issue number
Date of entry
Person entering the issue
Application/area affected
Issue description
Assigned responsible party
Status of the issue (e.g., entered, reviewed)
Status date
Issue priority
Notes
Resolution description
Resolution date

Closing the Project Closing the project is the final phase of project management. During this phase the project manager obtains formal consensus from the project team that the project has been completed and that the customer's needs, whether internal or external, have been met. The accomplishments and goals achieved from this project and key decisions made during the course of the project are formally documented. Pivotal corrective actions taken in response to deviations in the project plan are recorded. Project managers have commented on how useful the issues list and their project diary were in completing this final phase. Information compiled from the financial aspects of the project includes the human factors (such as the number of hours worked toward accomplishing the project plan); the methodology used; and the network, hardware, and software costs incurred. The ability to compare the actual project costs (human and monetary) with the planned project costs is perhaps most valuable for future projects. In project-driven organizations this analysis helps to establish the IS department's effectiveness in managing and executing projects from the combined financial and human perspective. The opportunity to make improvements in implementation methodology are equally as valuable for many organizations managing multiple IT projects on an ongoing basis.

AUTOMATED TOOLS TO SUPPORT PLANNING

Automated project management resources can come from a number of sources. Some are located on the Web; others are found in commercially available project management software.

The increasing complexity of projects and the need to manage multiple projects simultaneously has resulted in the development of project management software programs of increasing sophistication. At one time a distinct difference existed between "professional" project management software and "home computing" or desktop project management software. Technology and software advances have blurred that distinction. Some project management software programs specialize in the management of resources and schedules; others specialize in the accounting aspects of project costs, revenues, and billing. Although both can be considered project management software, the latter is perhaps more accurately termed project accounting software. For large organizations managing many large-scale projects, the project accounting and project management software systems communicate with the organizational accounting system. Increased ease of monitoring, highly accurate cost tracking, and greater responsiveness to ad hoc reporting requests can be accomplished through this integration. "Home computing" project management software contains the majority of the features and functions of the once-labeled "professional" project management software. Many large-scale projects have been managed, monitored, and controlled quite successfully with the use of "home computing" software. The reporting capabilities of the "home computing" software have also seen great advances; in addition to more robustly structured report offerings, some packages provide the flexibility of easily creating user-defined reports.

Two areas where project management software have provided added value are in the ability to do "what if" scenarios and the ability to produce graphical representations of the project. In the planning phase the "what if" capabilities can be used to compare the cost of different resource mixes to accomplish a single task or the entire objective. In one instance the "what if" scenario indicated that vast savings were possible if the experience qualifications for a category of project team members were lessened and specialized training in the areas of system testing and end user training were provided to the team. The costs associated with the additional training, both in terms of the project team member's time and the training fees for an outside resource, were minimal in comparison with the overall project's labor costs savings. A win-win situation was created; team members were honored to be chosen for the team and to receive specialized training. Team camaraderie was fostered, resulting in a highly successful project with final labor costs significantly less than original estimates.

The ability to produce graphical representations of a project is now considered a basic feature of project management software packages. The graphical representations depict three frequently used methodologies: critical path methodology (CPM), bar (Gantt) charting, and Program Evaluation Review Technique (PERT). These methodologies are explained as follows:

- CPM—The basis for this methodology is that there are certain tasks that must be completed on schedule to reach the target completion date. The sequence of these critical tasks becomes the determining factors for attaining the shortest duration of a project.
- Gantt chart—Named for Henry Gantt, who developed an intricate set of bar graph representations to depict the duration of tasks in a project, the Gantt chart provides a bar graph representing the amount of time assigned to complete a task in relation to the entire project. Representations are made in the graph indicating milestone events and task dependencies.
- PERT—PERT methodology was originally developed by the U.S. Navy and by the consulting firm of Booz, Allen & Hamilton during the development of Polaris missiles in the 1950s and 1960s. This methodology calculates the probability of a project event occurring on time and its relationship to the task to determine the length of time needed to complete a task and ultimately the entire project. Unlike the other methods, PERT uses the best, worst, and most likely completion time estimates to determine a project's completion.

CONCLUSION

Planning is a both a necessity and a predictor of success for any endeavor. In the health care IT arena it is imperative to complete quality planning in conjunction with IT projects. The benefits of quality planning include financial gains, staff satisfaction, and the consumer's perception of competence. Planning is required by all levels of the project team from the top down, with each level providing necessary information and support to the success of the project. Thoughtfully planning and documenting the plan require discipline from the beginning of the project's life cycle. Management and project teams must resist the temptation to just get started without having accomplished the planning process. A balance needs to be maintained between perfect initial detailed planning and the continuous planning required for those tasks with known uncertainties at the beginning of a project.

Communication and the selection of appropriate team members are two major factors in the success of projects. Online resources, automated tools, and structured methodologies are available to assist project managers and team members in gaining knowledge and competence in the field of project management.

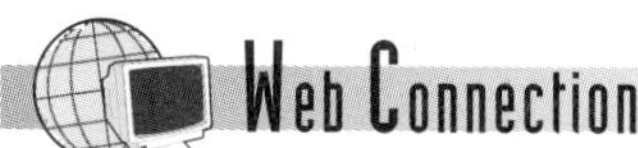

Project management involves sound strategic planning and competent management. It is the cornerstone of effective deployment of information technologies. The Web activities for this chapter are designed to review aspects of strategic planning and project management. Through applications available to support planning and project management processes, you will learn different perspectives of the processes and explore software and services available to facilitate effective management.

discussion questions

1. Describe three differences between strategic and tactical planning.
2. Develop a mission statement for a project you are working on, identifying the three major components of a mission statement.

3. Describe the four assessment areas of the SWOT methodology.
4. List and describe the eight topic areas to be included in a strategic plan.
5. List the five phases of project management, and discuss the major tasks to be accomplished in each phase.

REFERENCES

Austin, C.J., & Boxerman, S.B. (1997). *Information systems for health services administration.* Chicago: Health Administration Press.

The best-laid plans. (1998). *Government Executive, 30*(9), 20-25.

Fleming, Q., & Koppleman, J. (1998). Earned value project management: a powerful tool for software projects. *Journal of Defense Software Engineering, 11*(7), 19-23.

Fleming, Q., & Koppleman, J. (1999). Earned value project management . . . an introduction. *Journal of Defense Software Engineering, 12*(7), 10-14.

Jones, R.L. (1999, March 11). *Healthcare information security: Issues and solutions.* Presentation to the University health System Consortium, Philadelphia.

Laufer, A. (1997). *Simultaneous manager: Managing project in a dynamic environment,* New York: AMACOM.

LeRouge, C., & Davis, P. (1999). Managing by projects. *Strategic Finance, 81*(5), 69-80.

Lewis, J.P. (1997). *Fundamentals of project management.* New York, AMACOM.

Lidow, D. (1999). Duck alignment theory: Going beyond classic project management to maximize project success. *Project Management Journal, 30*(4), 8-14.

Mumma, F. (1998). *Team-work and team-roles.* King of Prussia, PA: HRDQ.

Pearce, J.A. II, & Robinson, R.B, Jr. (1988). *Formulation and implementation of competitive Strategy.* Homewood, IL: Irwin.

Simpson, J. & Ramsaroop, R. (1999, March 26-30). *Information technology—Linking business strategy with customer needs.* Presented at the 2000 Congress on Health Care Management, Chicago.

Standish Group. (1995). *Chaos.* West Yarmouth, MA: Author.

Standish Group. (1998). *Chaos.* West Yarmouth, MA: Author.

Tierney, W.M., Miller, M.E., & McDonald C.J. (1990). The effect on test ordering of informing physicians of the charges for outpatient diagnostic tests. *New England Journal of Medicine, 322*(21), 1499-1504.

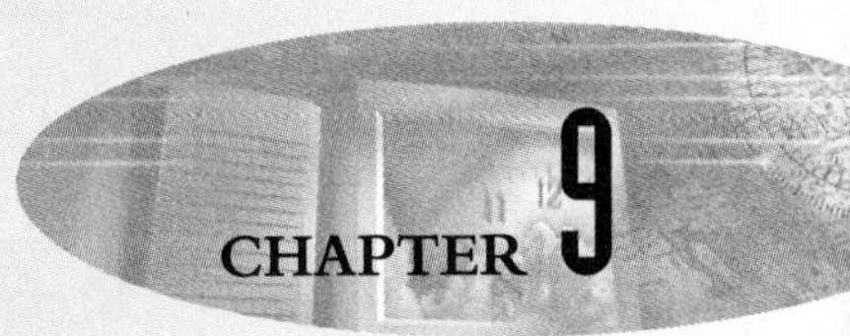

The Life Cycle of a Health Care Information System

JUNE BLALOCK CRAIG

Learning Objectives

Upon completion of this chapter, the reader will be able to:

1. ***Describe*** an effective, systematic approach for selecting a health care information system.
2. ***Develop*** a health care information system implementation plan.
3. ***Describe*** and ***compare*** two product evaluation methods.

Outline

Outline—cont'd

Support of Ongoing Product Development
- *Product User Group Activities*
- *Focus Group Design Projects*
- *Beta Projects*

A Decision to Change the Product

Key Terms

broken code
certified trainers
chief executive officer (CEO)
chief information officer (CIO)
deliverables
Gantt chart
go-live
information technology (IT)
matrix management
product evaluation
product implementation
product selection
Program Evaluation Review Technique (PERT) chart
request for information (RFI)
request for proposal (RFP)
return on investment (ROI)
rollout
stakeholders
strategic information plan (SIP)
suite of products
superusers
tactical information plan (TIP)
time line

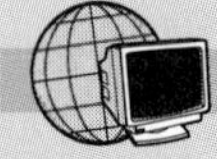

Web Connection

Go to the Web site at http://evolve.elsevier.com/Englebardt/. Here you will find Web links and activities related to the life cycle of a health care information system.

> *Computers in the future may weigh no more than 1.5 tons.*
> ***Popular Mechanics***
> (forecasting the relentless march of science, March, 1949)

The life cycle of a health care information system is made up of a logical sequence of events. The life cycle is initiated when a high-level vision or need is identified. The steps that follow describe the ever-increasing amount of specificity required to design or select a computer system. The design or selection is followed by the implementation process, which in turn is followed by an evaluation of the health care information system. The implementation of a health care information system is a complex and detailed set of work activities. Of the three subjects under discussion, only the management of an implementation project is reflected in a job title. This speaks to the standardization and precision for this one part of the work involved in the life cycle of a health care information system.

The question asked in system evaluation is "Has the need been met?" or "Has the goal been achieved?" Operational variables are identified and measured to determine the answer to the more global questions posed by the evaluation.

This chapter presents an overview of the processes and events in the life cycle of a health care information system. The steps in each major process are explained, and the skills necessary to complete each process are described. The major processes include the selection, implementation, and evaluation of a health care information system.

STRATEGIC INFORMATION PLAN

The vision or need that initiates the life cycle of an information system should be based on a **strategic information plan (SIP)**. The SIP presents the **information technology** (IT) mission and describes how IT will be used to address the specific information needs of an organization. It concentrates on the institutional goals of providing and promoting quality care for patients and the community while maintaining financial viability. The tasks needed to remain financially viable while providing patient care can be performed without a specific plan explaining how technology is to be used in the enterprise. However, the effective and efficient use of technology requires institutional planning. A SIP is a combination of a needs assessment analysis and problem/solution methods. The SIP is driven by the future plans for the organization, as well as by health care and IT trends. For example, the SIP should speak to the organization's policies and approaches concerning the use of evolving technology standards.

Goals

The goals of a SIP are as follows:

- Identify an overall IT vision that synchronizes with the mission and values of the organization.
- Formulate a logical series of product installations that result in integrated information access across the enterprise.
- Describe at a high level the necessary organization features, resources, and skill sets, with overall estimates of the time and money needed to accomplish the plan.

Consultants

The development of a SIP is a lengthy process that often involves the use of an outside consultant. An outside consultant can provide the plan with a high degree of objectivity. Consultants may be found in a number of ways, such as through the use of professional associations, networking, and referrals. All firms considered should be well established and known for the quality of their work. A proposal should be required, with site visits from the top potential consulting firms, before a consultant is selected.

Process

The process is driven by the **chief executive officer** (CEO) and other members of senior management, particularly the **chief information officer** (CIO). However, managers, physicians, nurses, allied health professionals, and daily operations people from all parts of the organization should be included in the process.

The primary staff members for the project are usually people who work in the IT division or department. Once upper management agrees on the need and general scope of the SIP, the assessment and planning process can begin. The assessment process begins by defining the questions to be asked and determining who will be asked the questions. If a consultant firm is to be used, consultants should be introduced and involved at this early stage of defining the key questions to be asked. Meetings and other "soft" technologies (the processes, approaches, or rules of an organization) are the primary tools employed by a consultant. The meetings can be with individuals or with groups, such as pharmacists or physicians. The meetings can also be drop-in meetings to accommodate the schedules of nurses, respiratory therapists, and others who work shifts and weekends. Written surveys and focus group sessions can be scheduled. The consultant can also be expected to review papers that describe a vision or a plan for a particular information system, as well as other formal planning documents.

Deliverables

The **deliverables,** or outputs from the consulting experience, should include multiple copies of the proposed SIP document, a copy of the document on a diskette, a summary of the SIP plus a graphical schematic of the plan, and a presentation to senior management and the board of directors. The senior management presentation emphasizes the identification of strategies, issues and concerns, and recommendations for solutions.

TACTICAL INFORMATION PLAN

The **tactical information plan (TIP)** breaks down the SIP into workable pieces, such as yearly budget projections, yearly product installation times, and a summary of the resources needed. The TIP can be organized by product, by what is called a **suite of products** (which are related products from the same vendor), or by a particular distinction, such as clinical products and business products. It is helpful if the organizational structure of the TIP is used to track budget dollars annually (e.g., by project or by suite). This is particularly necessary for large projects that cover two or three budget years. This information is used to project budgets for future projects.

The TIP is updated yearly, incorporating organizational changes and including changes in the SIP. For example, in the original TIP, a data warehouse for clinical information may be specified as part of "the clinical suite of products," along with an order entry system and a clinical documentation system. However, when the actual selection of these products is planned, it may be determined that a satisfactory clinical data mart product is not available in the marketplace. In this case the data mart for clinical information might be moved to a later time when it could be integrated with a financial data mart to create an institutional data warehouse. A planned data warehouse suite would be created to take advantage of this change. Changes such as these need to be updated and communicated to the CEO by the CIO. In turn, the SIP should be reviewed and updated annually to reflect changes in the TIP.

PRINCIPLES OF PROJECT MANAGEMENT AND ORGANIZATION

The successful implementation of the TIP is required to realize the goals of the SIP. To achieve this success, both project management and project organization are needed. Both project management and project organization are necessary, since neither is sufficient by itself.

Project management is the application of management principles to the administration of a project. No matter how small or how large the project is, following these principles can assist in reaching a successful outcome. These principles are shown in Box 9-1.

Project organization means that resources, both human and otherwise, are distributed effectively. When problems arise, swift action is taken to correct the problem. The first and most immediate step to be taken at the beginning of the project is the development of an organizational chart for the people assigned to the project. This chart illustrates where each person is in the chain of command and the reporting relationships. The chart also delineates how problems are escalated up the line of command. See Figure 9-1 for an example of a project organization chart.

Assignment of the Project Manager

In most IT projects, the CIO designates the project manager. The project manager will negotiate with organizational administrators to determine who will represent the project from specific areas and how these project members will fit into the project organization chart.

Box 9–1 Management Principles for Project Management

- Planning
- Application of sound "people skills," especially managing a group of people who may not report to the project manager (**matrix management**)
- Budget management
- Constant tracking of processes that make up the **time line** for the project, with special emphasis on projecting the next steps
- Identification of problems at any level as soon as possible and application of immediate solutions
- Good communication skills at all levels of the organization
- Coordination of skills across departments and divisions in the enterprise to get the job done

The effectiveness of the project manager has a major impact on the success of the project. A good project leader must be a good planner who requires planning at every level of the project organization, an excellent communicator who can express thoughts clearly and succinctly, a person who listens to people, and a person who can move successfully from the concept of a project goal to the smallest detail and back. Therefore a project manager should be an accomplished professional who has a long history of completing successful projects.

For clinical products, unlike with other areas of IT, the project manager should preferably be a person who has an in-depth understanding of the clinical processes unique to the specific health care setting. It is critical for the project manager to know the nature of the business being computerized. As a rule of thumb, clinical practice is best understood by individuals who have a clinical background (just as financial practice is best understood by individuals with a financial background). The learning curve of a nonclinician can be so steep that a clinical project managed by a person without a clinical background can be delayed or impeded. The appointment of a clinician as the project manager also increases the likelihood that the project manager will be able to understand very quickly the implications of clinically related implementation problems and have credibility with the clinical staff. A clinical project manager for a health care project will also provide a good sounding board when options for solving a problem are discussed. This give-and-take while trying to solve problems is often the most creative and fun part of the work of a project manager.

Organization of Resources

Once the project manager and staff are identified, the organization of resources can begin. The first step is usually a project team orientation in which the following items are discussed:

- Name of the project
- Goals of the project
- Overall reasons behind the project organization chart

When the project staff members are introduced, each person should be given the opportunity to give a brief overview of who he or she is and the details of his or her contributions to the project. It is recommended that members of senior management be present at this first meeting—to act as cheerleaders and supporters. Often, **stakeholders,** or persons who have a vested interest in the success of the project, come to this kickoff meeting to show their support of and interest in the project.

Management Planning

Management of Team Members

Another group of resources key to the success of the project are the various advisors from across the organization. Often, senior managers are

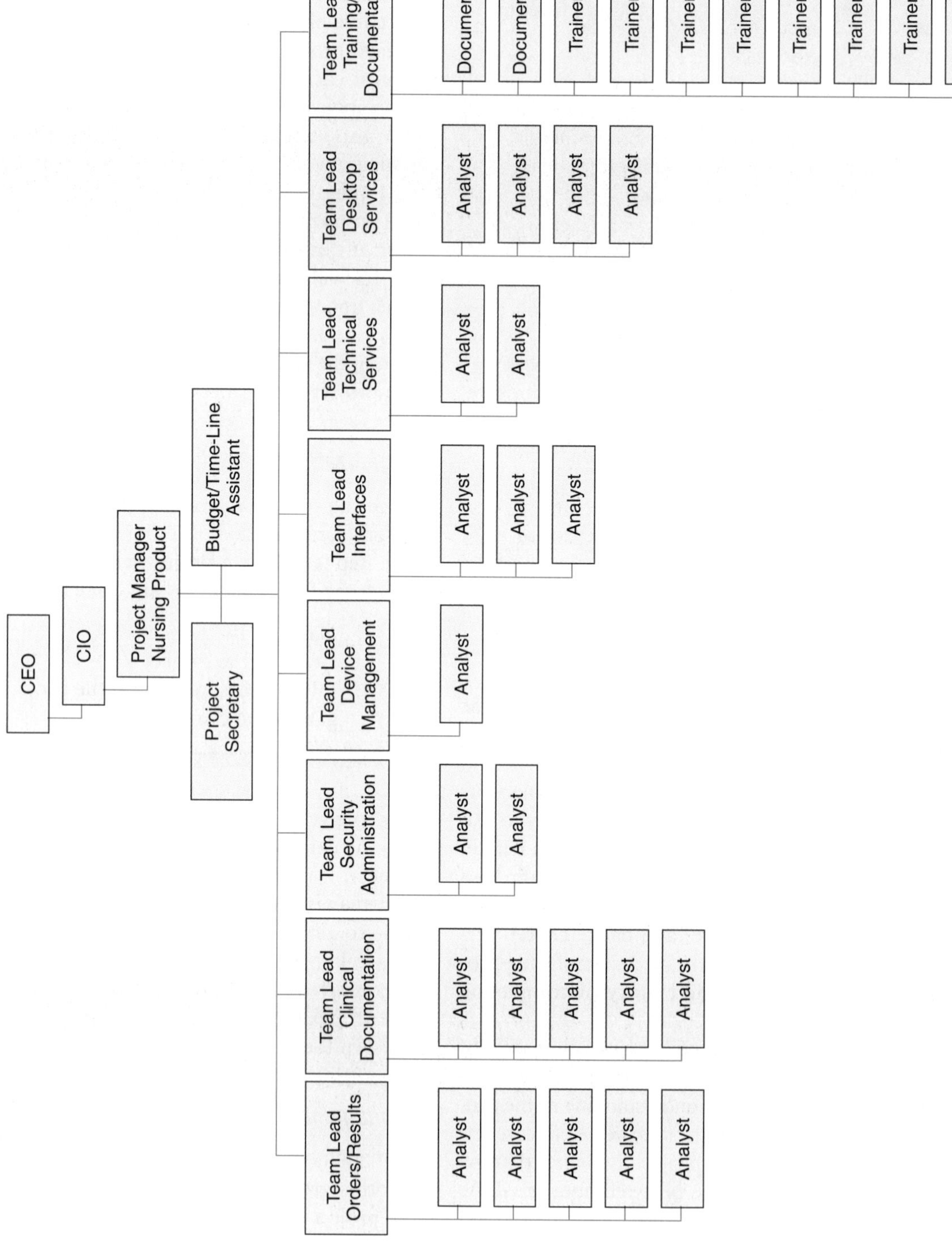

FIGURE 9–1 | Organizational Chart for the ACME Nursing Product Implementation

assigned to an information steering committee, which is the final escalation point for issues or problems related to the project. The CIO often chairs this committee. Steering committees usually focus on a specific area of the organization; for example, a clinical information steering committee provides oversight for all of the organization's clinical information systems. The committee provides a way for senior management to stay in the loop. Senior managers serve as advisors for the organizational areas that report to them. For example, the vice president for medical affairs can assist in organizing and training physicians concerning the new health care information system. Another example is that the vice president for public affairs, or in a smaller agency, the director of marketing, can assist in the promotion of the new information system.

People who are specialized in the work being automated are needed to help design the product and to solve problems that arise during the implementation. These people include general staff, department heads, and other directors. The IT staff members are organized to work with specific groups, depending on their specialties. A final chart is necessary to show how issues are moved up the organization's levels (i.e., escalated) until a final resolution is secured.

Medical staff is a special group who should have input into the planning process, including the design of the clinical information system, as well as input into the training plan. If there are other health care providers, including health care students, who will need to know how to use the product, then these groups should also be represented in the planning process. Small groups are usually more effective for gaining this type of input. A staff project member can set up and chair the meetings needed to gather the input.

The following are other groups that should be formed:

- An internal management group from which the project manager can seek guidance on specific project management problems. This group may meet weekly when the project is in full swing.
- A selection task force whose purpose is to select the product to be installed and implemented. The selection task force can also advise the project team on health care processes, as well as existing policies and procedures.
- Advisory groups who assist in the evaluation process.

The selection of the project members should involve other directors and the CIO. Usually project members are full-time IT staff members, but they could also include consultants, temporary employees for the project duration, clinical staff, or part-time employees. Any concerns about the management of IT staff members who report to another director should be discussed in full with the peer director before action is taken. For example, the implementation of a pharmacy information system should include a project team made up of IT professionals and members of the pharmacy staff who understand directly how the pharmacy operates.

Management of the Budget

Budget management policies, procedures, and workflow are defined early in the project. Some projects require changes from the usual procedures of the organization, such as when a vice president other than the CIO is responsible for the system. The following items could be included in the budget, and some of these may require that separate steps be delineated in the standards:

- Contract budget items
- Implementation costs, such as travel, training, and user group fees
- Hardware costs that are not included in the contract with the vendor for the health care information system, such as user workstations

- Operational items that are not put into the operating budget, such as printing costs, notebooks, telephone charges for projected analyst conference calls, and consultant fees

Monthly and yearly budget status summary reports must be done and distributed to senior management. A project team member may be assigned to assist in managing the budget.

Management of the Time Line

"Having a solid project plan is more that half the battle" (Weeks, 2000, p. 3). Management of the time line for the project may be easier if a software product management tool is used. MS Project is one such tool in general use that includes various presentations for the data, such as a time line, a **Program Evaluation Review Technique (PERT) chart,** and a **Gantt chart.** Information for the time line should be gathered quickly and put into the system so that the first meeting of the project team can be spent reviewing, changing, correcting, or adding to the proposed time line. The CIO usually has the final say on setting the **go-live** date, the date on which the system will be implemented at the health care institution; it is included in the composition of the time line. One way to ensure that this date is met is to emphasize early and repeatedly to all parties that the original date will be met, no matter what! Key to the successful management of a project is keeping the time line up-to-date. When the timeline is up-to-date, everyone can see where he or she is and where he or she is going.

When the first proposed schedule is being created, the following data are needed to provide complete documentation of the time line:

- A brief description of each task or subtask
- The number of days to complete each task or subtask
- Knowledge of who is responsible for the completion of each task or subtask
- Any concurrent tasks or subtasks

Once these items are entered and a start date is selected, the time line can be created. The end date may be identified, but it is more difficult to change the calendar of events when adjusting the schedule backward rather than forward. After the draft is complete, concurrent tasks can be organized.

After all parties have agreed to the time line, changes can be made only at the direction of the project manager. A project team member should be assigned to enter all updates and changes into the software.

METHODS OF SELECTING A VENDOR PRODUCT

Very few IT departments within health care organizations today actually develop (versus buy) a health care information system, although increasingly, IT organizations hire programmers to maintain purchased products. There are as many ways to select a vendor product as there are health care organizations. The key is finding the method that will bring the best results for the organization. Some of the ways to select a product depend on the way the IT function within the enterprise is organized (e.g., IT staff in each department versus IT staff organized into one enterprise-wide department or division).

The methods for selection, installation, and implementation of a product vary according to the number of user participants, the budget, and the time allotted to complete the selection. For example, a simple, niche software product for local use only may be needed to meet a minor but critical responsibility for one department. The system will not interface with any other system. Furthermore, IT has only to install the product on only a single workstation, with all other implementation tasks to be handled by the department. In this case the total cost of the selection, installation, and implementation is generally small, and the IT effort is for a short period of time. Contrast this niche product selection and implementation with a software product that is complex, with a large number of modules and functions that can be used enterprise-wide by a large number of clinical and business users with multiple interfaces. In this case the work done by the IT staff to support the users is significant with regard to selection, installation, and implementation processes, thus increasing the IT effort and lengthening the duration of the project. Also, in the latter case, the cost will be sizable, with the range of choices for selecting a product very wide as the organization continues to search for "the best way to find the best product."

INITIAL SEARCH FOR INFORMATION

The search for a product involves searching and evaluating information about potential products. Steps included in this process are shown in Box 9-2.

The selection of a viable product begins with a comprehensive search for information. The initial search process is usually directed by the project manager or by IT employees. One approach is to assign a person to research each potential vendor and report back to the members of the project team. Care must be taken to ensure that none of these "vendor liaisons" are co-opted by the vendor. Unfortunately, there is never a clear stopping point for research on a product; the quest for information can lengthen the process unless it is guarded against. The amount of information that is collected must be considered reasonable by the selection participants. Often the cost of the selection process provides a natural limit to what information can be collected.

Box 9–2 Steps of the Initial Search for Information

1. Literature, trade shows, and Internet search
2. Initial site reference calls and visits secured through informal networking or a literature search
3. Development of a request for information (RFI)
4. Market analysis
5. Development of a request for proposal (RFP)
6. Initial product demonstrations
7. Development of vendor and product requirements against which the various products can be compared and scored
8. Reference calls
9. Site visits to organizations that have experience with the product, talking with both IT personnel and end users (Curtin & Simpson, 2000)

Literature, Trade Shows, and Internet Review

The process starts with a search for the type of products that are sought by the organization. The purpose of this search is to acquaint the project management committee with the products currently on the market and to create a list of potential vendors. This search is important in that it can produce vital information about product types, actual products, or potential vendors. It is also important because it can assist the team in identifying superior background articles to be read by all members of the committee. This can include information on the selection process itself.

Other sources for information come from networked colleagues, Internet discussion groups, professional organizations (some recommend products), and publications that list vendors by type of product and present ratings by type of product. Some examples of journals that provide resource listings and ratings are *Health Management Technology* and *Health Care Informatics*. Each of these journals is also available in an online version. Trade shows and vendor booths at professional conferences can also be valuable sources of information. In these settings it may be possible to see several short demonstrations in a brief time. A serious effort should also include a search for new and relatively unknown Web-based products. If the selection process includes a search for newer types of hardware such as handheld or wireless technology, then the technical services area can provide leads or initiate another literature search for the specific type of hardware to evaluate (Nelson, 1999).

Request for Information

Once a final list of potential vendors is compiled, the process of elimination begins. Each vendor firm is sent a letter asking if it has a product that fits the inclusive functional model and technical standards (such as "Is the product HL7 compliant?") and if the firm would like to be included in this search. Often a "yes" to this query is followed by a request for information, allowing 2 to 3 weeks for responses. Vendors who do not respond or are unable to participate are removed from the list.

There is a significant difference between a request for information and a request for proposal (RFP). A **request for information (RFI)** is an official, written request to a vendor for general facts on a particular product. An RFI includes a general description of the health care organization, including key technical data and a brief description of the type of system needed. In addition, it asks for the following information: (1) product materials, including a list of modules, with the functions included in the modules relative to the type of product being selected; (2) financial reports, such as the company's annual report and any recent stock analysts' reports; (3) additional information about the firm, including any articles written about the firm or the product; (4) names of third-party consultants who are partners with the firm; and (5) a summary profile of the employees that describes how the employees' backgrounds are supportive of the product being offered. Sometimes the technical services section of the IT department asks for all of the detailed technical specifications for the software and hardware used by the vendor. Once this information is received, the technical staff members review these data to establish whether the technical specifications meet the standards of the organization's IT department. Products that do not meet technical specifications are eliminated.

Product information from the remaining vendors is reviewed for the breadth and depth of the product offering, and if even one of the areas does not meet the information needs of the organization, the vendor is eliminated from the product search. For example, if the health care institution is a large medical center and the vendor has focused on small community hospitals, the vendor will most likely be dropped. This step often reduces the size of the list to a workable choice of six or seven vendors, with a backup list of six or seven other vendors.

Market Review

The next step in selecting potential vendors is to perform a market analysis. The purpose of the market analysis is to identify those companies that can be expected to maintain financial viability for the long term. There is much more financial information available about publicly traded companies than about private companies, which are under no obligation to reveal the financial status of the company. Some health care organizations avoid dealing with private firms because they cannot establish financial viability. Public firms usually summarize their financial standing in reports to board members and stockholders. These reports should be included in the documents that are requested in the request for information. In addition, firms such as Standard and Poor's provide online analyses of vendor companies, as well as reports of mutual fund analysts who review vendors. A thorough financial analysis is imperative if one is to find a vendor that is expected to be fiscally sound for the foreseeable future.

Request for Proposal

A **request for proposal (RFP)** is an official, written request of a vendor for particular facts about a particular product, in this case an information system. The particular facts that are requested are stipulated in great detail in the request. Often the vendor is expected to comply with standards of content and form that are specified by the organization. RFPs often require a large investment in time and money by both the requesting organization and the vendor. Usually, government entities, as well as nonprofit organizations, require RFPs. Public agencies are often required to use an RFP process to ensure that there is no corruption in the process of vendor selection. These organizations usually have detailed guidelines that must to be followed. Many RFPs ask "yes" or "no" questions. One of the limits to this approach is that "yes" or "no" questions do not address serious issues such as how the system supports the organization's processes (Beinlich, 2000). For these reasons, some organizations do not send out traditional RFPs.

Initial Product Demonstrations

During the selection process there are two levels of product demonstrations. Initial product demonstrations are for the analyst staff—the staff members from IT who will be assisting the user selection task force. The second level of product demonstrations is to gain input from the end users. Initial product demonstrations for the analyst staff are helpful for several reasons. First, the demonstrations give the staff a chance to preview the product, and often it is this preview that reveals the product's strengths and weaknesses. This product information must be brought out in the demonstrations for the end users. Second, if the initial demonstrations are for 2 days or more, the analysts have time to test the system themselves and find any shortcomings. Third, this preview helps the analysts to identify any products that need to be eliminated from the vendor list. And fourth, these preview sessions allow the analysts to discern faults in the product that can be addressed on the more formalized site reference calls or visits.

Site Reference Calls and Visits

As part of the selection process, a survey of installed sites (organizations that have installed the system in question) should be done. If possible, site references should be identified in ways other than by simply asking the vendor. Vendors will usually provide the names of their most successful sites. The survey should be simple and not take too long to complete. The purpose of the survey is to determine other organizations' satisfaction with the selection of this vendor. Subtle but precise questions are required. Often this type of information can be obtained over the phone. Two sample questions are as follows: (1) "Are there modules that you bought from this vendor that you are not using, and if so, why not?" and (2) "If you had to do it all over again, would you choose this product; if yes, why, and if not, why not?"

Analysis of Findings

The analysts organize all of the background information into a summary report. This information is part of the material that is distributed for review by the selection task force. If done correctly, this initial collection of information shortens user learning curves and speeds up the entire process of selection. This investment of time is well worth the effort.

SYSTEM SELECTION TASK FORCE

The system selection task force is responsible for preparing a final report for senior management and/or the appropriate steering committee. This report includes recommendations concerning the product to be selected, as well as recommendations related to implementation of the product. The selection task force is composed of various representatives from each of the various communities of practitioners, who should be selected by their respective peer group. For clinical products, representatives should be selected from the medical staff community, from the nursing practice community, and from the ancillary services communities, especially from those ancillaries who will use the system for more than simply viewing the data. Representatives from other groups that support the practitioners who will use the product should also be included. Some examples include nursing secretaries or higher levels of nursing technicians. Other groups such as medical librarians, educators, and members of certain multidisciplinary committees such as patient education committees and adverse drug event committees are also helpful in the selection process. Sometimes one person can represent more than one group.

Clear expectations of task force members and an accurate estimate of the time involvement for such an effort should be presented to the candidates and their managers. If circumstances do not allow them to serve, they may be able to recommend an appropriate substitute who can. Reassuring candidates that they will be prepared by the IT staff to make the selection and that IT staff members will complete the documentation of the process may help allay worries about the time commitment.

A predefined structure for the task force is also helpful. The task force should have a chair who is a cheerleader in addition to being a member of the group; an executive director who actually leads the meetings; and members of the IT staff to support the task force as needed. The IT staff can support the task force in a number of ways, such as researching a product or type of functionality, planning site visits and making reservations, and documenting recommendations for senior management. The CEO, the CIO, and other organizational leaders who make it clear that there is administrative support for this group and their work should attend the first meeting.

Review of the Mission Statement and Problems to Solve

At the first meeting, the mission of the group is defined, and the problems to be solved by the selection of this product type are delineated. Both the SIP, which describes how IT will be used to address specific information needs, and TIP, which divides the SIP into workable pieces, should be helpful in meeting the mission of the task force, as well as in providing information about how the product that is eventually selected will solve organizational problems. The time line for the process is reviewed, with a reminder that the status of the project will be updated at every meeting to follow.

Preparation of Participants

It is important that the task force members operate at the same knowledge level when they begin to do their work. This can best be accomplished by the use of self-study units, which include pretests and posttests for use by the individual member. The self-study primer should be conceptual and include key terms that will be used by other participants and the vendors. Also included should be journal articles that describe the selection process as it was conducted at another organization. Although technical terms should be kept to a minimum, it is necessary for the novice user to understand the higher-level terms, such as *interface* or *clinical repository,* that should be included. These learning units should be pretested by a group of novice users to determine their effectiveness. Also, it is important to get input from experienced senior clinicians about the knowledge the end users need to participate effectively on the task force. This input should add variety to the type of information that is provided to novices as established by a study conducted by an informatics specialist at the North Carolina Memorial Hospital in Chapel Hill, North Carolina. The study found that the amount and type of information that is needed for a novice end user newly assigned to a selection task force depends on who is asked (Lytle, 1998).

Review of Findings

Once people agree to serve on the task force, they should receive a summary of the initial findings; the latest time line; and the dates, times, and places for all of the task force meetings, with an agenda for each meeting. Each task force member should be assigned to an analyst, and that analyst should be expected to follow up within 1 week of the mailing, indicating that the materials were mailed and asking if any questions need to be answered. If the selection process is not on a fast track, then a more collaborative approach can be used to develop the project tasks, time line, and calendar in discussions with the IT staff and end users.

Establishment of Agreements

Agreement on Vendor Expectations

One of the first activities of the task force is to agree on how the products will be evaluated, such as a list of expectations for the vendor, a list of functional requirements for the product, and a list of defined vendor support requirements.

A vendor expectation is an expected behavior of the firm (e.g., that the company spends a specific amount of money on research and development, thus indicating that the vendor is committing to the continual growth of the product). Another desirable vendor behavior is that a certain percentage of employees are health care professionals, indicating that software engineers did not develop the product in isolation. Along these same lines, it might be desirable for the firm to organize its resources into product management groups whose purpose is to develop and improve the software. This is another indication that the growth of the product is important to the vendor. Another example is an indication that the vendor is socially responsible. For example, a vendor may contribute a certain amount of money to an area of health care research.

Many vendors do not expect to be evaluated on more than their financial position. However, having additional expectations beyond financial viability demonstrates to the health care organization that the vendor is committed to the health care industry.

Agreement on Functional Requirements

One of the primary tasks of the selection committee is to develop a consensus on required and desired functional requirements. To expedite the group process, the supporting staff can develop an initial draft of the functional requirements. The easiest format for answers is a "yes" or "no" format, with a place provided for comments. The functional requirements that are developed will be used in writing the RFP and for planning vendor demonstrations. Sometimes different people in the same demonstration use a combination of the list and the scenarios. One way to test the initial draft is to present it to a focus group of users and add, change, or delete items as appropriate. There are also other ways to gather information about functions, such as by determining the number of clicks or screens it takes to perform a particular function or task. Each functional list of requirements should begin with general requirements about the user front end or computer interface of the product. This list should include such observations as "The graphical user interface (GUI) is fully Windows compliant," or "All reports are produced by an industry-standard, open system report writer."

Agreement on Vendor Support Requirements

Another criterion for evaluating vendors is based on the support that they provide to clients. This support includes methods of support during the implementation phase, as well as support provided once the system is implemented, when system and application maintenance is paid for.

Vendor support requirements for the implementation phase can include client training, client on-site support for events such as installation of hardware and loading of software, and actual analyst support during time periods when the product is being installed for use with real patients. One of the newer support offerings is a special way of developing the actual site data for building the product. This type of support is called a "fast-track implementation methodology" and includes schedules and techniques for interacting with practicing clinicians, as well as training schedules for the IT staff to learn how to take the data collected from practicing clinicians to build the system. Training support can be on site at the agency, or clients may need to go to vendor headquarters for training. These schedules and requirements are usually defined in the contract between the vendor and the health care organization.

Other requirements for support focus on when the product is implemented. Examples of these requirements include 7 × 24 × 365 support by analysts with backup for IT specialty areas such as system interfaces, application modules, or database administrators. Another support criterion is that maintenance payments, which are stipulated in the contract, should cover the cost of fixing **broken** programming **code** and the creation of specified enhancements to the current programming code.

Once the lists of vendor support requirements are completed, each member of the task force should receive a copy before the meeting in which the list is discussed. The final lists are distributed every time a new vendor presents its product.

Product Demonstrations

The product demonstrations for the selection task force and end users are scheduled and facilitated by the IT staff. The role of the IT staff is defined by the task force and can vary, depending on the confidence of the task force members and the amount of time needed for the demonstration.

Usually, task force members prefer that a health care professional employed by the vendor conduct the product demonstration. Two reasons for this preference are familiarity with health care terminology and knowledge of current procedures, trends, and issues in health care.

Ideally, a product demonstration should be on a live production system using the software that will be installed rather than demonstration software. The demonstration system should be able to produce reports during the demonstration and demonstrate live queries of the database. If these tasks cannot be demonstrated, then they are assumed to be unavailable and are marked "no" on the functional list for that particular vendor. Each vendor should be mailed the demonstration requirements; if they are unwilling to comply with the rules, this may be an adequate reason to eliminate them from the list of viable vendors.

Site Reference Calls and Visits

Vendors should also be prepared, at the end of the demonstration, to present a list of reference sites that may be called or visited. It is advisable to call and visit as many reference sites as possible, especially when the entire product has been tested at a large number of sites, module by module. Some reference calls will be made by the IT staff, but members of the task force must make the most crucial of the calls, especially when the call is to another health care professional. The same is true for the site visits. Standard forms for use in reference calls and site visits should ensure that the same information is gathered across vendors. The IT staff is usually prepared to create these forms once task force members provide the content. Furthermore, although staff members usually make calls to the IT people at a site, they may also be responsible for scheduling the calls for the task force's health care professionals.

Where possible, multiple site visits should be part of the selection process. This is particularly true when pieces of the product are in production at different sites. The task force needs to decide where to make site visits, the agenda for each site visit, and who from the task force and the IT staff need to go to which sites. Once all of the reference calls and site visits are complete, the IT staff can organize the forms and distribute copies of them to the task force members for their review. If there are questions about particular reference calls or site visits, follow-up conference calls can be scheduled with health care professionals at the site. Site visits can be costly, so these should be well planned in advance.

Final Review of Findings and Decision on the Product

Usually the decision is made on which product to purchase at the next-to-last meeting of the task force. The meeting should start with a general summary of the findings for each vendor and its product. Plenty of time should be given for discussion, as well as questions and answers. If there are members who want more information, then the decision can be delayed until the next meeting. If there are any major disagreements on which product to select, the CEO or the vice president for that department needs to get involved in the process.

Recommendations to Senior Management

At the final meeting of the task force, members should agree on the items to be placed in the contract and recommendations for the implementation of the product, including whether a pilot unit or the entire hospital should be undertaken. The final job of the IT staff for this product selection task force is to summarize the process and findings in a report for senior management. The final report includes the recommended product and vendor, as well as recommendations for the contract and implementation process.

NEGOTIATION OF THE CONTRACT

Contract negotiations are a series of very serious tasks that are usually performed by the CIO with approval by the CEO, the chief financial officer (CFO), and attorneys.

The final report from the selection task force may include recommendations for items to be placed in the contract. Examples of such items are the inclusion of a particular starter set for building screens and a database for specific clinical practices such as oncology or cardiology; the stipulation that the hospital or clinic will be a test site for new functionality that is very important to the hospital or clinic; and the provision of certain training classes during the implementation process. Other items that might be included are an agreement on the arbitration process and the placement of the actual programming code in a guarded location for the agency to access in the event that the vendor firm fails as a business. Also, it is wise to request a detailed explanation of all line items in the pricing schedule, especially those items that might be misinterpreted. All third-party software (software that is sold by another vendor but that is necessary to have in order to use the product being purchased) should be defined with a clear reason as to why it is required. It is also beneficial to require that the vendor define *all* vendor-specific terms and concepts referred to in the contract at the very beginning of the contract.

The most important items to the IT staff and the end users are those items that are necessary in order to get the implementation process started as soon as possible. Any time lines that are specified in the contract are usually discussed with the project manager and other project leaders. If the scope document is required to be completed before the contract is signed, then this is the first item on the immediate time line. No one wants to be held accountable for delaying the signing of the contract.

AGREEMENT ON THE SCOPE OF THE PROJECT

"The scope of a project" is the work that will be included in the project as defined by the limits of time, money, and resources. The scope may also include the content of the project as expressed by a list of modules or functions to be completed. The scope needs to be defined for implementation sites, interfaces between systems, and conversions of data from old systems to the new one. The more detailed the scope, the more protection is provided.

Defining the scope of a project is absolutely necessary to the success of the project. Within the predetermined limits of time, money, and resources, only a certain number of tasks can be accomplished. When requests are made for additional modules or functions, it may not be possible for them to be added, or there will have to be adjustments to the time, money, or resources allotted for completing the project. The term for adding items and not "paying" for them is called "scope creep," and it is a successful project's worst enemy. When the scope of the project is precisely defined, the rules are "etched in stone," and the rules cannot be changed in the middle of the game. Scope definition is an instrument of protection for the project manager.

The scope agreement includes the support schedule for each implementation date and time. Without a negotiated schedule for go-live, a project time line cannot be developed. Also included are the dates when the vendor staff will be available for certain tasks, such as installing the system's hardware and software, writing the interfaces, and preparing conversion data. This information is necessary for potential shortfalls in the vendor's support to be addressed while the time line is being developed.

The scope of the project may also include specific delivery and implementation dates for new releases. These releases bring new functionality. The client usually identifies which area needs the new offerings, either because this need has been defined in the contract or because certain characteristics are such that new functionality is required. For example, an update may include the delivery of code that allows automated patient records to be transferred among sites. Obviously, this code would have to be available for implementation at a second site. The vendor should also define the release frequency, the proposed numbers of releases per year, and when these releases will be delivered.

Product Specification Delivery

The contract includes an agreement between the vendor and the health care institution concerning the delivery of modules or functions from the vendor. The vendor should provide detailed specifications of these modules or functions to the client in writing, including the exact dates for delivery. For example, if the vendor has agreed to provide an order entry module, then detailed functions that are included in the module should be listed. Such a list might include "duplicate checking of an order upon entry, with a pop-up box that describes the duplicate order that is already in effect," or "the required entry and communication to the radiology department of the fact that a female patient who is scheduled for a radiological examination is pregnant." Once this list is provided to the health care institution, then negotiation and explication of the list usually ensue. Sometimes, functional specifications are grouped by module, and delivery dates are defined by module.

Multisite Delivery Agreement

The multisite delivery agreement defines when each site owned by an organization will receive the product. Often, this agreement uses the term *phase* to organize the delivery of programming code for each site. Additional sites can be added, and depending on the licensing agreement in the contract, additional money may be required.

Development of the Scope Document

The final scope document, when approved by both the vendor and the health care institution, is usually shared with all members of the project team. This enables the project team to answer questions and politely fend off attempts at scope creep. All persons who work on the project usually refer to this document throughout the life of the project.

FINALIZATION OF PROJECT DETAILS

On the basis of the information from the vendor contract, the implementation recommendations from the selection task force, the scope document, the experience of the people working on the project, and knowledge of current trends in health care implementation processes, the final planning for the **product implementation** can be completed.

Project Budget

The project budget is finalized to include the costs in the contract, as well as costs for additional hardware not included in the contract; costs for additional software products to supplement the product; costs for services from outside consultants and other resources; and operational costs, such as training fees, travel, and supplies. When budgeting is being done for both the selection and implementation of a project, a quick and simple method can be used to make sure that the budget is in line. See Figure 9-2 for a model of this method.

Project Time Line and Reporting

The project implementation schedule should be updated to include training for the analysts, travel time, training for the users, meetings that need to occur during the length of the project, and other tasks recommended by the vendor. The technical people may also need to add tasks after they have talked to the vendor. Weekly reporting on the status of the project includes a detailed review of the project time line.

FIGURE 9–2 | **Estimating the Amount of Time and Money Needed for a Project**

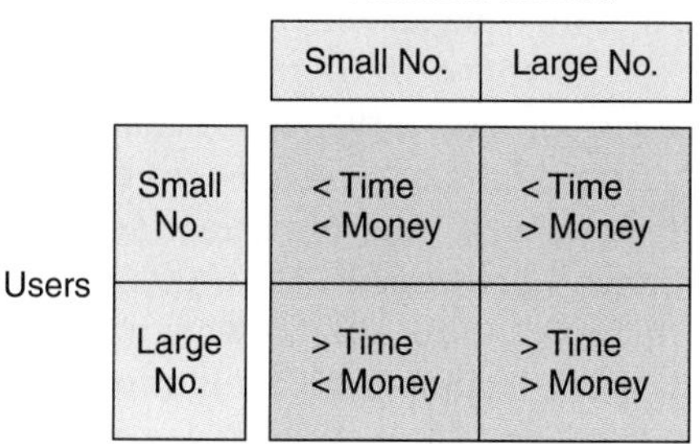

Project Members and Teams

The project organization chart should be reviewed for completion and to ensure that the various project areas and teams have been assigned the appropriate tasks and the needed resources. Vendors often provide their clients with charts that define the number of person-weeks needed for a particular task. Project roles and responsibilities are developed for each team leader and each team member. Included in the team leader's role is the responsibility for ensuring a consistent communication protocol among the team members, the vendor, and the entire project team. Examples of a communication protocol include weekly team meetings and weekly conference calls with the vendor.

Project Team Communication

The entire project team and the team leaders usually meet weekly. The continuity of the project is maintained by minutes taken at these weekly meetings. The weekly project team meetings are often held at the beginning of the week, early in the day, so that the activities from the previous week can be discussed and the current week's plans can be presented. The project time line is updated to reflect completed items, items that are now on the critical path for the project, items that need to be deleted, and items that need to be expanded, as well as any new tasks that need to be added to the time line. In addition to the weekly project meeting, the project manager will usually complete a conference call with his or her vendor counterpart, as well as a meeting with the internal management group director or CIO. The purpose of this last meeting is to coordinate the project with other ongoing projects. Sometimes concurrent projects create critical path issues. For example, the installation of a clinical documentation system may impact the concurrent implementation of a laboratory system or a radiology system.

Training of Team Members

The system analysts and programmers involved in the project usually require a training program to manage the software. For example, the training of the analysts on how to build the application screens, interfaces, or device tables must be scheduled and documented on the time line. Scheduling of training involves scheduling the individuals requiring the training, the trainer, and the resources needed to complete the training. These resources include identifying the training space, which should be secured early in the planning. If there are a number of projects or teams being trained at the same time, access to the training space can become very competitive. Training room preparation includes the loading of software and the requisitioning of audiovisual aids.

It should be noted that many of the practices outlined above will vary from institution to institution. What will not vary is the importance of tracking the budget, the time line, and the issues. Standardizing how each of these items is tracked early in the project in effect trains all project members on the correct procedure for each.

Issue Tracking

Each project will experience a list of issues or problems that develop as the project progresses. A systematic procedure is used to document and track each issue or problem. The first type of issues includes those that must be resolved by the vendor. Usually the vendor has special forms that are completed to track these issues. However, each team should always track its own issues and report them to the project manager as needed. The project manager relates the issues and any related problems in a call to a counterpart at the vendor company. The second type of issues that need to be tracked includes those that are internal to the health care organization. Examples of these issues include changes in required policies and procedures, work-arounds that are necessary because of software limitations, training issues, hardware problems, and internal issues that should be escalated to the appropriate information steering committee. Software is available for tracking these issues. Using software that will print out current status reports for each active issue can make it much easier to track issues. The software usually allows for the entry of a history for each issue. With this feature the person reviewing an issue can determine what has been done to date to solve the problem.

FAST-TRACK DESIGN-AND-BUILD METHODS

Once the software has been purchased, a significant amount of time will be spent designing, building, and customizing the application for the health care institution. Fast-track design-and-build methods have been developed to shorten the time required for collecting the information needed to build the software product. This method was devised by organization development professionals and assumes that the analyst team members can organize and facilitate the large number of groups that are needed to do these tasks in approximately 12 to 14 days. To be effective, these fast-track sessions require a serious commitment from the entire user population, especially the leadership who will have to cover for all those who are away from work. These sessions also serve as a forum to discuss the important human change issues that directly impact the success of information system implementations (Lorenzi & Riley, 2000).

With health care reimbursement shrinking and margins dropping, hospital administrators are requiring that large-scale implementations be completed more quickly. Fast-track design-and-build methods are one answer to this requirement. On the other hand, project managers also worry that speed will reduce the quality of the implementations to such an extent that there will be a negative impact on clinical user work and documentation.

The first step in using one of these methods is to gain the approval of the organizational leadership. For these methods to be successful, everyone involved, including the vendor, must understand the meeting attendance requirements. The IT staff should project the number of days that each participant must meet. The IT staff must also identify the dates and times for all of the meetings. The product vendor or the consultant should be able to assist with the development of these numbers and schedules.

Once the meetings are scheduled, the first session is opened. There may be changes in the numbers and schedules after the first meeting because "reality happens." A typical first meeting is described as getting a sense of that reality. The meeting is opened with support and "cheerleading" remarks from senior management. The project leader, who may be assisted by either a consultant or a vendor representative, will direct the meeting. The project leader, consultant, or vendor representative will describe the planned activities for the day. It is then that the work sessions begin. At the end of the day, users from each group describe the progress that their group has made and discuss how they think that the sessions can be improved on for the next meeting.

A generic example is a group charged with developing the screens and the database for a clinical documentation application focused on managing patients' pain. The group would first discuss the procedure and format for assessing a patient's pain. The group could decide to use a 10-point scale for assessing the degree of pain. Not only would the group define the meaning of each number on the scale, but also the group could ask that a place on the screen be allocated for documenting the exact words that the patient uses to describe his or her pain. The analysts would assist the users in drawing the screen and in defining the exact wording that would be required to support the assessment process. These words would make up the database portion of the design.

From the generic example it is very easy to see what other groups would need to be organized to help build a complete documentation system. For example, one additional group would be the radiology team. This group would be made up of representatives from the diagnostic services and radiology departments, as well as representatives from the nursing units where radiology orders are entered. This team would be responsible for standardizing the wording of each procedure; identifying the information that it is necessary for the radiology department to have in order to perform the test; and standardizing various codes such as frequency codes, transportation codes, and codes for why a radiology procedure has been ordered by the physician. Other teams could include a laboratory team with members from each section of the laboratory department; nurses and nursing secretaries; a skin care team with skin care specialists from across the enterprise, an ostomy nurse, and several nurses from various units that have patients with skin problems; a neurology team with neurologists, nurses from the neurology units, and a manager from a neurology unit; and a medications and intravenous team with nurses from a variety of nursing units and pharmacists who work in the pharmacy itself or on specific nursing units supporting specific protocols.

The purpose for all of the groups is to define the data, the screens, and the reports that should be designed and built into the system to meet their practice needs.

Once the needed information is collected, the system is designed and built. End users from the group return to validate that the system is what they designed. Usually the end users who validate the system participated in building the system, but sometimes it is good to have a fresh second group of end users validate the work of the first group. Senior management usually selects the people who participate in the fast-track design process. As a general rule, the more end users who participate, the better the product.

And finally, at the end of the meetings for the fast-track methodology, the analysts can begin to build the system, knowing that they have received an amazing amount of information in a very short period of time.

IMPLEMENTING THE PROJECT

While the application is being built, the implementation of the project is planned. Four specific plans should be developed: (1) the communication plan, (2) the training and documentation plan, (3) the command center plan, and (4) the go-live plan. In addition to these plans, downtime and recovery procedures should be developed by a small group of analysts and end users. The end users should be people who understand in great detail the functioning of the departments for which the procedures are being written. Once the analysts learn which application modules are going to be implemented, then this special team can begin to work on downtime and recovery procedures. The four plans and the downtime and recovery procedures should be validated by another group of users and then approved by management.

Developing Plans

Develop the Communication Plan

The communication plan describes how the project team will inform and explain the project across the health care organization. Basically, the plan describes in great detail how the system is going to be marketed to the end users. The plan should be developed with representatives from each user group who will be impacted by the implementation of the system, such as physicians, pharmacists, and nurses. The team leader for training and documentation is often responsible for developing the communication plan. Marketing personnel can also be helpful in developing the plan. Either the CIO or the CEO can approve the plan for implementation. Once the plan is approved, the actual tasks defined in the plan are added to the time line. In addition, any money that is approved for the implementation of the communication plan is transferred to the project budget. One way to kick off the communication plan is to have a contest to name the product.

Develop the Training and Documentation Plan

The training plan details when and how trainers, superusers, and end users will be prepared to use the application. The trainers may be supplied by the vendor, or there may be staff from the health care institution that are trained for this role. An additional quality control measure is to have **certified trainers** in the role of training others in the software being implemented. **Superusers** are unit-based professionals who assist with training and/or end user support for their units during implementation.

The training plan describes when training will start, when makeup classes will be held, how long training sessions will last, and what is included in the training. It also includes a summary of training requirements. This information must be shared early with the unit or department managers so that they can include the training costs in the unit budget and plan for the absence of the end users who will be trained. Training for personnel should be started no earlier than 4 to 6 weeks before go-live. Four weeks is optimal; however, depending on the number to be trained, the number of trainers, and the number of the training rooms, a 4-week time period is sometimes not possible. Most project managers are waiting for the ever-elusive "intuitive system" that will eliminate the need for training time, knowing that training time is one of the biggest time drains for implementations.

In developing the training plans, the leader for training and documentation is concerned with ensuring that the most appropriate learning methods for the people who will be trained to use the product are used. This includes the use of adult learning principles, since most of the health care professionals being trained on products today are adults (Draves, 1997). Web-based training as an alternative to more traditional methods should also be considered (Abernathy et al., 1999).

In addition to the training plan, the leader for training and documentation will also develop the training materials and user documentation required for the project. These documents are user reference manuals, frequently asked question (FAQ) sheets, training scripts for the trainers, classroom handouts, competency tests, and "quick help" documents. If these materials can be posted online, the "walk-the-units" work can be decreased (Pierson, Hesnard, & Hass, 2000). Even more important, end users, superusers, and trainers will have quick and easy assess to these materials when needed. Once the training plan is completed and approved by the project manager, all of the tasks from the plan are added to the project time line.

Develop the Command Center Plan

The project manager should develop the command center plan that details the requirements (or inventory) for a usable command center. With a multisite implementation, the number of command centers is equal to the number of sites where the product will be implemented. Sending an early alert to each of the sites as to when a room will be needed, the proportions of the room, and other criteria for the command center room is an excellent idea. The inventory may have to be estimated for the first go-live. After the first go-live, the inventory can usually be completely defined. The inventory may include office supplies, workstations, and telephone lines. The workstations may have to have special software loaded for those who will be working in the command center, such as interface engine software, software to view print cues, and software to view feeder systems such as registration systems. Network and power cables for the workstations and the telephone lines may have to be brought into the command center. Other necessary items include tables and chairs, food and drink, pagers, and forms for reporting issues and change-of-shift reports.

Develop the Go-Live Plan

The go-live plan is a subset of the project time line. Usually these steps are pulled out of the time line and copied for distribution and discussion with a variety of people. These items lead up to the day of go-live and the first few hours of go-live. Typically, these steps involve so many people that to copy the entire project time line would be prohibitive in cost. Examples of these items are as follows:

- Dates and times that the list of patients or census should be reconciled with the actual patient population. (This would be done, for example, to ensure that the census information from the registration system is being properly interfaced with the new laboratory or pharmacy system.)
- Lists of communication tools such as memoranda and eMail, and when they are to be distributed. (For example the memoranda sent to people who interact with the department that is installing a new system would let them know the dates, times, and process of installations and would include a list of activation meetings at which the details of the go-live plan will be reviewed, analyzed, and discussed until every detail is fine-tuned.)

At least three times before the go-live day, the plan is reviewed in meetings with any personnel who will be impacted by the implementation of the system so that everyone is clear as to what must be done and by whom. If the preparation for go-live is even more detailed than the plan states, then other handouts are developed. For example, during the go-live of the implementation of a clinical documentation system, the current data from the old system (be it manual or automated) must be input en masse into the new system. Handouts to explain how these data are to be entered are extremely detailed, and the coordination activities of many people have to be completed.

Finalize the Downtime and Recovery Procedures

The downtime procedure is written to give users guidance during system or network downtime. Downtime procedures for orders and results can be simple to write but must be developed in coordination with the interfaced ancillary IT departments. Clinical documentation is a much more complex procedure that usually requires the review of nursing leadership. Since there are differences among health care institutions, the procedures must be specific by site even in a multisite installation. Finally, the downtime procedure should be reviewed for any last-minute changes suggested at the go-live meetings.

Manage Multiple Rapid-Design Sessions

Usually the first two fast-track design-and-build meetings (lasting 2 days each) occur very early in the project, and most of the resources available to the project are included in the process. In addition, facilitators, timekeepers, and scribes are identified for each discussion group, and someone from each group is assigned to summarize the activities of the group for the day. The final activity of each day is an end-of-day session where the summary reports are shared. These end-of-day reports are helpful for making sure that the decisions of one group do not have a negative impact on the decisions of another group. It is important that everyone who is participating in the rapid-design session attend these end-of-day sessions, despite the fact that some groups may have completed their work before midday. Otherwise, the overall work of the groups may become disjointed. Summary reports of the work done on the preceding day should be reproduced in the form of a newsletter that is made available to all participants, as well as to the leadership of the organization.

Once the first fast-track meetings have been completed, the design-and-build information and decisions are organized. The project analysts who have been assigned to work on the related application modules usually complete this process. The information is organized into two groups: screen builds and tables of information (that will be the content of the drop-down boxes, the buttons, the lists of data, etc). Ongoing feedback is extremely important; most teams continue to work closely with the appropriate analysts to review and make improvements on the screens, in the information, and in the way in which the two flow. The process of reviewing and rereviewing the screens, the data, and the workflow processes is perhaps the most challenging part of the entire implementation. Attention to detail is required to ensure that the product is complete and consistent across all of the application modules.

Implementing Plans

Organize Design Requirements and Build the System

Once the design is complete, each of the analysts applies the user design-and-build aspect to the part of the vendor starter set for which each has responsibility. Sometimes starter set screens work, and sometimes they do not. This is why the design work done by the users is so important. If a starter set screen is unusable, then a new screen must be built from scratch. Also, whenever possible, everyone must use the same build conventions. This means, for example, that ideally the "close button" is at the same place on every screen and that the "date and time field" has only one format across all of the screens. The medical records committee defines commonly approved enterprise-wide abbreviations that must be used to build the tables that support the screen input process. Where possible, a standard health care nomenclature or terminology system should be used so that health care summary statistics can be easily compared with data from other entities. As the development and acceptance of such standards increase, health care institutions are better able to compare their outcomes with others across the country. After the screens and tables are built, they are compared with user recommendations to ensure that all items have been included.

Test the System and Conduct User Validation Sessions

The next step—testing of certain application and interfaces—is critical to the success of the first go-live. As the vendor releases upgrades, further testing will be done to ensure the success of future go-lives. Testing is the method used by analysts to ensure that the application actually works the way it was planned to work (Gibson & Hughes, 1994). All members of the project team are involved in testing some portion of the product. Detailed coordination and monitoring are required for the system to be thoroughly tested. End users are included in the testing of the product. This not only helps them to understand how the application actually functions but is also helpful in the identification of problems with the use of the application. The six different kinds of testing are shown in Box 9-3.

All testing should be recorded in detail on forms designed to provide for this documentation. Documentation of testing is tedious but very important. For example, a patient event could take place requiring risk management personnel to ask for validation that testing was done and by whom. Documentation also is used to alert analysts who are testing a new release as to how certain functions were tested in the past. Software testers who do not document test findings well or at random generally do not know how to test, except by a sort of "freelance" method, which is really just a unit test. A test plan should be developed by each team leader and submitted to the project manager for his or her review.

Box 9—3 Types of Testing

- Unit testing—tests within a module
- Program testing—tests between modules, such as testing the data entry screens and the output display screens
- Scenario testing—tests all of the modules (but without interfaces) in the product through the use of chart-based patient scenarios
- Integrated testing—tests the order entry screens, the departmental interfaces, and the results reporting output screens
- Report testing—tests all of the standard reports from the product
- User validation testing

Finalize the Build and Move the Product to Production

Once testing is completed, the fixes can be applied to the system for retesting and documentation. At some point after the testing has been completed and the required changes have been made, the database is frozen. No further changes are allowed unless approved by the project manager. The database on the test or quality platform is frozen in order to have a stable product running for at least a month before the go-live date. One month seems to be the optimum time because it is not so long as to hold up changes that are desired, and it is not so short that the actual programs do not get a chance to run and be determined to be stable. During the last month the test application—where the designing, building, and testing were done—is copied. The copy becomes the production application that eventually contains real patient data. Once the production database is ready, the interfaces are fed into the application, preparing the new system for the entry of current patient data on the go-live day. One final test of a system is the use of a pilot nursing unit where the system as well as the workflow changes and policies and procedures that support the application are given a "dry run" (Bush & Ebel, 1996).

Manage Go-Live Activities and Post–Go-Live Support

And finally, go-live day comes, the final pre–go-live activities are initiated, and the project command center becomes operational. The fact that these activities were planned for some time and reviewed in meeting after meeting increases the potential for a successful go-live day.

The length of around-the-clock post–go-live support is negotiated early on with the leadership of the department or the site. If training is done well and the system is stable, then 1 week of support after go-live is usually sufficient. After 1 week the staff is usually able to rely on their superusers and the on-call analysts for support. Besides providing user support, the first week after go-live is used for makeup classes and new-employee orientation. Once go-live support is complete, the command center is dismantled.

Manage Upgrades and Roll Out the System to Additional Sites

The first successful go-live is followed by system upgrades that come from the vendor and by **roll-out** of all of the modules to the remaining sites. The vendor should provide a list of scheduled upgrades. The contents of the upgrades are very important and sometimes determine if a module can be rolled out further. This part of the process is difficult to manage, but a skilled project manager can do it well by communicating effectively with the vendor, planning for the future changes, and monitoring to see that all of the expected product fixes and enhancements arrive on time with the promised code.

The installation of an upgrade is managed just as the original system installation was managed. Releases need to be moved to the test or quality database, tested, and implemented with training and/or documentation for the user.

For those sites that are 1 year beyond the fast-track design-and-build meetings, a current-state analysis is required. This determines if the current operations of the unit or the department have changed since the original meetings were held and whether the changes require a modification to the system that was designed and built. Despite the best efforts to standardize across an enterprise, sometimes such standardization cannot be done. With the use of detailed information from the project manager and the CIO, senior leadership determines the degree to which these changes are challenged.

PRODUCT EVALUATION METHODS

A **product evaluation** may be conducted in several ways. The most common method is to do a cost/benefit analysis, which establishes what the costs (direct and indirect) are for the product implementation and the benefits of implementing the product. Potential benefits are identified before the product is implemented. The potential benefits determine the baseline statistics to be gathered before and after the implementation for a comparison analysis. Benefits analysis addresses issues such as (1) productivity, (2) quality-of-care measures (which may be difficult to quantify), and (3) task performance levels for tasks performed now and after the implementation. Task performance measures deal with items such as "the number of medical records processed" or the "the number of charts completed by physician."

An evaluation of the **return on investment (ROI)** is a financial analysis that compares the outlay of dollars for the product, the **product selection,** and the product implementation with any reductions in the cost of doing business. Usually this type of analysis must be performed by an outside consultant to be considered valid. The vendor should not be allowed to participate in ROI activities because of the possibility of a conflict of interest.

Another way to evaluate the implemented product is to survey the users of the system, asking for feedback on the negative and the positive impacts of the product. These questions have to be worded carefully to avoid skewing the answers. The results from such a survey can help to identify problems that need to be fixed but have not yet been reported. This type of analysis should be done after the end users have completely adjusted to the new application.

The final type of analysis is system utilization studies. These analyses often focus on a particular problem area and are designed to identify possible solutions to the problems in that area. Another kind of system utilization evaluation is a current-state analysis of a particular combination of functions, such as clinical documentation, which can include documentation of intake and output, vital signs, allergies, advance directives, medication and intravenous line charting, assessments, interventions, flowsheet charting, and charting on a clinical path. In a current-state analysis of this type, the analysis is done not to find out how current operations have changed, but to determine if the users are using the functions as they were trained to do during go-live training. The comparison between a standard of practice and the actual work that is being done is informative for organizational decision makers and managers, as well as end users. Most hospital administrators wish to know that an application that the organization bought is really being used as intended. Once a current-state analysis is completed, a summary is presented to the operations manager, who then helps the analyst develop ways to improve utilization of the product for the area under study.

MAINTENANCE

The maintenance period in the life cycle of a health care information system should be one of stability, as well as steady but controlled growth and improvement for the software product. In return for maintenance fees, clients can expect two services. First, the system is expected to be stable and working well. Second, the software is expected to grow and improve through upgrades and rewrites.

Complete software rewrites might occur during a maintenance period. If a total rewrite of the product is necessary, then great changes should be anticipated. Even though a complete rewrite means planning for another large-scale go-live, the new product is usually worth it to the end users. During this time, training on the new product, as well as any needed remedial training, must be done. The users should also see growth in their skill sets during this time, which should lead to improvements in productivity and quality care or, at the very least, improvement in the documentation of the quality care.

If these changes do not occur, then the health care institution has every right to conclude that the product is not stable or is not growing to reflect the improvements in health care or patient management. Support issues should be discussed with the vendor. Negotiations often take place to ensure that the terms of the maintenance contract are being met. In extreme circumstances the vendor might be found to be in breach of contract and contractual binding arbitration or judicial remedies may be sought.

SUPPORT OF ONGOING PRODUCT DEVELOPMENT

To protect the investment of money and time in a health care information system, the product must continue to be supported and developed. The organization that purchased and implemented the system must support and develop the health care information system using change control processes to manage requested changes. The purpose of change control is to make sure that the implications and reasons for each request are evaluated before being approved. Changes should advance the product and add value to the work of the end user. The vendor must also support and develop the product by writing new programming code.

Product User Group Activities

One way to help the product to grow is to work with fellow users to provide group feedback and input to the vendor. The best way to do this is by working through a user group composed of health care institutions that are using software from the same vendor. Some professionals believe that a user group should be founded and organized as a separate entity from the vendor. Although the user group should work with the vendor to plan user group meetings, the vendor should not dominate and control the user group. The most effective user groups have successful interactive communication between the members and the vendor.

Ideally, health care informatics specialists should be able to attend at least one user group meeting over a span of 3 or 4 years. Their participation should be coordinated so that each of the attendees can contribute to the user group, as well as bring important information back to the health care institution. For example, an analyst could provide a presentation at the user group meeting or serve as an officer of the group. Many user groups also offer electronic mailing lists, which is an especially good way for users to help each other and communicate freely about common issues and problems. Sometimes users who are using the same series or release of the product work together even more closely to solve common problems with the product. Sometimes a small subgroup of users like this can exert a much greater influence on product development than its size might otherwise indicate.

Focus Group Design Projects

Another way to support the product is for informatics specialists to volunteer to participate in large- or small-scale efforts by the vendor to change the design of a module or to add additional modules to the product offering. A focus group on clinical path documentation or a focus group on new and improved flowsheet support are examples of this type of participation. In this way the analysts who work with the user groups can present how their organization uses paths or flowsheets. Sometimes health care providers from a specific practice group will also participate, especially if this allows them to influence the development of a new module in which they are interested. Participation in such a group might mean that the organization agrees to be a test site for the new module, but this is not a requirement of participation.

Beta Projects

A beta site is a health care institution where a new application is first installed and tested. The CIO must agree to the proposal to be a beta test site. Serving as a beta site obligates the organization to a substantial investment of time and effort. Both parties sign a beta test site agreement. Ideally, the vendor agrees to assume the same amount of risk as the health care organization. Often this means that the vendor will provide the final product to the organization for no charge. The organization has in fact paid for the product through the use of the health care site, as well as the time and expertise of the staff. Users usually like to be a beta site, since they have a great deal of input into shaping the product. Working on a beta site can also be exciting for analysts because it affords them opportunities to speak, to publish, and to gain even more influence over the product.

A DECISION TO CHANGE THE PRODUCT

Why would any organization decide to change from one health care information product to another? This step seems to be asking for more work on everyone's part, since it will result in a full go-live effort and a substantial expenditure of new resources.

Several reasons come to mind. First, the product could simply become out-of-date, with the cost of getting it up to speed being more than the vendor is willing to assume. Second, a clearly superior product may have reached the market, and financially and operationally the move to the new product may be determined to meet the organization's needs. Third, the IT used to support the product may be out-of-date, and thus it may be too costly to maintain and use. If maintenance costs are high enough, a new product using new technology may be a more viable solution. Fourth, the vendor may have financial problems or plan to go out of business. Fifth, the product may have been removed from the market by the vendor and therefore must be replaced. Sixth, the health care organization is in flux (a merger, a purchase, new leadership, etc.), and it may be exploring new products. Despite a change in the product, the most important directive for the organization always remains the same: to provide the best IT product for clinical users.

CONCLUSION

The life cycle of a health care information system is complex and involves many different kinds of work activities. The range and depth of knowledge and experience required by a health care analyst today varies from setting to setting. As the field of health care informatics grows and develops, standards of practice will emerge to enable health care informatics specialists to manage different kinds of work activities more efficiently and effectively. The outcomes will be better choices in health care information systems with improved implementations and more useful ways to evaluate the efficacy- and productivity-enhancing features of health care information systems.

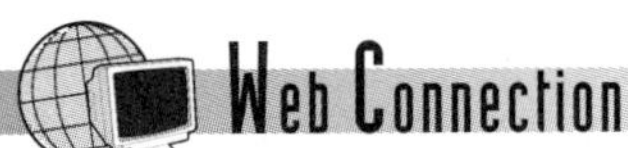

Web Connection

The life cycle of a health care information system is a complex sequence of events and processes that range from strategic planning for organizational information technology requirements to maintenance of the chosen applications and systems. The identification of organizational information management needs is the beginning of the life cycle of a health care system. Selection, implementation, and evaluation are the most common processes that occur during the life cycle of a health care information system. The Web Connection activities for this chapter will explore the resources available for systematically developing and managing the life cycle, while highlighting its different stages.

discussion questions

1. You are a newly hired health care informatics specialist in the IT department. Your first assignment involves an emergency department system selection. Your manager has asked that you do a literature search on the product selection process to identify the latest techniques being used by other health care organizations. Your manager also encourages you to interview your peers for any good tools and any good processes for selecting a product. You are welcome to come up with workable solutions yourself. List and explain those tools, processes, and items that you would recommend to your manager.
2. You are assigned to be the project manager for the implementation of a multidisciplinary critical path product. You helped select the product and have a basic understanding of the product. Your manager has asked that you develop a schedule for the implementation and rollout of this product to the seven sites in the enterprise, with special emphasis on the first site. Make the multiple sites as varied as you can, and make sure that you identify the first go-live site. Then develop the schedule, and explain why you made the decisions that you did.
3. The health care organization for which you work has had a clinical documentation product in use for over a year. In an effort to improve system utilization, you have been asked to lead a "special current-state analysis" to determine the quality of system utilization at the first hospital to implement the product. Explain how you will go about doing this evaluation.

REFERENCES

Abernathy, D., et al. (1999). Trenz. *Training and Development, 53,* 22-43.

Beinlich, J. (2000). Rescuing failing projects. *Advance for Health Executives, 4,* 101-104.

Bush, A.M., & Ebel, C.A. (1996). Testing an electronic documentation system. *Nursing Management, 27,* 40-42.

Curtin, L., & Simpson, R. (2000). . . . @ the speed of thought? Tips to help choose a productive clinical system. *Health Management Technology, 21,* 40.

Draves, W.A. (1997). *How to teach adults.* Manhattan, KS: The Learning Resources Network.

Gibson, M.L., & Hughes, C.T. (1994). *Systems analysis and design.* Danvers, Mass: Boyd & Fraser.

Lorenzi, N.M., & Riley, R.T. (2000). Managing change: An overview. *Journal of the American Medical Informatics Association, 7,* 116-124.

Lytle, K. (1998). *Assessing learning needs: Involving clinicians in computer system selection.* Chapel Hill: University of North Carolina School of Nursing.

Nelson, L. (1999). Step-by-step guide to selecting mobile wireless devices. *Nursing Management, 30,* 12-13.

Pierson, P., Hesnard, D., & Hass, J. (2000). Intranet systems offer fast access to policies and procedures. *Nursing Management, 1,* 13.

Weeks, A. (2000). Learn to juggle a project budget. *TechRepublic,* February 24, pp. 1-3. Retrieved March 1, 2000, from the World Wide Web: http://www.techrepublic.com/article.jhtml?id+r006200000244use01.htm.

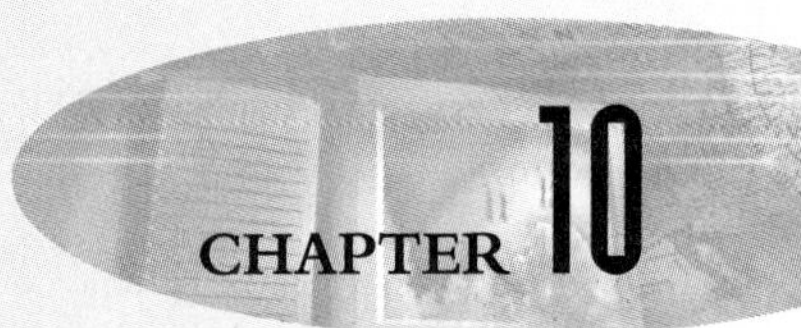

Electronic Health Records

KATHLEEN MILHOLLAND HUNTER

Learning Objectives

Upon completion of this chapter, the reader will be able to:

1. ***Describe*** current perspectives on the desired features of an electronic health record and an electronic health record system.
2. ***Identify*** the potential costs and benefits of an electronic health record and an electronic health record system.
3. ***Describe*** the relationships among the electronic health record, the Internet, and the growth of electronic health care (eHealth care).
4. ***Identify*** significant issues affecting the adoption of electronic health records.

Outline

The Electronic Health Record
Need for the Electronic Health Record
Historical Perspectives
- *Problems With the Paper-Based Record*
- *Early Solutions*
- *A Call for Action: The Institute of Medicine Report*
- *Public and Private Responses*

Functions and Features
Costs and Benefits of Electronic Health Records
- *Costs*
- *Benefits*

eHealth, the Electronic Health Record, and the Internet
Achieving the Vision: A Status Report
Factors, Forces, and Issues Affecting the Adoption of the Electronic Health Record
- *Informatics Standards*
- *Nomenclatures, Coding Systems, and Vocabularies*
- *Privacy and Confidentiality*
- *Federal Actions: The Health Insurance Portability and Accountability Act*
- *Organizational Cultures*
- *Accreditation Organizations*
- *Design Perspectives*
- *The Business Case for Developing an Electronic Health Record*
- *The Consumer*
- *Impact of Electronic Health Records on Clinical Practice*

Electronic Health Record Research

Key Terms

Agency for Health Care Policy and Research (AHCPR)
Agency for Healthcare Research and Quality (AHRQ)
American Health Information Management Association (AHIMA)
American Medical Informatics Association (AMIA)
American Society for Testing and Materials (ASTM)
chief nursing officer (CNO)
classification

Key Terms—cont'd

clinical data management system (CDMS)
clinical data repositories
code
Committee E31
Computer-based Patient Record Institute (CPRI)
confidentiality
critical care information system (CCIS)
data element
data set
data warehouses
database
electronic health record (EHR)
electronic health record system (EHRS)
eHealth
European Committee on Standards (CEN)
Healthcare Open Systems and Trials (HOST)
Health Insurance Portability and Accountability Act (HIPAA)
Health Level Seven (HL7)
Institute of Medicine (IOM)
integrated delivery system (IDS)
International Classification of Diseases, 9th Revision, Clinical Modification (ICD-9-CM)
Joint Commission on Accreditation of Healthcare Organizations (JCAHO)
MEDLINE
National Library of Medicine (NLM)
nomenclature
North American Nursing Diagnosis Association (NANDA)
Nursing Interventions Classification (NIC)
Nursing Minimum Data Set (NMDS)
original document
patient data management system (PDMS)
privacy
seamless
standards development organizations (SDOs)
Systematized Nomenclature of Medicine Reference Terminology (SNOMED RT)
trusted authority
unified terminology
uniform hospital discharge data set (UHDDS)
uniform nomenclature
vocabulary

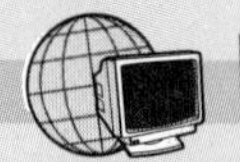

Web Connection

Go to the Web site at http://evolve.elsevier.com/Englebardt/. Here you will find Web links and activities related to electronic health records.

THE ELECTRONIC HEALTH RECORD

The **electronic health record (EHR)** is the core, essential component of electronic health (**eHealth**). eHealth is becoming the foundation for providing health care around the world. The continuous development and use of electronic-based technologies, such as computers, telephony, the Internet, and wireless communications, foster the rapid expansion and acceptance of eHealth. The EHR is the source of individual-focused health care data that makes it possible for practitioners and clients to interact in person and across distances in ways that expand the quality, quantity, and effectiveness of health care.

The EHR is defined as ". . . any information relating to the past, present, or future physical/mental health or condition of an individual which resides in electronic system(s) used to capture, transmit, receive, store, retrieve, link, and manipulate multimedia data for the primary purpose of providing health care and health-related services" (Murphy, Waters, & Amatayakul 1999, p. 5). This definition is the basis of this chapter.

The term *EHR* is used by major standards organizations and by many European groups. Other terms and acronyms have been used in the past, and some are still used today. These include *electronic medical record (EMR)*, *computer-based patient record (CPR)*, and *computer-based health record (CHR)*. Basically, they all refer to the same thing.

The vision of the EHR is not fixed. This is both its challenge and its strength. As informatics practitioners learn more about available technologies, as new technologies emerge, and as more is learned about the complex of meanings embedded in the EHR and eHealth, diverse concepts are developed, adopted, abandoned, and/or modified. A generally accepted view of the EHR is as an electronic database of health care data about an individual. This **database** is a record of all health-related activities in which the individual has been engaged and the health phenomena experienced by the individual. These activities may be focused on such things as health maintenance, the prevention of disease and/or injury, and the management of acute and chronic alterations in health. The individual may provide data for the record on his or her own initiative. Diverse health care practitioners and persons from other professions contribute much of the data and information, either directly or via interfaces with information systems, various electronic devices, and other sources such as the Internet.

Some groups want the EHR to contain all of an individual's health data from birth to death; others expect it to be prebirth and postmortem (Computer-Based Patient Record Institute, 1996). The EHR has been imagined on a more summary level, with detail data available as needed. Some envision the EHR as a virtual entity that is created on demand from numerous scattered data repositories (Kohn, 2000). Data may be stored in a central repository under the care of a **"trusted authority."** A core idea is that an individual's health data should be available on demand anywhere these data are needed and in sufficient detail to support health care–related decision making. For example, an electronic record consisting of data that are focused on the office visit is of great interest to physicians, psychologists, nurse practitioners, and others.

The electronic health record is just that—a record. By itself, it cannot do anything. A system is required to provide the functions that make the EHR useful. Naturally, this is known as an **electronic health record system (EHRS)**. The EHRS is made up of the applications that enable providers to add, delete, modify, view, copy, print, transmit, upload, download, and perform other manipulations to the data and information in the record. As may be expected, there are numerous perspectives about what these applications should be and how they should work. The EHR and the EHRS may be contained within a clinical or health care information system. It may exist as a unique system or may be part of some other system.

NEED FOR THE ELECTRONIC HEALTH RECORD

The personal computer (PC) and the Internet have profoundly changed the world. The Internet has had a major impact on both shrinking the world and expanding people's horizons. Today, it is possible to communicate visually, orally, and in writing across the globe with an ease unimagined even a short time ago. This ease of communication has created expectations.

At the same time, the health care delivery system in the United States has experienced rapid and astonishing changes. New and modified payment systems have affected the use of physical and human resources. There is increased emphasis on quality, effectiveness, efficiency, and cost control. The need to substantiate that these factors are being addressed successfully, or to learn why they are not, has led to unrelenting and growing demands for health care data. Whether they are solo practitioners, members of a group practice, employees of a health care provider organization, or any other arrangement, health care professionals are inundated with demands for data.

Practitioners have their own needs for data as well. The knowledge explosion in health care places incredible demands on the human ability to acquire this new knowledge and to integrate it into practice. A well-designed EHR supported by an EHRS brings an individual's health data and information to practitioners while providing a **seamless** link to new and old knowledge. That is, the links to the knowledge do not require any special action by a user or program in order to access that needed information. Clinical decisions can be better informed and clients can receive more timely and effective care.

HISTORICAL PERSPECTIVES

Problems With the Paper-Based Record

The challenges of working with the traditional paper-based clinical record have been noted and discussed for decades (Milholland, 1989). This record, "the patient chart," is an **original document** (i.e., there is only one copy) used for many purposes by many people over varying lengths of time. This original document is the primary source of current data and information about the individual seeking and receiving health care. When one person is reviewing or recording in the chart, no one else has access to it. If the chart accompanies the client to a diagnostic test or therapy session, access is lost again. Data are accumulated in the chart through a combination of handwritten entries and the insertion of printed documents (e.g., laboratory reports, surgery reports). Poor-quality writing instruments and illegible handwriting increase the risk of misunderstanding what is written. Misunderstanding, in turn, increases the risk of errors and potential harm to the client. The traditional approach to the chart often means that updating requires that the same data be written on several different forms. Because of the nature of human perceptions, different practitioners may record different values for the same parameter for the same time frame. The loose-leaf, unduplicated structure of the paper-based clinical record makes it vulnerable to security and confidentiality breaches. Because different practitioners use different parts of this paper record, they often remove the sections on which they want to work. Thus it can be difficult to assemble and maintain a complete set of the documents. As it exists today, the traditional chart impedes the efficient delivery of health care. Determining the effectiveness of care via analysis of these records is time consuming, costly, and often daunting (Barnett, 1984; Weed, 1971; Wilson, McDonald, & McCabe, 1982).

Early Solutions

Along with the recognition and articulation of the problems of the paper-based clinical record, visionaries and innovators recognized the power of computer-based systems to solve these problems (Milholland, 1989). Systems designed for use in critical care units were among the first to incorporate the features and functions intended to replace the paper chart. These systems were known by various names, such as **patient data management systems (PDMSs)**, **clinical data management systems** (CDMSs), and **critical care information systems** (CCISs). The systems were designed to collect, store, organize, and retrieve data related to direct patient care. The concern of these systems was with individual patients, and the primary focus was organizing clinical data for use in daily patient care (Milholland & Cardona, 1983). It was the focus on clinical data that set these systems apart from preceding generations of health care–oriented computer systems, such as hospital information systems. The goals of these early data management systems are resonant with those of today's EHRSs—to increase the quality of patient care. To achieve this goal, the system seeks to meet the information needs of clinicians through improved timeliness, accuracy, reliability, integrity, and availability of data; improved data organization; increased diagnostic value from collected data; and reduction of repetitive work and of costs (Manzano et al., 1980; Stega, Pollizzi, & Milholland, 1980).

A Call for Action: The Institute of Medicine Report

In 1991, the **Institute of Medicine (IOM)** released the results of a study on the problems of the paper-based patient record and the IOM's recommendations for solving those problems. This landmark report, *The Computer-Based Patient Record: An Essential Technology for Change,* became a call for action to stimulate the development and adoption of the EHR throughout the United States (Dick & Steen, 1991, 1997).

The IOM study reiterated the well-known problems of the paper-based, traditional medical record, identified the need for an electronic patient record, and advocated the creation of a computer-based patient record institute that would bring together public and private entities to carry out the vision articulated in the report. This vision is of a computer-based record and a computer-based system to support that record. The computer-based patient record is "an electronic patient record that resides in a system specifically designed to support users through the availability of complete and accurate data, practice reminders and alerts, clinical decision support systems, links to bodies of medical knowledge and other aids" (Dick & Steen, 1991, p. 55). Twelve essential components of a comprehensive EHR are identified in the report. These 12 attributes, listed in Box 10-1, have guided the work of the organizations and companies involved in developing, studying, promoting, and selling EHRs and EHRSs. The committee also identified seven recommendations for activities needed to achieve its vision. These recommendations, with some adaptations to reflect current terms and perspectives, are provided in Box 10-2.

Features of the IOM committee's envisioned EHR and EHRS include the following:

- Complete and accurate patient data
- Practitioner reminders and alerts
- Clinical decision support systems
- Ability to study patient outcomes
- Electronic links to bodies of scientific knowledge, institutional databases, registries, and other external sources
- Standardized coding systems and formats
- Integration of data and information from multiple health care disciplines and multiple sites
- Continuous access to the record, 24 hours a day
- Standardized and customized reporting
- Ease of use
- Easy access for patients, families, and practitioners
- Strong protections for confidentiality and data security

Public and Private Responses

The excitement generated by the IOM report led to the development of the **Computer-Based Patient Record Institute (CPRI)**, an organization of private-sector organizations devoted to facilitating the achievement of the IOM study's vision. Interested federal agencies attend CPRI meetings but are not members. The CPRI educates the public, policy makers, and the health care community about the EHR, awards national recognition to exemplary EHR developments, and publishes monographs, guidelines, position papers, and White Papers (detailed or authoritative reports) on various aspects of the EHR. The CPRI has asserted that "a computer-based patient record is electronically maintained information about an individual's lifetime health status and health care" (Work Group on CPR Description, 1996, p. 5).

In 2000 the CPRI merged with the **Healthcare Open Systems and Trials (HOST)** organization

Box 10–1 Attributes for a Comprehensive Electronic Health Record and Electronic Health Record System

The computerized patient record (CPR):

1. Contains a problem list that clearly delineates a client's clinical problems and the current status of each problem.
2. Encourages and supports systematic measurement and recording of a client's health status and functional level to promote more precise and routine assessments of the outcomes of health care.
3. States the logical basis for all diagnoses or conclusions as a means of documenting the clinical rationale for decisions about the management of a client's care.
4. Can be linked with other clinical records of a client to provide a longitudinal record of events that may have influenced a person's health.
5. System addresses client data confidentiality comprehensively.
6. Is accessible for use in a timely way at any and all times by authorized individuals involved in direct client care.
7. System allows selective retrieval and formatting of information by users.
8. System can be linked to both local and remote knowledge, literature, bibliographic, or administrative databases and systems.
9. Can assist, and in some instances guide, the process of clinical problem solving by providing clinicians with decision analysis tools, clinical reminders, prognostic risk assessment, and other clinical aids.
10. Supports structured data collection and stores information using a defined vocabulary.
11. Can help individual health care practitioners and health care provider institutions manage and evaluate the quality and costs of care.
12. Is sufficiently flexible and expandable to support not only today's basic information needs but also the evolving needs of each clinical specialty and subspecialty.

From Dick, R.S., & Steen, E.B. (Eds.). (1997). *The computer-based patient record: An essential technology for health care* (rev. 2nd ed.). Washington, DC: National Academy Press.
NOTE: *Patient* has been replaced with *client* to reflect a broader view of health care delivery and recipients. *Computer-based patient record* is the term used by the IOM committee in 1991.

to form the CPRI-HOST. This new organization aims to provide vision and leadership to promote the universal and effective use of electronic health care information systems to improve health and the delivery of health care. It has expanded from a focus on the computer-based patient record to a focus on health care information systems to keep pace with changing technology.

The **Joint Commission on Accreditation of Healthcare Organizations** (**JCAHO**) is the primary agency for accrediting hospitals and other health care organizations. It is a private entity whose actions and policies influence practitioners, providers, governments, and third-party payers. An institution that receives a poor accreditation rating or that fails to receive accreditation may lose its ability to receive Medicare reimbursement and may no longer be acceptable to health insurers. The JCAHO recognized the importance of EHRs and electronic information systems by including an entire chapter on information management in its *Accreditation Manual.*

Box 10–2 Institute of Medicine Recommendations for Advancing the Electronic Health Record

1. Health care professionals and organizations should adopt the computer-based patient record (CPR) as the standard for all records related to client care.
2. To accomplish the first Recommendation, the public and private sector should establish a Computer-based Patient Record Institute (CPRI) to promote and facilitate development, implementation, and dissemination of the EHR (formerly CPR).
3. Both the public and private sector should expand support for the EHR and EHRS implementation through research, development, and demonstration projects.
4. The CPRI should promulgate uniform national standards for data and security to facilitate implementation of the EHR and its secondary databases.
5. The CPRI should review federal and state laws and regulations for the purpose of proposing and promulgating model legislation and regulations to facilitate the implementation and dissemination of the EHR and its secondary databases and to streamline the EHR and EHRS.
6. The costs of the EHRS should be shared by those who benefit from the EHR's value.
7. Health care professional schools and organizations should enhance educational programs for students and practitioners in the use of computers, EHRs, and EHRS for client care, education, and research.

From Dick, R.S., & Steen, E.B. (Eds.). (1997). *The computer-based patient record: An essential technology for health care* (rev. 2nd ed.). Washington, DC: National Academy Press.
EHR, Electronic health record; *EHRS,* electronic health record system.

A corollary recognition of nursing's importance in information systems is the requirement that the **chief nursing officer (CNO)** or designee have an active role on all information systems committees. Additional information concerning the JCAHO is included in Chapter 19.

The federal government's main responses to the IOM report were through the **Agency for Health Care Policy and Research (AHCPR)** and the **National Library of Medicine (NLM).** The AHCPR was created in 1986 to improve the quality of, appropriateness of, effectiveness of, and access to health care. One of the major approaches used by the AHCPR was the development and dissemination of clinical practice guidelines. The agency recognized early on that EHRs are critical to collecting the data needed to support the development of guidelines, to integrating guidelines into daily clinical practice, and to providing data for evaluating the use and effectiveness of guidelines. Reauthorizing legislation passed in November 1999 renamed the AHCPR as the **Agency for Healthcare Research and Quality (AHRQ)** and established the AHRQ as the lead federal agency on quality research. The AHRQ, part of the U.S. Department of Health and Human Services, is the lead agency charged with supporting research designed to improve the quality of health care, reduce its cost, and broaden access to essential services. As the AHCPR, and as the AHRQ, this agency provides substantial support to private-sector activities related to the development, adoption, and evaluation of EHRs (AHRQ, 2000).

The NLM has a long-standing interest in health care information and its management, both during clinical care and afterward. **MEDLINE** is the Library's extensive bibliographic database and retrieval system for medical literature (here "medical" encompasses the broad spectrum of health and illness). MEDLINE is available free to the public online (Murphy, Waters, & Amatayakul, 1999).

FUNCTIONS AND FEATURES

The initial report from the IOM identified the essential features of the EHR and the necessary functions of EHRSs (described earlier). These features and functions have proved to be enduring. Over time, the list has changed very little. Different authors may have put more detail in a list of desired features, or there may be different ways of describing these features. For example, the abilities shown in Box 10-3 are among those proposed in current literature for the "ideal" EHR.

Box 10–3 Features of an Ideal EHR

- Review all client records
- Measure expected improvements in a client's functional ability
- Measure cost-effectiveness
- Document the evidence of quality care for third parties
- Track client status postdischarge
- Identify "best practices" from data in the records
- Identify appropriate care for a specific client
- Identify the immediate and long-term impact of treatments
- Assess various indicators of quality, safety, and effectiveness
- Benchmark client types
- Benchmark individual client progress and health outcomes

From Barrett, M.J. (2000). The evolving computerized medical record. *Healthcare Informatics, 17*(5), 85-92.

Looking back at the IOM list, it can be seen that the features listed in Box 10-3 are extensions of that list, further details of an item on that list, or just different terminology for the same feature.

COSTS AND BENEFITS OF ELECTRONIC HEALTH RECORDS

Although the EHR concept has been discussed and has been under development since the early 1970s, the ideal model proposed by the IOM is rarely seen. The clinical component (the caregiving part) of health care is complex, especially because it involves people, and our understanding of the processes involved in this component is limited. The limited understanding of the processes of health care, combined with the costs of EHRs, has contributed to the slow adoption of this technology. Despite the slow rate of adoption, the potential benefits of the EHR, together with the research that is demonstrating actual benefits, have kept interest and enthusiasm high.

The cost of the EHR refers to more than the cost of acquiring and implementing a system. Costs also involve such things as time expenditures, energy used, opportunities lost, work not done or not done well, and stresses on people and organizations. EHR benefits or values are viewed in a similar fashion. Although direct savings for an organization may be calculated, dollar savings are only a portion of the benefits. There are strategic, operational, and direct client care benefits as well. For the organization and the people involved, costs and benefits are both quantitative and qualitative.

Costs

When contemplating the implementation of an EHR, some costs are obvious immediately. The vendor selection process is complex, is time consuming, and uses extensive personal and organizational resources. Once a system is selected, hardware and software maintenance is an ongoing, significant, and necessary cost. Implementation of the EHRS often involves hiring a consultant to manage the project. The users of the system must be taught how to operate the system, which means they are not available for work during training time. Sometimes extra staff must be found (and paid) to cover essential clinical care areas.

Less obvious costs pertain to infrastructure, technology overhead, and the impact of collateral projects. As health care organizations become more physically distributed, the costs of obtaining high-speed connections between facilities become significant. Failure to spend money on this function, however, results in systems with slow response time. Inadequate response time leads to nonacceptance by the end users and the waste of a very large investment. An organization does well to obtain the best information system infrastructure it can afford.

Technology overhead refers to the costs incurred by an organization in ensuring that hardware, software, and related technologies can be maintained and updated. Although an organization may purchase external support contracts, inevitably there is a need for in-house experts. Providing current staff with the ongoing education to acquire and maintain this expertise is one of the overhead costs. The current shortage of appropriately educated and experienced information technology staff increases the costs of hiring and keeping experts (Fox & Jesse, 1999).

EHRs have an impact on ancillary information systems, such as laboratory, pharmacy, and radiology systems. A new EHRS may require the purchase of new interfaces for existing systems. Sometimes, to take advantage of all of the capabilities of an EHR, older ancillary systems need to be replaced. These collateral projects, brought on by the EHR, have significant financial costs, as well as long-term savings.

Benefits

Fully implemented EHRs still are rare, although there are increasing numbers of organizations that are building their EHRs through gradual introduction of various components and features. The small number of EHRs and the short duration of these implementations mean a lack of definitive evidence of the benefits of the EHR. Thus most discussions of EHR benefits are about potential benefits—what is expected to happen as a result of using an EHR and related systems. Predictions of EHR benefits range from grand views of a new era in health care to listings of specific client-centered results.

Always, the EHR is expected to improve the quality of health care provided to individuals, communities, and the nation. This improvement in quality comes about through fostering new care delivery methods and through better management of health care information. The EHR supports innovations in clinical processes and care models that would not be possible without it (Fox & Jesse, 1999).

Documentation benefits are an important and highly touted benefit of the EHR. In the early days of electronic records, the primary benefit predicted from electronic documentation was time savings. Predictions were made that documentation via computer would reduce staffing needs because so much time would be saved. Reality has shown that the time savings are small, if any. The emerging benefits are more complete, better organized, less redundant, more legible documentation and the ability for multiple practitioners to have simultaneous access to clinical information. An additional benefit is the storage of the documented data as discrete data elements, which can be used for clinical, operational, and strategic studies.

eHEALTH, THE ELECTRONIC HEALTH RECORD, AND THE INTERNET

As noted at the beginning of this chapter, the EHR is central to successful eHealth. eHealth also depends on the Internet (and its main application, the World Wide Web [WWW]).

Health care is as involved as any other domain or industry in using the Internet for many purposes. In some ways, health care consumers may be the biggest beneficiaries of all this activity.

There are Internet sites offering such resources as information on specific diseases, ways to evaluate one's health lifestyle, ways to change a health lifestyle, ways to find health care practitioners, and directions to support groups. A consumer can search the WWW at any time or place to find information on almost any health-related topic. Consumers regularly bring Web site printouts to their practitioner's office. Practitioners are beginning to develop their own Web sites as a means of connecting with their clients and providing accurate information. Additional information about this topic is discussed in Chapter 12.

A recent innovation in eHealth is Web sites offering consumers a place to keep a personal EHR. This is a compendium of one person's health and illness information. There are different approaches to this personal health record (PHR). One approach is for the individual to provide all of the information in the record. Another is for the primary health care practitioner to provide the substantive portion of the information with the client providing additional perspectives. When it is envisioned that the practitioner provides the information, most often an electronic transfer of selected data from an EHR is proposed. At this time, PHRs on the Internet are provided mainly by managed care organizations and other health care insurance organizations. They are offered as a member benefit, and members are encouraged but not required to participate. Along with the PHR, the Web site usually offers health information individualized to each consumer, based on information in the health record and consumer questionnaires. The long-term commercial success of these ventures is unclear. The impact of such sites on individual health and on population health is unknown as well. The term *population health* is a public or community health term that is used when the client is a population rather than an individual or family.

Protecting the privacy of the individual who has placed personal information on a Web site is an important issue. Consumers need to know what policies and practices a given PHR site follows for protecting information and for sharing information. Interestingly, not every PHR site on the Web makes the information regarding these policies and practices available to their customers. Undoubtedly, the average consumer has an expectation that no one else will see his or her information, but there are no guarantees that this expectation will be met. There are, at present, no government regulations addressing PHRs. Standards organizations are beginning to address issues such as this, but no standards exist as yet.

As tools for the Internet continue to be developed, refined, and proven, health care enterprises are exploring using the WWW to implement components and functions of the EHR. The use of the WWW for this purpose is perceived as cost-effective and expedient. On the Web, information exchange is rapid and dynamic, allowing for immediate feedback between information providers and receivers. New and improved Web browsers (the software programs that allow users to access, retrieve, and display multimedia information from the WWW) contribute to the emergence of the Internet-based EHR (Murphy, Waters, & Amatayakui, 1999). Some of the features and functions of EHRs that are being implemented (or are being considered for implementation) via the Internet include the following (McCormack, 2000):

- Remote access to EHRs from a health care practitioner's home or office
- Access to multiple clinical information systems in lieu of purchasing a standalone electronic records system
- Creation of a virtual EHR by bringing together information from multiple systems in a way that appears seamless to the end user
- Use of application service providers to provide access to the EHR
- Direct client access to the official version of the client's EHR

The Internet of the future, like the EHR of the future, cannot be predicted accurately. The lessons learned from technological innovations as well as the responses to those innovations facilitate new innovations that cannot yet be imagined. It seems clear, however, that eHealth and Internet-connected EHRs will be strong elements of the future of health care. Additional information about eHealth can be found in Chapter 13.

ACHIEVING THE VISION: A STATUS REPORT

Although there has been much activity since the original publication of the IOM report on the electronic patient record, the IOM vision remains a guide and a goal.

Vendors and users have built on the IOM vision by creating clinical data repositories, clinical workstations, clinical applications, clinical decision support, clinical data warehouses, and master person indexes. Clinical information systems (CISs) are now envisioned as, and are being built as, systems containing an EHRS (which contains the EHR), as well as numerous clinical specialty systems, such as laboratory, radiology, pharmacy, nursing, dietary, and occupational therapy/physical therapy information systems. Health care–related systems that are external to CISs are being integrated with each other and with the CIS. These include managed care systems, financial systems, administrative/executive systems, local and national databases, national knowledge systems, accrediting and regulatory systems, research systems, and other EHRSs (Blair, 2000). The integration and/or connection of these various information systems enrich the clinical database used by the EHR and subsequently enrich the data and information available to the user. At the same time, the contributing systems are recipients of important clinical data from individual clients and/or populations.

In the 1999 EHR Survey of Trends and Usage by the Medical Records Institute (MRI) the respondents indicated that the top seven driving forces for an EHR are (in descending order) the need to (Blair, 2000):

- Share data
- Improve the quality of care
- Improve clinical processes
- Provide a competitive advantage
- Improve decision support
- Improve documentation
- Contain or reduce health care costs

One measure of progress toward the IOM vision is continued market acceptance of the EHR. That is, how many organizations have purchased an EHRS or are thinking about purchasing such a system? The Leadership Surveys for 1999, 2000, and 2001 by the Healthcare Information and Management Systems Society (HIMSS) provide some answers. The number of health care providers who have no investment in EHRs has decreased from 60% in 1996 to 29% in 1999. An increased number of providers are beginning to adopt EHR components, if not an entire system. When asked about plans for 2000, respondents indicated that 27% had no plans for doing anything with an EHR, 24% had developed a plan, 28% planned to begin installation of some form of an EHR, and 11% expected to be fully operational (HIMSS, 1999, 2000). The 2001 Leadership Survey demonstrates that this progress is continuing. Two thirds of health care provider organizations have already installed EHR systems or are in the planning or implementation phase. In 2001, 13% of providers have a fully operational CPR system in place, compared with 12% in 2000. Only one in four respondents reported that their organizations have not yet begun to plan for the use of an EHR. Also, 45% of respondents ranked an EHR number four among health care applications areas considered most important during the next 2 years (HIMSS, 2001). A master person index or enterprise directory; a clinical data repository supporting text, data, and reimbursement codes; and a network connecting the data repository to clinical workstations and departmental systems are the most frequent EHR components that MRI survey respondents have installed already (Blair, 2000).

FACTORS, FORCES, AND ISSUES AFFECTING THE ADOPTION OF THE ELECTRONIC HEALTH RECORD

How has health care moved this far between 1996 and 2001, and why didn't the movement toward an EHR go further in the preceding decades? These are two ways of looking at the information on the current status of the EHR. To begin to answer either question, an understanding of the influences on the adoption of the EHR is necessary.

The following is by no means the complete, exhaustive list of influences that had an impact on the acceptance and progress of the EHR. However, these are the items that most experts agree have a strong impact on organizational decision making about the EHR:

- Availability of usable informatics standards
- Nomenclatures, vocabularies, and coding systems to be used in EHRs
- Protection of privacy and confidentiality
- Congressional legislation and government regulations
- Cultures of health care practitioners and health care organizations
- Requirements of accreditation organizations
- Design perspectives of EHRs
- The business case for and against EHRs
- The consumer

Informatics Standards

Chapters 17 and 18 address the concepts and development of health informatics standards in detail. However, two standards organizations are of particular importance to the EHR and are also discussed here. These are the **American Society for Testing and Materials (ASTM)** and **Health Level Seven (HL7).**

The standards published and in development by **Committee E31** of the ASTM, known as ASTM E31, are very important to the developers of EHRs and EHRSs. Because published standards are revised regularly and new standards emerge throughout each year, it is not possible to provide a complete current list of relevant standards. These can be found on the ASTM Web site. It is hard to select any one or even a set of these standards as the most important. Later standards are built on the work of earlier standards and often are tightly integrated. ASTM E31 has focused its work on the content of the EHR. Standard E1384 is the *Standard Guide for the Content and Structure of the Electronic Health Record.* This important work strives to identify, define, organize, and code data elements to be used in the EHR. Specific views, such as a diabetic health record or an anesthesia record, may be built from the set of data elements in E1384.

Until recently, the work of the ASTM, HL7, and other American **standards development organizations (SDOs)** has been oriented to the needs of American developers, sellers, and users of health care information systems. In Europe, the separate national efforts at developing and adopting standards were brought together into the **European Committee on Standards (CEN).** The CEN organizes and directs the development of standards for EHRs and EHRSs in Europe. During the last decade of the 1900s, there was active effort to coordinate the standards work of Europe and the United States. Although this is challenging, considering the multiple cultures, languages, personalities, and politics, the efforts are bearing fruit.

Nomenclatures, Coding Systems, and Vocabularies

Chapter 18 on professional informatics standards addresses in detail the concepts of standardized nomenclatures, coding systems, and vocabularies. These systems are important to effective functioning and use of EHRs, so some discussion takes place here as well.

Data elements are the entities in an EHR to which values are assigned. These values may be numerical, alphabetic, or alphanumeric. The **data element** gives a name to the entity. For example, *heart rate* is a data element. The number *88* is a value assigned to heart rate. The name of a client's *significant other* is another data element. *Tom Jones* is the assigned value.

As demonstrated with the traditional paper charts used in health care settings, there are many different ways to name the same data element. Different names may be used within the same setting. The practice of naming the same things differently makes it very difficult to make reliable comparisons. The EHR has brought this difficulty into sharp focus.

To be easily used and to be useful, an EHR must capture data in a consistent and valid way. Standardizing the terms used in naming data elements makes it easier to achieve this consistency and validity. At the same time, the use of standardized terms can smooth out the learning process. The data collected within the EHR can be used to analyze trends in an individual client and trends in client populations, monitor the quality of care, identify best practices, and support other operational and clinical investigations.

Once data elements have been identified, definitions are established and the data elements are organized in some fashion. (Note that an alphabetic listing is a form of organization, albeit not a very useful one.) One form of organization is a **data set.** A data set is a collection of data elements organized for a specific purpose. For example, the **Nursing Minimum Data Set (NMDS)** contains 16 data elements brought together to capture nursing practice. The **uniform hospital discharge data set** is a set of data elements used by every acute care hospital to serve as a summary of a client's hospital experience. A database is a structured collection of data elements, associated data values, and data relationships stored on computer-readable media (Degoulet & Fieschi, 1997). Many different data sets can be drawn or created from the data elements in a database. Chapter 3 includes a detailed discussion of databases.

More complex collections of data elements are found in classifications, nomenclatures, coding systems, and vocabularies. **Classification** is the process of grouping similar items together according to a specific scheme or model. In a nursing intervention classification, similar interventions (which may be considered data elements) are grouped together under a single heading. Sometimes the heading and the group members are assigned a code. A **code** is a numeric or alphanumeric representation of a data element or classified item (Murphy, 1999). A **vocabulary** is a list of standard terms with specific definitions that have been accepted by a discipline, group, or organization to express, organize, and index the concepts and phenomena of interest. The **Nursing Interventions Classification (NIC)** is an example of a classification system used in nursing (McCloskey & Bulechek, 2000). Structured into categories and levels, the NIC is an organized collection of interventions that nurses may perform. The ***International Classification of Diseases, 9th Revision, Clinical Modification* (ICD-9-CM)** is a classification system used in the United States to capture the medical reasons for health care (National Center for Health Statistics, 1998). The ICD-9-CM is used by practitioners to codify a client's medical diagnoses. The government and third-party payers use these codes to determine if a client's diagnoses are eligible for reimbursement and to analyze patterns of diseases in various populations.

A **nomenclature** (also known as a terminology) provides a systematic listing of the proper names for concepts, items, actions, and other aspects of a particular knowledge domain or a particular area of interest. Definitions are provided for each term in the nomenclature. Nomenclatures can be very narrow or have a broad focus. The nursing diagnoses of the **North American Nursing Diagnosis Association (NANDA)** are a listing of the proper names and code numbers of the nursing diagnoses accepted by NANDA (NANDA, 1999). The **Systematized Nomenclature of Medicine Reference Terminology (SNOMED RT)** is a broadly focused collection of terms that encompasses diagnoses, interventions, outcomes, signs and symptoms, and other aspects of human medicine, nursing, veterinary medicine, and related health care practices (SNOMED International, 2000).

Health care has many nomenclatures, classifications, and coding systems. Some are specific to one domain (e.g., medicine, nursing, and dentistry). Others are multidisciplinary in nature and encompass most of the health care processes (examination, diagnosis or problem, intervention/action, outcomes). These different systems and the capabilities of the EHR have stimulated discussion on the need for and feasibility of a single nomenclature for a single discipline such as nursing or medicine. Informatics practitioners and others continue to debate the benefits of a unified versus a uniform terminology for describing health care.

A **unified terminology** is one in which separate nomenclatures are kept intact but are linked together through a mapping of the relationships between terms. For example, the diagnostic terms in NANDA are mapped to the problem statements in the Omaha System. Thus a unified nomenclature allows practitioners in a health care setting to use the terms with which they are most familiar. The terms used by health care practitioners in one setting to describe their practice can be compared with the terms used by practitioners in another setting. A unified terminology really is workable only with an EHR and its related functions.

A **uniform nomenclature** is a single set of terms with definitions and codes intended to describe all of the aspects of a domain. The terms may be drawn from existing nomenclatures and developed as new entities. A uniform nomenclature does not exist for any of the practice disciplines in health care. Among those studying the issues of nomenclatures, classifications, and coding systems in health care, there seems to be an emerging sense that it may not be possible to develop a single standardized system to meet the complexities of capturing health care data in all settings and across all domains and health phenomena.

Table 10-1 is an alphabetic list of many of the most well known or well established nomenclatures used in health care today. Several of these naming systems were developed before the advent of the EHR and are now being adapted to accommodate the EHR. Most do not have a substantive empirical research base but have been developed using a consensus process. This consensus process can be very rigorous. The nursing terminologies have a strong research base underlying the content and structure.

No one coding, classification, or vocabulary system is sufficient for capturing the richness of the clinical setting, as well as the extended health care environment, which supports clinical practice. Nursing systems recognized by the American Nurses Association (ANA) have been deemed necessary but not sufficient for representing the work of nurses and the scope of nursing practice (Henry & Mead, 1997). Performance studies of existing vocabularies have led to the conclusion that a combination of these vocabularies provides the best coverage of clinical concepts, research needs, and administrative information (Murphy, 1999).

Privacy and Confidentiality

The terms *privacy* and *confidentiality* are often thought of as being synonymous, and sometimes the terms are used interchangeably. This is an error. **Privacy** is the concept that an individual has the right to decide what information he or she will disclose. Although there is no constitutional right to privacy, over the years laws and customs have established that individuals do have certain privacy rights.

Confidentiality means that information and data, once disclosed, will not be shared without

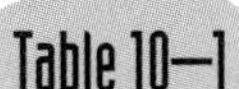

Table 10–1 Health Care Nomenclatures, Classifications, and Coding Systems

System	Content Focus
Arden Syntax	Encoding health care knowledge for making decisions
Current Procedural Terminology (CPT)	Procedures and treatments primarily performed by, but not limited to, physicians
Home Health Care Classification (HHCC)	Nursing diagnoses, interventions, and outcomes related to home care
Diagnostic and Statistical Manual of Mental Disorders (DSM)	Psychiatric diagnoses
International Classification of Diseases (ICD), 10th Revision	Reasons for morbidity and mortality; not available yet in the United States
International Classification of Diseases, 9th Revision, Clinical Modification (ICD-9-CM)	Version modified for use in the United States; used for indexing diseases, injuries, and procedures
Logical Observation Identifier Names and Codes (LOINC)	Nomenclature of laboratory and clinical observation terms and codes
National Drug Codes (NDC)	Pharmaceuticals
North American Nursing Diagnosis Association (NANDA) list of nursing diagnoses	Client health problems and client responses to health problems that are treatable by nurses
Nursing Interventions Classification (NIC)	Actions that nurses may do to manage nursing problems
Nursing Outcomes Classification (NOC)	Results of nursing interventions for nursing problems (resolution of nursing problem)
Omaha System	Nursing problems, actions, and outcomes for home care
Perioperative Nursing Data Set	Perioperative nursing problems, interventions, and outcomes
Read Codes	Multidisciplinary health care terms for use in the United Kingdom
Systematized Nomenclature of Medicine Reference Terminology (SNOMED RT)	Assessment, diagnosis, and treatment of humans and animals

the permission of the information's originator (the person). Sharing of personal information is limited to those with a need to know the information. In health care, individuals share a large amount of intimate information with health care practitioners. Practitioners have a deeply ingrained ethical responsibility to keep this information confidential. Health care clients expect this.

One of the most positive features of the electronic record is the ease of access to client data and information. However, this same ease of access increases the risk of breaches of confidentiality. Computer hardware and software, however, offer sophisticated approaches to fortifying data and system security. When properly designed (i.e., when these sophisticated approaches are applied), the EHRS can be far more secure than the paper health record system. Chapter 20 provides additional information on this topic.

ASTM Committee E31 on Healthcare Informatics has published several standards and guidelines related to data and system security. Other organizations, such as the **American Health Information Management Association (AHIMA)**, the CPRI-HOST, and the **American Medical Informatics Association (AMIA)**, also have publications that are intended to help individuals and organizations keep their commitment to client and practitioner privacy and confidentiality.

The most important element in maintaining the security of EHRs is the human element. People are the weakest link in any security system. For example, the ubiquitous paper printout enables common breaches of confidentiality and probably is rarely thought of in those terms. Signing on to and signing off of an electronic system using identifiers and passwords can be irritating, and people may become lax about this. Sharing identifiers and passwords often is a problem when a system is new and people are adjusting to the new way of doing things. All persons having access to client data and information need to be taught the importance of maintaining data and information security. It is a good idea to regularly remind EHRS users about their responsibilities in this area.

Federal Actions: The Health Insurance Portability and Accountability Act

The Health Insurance Portability and Accountability Act (HIPAA) of 1996 was passed by Congress to protect individuals from losing their health insurance when they changed employers and to simplify the administration of health insurance claims and payments. These administrative simplification provisions were passed in response to private sector requests for government assistance in accelerating the standards development process for health care information systems. The publication in 2000 of the final regulations for the various aspects of information standards within the HIPAA started a 2-year clock for organizations and information systems vendors to implement what some see as some very radical changes in how health care systems will work. There are substantive financial penalties for failure to comply with the HIPAA standards. To effectively, efficiently, and economically meet the HIPAA regulations, health care providers will need to collect data from individual records for direct reporting to select government agencies and for aggregating data to prepare other government reports. The HIPAA is discussed in greater detail in Chapters 19 and 20.

Organizational Cultures

The EHR and health care information systems have profound effects on the cultures and on the many subcultures within an the organizations that implement them. At the same time, these cultures influence the success or failure of an information system in an organization. Each group of health care professionals has its own culture, philosophical background, beliefs about the profession's primary roles and place in the health care team, and beliefs about information technologies. When health care professionals see that computer systems are of practical help, they are more willing to accept the systems. If a system is perceived as an added burden without significant payback, resistance is a common response.

Informatics practitioners involved with EHRs need to be sensitive to the cultural aspects of the multiple groups within an organization. There can be significant role changes within a professional group when an EHR is adopted. Whole ways of interacting between cultural groups can change, leading to both positive and negative consequences. Lorenzi and Riley (1995) have provided a classic example of these phenomena in their discussion of the results of having physicians enter orders directly into a clinical computer system (Box 10-4).

Accreditation Organizations

Accreditation organizations influence various aspects of the EHR, such as the content of the

Box 10–4 Relationship Between Organizational Culture and EHR: One Example

Nancy Lorenzi and Robert Riley (1995) have illustrated how professional conflict can arise during the implementation of an electronic information system because of changes in cultural roles. In their example the nurses on an inpatient unit used a manual system to enter physician orders. The nurses perceived their roles in the order entry process to be integrators and reviewers of orders. The nurses were the conduits for the transfer of information around physician orders. By filling this role, the nurses had a total picture of the care processes surrounding their patients. The physicians depended on the nurses to interpret their individual "shorthand" and, by conducting the review of orders, to catch any mistakes. Then an electronic order entry system that required the physicians to directly enter their orders was introduced onto the nursing unit. The nurses experienced a significant loss of their roles as integrators and reviewers of care. They no longer had the total picture of the patient. Physicians had to be very specific in the orders they wrote, and they wrote them in isolation from the nurses, forcing a change in how they interacted with the nurses. Physicians made mistakes when entering orders, and the nurses no longer caught those errors. Coordination between the nursing plan of care and the medical plan of care decreased. Nurses began to show less initiative in making treatment suggestions.

health record, and often provide a subtle push toward the adoption of the EHR and EHRS. The JCAHO provides one example. The JCAHO specifies in its accreditation standards that each client should have a written treatment plan. The treatment plan must identify client goals and objectives, including a time frame for achieving each objective. However, the JCAHO does not specify the terms or data elements that must be included in the record (Hanken, 1999). The agency supports, but does not mandate, the use of electronic information systems and health records. The challenges of compiling the evidence for an accreditation visit by the JCAHO can be a strong argument for computerization of clinical and nonclinical processes.

Design Perspectives

There are many ways to approach the design of an EHR and its system. One can focus on the hardware and the multiple configurations for choosing and placing different kinds of computing devices. Certainly, devices that are hard to use or that are not sufficiently or conveniently distributed will deter persons from using a system. The technical structure of the system is important as well. For example, if the EHR depends on data from diverse information systems, smooth communications between these systems is essential. Delays in obtaining information or information that may be corrupted by the messaging process will lead to distrust of the system's reliability.

The most important design issues center around the clinical users and other end users. Fundamental principles that may help achieve successful EHRS implementation include the following (Teich, 1999):

- Improving information access for existing processes
- Presenting information needed for specific work scenarios
- Organizing displays so that all of the information needed to support a clinical process is on one screen

- Organizing entry forms in the same way
- Analyzing existing data in the context of current knowledge to monitor a client's condition
- Providing clinical users with the assurance that expert clinicians are involved in the development of the computer system's analysis of client data

The Business Case for Developing an Electronic Health Record

Computer systems can be very expensive. Not only is there the cost of the equipment and the software, but also there are expenses associated with the physical preparation of a facility; the extensive staff planning; the need to teach everyone how to use the system; troubleshooting; ongoing maintenance of hardware and software; and the many other aspects of the selection, implementation, and evaluation process. In the early days of EHRs, there were demands for evidence that these systems were worth the expense. Such evidence was often hard to find, especially when the benefits of EHRSs, such as improved clinical decision making, are not easily quantifiable. Absence of a direct, immediate, and positive financial benefit made a formidable barrier.

Now, the health care industry has recognized the value of data and information. **Clinical data repositories** provide an electronic place to house the data and information from individual client health records. The repository enables an organization to assemble and reorganize information from a variety of internal systems, including digital images (Murphy, Waters, & Amatayakul, 1999). Workstations enable practitioners to access data repositories, construct ad hoc reports, and conduct real-time analyses of a client's health status. **Data warehouses** are electronic storage devices for clinical, financial, administrative, and other categories of information from one or more facilities. These warehouses enable organizations to aggregate discrete data elements in order to study clinical and business practices for a variety of purposes. Additional information on these processes is provided in Chapters 4 and 5.

Experiences with EHRSs have demonstrated that as clinicians come to trust the client information available from the EHR, the EHR becomes a significant supporter of the care process. Support for the care process can mean increased revenues if clients receive better care more effectively and efficiently. Increased revenues can mean organizational survival in today's competitive business environment.

The business side of health care recognizes that more efficient methods are needed to manage the explosive growth of client and business information. EHRSs are being purchased as the understanding grows that client-originated information is the foundation for meeting clinical needs in health care. This foundation is the significant basis for meeting the information needs of national health initiatives, economic imperatives, managers, researchers, and consumers (Murphy, Waters, & Amatayakul 1999).

The emergence of the **integrated delivery system (IDS)** in the 1990s was a force that supported the use of EHRs. An IDS results from the merger and acquisition of diverse health care delivery organizations. These previously separate entities are combined into a single, multiservice enterprise with the mission of offering health services from cradle to grave. The IDS is intended to provide services across the entire spectrum of health care (ambulatory, acute inpatient, long-term, home health, behavioral health, rehabilitation, complementary, hospice, etc.). With such a broad scope, the IDS must focus on aggregate data to manage the client population (Murphy, Waters, & Amatayakul 1999). Aggregate data are effectively derived from EHRs.

The Consumer

From birth to death, most individuals are consumers of health care services. Up until recent times, most health care consumers were passive consumers—patients. Patients depended on health care practitioners to provide the information needed for decision making about health care and often for making the decisions themselves. Much of this pattern has been due to the consumer's difficulty in obtaining such information, a primary focus on pathology and its treatment, the tradition of the physician's being more highly educated than most of his or her patients, and the corollary belief that patients would not understand medical information.

Today, consumers are better educated, information of all kinds is available from many different sources (e.g., books, magazines, radio, television, movies, and the Internet), and there has been a shift to an emphasis on health and wellness and individual responsibility for health. Consumer empowerment has moved from the traditional commercial sector to the health care sector. There are many more terms now for the recipient of health care services: *client, consumer, recipient, individual,* etc.

Consumers use the Internet to research issues affecting their health. They bring printouts of Internet-based information with them when visiting health care practitioners. The Internet is becoming a repository for personal health information through a variety of sites. This increasing computer and information sophistication of consumers means that they have greater expectations that their health care practitioners will have the same sophistication and will make use of the information technologies available.

Impact of Electronic Health Records on Clinical Practice

Research is only beginning to be conducted that will tell how the EHR really affects the thinking-and-doing components of health care practice. The primary work of health care practitioners is a thinking process in which data are collected, analyzed, converted to information, and used to support decisions. A practitioner's decisions guide every aspect of operational activity (i.e., the verbal and physical actions they take on behalf of the client or on behalf of an organization).

The EHR brings major changes in the ways that data elements are determined, data are collected (manual and automatic), data are stored and organized, data are transformed into information, information is organized and displayed, and knowledge is generated from clinical practice. Health care practitioners have more data available (organized in ways that support each profession's approaches to interpreting data and understanding multivariate information) and have active interactions with decision support functions that enable them to manage a wealth of data and information more effectively and efficiently.

As discussed earlier, when an EHR is implemented in a health care setting, the traditional ways of managing the collection and distribution of information are altered. For example, nurses working on clinical care units may no longer have to monitor or enter physician orders. Nurses may gain more time to be with clients. Along with the EHR, a more professional mode of nursing practice may be introduced more easily (e.g., the use of nursing diagnoses, nursing orders, a standardized nomenclature, measurement of client outcomes, and multidisciplinary plans of care) into a culture that has not previously practiced in this way. More accountability for individual practice becomes possible. This accountability may be viewed as a positive, growth-enhancing step or as a high-risk, potentially punitive action. Informatics practitioners must be prepared to deal with the positive, negative, and unexpected consequences of EHRs for nurses and nonnurse practitioners.

ELECTRONIC HEALTH RECORD RESEARCH

The relative newness of the EHR means that valid empirical evidence of its costs and benefits is just beginning to emerge. Because there are many variations on what constitutes an EHR, because many record systems are implemented gradually, and because the EHR is so totally different from the paper record system it replaces, classical experimental studies are very hard to design. Thus there usually is a lack of a true control group, and comparison of before and after (pretrial and posttrial) data are difficult.

Major funding from studies of EHRs and the supporting systems comes from the federal government. Foundations, system vendors, professional associations, and health care organizations also support EHR research.

Throughout this chapter, areas where there is a lack of research have been identified. In essence, because electronic records and the related information systems are new phenomena in the practice environment, there are myriad questions to be asked and answered. A few examples published in 2000 are provided to stimulate discussion and thinking. Myers et al. (2000) studied the development, implementation, and uses of an integrated data warehouse. In Nottingham, England, researchers used the electronic records in an emergency department to describe the characteristics of children and adolescents who came to that department after inflicting deliberate self-harm (Nadkarni et al., 2000). A qualitative study in Australia suggested that nurses were critical of patient information systems with respect to "user-friendliness" (Darbyshire, 2000). At the University of Minnesota in Minneapolis, a work-sampling tool was used to collect productivity data before the implementation of an EHR (Fontaine et al., 2000).

CONCLUSION

The EHR and the systems that make the EHR functional are increasingly necessary to the delivery of effective and affordable health care. In the current competitive environment, the data and information found in the EHR are necessary to the success (survival) of health care organizations. The cognitive work of health care practitioners demands the immediacy, comprehensiveness, accessibility, and readability that the EHR brings to clinical data used in decision making. Consumers expect their health care practitioners to use information technologies as tools for providing the best quality and most current care possible. No one can predict exactly where EHRs and record systems will take health care in the future, but if "the past is prologue" the journey will be exciting and enlightening.

Web Connection

An electronic health record is a dynamic idea in health care. Never before has the documentation of health care data been so critically needed and so difficult to accomplish. Data repositories compiled from the data of individual care episodes offer the potential for learning about relationships of physical, psychological, social, and environmental factors that may lead to improved interventions and outcomes. Paper records have been cumbersome and are inadequate for making inferences about relationships that can lead to improved care. The electronic health record is perceived as a core source of relationship data and information that can be manipulated. As technologies change, so does the vision of a comprehensive health record. The Web Connection activities for this chapter review the vision of an electronic health record held by various health care experts. Additionally, you will learn about the complexity of developing a comprehensive electronic record due to the numerous variables involved in its development.

discussion questions

1. You are a member of the EHR project team whose mission is to introduce EHRs into your facility. The team is using a series of debates to educate the future users of the system. Decide if you will be on the "pro" or the "con"

side of the debate. Prepare a 10-minute argument supporting your position.

2. eHealth has many enthusiasts, and there are predictions that soon all EHRs will be on the Internet. With the knowledge you have gained about the history and current state of EHRs, what position do you take regarding the Internet and EHRs? Provide at least two supporting arguments for your position.
3. You are a senior member of an informatics consulting firm. You are responsible for helping the marketing staff develop effective sales techniques. Decide which of the factors influencing the adoption of EHRs is most powerful. Defend your position, and explain how the positive aspects can be enhanced and the negative aspects minimized.
4. As an informatics researcher, you have the opportunity to pursue a funding opportunity focused on the EHR. Identify one researchable question, and explain how answering this question will help promote the EHR and have a positive impact on the delivery of health care.

REFERENCES

Agency for Healthcare Research and Quality. (2000). *About AHRQ*. Retrieved November 10, 2000, from the World Wide Web: http://www.ahcpr.gov/about/overview.htm.

Barnett, O.G. (1984). The application of computer-based medical record systems in ambulatory practice. *New England Journal of Medicine, 310,* 1634-1650.

Barrett, M.J. (2000). The evolving computerized medical record. *Healthcare Informatics, 17*(5), 85-92.

Blair, J. (2000, May 21-24). *On the road to the electronic patient record.* American Telemedicine Association Symposium, Phoenix, AZ.

Computer-Based Patient Record Institute. (1996). *Description of the computerized patient record.* Bethesda, MD: Author.

Darbyshire, P. (2000). User-friendliness of computerized information systems. *Computers in Nursing, 18*(2), 93-99.

Degoulet, P., & Fieschi, M. (1997). *Introduction to clinical informatics.* New York: Springer-Verlag.

Dick, R., & Steen, E. (1991). *The computer-based patient record: An essential technology for change.* Washington, DC: Institute of Medicine.

Dick, R.S., & Steen, E.B. (Eds.). (1997). *The computer-based patient record: An essential technology for health care* (rev. 2nd ed.). Washington, DC: National Academy Press.

Fontaine, B.R., et al. (2000). A work-sampling tool to measure the effect of electronic medical record implementation on health care workers. *Journal of Ambulatory Care Management, 23*(1), 71-75.

Fox, C.S., & Jesse, H. (1999). Electronic health record costs and benefits. In G.F. Murphy, M.A. Hanken, & K.A. Waters (Eds.), *Electronic health records: Changing the vision* (pp. 329-344). Philadelphia: W.B. Saunders.

Hanken, M.A. (1999). Laws and security standards. In G.F. Murphy, M.A. Hanken, & K.A. Waters (Eds.), *Electronic health records: Changing the vision* (pp. 6-86). Philadelphia: W.B. Saunders.

Healthcare Information and Management Systems Society. (1999). *Leadership survey.* Chicago: Author.

Healthcare Information and Management Systems Society. (2000). *Leadership survey.* Chicago: Author.

Healthcare Information and Management Systems Society. (2001). Leadership survey. Retrieved June 18, 2001, from the World Wide Web: http://www.himss.org/2001Survey/surveyfinal/7.htm.

Henry, S.B., & Mead, C.N. (1997). Evaluating standardized coding and classification systems for clinical practice: A critical review of the nursing literature in the United States. In U. Gerdin, P. Wainwright, & M. Talberg (Eds.), *The impact of nursing knowledge and healthcare informatics* (pp. 15-20). Stockholm, Sweden: IOS Press.

Kohn, D. (2000). Caught in the web by the killer app! An update. *Journal of Healthcare Information Management, 14*(1), 7-15.

Lorenzi, N.M., & Riley, R.T. (1995). *Organizational aspects of health informatics: Managing technological change.* New York: Springer-Verlag.

Manzano, J.L., et al. (1980). Computerized information system for ICU patient management. *Critical Care Medicine, 8,* 745-747.

McCloskey, J.C., & Bulechek, G.M. (2000). *Nursing interventions classification (NIC)* (3rd ed.). St. Louis: Mosby.

McCormack, J. (2000). The Internet reroutes electronic records. *Health Data Management, 8*(5), 50-62.

Milholland, D.K. (1989). *A measure of patient data management system effectiveness: Development and testing.* Unpublished Dissertation, University of Maryland, Baltimore.

Milholland, D.K., & Cardona, V. (1983). Computers at the bedside. *American Journal of Nursing, 83,* 1304-1307.

Murphy, G.F. (1999). The role of vocabulary in electronic health record systems. In G.F. Murphy, M.A. Hanken, & K.A. Waters (Eds.), *Electronic health records: Changing the vision* (pp. 157-182). Philadelphia: W.B. Saunders.

Murphy, G.F., Waters, K.A., & Amatayakul, M. (1999). EHR vision, definition, and characteristics. In G.F. Murphy, M.A. Hanken, & K.A. Waters (Eds.), *Electronic health records: Changing the vision* (pp. 3-26). Philadelphia: W.B. Saunders.

Myers, D., et al. (2000). An integrated data warehouse system: Development, implementation, and early outcomes. *Managed Care Interface, 13*(3), 68-72.

Nadkarni, A., et al. (2000). Characteristics of children and adolescents presenting to accident and emergency departments with deliberate self harm. *Journal of Accident and Emergency Medicine, 17*(2), 98-102.

National Center for Health Statistics. (1998). *International classification of diseases, 9th revision, clinical modification* (CD-ROM). Washington, DC: Author.

North American Nursing Diagnosis Association. (1999). *NANDA nursing diagnoses: Definitions and classifications 1999-2000.* Philadelphia: Author.

SNOMED International. (2000). *Systematized nomenclature of medicine reference terminology.* Northfield, IL: American College of Pathologists.

Stega, M., Pollizzi, J., & Milholland, A. (1980). *A successful clinical computer system.* Paper presented at the Fourth Annual Symposium on Computer Applications in Medical Care, Los Angeles, CA.

Teich, J.M. (1999). Development of the EHR for Brigham and Women's Hospital and Partners Healthcare System. In G.F. Murphy, M.A. Hanken, & K.A. Waters (Eds.), *Electronic health records: Changing the vision* (pp. 27-41). Philadelphia: W.B. Saunders.

Weed, L.W. (1971). *Medical records, medical education, and patient care.* Cleveland: The Press of Case Western Reserve University.

Wilson, G., McDonald, C., & McCabe, G. (1982). The effect of immediate access to a computerized medical record on physician test ordering: A controlled clinical trial in an emergency room. *American Journal of Public Health, 72,* 698-702.

Work Group on CPR Description. (1996). *Computer-based patient record description of content.* Bethesda, MD: Computer-Based Patient Record Institute.

PART THREE

Using Technology to Deliver Health Care and Education

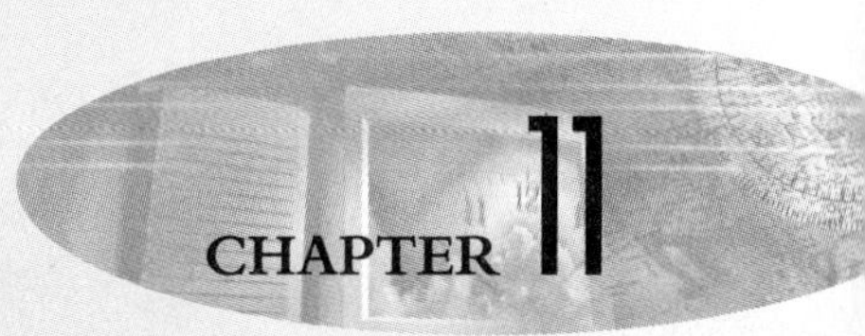

Technological Approaches to Communication

ROBERT G. HENSHAW

Learning Objectives

Upon completion of this chapter, the reader will be able to:

1. ***Develop*** a general understanding of common communications applications and technologies.
2. ***Assess*** both the potential and the limitations of the underlying communications technologies driving new approaches to health care delivery and education.
3. ***Gain*** perspective on the evolution and convergence of communications technologies over time.

Outline

A Framework for Following Technology Trends
- *Standards*
- *Technology Adoption*

Wringing Out the Old: The Static and Changing Roles of Traditional Technologies
- *Telephony*
- *Paging*
- *Fax*
- *Voice Recording*
- *Document Production*
- *Personal Information Management*
- *Television*
- *Videoconferencing*

The Internet: How Data Networks Are Driving Communication
- *Network Primer*
- *Internet History and Development*
- *How the Internet Works*
- *Internet Applications*
- *Toward a User-Friendly Internet*
- *The Internet: A Look Ahead*

Communications Integration: Bringing It All Together
- *Linking Old and New Applications*
- *Enterprise Computing*
- *Case Study*
- *Outlook on Integration*

Key Terms

analog
asynchronous
bits
circuit-switched network
client server computing
communications
contact centers
database
defacto standard
digital
dynamic content
encryption
enterprise computing
fat-client computing
firewall
Internet
intranet
legacy system
open standards
packet-switched network
personal digital assistant (PDA)
portal
proprietary standards
protocol

Key Terms—cont'd

synchronous
telemedicine
thin-client computing
transmission control protocol and Internet protocol (TCP/IP)
World Wide Web

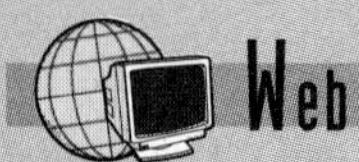

Web Connection

Go to the Web site at http://evolve.elsevier.com/Englebardt/. Here you will find Web links and activities related to technological approaches to communication.

Roughly a century after the beginning of the Industrial Revolution, digital technologies are ushering in a new construct that is fundamentally changing the way people interact with each other and with information. Data stored as electrical signals on small pieces of semiconducting material serve as the foundation for what many are calling the "Digital Age." The ability to transmit electrical signals between devices over networks such as the Internet is moving the world closer to a ubiquitous communications environment. In the home, in the workplace, in schools, and in hospitals, the impact of digital technology is undeniable. Digital technology is providing new options for achieving objectives; it is also helping to give rise to new objectives, opening up worlds and possibilities that could not be envisioned before.

In light of the enormous advances in communications technologies in recent years, it is easy to overlook how young the Digital Age is. In many ways, an era of transition has just begun. This era of transition is either complementing or replacing many of the tools and methods born of the Industrial Revolution with digital technologies. This change process is not seamless and is hampered by a number of impediments that include the uneven maturation of the technology itself, competing standards, inadequate infrastructures, and a reluctance to change on the part of the cultures that are being driven to integrate the technology. Perhaps more important than the evolution of the technology itself are the decisions being made at this time about the appropriate role of technology in our lives. These decisions will have profound implications on the delivery of health care and health care education.

By its very definition, *transition* denotes a continuum. The integration of digital technologies into the fabric of society is a gradual process. Thus this current period is marked by a convergence of old and new technologies. In some cases technologies represent the future; in other cases they are placeholders for technologies yet to come. This chapter will begin by examining some of the technologies that have served the communications needs of health care for many years and by exploring their changing roles in the context of emerging technologies.

For the purposes of this chapter, **communications** is defined broadly to include not only interpersonal interaction but also the retrieval and dissemination of information.

A FRAMEWORK FOR FOLLOWING TECHNOLOGY TRENDS

During the consideration of various technologies in this chapter, several common themes emerge that serve as a useful framework to help the reader understand how communications technologies have arrived at their respective places in society. First, most successful technologies are based on some kind of widely accepted standard that helps to ensure that competing implementations of the technology can be used interchangeably. Second, most technologies become successful only when they support a popular use or application. Finally, communications technologies and applications are converging. The implications include changing roles for familiar applications and devices and movement toward a more seamless communications network and infrastructure. This trend is considered in more detail in the last section of the chapter.

These three themes are explored in this chapter, along with a survey of specific technologies. As readers strive to keep up with technological trends of the future, this framework for considering the viability of new technologies will be useful.

Standards

A standard is a definition, or set of widely accepted rules, for how a particular system or technology works. English and metric measurements, for example, are two different standards for systems of measurement. The existence of a standard for measurement ensures that 1 cup of sugar in a shared recipe will be roughly the same, regardless of who is doing the baking. It means that an auto parts maker can design parts with the assurance that the tools in most garages will fit them. On the other hand, the fact that there is no single universal standard for measurement creates a number of inconveniences and incompatibilities. How many readers have been frustrated to find that their metric wrench or socket set was incompatible with the nuts and bolts they were trying to manipulate? The world of communications technology yields the same mixed results. Hardware and software producers would have no way to ensure that their products worked together without many of the important standards that are in place today. However, standards in many areas are either nonexistent or embroiled in fierce competition.

How are standards created? Some standards are created by organizations established solely for the purpose of creating standards. These quasi-government organizations often comprise a variety of partners representing both nonprofit and commercial interests. Many of the important standards that make the Internet possible were developed by standards organizations such as the Internet Engineering Task Force (IETF) and the Internet Architecture Board (IAB). Most of the Internet standards are **open standards,** which means that the blueprint for how a system works is public information. There is a published standard, for example, for how electronic mail (eMail) programs should be written. Based on the publicly available standard, anyone who is interested can write his or her own basic, functional eMail program. In the eMail program market, software companies compete by adding value (features and functionality) to the underlying standard.

In contrast to open systems, closed standards, or **proprietary standards,** represent intellectual property that is not publicly accessible. Microsoft Windows is an example of a system based on a closed standard; the Linux operating system, on the other hand, is known as open source software. In cases where a standard for a particular technology has not been created by a recognized standards organization, an open or proprietary standard may become the **defacto standard** in the industry. That means that it is unofficially recognized as the standard because it is so widely used or because there is no viable alternative. With many communications technologies in their relative infancy, companies are often embroiled in fierce competition in an effort to have their particular solutions become the defacto standard.

While competition promotes innovation on the one hand, on the other hand it can be very frustrating for consumers when a standard, defacto or otherwise, is no longer in vogue. Selecting technologies based on open standards can help to ensure that data remain portable in the event that a particular hardware or software vendor goes out of business. Readers involved in organizational decisions regarding technology adoption and implementation may want to ask whether the technology under discussion is based on a widely accepted standard.

For additional information related to technical and professional standards, see Chapters 17 and 18.

FIGURE 11–1 Gartner Group's Hype Cycle

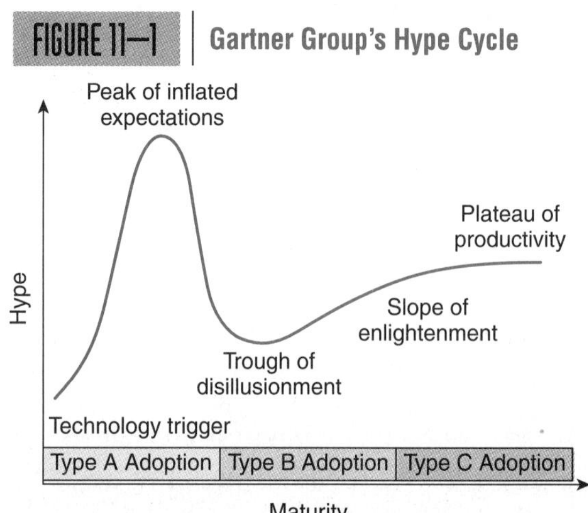

(*From Fenn, J., & Hieb, B. [1999]. How should healthcare jump onto the hype cycle?* Gartner Strategic Analysis Report: DF-08-9287. Gartner Advisory Intraweb, *p. 1. Retrieved February 6, 2000, from the World Wide Web: http://help.unc.edu.gartner/.*)

Technology Adoption

A technology is only used if it is useful. Although this seems intuitive, the history of technology is littered with examples of technologies that never really found a popular use, or application, and thus faded away. It is often said that eMail was the "killer application" for the Internet, meaning that it was the application that drove the initial use of the Internet. Why do some technologies fail to make it? The technology may be superseded by a superior new technology, or it may not be stable enough to garner widespread adoption. It may simply never find an application that generates sufficient interest.

In any case, readers may be faced with decisions regarding technology adoption and implementation. Knowing when to adopt a particular technology or application can be like playing the stock market. One way to look at the evolution of a particular technology is to think about it in terms of a predictable cycle. Gartner Inc., a research and information technology consulting firm, offers a model for looking at the evolution of technologies that Gartner calls the Hype Cycle (Figure 11-1). In the Hype Cycle, the "technology trigger" signifies the launch or public introduction of a particular technology (Fenn & Hieb, 1999). This initial stage ("peak of inflated expectations") is often characterized by high expectations and hype about the product as proponents try to build support and market share for the technology. During this time there may be some successes, but an equal number of failures occur as the limitations of the technology become more apparent. Technologies that are unable to gain a critical mass following are likely to fall into a period where there is little media attention, and market share stagnates or decreases ("trough of disillusionment"). Some technologies never rebound, but some get renewed attention as the technology matures, third-party companies develop authoring or implementation packages that make the technology easier to use, and some of the early adopters begin working through the obstacles to effective utilization. If enough successes are demonstrated at this point, the technology may enter a stage ("plateau of productivity") where the benefits of the technology are clearly demonstrable. The actual level of use will vary according to what applications are driving it.

Not all organizations and individuals adopt a technology at the same stage in the cycle. Decisions concerning technology adoption are affected by a number of factors, including strategic goals and objectives, cultural climate, and available resources. In the Hype Cycle model, type A adopters are technologically aggressive and more likely to adopt a technology early in the cycle. Type B adopters minimize risk and emphasize competitiveness, whereas type C adopters emphasize cost reduction and generally take a very cautious approach to risk. Most health care organizations approach technology adoption from a type C perspective, waiting until late in the cycle. However, in the increasingly competitive environment that characterizes today's health care industry, a new technology may be of strategic importance to an organization. High-impact technologies often require significant financial and time investments for effective implementation. Waiting until too late in the cycle may come at a competitive cost.

WRINGING OUT THE OLD: THE STATIC AND CHANGING ROLES OF TRADITIONAL TECHNOLOGIES

Traditional and new communications technologies can be distinguished in a number of ways, but one of the keys to appreciating their differences is understanding the difference between *analog* and *digital.*

Just about everything in the world can be represented as either digital or analog. To say something is **analog** means that it can be perceived on an uninterrupted continuum. A turntable is an example of an analog system because the turntable's stylus follows the grooves in a vinyl record, converting the signal to sound in one continuous motion. Sensory signals such as human vision are processed continuously. All things **digital,** on the other hand, consist of values measured at discrete intervals. At the most basic level, these intervals are electrical signals set at either "on" or "off," represented by *0* and *1*. These signals are stored on semiconducting chips, or semiconductors, that handle storage and processing of the data. A computer is a collection of semiconductors programmed to carry out specific tasks.

Remember that data represented digitally are broken down into discrete, measurable units. The ability to break down an object into smaller units provides more control over the storage, transmission, and manipulation of specific elements within the object. For example, consider a photograph of a friend. In its digitized form on a computer screen, the digitized photograph appears to be a continuous analog image. However, when the image is made larger, it becomes apparent that it actually consists of thousands of component squares, or pixels. Each one of these tiny elements can be edited, deleted, or reproduced. So, for example, with the proper software, the pixels representing the color of a friend's eyes could easily be modified. This is a very simple example, but it underscores how the ability to represent data digitally is changing the way people interact with information.

Telephony

Traditional communications technologies such as telephony have been the backbone of the telecommunications sector for many years. For most people, plain old telephone service (POTS) remains the preferred option for interpersonal communication. Telephony has seen a number of important advances since Alexander Graham Bell's breakthrough, all which have helped make the telephone a reliable, high-quality communications device.

Telephone networks are owned and maintained by the telephone companies. Also known as the public switched telephone network (PSTN), this analog technology was initially designed to support voice alone. In the wake of the Internet's popularity, demand for transmission of nonvoice signals, often referred to as data services, sent the telephone companies scrambling to redeploy their networks for expanded uses.

Telephony is designed to support real-time, or **synchronous,** communication. That is, the communication takes place between two people at the same place in time. **Asynchronous** communication, on the other hand, does not require that two people occupy the same space in time. Postal and electronic mail are well-known examples of asynchronous communication. A number of efforts have been made to make the telephone a more well rounded communication device by building in asynchronous functionality. The home answering machine is a common example of voice messaging options that provide asynchronous functionality. However, the coupling of telephony and computer technology is taking voice messaging services to new places.

Call Centers

Human beings have performed the tasks of properly routing incoming calls and making outgoing calls in the past, but much of that work can now be done with computer software. Computer-based solutions for handling common telephone-mediated tasks are also known as call centers. Call centers can be programmed to handle a variety of incoming patient calls. If the call center can link patient records with a caller's phone number, it can route the call to the specific department or health care provider with whom that patient has been interacting. The call center may interact with the patient by first requesting information verifying his or her identity. The patient might also be presented with a list of prerecorded options from which to select and, using keys on a touch-tone phone, the patient can enter that information. If the call center is using interactive voice response (IVR), the patient can interact with the call center verbally. In either case, the patient is able to provide information that helps ensure that his or her call will be routed to the most appropriate agent. If the caller's needs are purely informational, the appropriate agent may simply be another piece of voice processing software that stores prerecorded information and messages. If the appropriate agent is human and the call center's telephony and computer networks are closely integrated, the patient's records may be automatically called up at the agent's computer terminal when the call comes in (Straub, 1998).

Call centers are also being used to automate many outgoing calls. Computer software programs, for example, increasingly handle patient reminders about upcoming appointments or calls to provide them with laboratory test results. A number of health care organizations have reported reductions in their no-show rates after implementing outgoing IVR solutions. The savings in health care costs for patients who fail to show up for appointments is also potentially significant (Steele, 1999). Overall, health care organizations are beginning to look at telephone systems as strategic tools. Call centers have the potential to provide cost savings in administrative overhead and improve customer service and retention.

Contact Centers

Contact centers, based on the same concept of computer-intermediated services, build on voice-only call centers by including eMail, Web-based, and videoconferencing options. Where personal patient information is available through contact centers, the issues surrounding the authentication of the patient requesting information through the contact center is all-important. That is, the system needs to ensure that a request for personal information is being made by a person with rights to that information. There is no global standard for caller authentication at this time, although recommendations have been made in several countries (Flynn, 1999). For more information on security standards, readers should also refer to Chapter 17 for a discussion of specific technical standards related to security as well as Chapter 20 for a more general discussion of security issues, which covers the 1996 Health

Insurance Portability and Accountability Act (HIPAA).

Cellular Telephony

Until recently, telephone service for most consumers has been restricted to devices wired to the physical network. The availability of affordable mobile, or wireless, telephone service has unshackled callers from the hardwired wall plate. An antenna, or transponder, is required to facilitate communication between two wireless devices. The geographic coverage of each transponder defines a particular "cell" within the radio spectrum. Thus wireless telephone service is often referred to as cellular phone service. A mobile telephone switching office (MTSO) handles the switching of signals between the PSTN and wireless cells. Many cellular telephone systems are analog, but digital systems have been developed. The digital systems provide for more error checking and reduced noise during transmission. The earliest use of the radio spectrum for interpersonal communication dates back to the 1920s. Its use was limited to local police, government, and military officials. In the late 1970s the spectrum was divided into smaller cells to encourage the reuse of signals, and in 1981 the Federal Communications Commission (FCC) issued new rules outlining commercial use of the radio spectrum (Cellular radiotelephone, 2000). These events spawned the cellular telephone industry, and by the turn of the century over 40 million cellular devices were in use.

The ability to contact transitory health care workers directly, bypassing asynchronous voice messaging and paging systems, has translated into substantial savings for many health care organizations. However, today's mobile telephony should not be confused with ubiquitous telephony. To access cellular services, a cellular user must be within proximity of a transponder to transmit the signal. Although uninterrupted service is common in most urban areas, service is unreliable in many suburban and rural areas. Cellular signals are also subject to physical obstructions, such as heavy concrete walls. A number of concerns have been raised about the security of cellular transmissions. The implications for patient-sensitive information are obvious. Furthermore, demand in many urban areas is close to exceeding the capacity of the present cellular technology. Fortunately, new standards based on digital technology are expected to increase cellular capacity.

The use of the radio spectrum to deliver voice foreshadows the convergence of voice and data transmissions that will likely make mobile communication devices a single point of contact for health care professionals and patients. Personal digital assistant (PDA) technology, covered later in this chapter, is moving in a similar direction from its current emphasis on data storage and transmission. Not surprisingly, the rush to bring voice and data together is currently marked by intense competition in the telecommunications industry.

Paging

Another very well known communications application that uses the radio spectrum is the pager, a standard appendage for many health care professionals. Some beep, some flash a light, and some vibrate. These familiar palm-size devices provide another purely asynchronous option for reaching health care workers and patients who are on the move. In its earliest incarnations in the 1920s, paging services consisted of one-way, voice-only broadcasts (History of pagers, 2000). The messages were received and recorded by an intermediary operator, who then broadcast the messages to the mobile paging units. To receive the broadcasts, subscribers had to tune into the appropriate frequency at designated times.

The assignment of addresses for each paging device now allows selective paging, or the ability to designate messages for a particular device. As with phone systems, the switching, routing, and conversion of messages is fully automated. Finally, with the option of cellular phone service for voice messages, paging has developed into a lower-cost, asynchronous alternative to cellular telephony. The standards that laid the groundwork for advances and growth in the wireless network were the Post Office Code Advisory Group (POCSAG) in 1981 and its successor, FLEX, which was developed in 1993 (FLEX, 2000).

Most of the messages received by today's pagers are short numeric messages, usually telephone numbers that read out on the pager's digital display. Numeric pagers are efficient, affordable, and the most commonly used paging devices. Alphanumeric pagers can display alphabetic characters as well. These devices are being used to receive a variety of text messages originating from fax services, eMail, etc., and often eliminate the need for the party being paged to respond for additional information. Pagers supporting ideographic languages are common today. Alphanumeric pagers require more memory and display capacity and thus are more expensive than numeric pagers and even cellular telephone service. Much like cellular service, MTSOs convert calls from the PSTN into radio waves that interact with the paging devices. Pagers are also subject to many of the same restrictions governing cellular use (e.g., proximity to MTSOs and physical structures that impede signal transmission).

Paging services and cellular telephone services are examples of applications that began by pushing a single underlying technology in two different directions. Over time, with technological advances in digital display and standards integration, it appears that data and voice transmission from a single device will move toward convergence.

Fax

Fax, or facsimile, technology is based on the same technology that makes scanning possible. As a piece of paper is fed through the fax machine, an optical scanner in the fax machine digitizes the image on the page. It does not matter what is printed on the page; the optical scanner treats images and text the same. The image on the page is sent electronically over the telephone line. The fax machine on the receiving end then reproduces the incoming bitmap and prints it. The idea for fax machines has been around since the mid-1800s, but it was not until adoption of the Comite Consultatif Internation Telephonique et Telegraphique (CCITT)—an organization that set international communication standards—Group 3 standard of 1983 that fax machines became widely available (Federal standard, 1981). Fax machines vary according to their features and functionality. Some models allow the image scanned to be broken down into a larger number of dots per square inch (dpi). This is also known as the image's resolution. The higher the resolution, the greater the clarity. Fax machines also transmit data at different rates, with 9600 bits per second being the highest supported by the Group 3 standard. Other variables include printer type, paper type, paper feeding and cutting options, and the ability to program the fax machine to send or receive documents at specific times.

Fax technology was one of the first common examples of telephone lines being used for data transmission. Data networks such as the Internet have made many health care providers less dependent on fax technology, since digital copies of data transmissions can be easily sent from computer to computer and then stored or printed by the recipient. However, fax technology will likely remain an important part of the global communications infrastructure, if for no other reason than its ubiquity. A hybrid approach is made possible by the fax modem, which can be used with a personal computer (PC) to send documents residing on the computer directly to another fax machine. Other advantages of fax technology, at least in the short term, include accommodating prevailing attitudes on authentication and verification. For example, a faxed copy of a signed document is still more likely to be accepted in many transactions than an eMailed copy with an appended digital signature (Gilbert & McCoy, 1999).

Voice Recording

Voice recording has long been a widely employed communications technology in health care. The dictaphone, one of the earliest popular solutions for portable voice recording, is a handheld recording device used to dictate notes and messages (Deutsch, 1999). The voice is recorded on a magnetic tape medium, generally in small-cassette format, and played back for listening or transcription. Transcription, the process of entering data via a typewriter or computer keyboard, has traditionally been labor intensive. Digital technology now makes it possible to convert voice directly into text and then to manipulate the text with a word processing program on a computer. Voice recognition technology has been available to the health care community since the 1980s, but early implementations were very unreliable (Noble, 1999). Advances in the technology have made it a driver for a number of successful communications applications. The IVR systems mentioned earlier use voice recognition technologies. Increasingly, voice recognition packages are being integrated into computer operating systems and specific software applications that enable command and control functions by voice. Consumers with physical disabilities are among those realizing enormous benefits. In dictation, voice recognition software has found another application that represents potential cost savings and time savings for health care providers.

Voice recognition technology is still maturing. Even after "learning" the voice of the user, the software generally has about a 98% accuracy rate at recognizing human speech (Essex, 2000a). Although that may suffice for some tasks, others will continue to require correction and editing. Ambient noise during the recording process is also likely to be an issue in many settings. However, as accuracy increases, the microphone becomes a viable new alternative to the mouse and keyboard for data input.

Speech-to-text applications have driven this technology thus far, but applications for text-to-speech conversion are not far behind. Although the notion of synthesized speech may bring to mind Hal, the rogue computer in Stanley Kubrick's *2001: A Space Odyssey,* advances in digital synthesis now offer options for making computer-generated voice very natural sounding. Applications driving this technology include common voice messaging systems that use computer-generated speech for standard voice prompts. Some health care providers are exploring the use of this technology in clinical settings. For example, the ability to access medical records and notes audibly may be liberating for physicians during certain patient-provider interactions. Patients with speech and hearing impediments may find new "voices" through this technology.

Document Production

In some health care agencies, pen and paper still function as the core technologies for many everyday applications such as patient records, dictation, address books, and messaging. Even with the plethora of new technological options for communicating, there remains a place for the common sticky note. Still, new technology has introduced efficiencies that the paper-based notepad will never match. Word processing and printing technologies allow for almost unlimited control and flexibility, surpassing that of office memos, reports, and other documents. These core technologies are used to support data entry and manipulation in databases, spreadsheets, and a wide range of other applications.

Word Processing

The invention of the typewriter during the late 1800s (Rehr, 1996) made it much easier to produce customized, accurate text documents "on the fly." Subsequent advances in technology led to the electronic typewriter, which incorporates digital technology to allow for easy editing, the digital display of documents on a small screen for previewing, and other major improvements over the original typewriter.

The demand for electronic typewriters began falling off dramatically as the prices of PCs and personal printers plummeted throughout the 1980s. Computer-based word processing and desktop printing have revolutionized custom document production. The author now has complete control over text formatting and style. The features, functionality, and overall print quality afforded by word processing programs vary. At the top end of the scale are desktop publishing programs that are used to produce high-quality print documents such as newsletters and publications. The quality of most word processors today is blurring the line between desktop publishing and word processing software.

Printing

Where word processors have facilitated the input and manipulation of text and other objects, desktop printers have done the same for physical output. In a break from the model represented by the typewriter and the traditional printing press, input and manipulation are now divorced from the physical printing process. Printing a document is only one of many options for output in a digital environment. Furthermore, desktop printers can now produce documents with the quality once available only through publishing shops.

Typewriters are based on the concept of impact printing, which involves the physical striking of a key against an ink ribbon. Dot matrix printers, popular early desktop printing devices, operate similarly but use pins that create characters as a series of dots on the page. The 1980s saw the emergence of laser printers. Based on the same technology found in photocopiers, laser printers use a laser as their primary light source for optical scanning (Anderson, 2000). Laser printers are easy to maintain and can be used to produce high-quality output. Resolutions of 600 dpi are now common. In the 1990s ink jet technology emerged as a popular alternative to laser printers. Ink jet printers force ink onto a page by applying heat to the ink cartridges. Although they are more costly to maintain than laser printers, their appeal is their support for four-color printing. Inkjet printers have helped make high-quality color printing affordable to the average computer user.

Personal Information Management

A digital solution is now available for almost any application that has historically involved the use of pen and paper. Consider, for example, the printed calendar, a staple in most offices and homes. The software version of such a calendar may look very similar on a computer screen, but it provides a host of functionality that the printed calendar never could. For example, regularly scheduled patient visit events can be entered automatically across weeks, months, or years. The software may be used to produce reminders (beeps, eMail, etc.) about an upcoming administrative meeting 10 minutes before the meeting begins. Entries can be easily added or deleted. Most calendar programs also function as schedulers. Multiple individuals who are using the same calendaring system can use the software to check on their colleagues' availability, schedule meetings for them where appropriate, and notify them about events via eMail. For example, a physician wishing to schedule a consultation with two other colleagues can check on their availability without having to consult a third party. Rooms, equipment, and other resources can also be reserved through such software.

Electronic address books are standard on most computers. In addition to storing the same kind of contact information contained in any paper-based address book, such programs provide a variety of output options. For example, names and addresses can be printed directly to paper or envelopes. Phone numbers can be used to interact with external communications devices such as fax modems or telephones.

Financial and numeric data, once relegated to the paper ledger sheet, has also migrated to a digital format. Calculators have long employed computer technology to automate a variety of calculations. Spreadsheet programs on computers expand on that application by allowing calculations and formulas to be saved, stored, and edited. Separate spreadsheets can be linked, which means that changes to formulas or numbers in one spreadsheet can automatically trigger the desired changes in other spreadsheets. Many spreadsheet programs also make it easy to generate graphical representations of the data, such as charts and graphs. These and other applications that involve small amounts of information are commonly referred to as personal information management (PIM) applications (PIM, 2000).

Although the PC has produced exciting new breakthroughs for managing communications and data, it has one very practical disadvantage for anyone on the go: its lack of mobility. Even today's lightest laptop computers are awkward to tote and deploy rapidly in most health care settings. Many consumers are looking for something closer to the size of the traditional address book, a handheld device that can be easily transported and used with minimum preparation. Easily transportable devices are called personal digital assistants (PDAs).

Personal Digital Assistants

The intent of a **personal digital assistant (PDA)** is to offer as much of the power and functionality of a PC as possible in a device that can be handheld and easily transported. In the 1980s the first generation of PDAs featured common PIM applications such as address books, calendars, calculators, and games (Anderson, 2000). By the end of the 1990s, many of these devices were emulating "lite" versions of desktop applications such as word processing and spreadsheets, as well as providing Internet services such as eMail and limited Web browsing. One of the first challenges facing manufacturers of handheld computing devices was how to provide for easy entry and manipulation of data on such a small device. Today, two solutions are represented in the market. Some PDAs use a tiny keyboard that while too small for touch-typing with fingers, can be easily manipulated by some kind of stylus. The second option is a stylus-based system that uses handwriting recognition software. The latter uses a very simple graffiti-like system of symbols for representing alphanumeric systems. Without having to recognize an infinite variety of personal handwriting styles, this handwriting recognition software performs nearly flawlessly.

Another challenge facing manufacturers was how to ensure that data entered in a portable PDA could be transferred to or synchronized with software applications residing on a user's PC. For example, if a health care worker uses a PDA to schedule a patient appointment, he or she will want to ensure that the meeting is also in his or her organization's online calendaring system. Easy synchronization is now a standard feature of PDAs. In most cases it is as easy as placing the PDA in a docking station that automatically carries out synchronization commands. Synchronization can also be achieved remotely, either through traditional network access models (e.g., dial-up modems) or through wireless protocols such as the wireless application protocol (WAP).

Although great strides have been made in maximizing PDA technology, limitations on memory, battery life, and input and display options will likely ensure that it remains a complementary technology to the PC in the near future. Still, demand for mobile computing devices in the health care industry should continue to increase. Open standards such as WAP provide for secure transmission of wireless communications and options for the formatting and display of data on small PDA screens. Increasingly, health care providers and students are using PDAs to access drug and other reference information, as well as to record clinical observations. Common personal communications devices such as telephones, pagers, and PDAs will continue to overlap in functionality. Meanwhile, PDAs will be integrated with a variety of new systems. For example, users will be able to determine their locations and chart their destinations by linking in with the Global Positioning System (GPS), a system of satellites that broadcasts high-frequency information on time and location.

Television

The ubiquitous television has long been a popular medium for health care education programming and advertising. It remains an important tool for disseminating health advisories and information to the public. Since the 1950s the television industry has been searching for ways to make television programming more interactive (Brinkley, 2000). "Interactive television" is a generic phrase used to describe a range of past and current initiatives in this area. The idea is to allow viewers to be more than just passive recipients of a broadcast. For example, they may be able to order a product via an interface on the television during a commercial or access a Web site for additional information on a particular program. Time Warner's video on demand initiative in the 1990s is one of many ambitious projects that failed to catch fire. Although some say that these initiatives have failed largely because of poor implementation, it is not clear to what degree viewers are interested in making their regular television programming more interactive.

Interactivity in other video formats is certainly gaining popularity. Digital video disks (DVDs) are a type of CD-ROM with enough storage capacity for full-length feature films. Unlike analog video formats such as VHS and beta, DVDs give viewers maximum control over their viewing experience. For example, they can jump back and forth quickly between scenes, or step through a video sequence frame by frame. DVDs can support a variety of media, including video, audio, text, and animation. Filmmakers using the DVD format may include behind-the-scenes footage or scripts that can be accessed at any time during the film. Viewers can choose what language they would like to use for subtitles. Until the popular use of applications such as DVDs, the digital technology supporting this level of interactivity has been accessed primarily through PCs in the form of installed software or CD-ROMs. Many patients, providers, and students in health care have been using such software for reference and educational purposes for years.

The use of television to access services such as the Internet is yet another example of how various communications technologies converge. Many of these early experiments simply allow users to switch back and forth between a computer and television interface, whereas others are actively exploring the potential of advanced digital television services. High-definition television (HDTV), which greatly enhances the picture quality of programming, is one of the first features of digital television to be developed and marketed. Digital television still has many obstacles to overcome, including competing standards, programming costs, and the cost of new services to viewers. The full digital television package is still early in the Hype Cycle model.

Videoconferencing

Telemedicine is the use of telecommunications to provide for consultations between medical providers and patients who are separated geographically. Communication may happen over short distances within a single building or between providers and patients separated by thousands of miles. Videoconferencing is the backbone of most telemedicine initiatives, and in fact the Health Care Financing Administration (now known as the Centers for Medicare & Medicaid Services) published new telemedicine rules at the beginning of 2000, stating that it would only reimburse practitioners for real-time videoconferences (Essex, 2000b). Videoconferencing also plays an important role in many health care education programs.

Today's options for videoconferencing are a tale of two approaches: traditional room-based videoconferencing and desktop videoconferencing. Another dichotomy has emerged with the transmission of video signals. Traditional videoconferencing has used expensive leased analog networks to ensure high-quality video, whereas public packet-switched networks such as the Internet are beginning to support video quality that may be sufficient for many applications.

Not surprisingly, quality is a key variable in any consideration of videoconferencing solutions. It may be helpful to provide some frame of reference for gauging video quality. Video is essentially captured as a series of images, or frames. The rapid sequencing of these frames across a screen conveys motion. Television generally displays video at 30 frames per second (Kuhn, 1999). Video display under 24 frames per second is usually perceived by the viewer as jerky movements. Common computer video formats such as AVI run at about 15 frames per second.

Video in its purest form constitutes a very rich signal. Compared with text or audio alone, video requires much more network capacity, or bandwidth. To make the signal less dense for transmission over a communications network, it is compressed before it is sent and then decompressed again at the receiving end. The devices used for compressing and decompressing video on each end of the network are known as codecs. Compression technology is an essential part of any video transmission strategy.

Both analog and digital technologies are used to transmit video. At this point in time, analog transmission offers the most reliable and highest-quality signal for videoconferencing. Analog service establishes a continuous, dedicated line between one or more sites. These dedicated, high-capacity lines are very expensive. Expenses are often shared among large companies and other institutions such as universities and hospitals.

Video transmitted over digital networks is divided into packets. Packets may be lost or delayed during transmission as the video signal competes with other packets. The resulting latency often impacts the quality of the video received. H.323 is the standard for transmitting real-time video signals over digital networks (A primer, 1999). It is part of the H.320 series that governs the transmission of video over digital switched telephone lines. Digital network transmission standards are discussed in more detail in the next section of this chapter.

Although these components represent the basic architecture of real-time videoconferencing solutions, there are a number of other issues to consider. For example, the number of people involved in a videoconference at any given site has a major bearing on associated costs. Consider a teleclass on health care education. What is the optimal seating arrangement for students? How many microphones are necessary to ensure a good audio signal, and what is their optimal placement? How many cameras are necessary? Will it be necessary for someone to adjust cameras during the teleclass? Is lighting in the room adequate? Another variable to consider is the number of remote sites involved in a videoconference. In a multipoint conferencing environment, there must be some way to facilitate floor control (access to the microphone). A number of strategies are being used to accommodate floor control, including voice-activated selection that automatically displays the site of the current speaker.

Although it is not appropriate for all videoconferencing needs, it is easy to see why desktop videoconferencing has the potential to become a popular application. Room-based conferencing solutions generally involve substantial overhead in initial startup and production costs. Furthermore, use is restricted to participants' proximity to the videoconferencing site. The ability to participate from any site with a desktop computer and appropriate Internet connection allows for a more distributed model. Desktop videoconferencing, especially one-to-one, can be done with inexpensive cameras and headsets. Compression/decompression is handled by software on the PC. The industry is beginning to respond to the H.323 standard as it matures. Bandwidth limitations over the public Internet will continue to impede videoconferencing applications where high quality is essential. There are also few viable solutions for supporting simultaneous audio and video multipoint conferencing from the desktop.

By freeing health care providers from the costs and limitations of room-based conferencing, the emergence of high-quality desktop videoconferencing should expand the use of this technology for remote consultation, resource sharing, health education, and continuing education of health care professionals.

THE INTERNET: HOW DATA NETWORKS ARE DRIVING COMMUNICATION

The Internet became a household word during the last several years of the twentieth century. In fact, the Internet has been around since the 1960s but has only recently developed a mass appeal. The essence of the Internet can be summed up in one word: *network*. The **Internet** is a huge network of networks linking computers and other electronic devices. In addition to the many miles of copper wire, fiberoptics, and other physical media that make up this network, it is the use of open communications standards that link the millions of computers and their users together. Standards are what make the Internet a single network of networks. Before learning more about the Internet and some of the applications driving it, readers should familiarize themselves with some key concepts in the world of digital networks.

Network Primer

An important part of assessing the potential of any network-based application is knowing its required throughput. Throughput is the rate of data transmission that is actually realized between two devices on a network. When connecting to a network through computers, data are sent and received at a certain rate. Understanding the rate at which connectivity is measured is a matter of bits and bytes. Bits were discussed briefly earlier in the chapter. **Bits** are the most basic unit in the digital world, analogous to atoms in the physical world. Each bit has a value of either 0 or 1. A byte consists of 8 bits, and metric prefixes (such as *mega, kilo,* and *giga*) are used to scale the concept. For a better idea about what bits and bytes mean in a data context, consider one or two pages of plain text on a computer screen. Those pages consist of roughly 32,000 bits, or 4000 bytes, or 4 kilobytes (KB). Bytes are most commonly used to measure storage capacity on computers. Bits are used in a variety of computer-related measurements, including network throughput. For example, a 56K modem is capable of transmitting and receiving data at 56,000 bits per second (Kps).

The speed at which data will be transmitted over a network depends on a number of factors. The physical medium does make a difference. Thin copper wire, for example, is a more resistant medium than glass. Glass, the medium that makes fiberoptics possible, can transmit data as bursts of light up to 155 megabits per second (Mbps). Because of its superior speed, fiberoptics has replaced satellite and other radio-based technologies as the preferred medium for transmitting data over long distances.

There may be a variety of transmission technologies available to optimize any given physical medium. Consider, for example, the numerous technologies available now for transmitting data over standard copper wire. An Ethernet, a popular network technology for connecting computers over a local area network (LAN), may transmit data at a rate of 100,000,000 bits per second (bps), or 100 Mbps. In a wide area network (WAN) environment, network speed is considerably less. Most people depend on WAN transmission technologies to access the Internet. There are now a variety of options for connecting to the Internet (Table 11-1). An integrated services digital network (usually referred to as ISDN) has the capacity to receive data at twice the rate of a 56K modem. Digital subscriber line (DSL), another popular technology at this time, supports rates of up to 8 Mbps. These technologies are especially popular because they are able to squeeze

Table 11–1 Comparison of Popular Options for Connecting to the Internet

Internet Access Method	Maximum Speed
Phone line (Analog)	56 Kbps
ISDN	128 Kbps
DSL	1.5-8 Mbps download; 640 Kbps upload
Cable modem	1-10 Mbps download; 768 Kbps upload
T-1 line	1.54 Mbps

ISDN, Integrated Services Digital Network; *DSL*, digital subscriber line.

more bandwidth out of an existing infrastructure, in this case common telephone wire. For that same reason, the cable television industry is using the coaxial cable to bring cable television services to many of the world's households to provide Internet services.

The maturation of wireless technology may help ease the burden on the physical infrastructure of the future. High-frequency radio waves have for many years served as vital links in the global communications network, especially for satellite-enabled transmissions. Now, wireless technologies are freeing computer users from the shackles of the physical network infrastructure, fueling the use of devices such as cellular telephones and PDAs for data transmission. Although the latest wireless network cards for PCs support very fast throughput, most wireless computing is limited to LAN environments. The creation of IEEE standard 802.11 in 1997 has greatly enhanced interoperability among wireless devices and will likely serve as a foundation for continued advances in this area (Introduction to wireless LANS, 2000).

The Internet has indeed become a network of networks that makes use of a wide variety of physical media. A message from halfway around the world may travel most of the way on a high-speed segment of the Internet, or backbone, but at some point it will still have to make its way from the Internet service provider (ISP) to the home computer. It is that "last half-mile," as noted often in the industry, that is likely to be the biggest impediment to high-speed network access. In other words, the speed of a network is only as fast as its slowest link. Other impediments to network speed include network congestion over limited-capacity networks and other unexpected interruptions in network performance. These issues are especially problematic for home users and small businesses that depend on dial-up connections over phone lines to access the network. Most large institutions use leased lines that guarantee a permanent, dedicated connection to the network at higher throughput rates than dial-up connections can offer.

Pre-Internet Networking

A number of networks have already been discussed in this chapter, including the telephone network. Telephone networks have been in place for many years. Most of those transmission technologies were based on proprietary standards created specifically for transmitting voice. With the increasing use of computers beginning in the 1960s, the need arose to share data, or nonvoice signals, between computers. The physical transportation of tape, floppy drives, and other storage media between computers, also known as a "sneakernet," was wholly inadequate and inefficient.

The move toward linking computers together developed on two roughly parallel tracks. LAN technologies were developed to link computers residing in close proximity—in an office or building setting. Key LAN technologies such as the Ethernet were developed in the 1960s and 1970s. The demand for LAN solutions skyrocketed as the number of PCs began to proliferate in the 1980s.

With speeds that impressive, why couldn't LAN technologies be used to transmit data over longer distances, or WANs? LAN technologies have their own limitations. For one thing, there are physical limitations about how far a signal can be transmitted over a LAN. In addition, LAN technology is based on best effort delivery, meaning that there are few mechanisms for ensuring successful delivery of messages. Finally, in the early days of networked computing there was no agreed-on standard, so there was no easy way for competing LAN technologies to communicate with one another.

Meanwhile, the creation of duplicative wide area data networks was plagued by high costs and slow speeds. Standards were again a problem, since WANs had no specified protocol for communicating with LANs. What was needed was a standard **protocol,** or set of rules, for communicating that would optimize trade-offs between speed and distance and provide homogeneous communication between heterogeneous hardware (Comer, 1995).

Internet History and Development

The Internet began as a networking research project in the U.S. military's Advanced Research Project Agency (ARPA) in the late 1960s. This original network linked a small number of geographically dispersed government research facilities and universities. The project was driven in part by the realities of the Cold War. Military officials were concerned that in the event of a nuclear attack on the United States, transcontinental communications dependent on voice lines could easily be disrupted. The telephone network is a **circuit-switched network,** which means that a dedicated connection is established between two points in real time. If that connection is broken, it must be reestablished. To address this concern, researchers began experimenting with a technology called packet switching. In a **packet-switched network** the data are first broken up into smaller packets of information. During transmission from point to point, the packets can easily be rerouted if there is a bottleneck or disruption between two points on the network. Packets making up a single message might take different routes, but they are reassembled by the computer receiving the message. The world's largest packet-switched network today is the Internet.

Circuit-switched and packet-switched networks both have their place in today's communication environment. Because circuit-switched networks guarantee a high-quality, consistent connection, they are ideal for real-time, synchronous communications such as voice and video conferencing. For that reason, they are also more expensive and less efficient. Two people on either end of a circuit-switched connection are reserving network capacity whether they are speaking or not. Packet switching makes more efficient use of networks because the network is being used only when packets are in route. More people today are experimenting with the use of voice and other applications over the Internet, but higher rates of throughput must be guaranteed before packet-switched networks can provide the quality of real-time voice communications available through circuit-switched networks.

The concept of packet switching satisfied the military's contingency concerns and formed the foundation for today's Internet. What was needed next was a standard set of rules and conventions for transmitting packets between networks. For example, how would errors during transmission be checked for and addressed? How would the data be compressed? When packets took different routes to a destination, how would they be put back together in the appropriate order? How would the device sending data know that it had been received on the other end? All of these issues and more were addressed by the **transmission control protocol and Internet protocol (TCP/IP).** TCP/IP provided reliable, in-order, end-to-end transmission of data. Equally important, it could be used in combination with a variety of LAN and WAN technologies to guarantee interoperability across different networks.

Although the creation of TCP/IP marked the first important step, only the dissemination and widespread adoption of this open standard made today's Internet possible. In fact, there were other internetworking protocols serving similar missions. BITNET, based on internetworking protocols developed by IBM, was used by many universities beginning in the 1980s (Cerf et al., 2000). CSNET, initiated by the National Science Foundation (NSF) in the early 1980s, was another. However, the use of TCP/IP in government and university networks throughout the 1970s provided a stable test bed and led to a proliferation of applications based on education and research. When the NSF took over funding and management of the Internet from the ARPA in 1986, it heavily promoted the use of TCP/IP and began enhancing the Internet's capacity. Network throughput and performance began to improve dramatically. During this time, connectivity to the Internet began to increase exponentially. Since 1988, the number of Internet users has doubled each year. By the end of 2002, the number of Internet users is expected to be more than 673 million and will likely exceed 1 billion by the end of 2005 (Juliussen, 2001).

Today, TCP/IP remains the glue that holds the Internet together. Networks that were part of BITNET now route their data through TCP/IP, and CSFNET became part of BITNET in the early 1990s. Still, accommodating the ever-growing demand for Internet access and bandwidth is an ongoing challenge for the loose confederation of public and private organizations that oversee the operation of the Internet. The limitations of the architecture and technologies that underlie today's Internet will give way to a new generation of protocols and networking technologies that are already being developed. A consortium of universities, corporations, and government agencies are working together on the next generation Internet (NGI) (also known as Internet2) and vBNS research networks—projects that may serve as the foundation for the public Internet of the future. Additional information about Internet2 can be found in Chapter 23.

Both the private sector and the federal government currently provide funding for the Internet. The trend has been to push the funding model toward the private sector. The NSF stopped supporting the Internet backbone in 1994. Some worry that private sector funding promotes narrowly focused research on commercial applications at the expense of the kind of basic government-funded research that led to the initial development of the Internet. A loose federation of nongovernment, nonprofit organizations govern the Internet. The Internet Society (ISOC), a professional membership society with representation from over 100 countries, leads efforts to maintain and promote the Internet (All about the ISOC, 2000). It charters a number of organizations created to address specific goals of the ISOC, including the IETF and IAB.

How the Internet Works

Knowing a little more about how the Internet works will help readers appreciate some of the challenges associated with sustaining this important network over time, and it may also give them a foundation for troubleshooting Internet applications. To transmit data from one computer to another over the Internet, the data source and destination must be identified in some way. Every computer, printer, or other device that is connected to the Internet is known as a host. As specified by TCP/IP, every Internet host must have a numeric Internet address, or IP number. IP numbers typically consist of four sets of numbers, separated by periods (e.g., *777.33.55.333*). The Internet Assigned Numbers Authority (IANA) assigns these numbers. The IANA often assigns them in blocks to organizations that administer many network devices. There the local network administrator assigns them to organizational network devices. Readers dialing in to the Internet through an ISP at home may be assigned an IP number dynamically, meaning that the IP number used identifies their computer for only as long as they are connected.

In any case, every device uses an IP address while it is a host on the Internet. Whereas machines use numbers to identify themselves, humans prefer names. To get around the difficulty of trying to remember numbers, a name can also be assigned to a particular IP address. This is known as the domain name system (DNS). Domain name servers manage such name/address pairs. For example, to connect to the University of North Carolina Web site, one would type in the user-friendly domain name *www.unc.edu*. However, the only way that the Web browser being used can actually communicate with the computer in Chapel Hill is to have its IP number, which might be *152.2.1.137*. The software goes out on the network and queries a domain name server to "resolve" the domain name. It returns the IP number to the local computer. The Web browser then uses it to establish a connection with the destination computer. The DNS is a hierarchical system. Top-level domain names include *.edu* (education), *.org* (organizations), *.com* (commercial), *.gov* (government), or country codes, such as *.ca* (Canada) and *.au* (Australia).

Client Server Computing

Another concept important to understanding how Internet applications work is **client server computing.** In the simplest terms, a client is a user of a service, and the server is the provider of a service. The client makes a request of the server, and the server provides the client with the requested service. Again, the protocol defines the set of interactions between the client and the server. Although TCP/IP and its related suite of protocols specify the transmission of data over the wires and other physical media of the Internet, there are also protocols that determine the way specific applications will interact. For example, a Web browser is a client application. A Web server is software on a host computer on the Internet that "serves" files requested by Web browsers. In the Internet world, most applications operate on this paradigm. Multiple clients can request copies of files from one server. With standard protocols in place, a variety of clients running on different operating systems can request services from the same server.

Readers may have heard references to "thin" clients and "fat" clients. Most software applications today are installed on local computers and take up disk space whether they are being used or not. Today's feature-rich applications require more and more disk space and computer memory to run. This is often referred to as a **fat-client computing** environment. Microsoft Windows is a popular computing environment based on this model. **Thin-client computing,** or network computing, is based on the idea that software can be delivered over the network on an as-needed basis. For example, an office manager in a medical practice who needs to type a memo might download a scaled-down version of a word processing application, or applet, and store it temporarily on the computer for as long as it takes to complete the memo. Before the applet is downloaded, the local client computer communicates with the server to determine if there is enough memory to run the applet locally. There is no standard definition for a thin client, but this is an example. Many thin-client computers, or Internet only PCs have minimal hard drive storage space.

For computer users who travel frequently, it may be advantageous not to be tied to a specific machine. Moving applications and files off of the client machine into a server environment means that files and applications can in theory be accessed from any computer connected to the network. In addition to the inefficient use of computer storage and memory, applications in a fat-client environment must be updated and configured on each machine. A hybrid solution is the application server in a LAN environment, where the local client uses applications housed on a server, so that only the single server application needs to be updated and configured. Still, this solution does not generally scale in a WAN environment. Scalability refers to the ability of a technique to work when applied to larger problems or environments. The obstacles facing the thin-client computing revolution at this time include a limited number of appealing applets and the absence of a cost-recovery mechanism for supporting their development, the lack of widely accepted standards for distributed file storage, limited bandwidth, and a mass computer culture that is more accustomed to the fat-client environment.

The emergence of thin-client computing as an alternative to common fat-client environments has been driven to some degree by the growing use of network-portable programming languages, such as Java. Java was developed by Sun Microsystems in the early 1990s as a computer programming language that could be used with handheld computing devices. As a programming language, it has several characteristics that make it easy to port over networks in the form of applets. Java embodies the "write once, run anywhere" concept of server-based applications (The enterprise Java platform, 1998).

Intranet

The appealing features of the Internet and its client server architecture have led many organizations to create their own internal Internet, or **intranet.** The idea behind an intranet is to restrict external access to the organization's internal Internet to users with the proper authorization. The organization's intranet may or may not allow access to the external Internet. The hardware or software that serves as the protective gateway on a network is often referred to as a **firewall.** There are a variety of strategies for restricting access. For example, some firewalls may be configured to restrict packets generated by specific applications. A firewall may be configured to restrict the organization's access to a specific external site on the Internet.

Many organizations are discovering that those now common applications that the Internet made popular (Web browsers, eMail, chat, conferencing) can be just as effective a solution for communicating and sharing information within the organization as proprietary groupware products. The interoperability across computer platforms made possible through the use of standard interfaces and open protocols such as TCP/IP has provided many organizations with substantial cost savings and flexibility.

Internet Applications

During the early development of the Internet, researchers and scientists quickly discovered they had some basic needs with regard to the use of the network. For example, they needed to share files across the network, to control software and manipulate data remotely, and to communicate both asynchronously and synchronously. These basic needs led to the development of a number of applications that drove early use of the Internet and remain important today.

File Transfer Protocol

For example, the file transfer protocol, popularly known as FTP, was developed for the sole purpose of transferring large files between two computers on the Internet. The baseline standard for FTP over TCP/IP networks was finalized in 1985. Using an FTP client, or program, the user can establish a connection with an FTP server on the Internet and transfer files either to or from the server. FTP does not care what kind of file it is. An FTP server administrator may want to restrict the number of people who can access files on the server or upload files to the server, so FTP access requires user authentication. Authentication is generally linked to a user's account, or user name and password, on the server. Some individuals and organizations prefer to make files available to the public without having to administer individual accounts for every person who might wish to access the server. These sites are popularly known as anonymous FTP sites.

Telnet

One of the big advantages of networked computing is the ability to interact with applications and files on one computer without having to physically interact with that computer. What is needed is a way to interact remotely with a host computer as if the user were sitting in front of it. The application most commonly used for these purposes is known as Telnet. The Telnet protocol became a standard in 1983. A Telnet client program is used to establish a connection with the host computer, or Telnet server. Once the connection is established, there is no actual processing of data on the client end. It simply displays screen text as it would appear on the host computer. For this reason, Telnet service is "dumb terminal" access. Like FTP, Telnet requires some kind of authentication, either private or public. In addition to being used for accessing personal server accounts, Telnet is still used to access some text-based database services, although increasingly such services have migrated to the World Wide Web.

Electronic Mail

The desire to share short messages across the network is embodied in the popular application known as electronic mail, or eMail. Among the early Internet applications, eMail is generally recognized as the application that generated popular interest in the Internet and similar public networks such as BITNET throughout the 1980s. eMail can be used to send messages to one or more individuals. Messages received can be forwarded, stored, printed, etc. A separate file can be attached as part of the eMail message. eMail features and functionality vary among clients.

eMail makes use of a variety of protocols, clients, and servers. The simple mail transport protocol (SMTP) was developed in 1982 as a standard for ensuring the effective transfer of an electronic message. Consider a simple eMail transaction. The eMail client application is used to create a message, and the message is transferred from the client to an SMTP server. Using SMTP, the server then sends the message out over the network to the message access server specified in the target eMail address. The eMail message resides on that message access server until the recipient connects with the server through a client eMail application and retrieves the messages. In some ways, electronic mail is bigger than the Internet. Gateways between the Internet, BITNET, and private networks have been established to allow the sharing of eMail messages. Although these underlying protocols have been effective for basic delivery and retrieval of messages, standards for other important functionality such as attachments and address books in eMail have been more elusive.

When a group of users with common interests wish to communicate with each other via eMail, electronic mailing lists are often employed. Also commonly referred to as a *listserv,* this application stores the names and eMail addresses for a particular group on a server instead of depending on each user to enter the eMail addresses into their respective eMail programs. A single eMail address is designated for the group (e.g., *healthtech@listserv.unc.edu).* When a message is sent to that address, it is delivered to the listserv server, which then distributes the message to all of the eMail addresses that have "subscribed" to the list. In open subscription lists, users can join or leave the list as they wish. The administrator of the list monitors participation in closed subscription lists.

Newsgroups

A similar application for facilitating communication among groups of users is the newsgroup, also known as a forum. Rather than receiving messages in an individual eMail account, a newsgroup is more like an electronic bulletin board that is shared by users who have subscribed to a particular newsgroup. Each newsgroup is named according to a hierarchical naming convention (e.g., *rec.hobby.painting, alt.music.cheaptrick*). There are literally thousands of newsgroups available on almost every topic conceivable. There is a process for establishing a public newsgroup. Organizations can also set up their own internal newsgroups.

Chat and Synchronous Document Sharing

eMail and newsgroups are both examples of applications supporting asynchronous communication. Early users of the Internet also found it useful to be able to communicate synchronously with short text messages. The Unix operating system supported an early version of real-time text-based conferencing, but it was limited to one-to-one communication. Later client server implementations expanded on the concept by enabling many parties to participate at once. One of the earliest real-time "environments" to emerge was MultiUser Dungeon (MUD), a fantasy genre game created by two students at Essex University in 1980 (Lehnert, 1998). Players would log in to the server through a Telnet client, and their characters would wander through a series of virtual rooms, reacting to situations imposed by the game. MUD players could also talk to one another in real time, or chat. MUDs gave rise to a number of similar virtual environments (e.g., MOO [MUD Object Oriented], MUSH [Multi-User Shared Hallucination], MUCK [Multi-User Chat Kingdom]).

Synchronous online communication got a big lift in 1988 with the creation of Internet Relay Chat (IRC). Users log on to an IRC server and join or create a channel. A channel is similar to the virtual rooms made popular by MUDs, except that channels can be shared across multiple IRC servers. This is the model for a wide variety of chat environments available on the Internet today. Chat programs are still predominantly text based, but an increasing number of chat clients support voice conferencing as well.

There are a number of software products that allow the joint manipulation of a single document or interface from more than one computer. For example, an instructor teaching students in a distance learning environment might use an electronic whiteboard to draw a diagram during class. All of the remote students accessing the whiteboard application can see the diagram on their computer screens as it is being drawn. Document-sharing software might be used to collaborate on a medical report by recreating a local interface on a remote computer, so that two or more parties can take turns editing the document in real time. These tools are often used in conjunction with traditional audio and video conferencing technologies.

Internet Telephony

Internet telephony, or "voice over Internet protocol (IP)," represents the convergence of two significant communications applications. More consumers are using the packet-switched Internet for synchronous voice communication, allowing for the integration of voice and data applications around a common device and interface. A variety of vendors are emerging with services and software to facilitate Internet telephony. Audio input and output devices are now standard components on most new computers. As the speed and reliability of local Internet access options improve, so will Internet telephony services. Telecommunications companies that have historically counted on traffic over voice lines for most of their revenue are revisiting business models as demand for voice over data lines grows (Darrow, 2000). Data service is usually charged at a flat monthly rate for the connection, rather than the number of minutes a voice line is being tied up. The voice quality of Internet telephony does not rival that of the circuit-switched voice networks, but many consumers are willing to forego some degree of quality for savings on traditional long-distance telephone calls.

Toward a User-Friendly Internet

Client applications in general have come a long way since the early days of the Internet. Clients left much to be desired in the way of user interfaces. Those interfaces were command-line interfaces, meaning that the user interacted with the application by typing a series of often arcane commands. Most of the commands were specific to a particular application. Many early clients for eMail, FTP, and chat services ran on the same computer as the server. Users accessed the client applications on the server from a remote machine through Telnet. This environment did not support graphics of any kind, so the only thing users saw on the screen was text. This environment mirrored early computer operating systems. Eventually, operating systems began to adopt a graphical user interface (GUI). As GUI operating systems such as Macintosh and Windows 3.0 began to proliferate, Internet application clients began to take on more GUI characteristics. With a GUI client, users could simply point a mouse and click on the appropriate icon, button, or drop-down menu, instead of depending on a command-line interface. More clients began making their way off of servers and on to PCs. In short, the Internet was beginning to become much easier to use.

Gopher

Early Internet applications discouraged Internet use in many ways. For one, access to various information resources was very disjointed. To access information on four different Internet servers, users had to authenticate four separate times. There was no convenient way to move from server to server. Users were forced to use multiple client applications. Data on an FTP server could be accessed only with an FTP client; a database on a Telnet server could be accessed only through a Telnet client. One of the first Internet applications to provide a more GUI interface was Gopher, a system of file storage and access developed at the University of Minnesota in 1991. It featured a hierarchical menu of point-and-click folders. By opening a hierarchy of folders through a Gopher client, a user would eventually reach a collection of files. Text files could be opened and displayed on the screen immediately. In addition, Gopher could also support links to other services. For example, it was possible to imbed a command to open an FTP connection in a Gopher menu item. In this way, Gopher supported multiple protocols. Finally, a Gopher menu could also link directly to another Gopher server. The Gopher protocol did not require user authentication, negating the need to enter a user name and password every time information on a new server was requested.

World Wide Web

In many important ways, Gopher set the stage for the **World Wide Web,** which was poised to make the Internet a household word. As it turns out, the foundations of the World Wide Web were being laid about the same time that Gopher was being developed. Tim Berners-Lee was a graduate research scientist at the Swiss research laboratory CERN in 1989 (Zakon, 2000). He was working on a hypertext project that made it possible to build a link into an object (text character, image, etc.). With a click of the mouse, that object could then be used to call a new file or service. Each file or service had a unique address, or uniform resource locator (URL). It offered a nonlinear way of linking and presenting information that was coined the *World Wide Web.*

Berners-Lee used hypertext as the centerpiece for his first Web browser, developed in 1990. The browser was the client application used to call up files from a Web server. The hypertext transfer protocol (HTTP) was created to provide for the client-server interaction. Like Gopher, HTTP is connectionless and does not require user authentication, although authentication can be imposed on a file transaction for purposes of security. In addition to reading text files and supporting other protocols as Gopher had, the browser also supported and displayed images natively. Before the browser, images and other media files would have to be opened with separate applications. Berners-Lee also included a set of tags and syntax for formatting content for display on the Web, called hypertext markup language (HTML). It was borrowed from the standard generalized markup language (SGML), one of the early efforts at creating standards for document formatting. In comparison, HTML depended on a much smaller tag set and thus promoted a much larger authoring community. The ability of laymen without computer programming skills to create HTML documents is one of the primary reasons for the explosion of information on the Web today. Web server software was distributed in 1991, and the first widely distributed browser, called Mosaic, was developed in 1993 by the National Center for Supercomputing Applications. Netscape, one of the leaders in today's browser market, was established in 1994. In 1995 Microsoft entered the browser market to compete with Netscape via its Internet Explorer.

Dynamic Web Content Most of the content on the Web today is static. A file is created in HTML, loaded on a Web server, and sent out on request. To change the document, the author must manually edit it. **Dynamic content** is becoming much more prevalent on the Web. There is no standard definition for *dynamic,* but it can generally be defined as information that is customized in response to input provided by the user or information that is updated automatically. One example would be a Web site that offers information on competing health insurance plans. A consumer visiting that site might be asked to complete a brief online questionnaire and then submit the questionnaire. The input would be sent to a server where another program might parse and process it. On the basis of the information provided, a new Web page containing links to appropriate plans would be generated "on the fly" and returned to the consumer. A local weather site is another example. Data from the weather station's instruments can be collected periodically and used to dynamically update a Web page as the weather conditions change. These are very simple examples of a more interactive environment possible via the Web. As mentioned earlier, the markup language used to format the display of Web page content, HTML, is not a programming language. A Web server must make use of an external program to provide dynamic content. The common gateway interface (CGI) is a common protocol that specifies how data will be shared between a Web server and an external program. These instructions are often referred to as CGI scripts. There are other ways to call up dynamic content, including the use of Java-based servlets, or applets that run on a server.

Media on the Web There is almost no limitation to the type of content that can be delivered via the World Wide Web. The ability to enrich a Web page with digitized photographs, clip art, drawings, graphical buttons, and banners has greatly spurred the interest in Web authoring. At the appropriate resolution (72 to 100 dpi), most image files can be downloaded and displayed in an acceptable period of time, even through a dial-up modem connection. Unfortunately, some images require that very high resolutions be maintained to be of practical use. An x-ray image of a minor fracture of the hand is an example. Compression and bundling technologies and the use of leased high-capacity lines must be considered when transmitting such images over a WAN. Similarly, the use of audio and video (AV) is also problematic because of the large size of these files. AV files used to be downloaded via FTP and then opened locally with a separate application. The Web browser industry began exploring ways to integrate AV files into the Web. One of the keys to the Web's success is the way Web browsers make use of helper applications to display content that is not supported natively by the browser. Browsers can easily be configured to launch the appropriate helper application when they recognize that they cannot support file types or protocols natively. Plug-ins are similar in concept, except that they are much smaller modules and exist as part of the browser. One of the challenges facing today's users is keeping up with all of the plug-ins and helper applications necessary to support the rich variety of content types available through the Web.

One approach to delivering AV files over the Web is to download the entire file and then have it played with a helper application. The problem with this approach is the download time for larger files. Some formats cannot be played until the entire file is downloaded. In addition to improved compression algorithms, the industry has also made great strides in streaming solutions. With streaming technology, the client can begin playing the AV file as it begins downloading without having to wait for the entire file. Although proprietary solutions have acted thus far as defacto standards, the Moving Pictures Expert Group (MPEG) is likely to provide the foundation for AV standards of the future.

Push Technology Earlier in the chapter the client server architecture, on which most Internet applications are based, was discussed. In most transactions on the World Wide Web, the client makes a request of the server and then the server responds to the request. Most of these requests are made manually. For example, during a session on the Web, a page from a new site is not downloaded unless the user selects a particular link or a new Web address is entered. These interactions are often referred to as "pull" transactions because the client must first make a request. Another mechanism used on the Internet is known as "push" technology, which is the automatic delivery of data from a server. In this chapter we have already discussed several forms of push information delivery. One was the television broadcast. The information is always being delivered; the user need only tune in to the appropriate channel. eMail is another example of push delivery, where messages are delivered to the end user's mailbox, although it is up to the end-user to check his or her account for messages. The use of Java servlets to update Web content dynamically is an example of push technology.

On the Web, push can be achieved by either automating the pull process on the client side or by broadcasting data from the server. In either case, the result for the end user is data that are automatically updated at specified intervals. Another example of a case where push delivery might be useful would be a health care worker who wanted to monitor a patient's vital signs remotely. Push technology on the Web is an example of a technology that entered public consciousness high on the Hype Cycle (Richtel, 1998). In 1997 it was heralded by some as the technology that would mark the end of the pull-based Web browser. Unfortunately, many early push implementations transmitted continuous streams of data at a steep cost in bandwidth. Perhaps more important, the industry discovered that applications for the technology were limited. Although no longer seen as a revolutionary concept, push delivery is being used very effectively and is playing an important role in making the Web a more interactive, flexible medium for information manipulation.

The Internet: A Look Ahead

With Web browsers providing a standard user-friendly interface, the Internet is hosting a revolution of information dissemination that is unprecedented since the invention of the printing press. It is providing countless new options for interpersonal communication, expression, and commerce. Content that was once available only through special applications is now part of a unified Web-accessible world of information. Most Gopher, FTP, and Telnet-based information services have migrated to the Web. Web-based versions of eMail, newsgroups, chat programs, and other communications tools are all commonplace.

The Internet has its limitations, and there are experts in both the nonprofit and commercial world dedicated to addressing those shortcomings. Unfortunately, the enthusiasm to add value to the Internet often results in additional problems. Perhaps nowhere is the tension between innovation and standards more pronounced than in the Web browser industry. For example, how many readers have come across Web sites with the disclaimer that the site is best viewed with a particular browser? Proprietary tag sets pushed by the browser companies often result in content that can be fully appreciated only with a single browser (Caruso, 1998). There has also been a proliferation of plug-ins necessary to access Web content. Too often, content is accessible only through a proprietary application. To some extent, these developments represent a move away from the interoperability that gave rise to the Internet in the first place. On the other hand, the intense competition that characterizes the development of the Internet at the turn of the twenty-first century may benefit users in the long run.

Many promising Internet applications will continue to fall short of their potential because of network limitations. The rush to provide an affordable, scalable mechanism for high-speed Internet access is the golden calf of the telecommunications industry. The frenzy of merger and acquisition activities that marked the industry in the late 1990s reflects the intense competition among media giants to position themselves as "one-stop-shop" providers in the media access market. In a world of unlimited bandwidth, the potential for true interactivity over the public Internet would be boundless. In the real world, bandwidth will remain a precious commodity for the foreseeable future. Research money continues to pour into efforts to squeeze more and more out of our existing infrastructure while advances in wireless technology hint at a more scaleable infrastructure for the future. Thus far, the world has shown an impressive propensity to saturate network capacity whenever it is increased.

Discrepancies among user populations in their access to the Internet are another issue without easy answers. World citizens who live in rural areas and developing countries where infrastructure investments have not been made are less likely to have convenient access to the Internet. Much work remains to be done to make software and hardware more accessible to populations with physical disabilities. The so-called "digital divide" surfaced as a second-tier issue in U.S. presidential politics in the early part of the twenty-first century.

Although the Internet has in many ways democratized the ability to share information with the world, it has also placed certain information at risk. There are few guarantees to security and privacy in today's online communications environment. The Internet is still an untamed frontier with respect to many of these issues. Safeguards for the protection of consumer information are spotty and mostly self-imposed by commercial interests. Sensitive data will always be an attractive target for hackers who take sport in compromising firewalls. There is widespread disagreement about what level of **encryption** technology should be available to the public and how the availability of encryption software impacts other public missions such as law enforcement. A more detailed consideration of security in the health care industry is covered in Chapter 20.

COMMUNICATIONS INTEGRATION: BRINGING IT ALL TOGETHER

A common thread in this chapter has been the convergence of various technologies. Rather than think of a range of communications technologies and applications as separate, finite approaches, it is perhaps more realistic to think of them as part of a continuum. Technologies that began as hardware and software solutions customized for very specific uses are being subsumed under the broader umbrella of applications integration. This chapter has noted numerous examples of technologies and applications converging in a single direction. For example, the lines between PDAs and telephones are becoming harder to distinguish. In this case the world of mobile voice and data are beginning to converge. Cellular telephones can now be used to transmit data messages. The Internet can now be used to transmit voice messages. Another example is the blurring of lines between devices such as the television and the computer. Televisions in many homes now have set-top boxes that can be used to change the broadcast television signal into a thin client supporting two-way Web access. The underlying technologies are being applied to a plethora of new applications and devices, breaking down artificial barriers that have largely been associated with prevailing definitions of physical objects. Today many vending machines are equipped with network cards so that their stock can be monitored via the Internet. Early incarnations of Java were used in light switches. The rash of historically analog devices that are now preceded by the word *smart* (e.g., smart board, smart house, smart room) reflects the growing reach of technology and the way it is transforming many traditional technologies. It also suggests an infrastructure in transition.

Linking Old and New Applications

Consider the unassembled jigsaw puzzle as a metaphor for the communications applications and systems in a typical health care organization today. This is not a typical, static jigsaw puzzle. In this puzzle, new pieces are constantly being thrown onto the pile. The new pieces fit nicely with some of the older pieces, but not with all of them. As enough new pieces are added, the puzzle begins to take on a new character. Suddenly, some of the older pieces no longer seem to fit. Such is the case with communications systems in which the organization has invested substantially (which are also known as **legacy systems**). Sometimes a legacy system can be made to fit into a changing communications environment with minimal reworking. Software can often be written to serve as a gateway between incompatible systems. The gateways developed to accommodate data exchanges between the Internet and BITNET are one example already mentioned in this chapter. Many new applications are written with legacy systems in mind. Although ensuring compatibility between old and new systems may compromise design and functionality to some degree, the organization may decide that the cost of compromise is less than the cost of replacing established communications technologies outright. Ultimately, however, most legacy applications must be replaced or migrated to new systems.

Enterprise Computing

Some pieces of the puzzle are simply missing, which means that key sections of the puzzle often remain disconnected. Consider the following example of a hospital's employee database. Over the years it has served traditional administrative functions, such as generating a variety of periodic reports and payroll information. The organization's professional development team has now decided to set up a number of internal electronic mailing lists. The eMail addresses are part of the employee database, but there is no way to download them directly into the listserv software. The systems and applications in this case have not been integrated. Although they are certainly useful as independent applications, their interoperability would benefit the organization in new ways. The pieces of software that integrate such applications are being written hundreds of times daily in organizations throughout the world. This piecemeal approach to integration has led to the call for more comprehensive solutions, or **enterprise computing.** Enterprise solutions are taking the communications technology puzzle and giving it a more clearly defined framework.

The effective integration of once-disparate systems is giving rise to new communications opportunities. Many organizations are providing their employees and clients with new options for customizing the way that they interface with the organization. Using a common Web interface and some of the permissions management strategies employed by intranets, organizations are taking advantage of their integrated systems to provide a single point of client access, often referred to as a **portal.** A Web portal for patients, for example, might require that the patient enter the system with a unique user name and password. Appropriate user authentication and verification standards for online systems are among the issues addressed by the HIPAA (see Chapters

17, 19, and 20). Once authenticated, the patient may be presented with a variety of personal information, including appointment reminders, information about prescription drugs that he or she is currently taking, medical records, and financial statements. The system that provides such information to the patient may be pulling data from a variety of databases throughout the organization, but those transactions are transparent to the patient. Through the use of a common interface and accepted protocols for sharing information across systems, organizations are discovering scalable ways to further personalize their interaction with customers.

Integrated systems are also changing the way that people collaborate. For example, think about what kind of interaction goes into the creation of a typical medical report. A variety of people in the organization may need to see the report at different stages of its production. The person who works on the first draft may be required to send it on to two other authors. Subsequent authors may need to look back at all of the earlier drafts. This is an example of a series of tasks required to accomplish the goal. This process is referred to as workflow. Communications technologies are now automating workflow in many organizations. In the example described here, the system may be set up so that all involved parties are automatically notified each time a draft is sent on to a new author. Each draft may be saved in a database that can be accessed via the Web by any of the involved parties with proper access rights. Changes to each draft can be tracked within a document over the course of its creation.

Databases

The use of **databases** as vessels for content that can be accessed via a Web server to produce dynamic Web pages is mentioned earlier in this chapter. Databases are discussed in greater detail in Chapter 3. Database technology plays an increasingly important role in today's communications systems. Conceptually, it may be helpful to readers to think of a database as a strategy for storing information. One way to record and store information is in a standard text document produced with a word processor. The word processor provides many options for formatting and displaying information but no easy way for a computer to recognize different elements of the document. To write a software program, for example, that would identify all instances of a prescription drug mentioned in a patient record, the software would need a way to identify a particular word as a prescription drug. In a database all drugs might be entered in a table labeled "Prescription Drugs." With the use of technology that makes it possible to distinguish among different elements in a patient record, specific pieces of information can easily be accessed. A hospital administrator may ask for a report listing the names and addresses of all patients admitted to the hospital in the last 3 days. The database(s) that store that information can be queried to sort patient records by date of admission and copy the desired elements from each patient record—in this case the first and last names. The more specifically data are defined, the more flexibility there is for manipulating the data. Within a database, information is often stored in separate tables. Updating a record in one table may automatically result in updates in many tables or across databases. The ability to define relationships within a data structure is often referred to as a relational database.

The overwhelming majority of communications are not recorded. Copies of written communications can be stored, but there is no easy way to link documents across file cabinets without digitizing them. Even though eMail messages are in digital form, most eMail systems are not set up for searching or analysis. By storing interpersonal communications in databases, many organizations are exploring new ways to add value to their communications. Consider a hospital setting in which numerous communications take place between providers and patients about the effective use of dietary supplements. A record of patient and provider experiences with dietary supplements can serve practitioners in the field or serve as the foundation for creating a list of frequently asked questions (FAQs) for patients. As content in a database, it may serve as a knowledge base that can be used as an information and contact resource. Many organizations maintain information over many years. Most of these data are used for specific purposes, and organizations generally look at a limited set of indicators in reports generated from a particular data source. Advanced algorithms for analyzing data have resulted in new efforts to discover hidden patterns in data that may yield important strategic indicators. Known as data mining, it holds great promise for helping health care organizations see the forest for the trees in the world of data. Additional information about data mining can be found in Chapters 4 and 5.

Extensible Markup Language

Similarly, the increasing use of exstensible markup language (XML) is making it possible to apply a database-like structure to information formatted for the World Wide Web. Both XML and HTML are subsets of SGML. Although SGML is still used by the library community and other organizations managing large documents, it is too complex for the average user. HTML does provide for some logical treatment of formatting, but it is a very limited and awkward content descriptor. XML swings the pendulum back toward SGML by emphasizing the importance of defining and tagging the document content. Style sheets can handle the actual formatting of the document. Style sheets consist of a set of rules defining how various elements within a document will be displayed. Style sheets can exist external to the actual document, making it very easy to switch between formatting options.

Standards for Interconnectivity

At this point in time, enterprise computing is still loosely defined, but the overarching goal of most enterprise solutions is to facilitate tighter integration of technology applications and systems. Custom programming will likely remain necessary for some time, but great strides are being made to integrate systems in a networked environment. Standards such as open database connectivity (ODBC), which makes it possible to access data across different databases from any application, have gained wide acceptance. XML is supporting the schema for flexible data exchange between organizations. Java and other programming tools are being used to program the building blocks for many enterprise solutions. These and many other standards and technologies will comprise the gateways needed to pull all of the pieces together.

Case Study

Diane is a physician in a medium-size U.S. city. She works part-time in a private practice and also does rounds at a local hospital. One evening while Diane is relaxing after dinner at home, she comes across an article in the local newspaper on the announcement of a new drug shown to be effective in fighting high blood pressure for people who meet a certain demographic profile. Right under the title of this brief article is a small bar code. Diane takes her handheld PDA out of her pocketbook, turns it on, and scans the bar code on the newspaper. The bar code represents a Web address that contains additional information on the new drug. The PDA automatically establishes a wireless connection to the Internet and launches a Web browser configured to display Web content on the PDA's small screen. The Web site contains more detailed information about the new drug not included in the newspaper article.

Diane scans the list of frequently asked questions about the drug and determines that it is probably suitable for one of her new patients. She prepares her PDA to send a message to the nurse's station at the hospital where the patient has been admitted. She enters all of her system commands verbally, including the content of her message. She requests a secure connection with the nursing station's patient record system. She provides her name verbally and then is asked to manually enter the password and pin information required by the HIPAA. All transmissions via the wireless unit are translated into secret code, also known as encryption.

To begin her message, Diane assigns it a priority status with the words "Priority . . . Normal." This means that the new drug can be administered after the next physician on rounds has approved the new prescription. She also assigns it a code with the words "Code . . . Prescription." She follows a similar syntax for all of the information that is part of her message, including the name of the drug, dosage, and frequency. All of her voice commands are translated into text by voice recognition software in her PDA. To allow for error checking, the message is displayed in text on her screen before she sends it. At the hospital nursing station, the station's communication server receives the contents of the message. Software running on the server automatically parses the message, recognizing fields called in the message (e.g., *code, priority*) and matching them with corresponding fields in the patient record database. The variables in the message (e.g., *normal, prescription*) are entered as a new record in the database.

The workflow for the system is set up to automatically initiate a number of other communications. First, the prescription appears as a new entry on the patient's eChart. If the priority status were urgent, the attending nurse and head nurse at the station would be contacted via pager, eMail, and voice mail with the new prescription. The system would continue to initiate a series of messages to hospital personnel on duty until someone responded.

The message is also sent to the pharmacy, appearing as a new entry in its database and listed on work orders as a new prescription to fill. The priority status, time sent, and time of the next scheduled rounds are part of an equation calculated to determine when the prescription should be delivered. The prescription is moved up in the queue according to the required time of delivery. The contents of the message are also run against the hospital's knowledge base. The knowledge base contains general information about the drug, links to information on the Internet and proprietary databases, contact information for local physicians and pharmacists who may also serve as references, etc. If the drug is recognized by the system, a selected menu of resources will be included as links in the patient's eChart. In this case the drug has not been used in the hospital, so the knowledge base queries a regional knowledge base for additional information about the drug. Because the drug has never been prescribed at the hospital, a message is also sent to the chair of the department. If the chair has any concerns about use of the new drug, he or she may follow up with the prescribing physician.

This case study is fictional, but nothing described in it falls into the realm of science fiction. All of the technologies used in this example exist. In fact, many of these technologies are mature and stable. What makes the communications system in this example seem far-fetched today is its seamless integration.

Outlook on Integration

Although the terms *stable* and *mature* can be applied to many communications technologies, it is important to remember that many organizations are still grappling with technology adoption, much less integration. Given the fact that the first commercial Web browser was introduced in 1994, it is easy to understand why the initial ripples of the Internet revolution are still resonating. Everyone involved in the health care industry, from the average patient to the hospital administrator, is still trying to determine his or her role and his or her organization's role in a networked world. Entire industries are redefining themselves. It is a period of marked transition from a local, predictable environment to a distributed computing environment where access points to the network are commodities and bandwidth and integration are the critical factors.

The fertile ground of networked computing has seen a proliferation of services, devices, and applications all competing to find a foothold on the new frontier. For every successful new application, there may be two or three that fail. Many IT consumers find themselves in the position of betting on horses at the track. Each product sponsor is confident and will do (and say) almost anything to remain competitive. The antitrust case involving software giant Microsoft only hints at the vulnerability of consumers in this market. In this environment of competing ideas and wills, standards remain elusive in many areas of the information technology (IT) industry. The absence of standards will continue to hinder the integration of communications technologies.

The degree to which even standards can help make technology more extensible is debatable in today's rapidly changing world. Moore's law, named after Gordan Moore's 1965 prediction that the processing power of computer chips would double every year, has played out largely as he predicted and raises important questions about the shelf-life of consumer investments (Mann, 2000). The cost of upgrading recently purchased systems or replacing obsolete systems is now part of the cost of doing business, but many organizational budgets do not reflect this fact. Operating under tight IT budgets, many organizations will continue to approach integration in a piecemeal fashion.

Perhaps the biggest obstacle to technology adoption and integration has nothing to do with the technology itself. Organizational cultures and personal attitudes about technology often shape a reluctance to adopt new communications tools, even in cases where their adoption would clearly pay dividends. During consideration of the Hype Cycle model earlier in this chapter, health care organizations were identified as taking a very cautious approach toward technology adoption. Given the life-critical nature of many health care settings and concerns about patient privacy, a cautious approach is certainly understandable. However, in an era where managed care arrangements are prevalent, the organizational drive to remain competitive is likely to clash with traditional cultures and attitudes toward change.

CONCLUSION

With a basic understanding of common communications technologies, readers should be in a better position to (1) keep up with what is certain to be ongoing change in this field and (2) assess the appropriate role of technology in various settings.

In the information technology industry, the announcement of a technological breakthrough or a new product seems to occur daily. Meanwhile, communities of all sizes continue working to craft effective policies and laws governing the use of technology. Following news and trends associated with a particular technology may have a direct impact on a personal or organizational decision concerning technology use. For example, a wireless networking card that supports throughput of only up to 2 Mbps may be a prohibitive factor in a health care organization's plans to use wireless laptops to transmit high-resolution x-ray images in a timely fashion. A subsequent industry announcement about affordable cards supporting 11 Mbps throughput may signal to the organization that its original plans for wireless networking are now worth revisiting. Attempting to keep up with today's technologies may seem like a daunting task to most readers. Fortunately, there are a number of resources available that do a good job of summarizing important developments.

Readers are reminded that they need not be technical experts to contribute to discussions in their respective health care settings about the appropriate roles and uses of technology. The understanding that readers are developing through their studies or personal interest may enable them to make technical recommendations in a problem-solving environment or, at the very least, ask important questions about technology recommendations being made. It would be a serious mistake to discount the value of questions raised about technology from a user's perspective. Too often, in organizations of all kinds, technical applications and systems are developed without the proper input of the people who will actually be using them. The results are usually not only disappointing but also a waste of valuable time and resources.

Web Connection

Information and communication technologies are changing the way we interact with clients and with other health care professionals. The development of industry standards, the relative advantage of the technologies and applications, and the convergence of information and communication technologies toward integrated systems are themes in this chapter that describe how technology has facilitated communication. In the Web Connection activities, you will identify current communication technologies that might be used in health care and learn about practices that facilitate or hinder the use of these technologies in clinical settings.

discussion questions

1. Identify several tools or technologies that you use that are *not* digital. Are there digital counterparts for those tools? How do they compare in regard to functionality?
2. How would you explain the popularity of the World Wide Web? Compare it with earlier Internet applications.
3. Think about the use of communications technology in your workplace or school. What are some of the potential obstacles to technology adoption there? Are they technical, financial, or cultural?
4. Consider health care providers whom you know. How are they using communications technology? If they are using communications technology, is it for personal or professional activities?

REFERENCES

All about the ISOC. (2000). Reston, VA: The Internet Society. Retrieved May 28, 2000, from the World Wide Web: http://www.isoc.org/isoc/.

Anderson, D. (2000). *The PC technology guide.* Retrieved May 26, 2000, from the World Wide Web: http://www.pctechguide.com/io.htm.

Brinkley, D. (2000). Do viewers even want to interact with TV? *New York Times Technology Supplement,* February 7. Retrieved April 1, 2000, from the World Wide Web: http://www.nytimes.com/yr/mo/day/tech/.

Caruso, D. (1998). Internet is snagging on free-market appetites. *New York Times Technology Supplement,* August 3. Retrieved April 1, 2000, from the World Wide Web: http://www.nytimes.com/yr/mo/day/tech/.

Cellular radiotelephone service fact sheet. (2000). Washington, DC: Wireless Telecommunications Bureau. Retrieved February 10, 2000, from the World Wide Web: http://www.fcc.gov/wtb/cellular/celfctsh.html.

Cerf, C., et al. (2000). *A brief history of the Internet, version 3.31.* Reston, VA: The Internet Society. Retrieved May 28, 2000, from the World Wide Web: http://www.isoc.org/internet-history/brief.html.

Cerf, V. (1999). *The Internet is for everyone.* Given April 7 at Computers, Freedom, and Privacy, Washington, DC. Retrieved May 28, 2000, from the World Wide Web: http://www.isoc.org/isoc/media/speeches/foreveryone.shtml.

Comer, D. (1995). *Internetworking with TCP/IP* (Vol. 1). Englewood Cliffs, NJ: Prentice Hall.

Darrow, M. (2000). If you bill it, they will come. *Internet Telephony,* May 1. Retrieved May 28, 2000, from the World Wide Web: http://www.internettelephony.com/.

Deutsch, C. (1999). Take a memo: Dictaphone is still in business. *New York Times Technology Supplement,* December 27. Retrieved April 1, 2000, from the World Wide Web: http://www.nytimes.com/yr/mo/day/tech/.

The enterprise Java platform: a Java adoption white paper for developers. (1998). Palo Alto, CA: Sun Microsystems. Retrieved May 28, 2000, from the World Wide Web: http://www.sun.com/swdevelopment/whitepapers/enterprisejava wp.pdf.

Essex, D. (2000a). Nine hot technology trends: Continuous speech recognition. *Healthcare Informatics,* February. Retrieved January 22, 2000, from the World Wide Web: http://www.healthcare-informatics.com/issues/2000/02_00/cover.htm.

Essex, D. (2000b). Nine hot technology trends: telemedicine. *Healthcare Informatics,* February. Retrieved January 22, 2000, from the World Wide Web: http://www.healthcare-informatics.com/issues/2000/02_00/cover.htm.

Federal standard telecommunications: Group 3 facsimile apparatus for document transmission. (1981). Washington, DC: National Institute of Standards and Technology. Retrieved May 29, 2000, from the World Wide Web: http://www.itl.nist.gov/fipspubs/fip147.htm.

Fenn, J., & Hieb, M.B. (1999). How should healthcare jump onto the Hype Cycle? Gartner Strategic Analysis Report: DF-08-9297. *Gartner Advisory Intraweb,* August 9. Retrieved February 6, 2000, from the World Wide Web: http://help.unc.edu/gartner.

FLEX technology overview. (1999). Motorola. Retrieved May 28, 2000, from the World Wide Web: http://www.motorola.com/MIMS/MSPG/FLEX/.

Flynn, H. (1999). What is the best way to authenticate callers? *Gartner Advisory Intraweb,* March 3. Retrieved February 6, 2000, from the World Wide Web: http://help.unc.edu/gartner/.

Gilbert, M., & McCoy, D. (1999). Fax: Life beyond the Internet? *Gartner Advisory Intraweb,* March 16. Retrieved February 10, 2000, from the World Wide Web: http://help.unc.edu/gartner/.

History of pagers. (2000). *About the human Internet.* Retrieved May 28, 2000, from the World Wide Web: http://inventors.about.com/science/inventors/library/inventors/blpager.htm.

Introduction to wireless LANS. (2000). Willoughby, OH: WLANA. Retrieved May 28, 2000, from the World Wide Web: http://www.wlana.com/intro/introduction/summary.html.

Juliussen, E. (2001, February 6). *Internet users will surpass 1 billion by 2005.* Buffalo Grove, IL: eTForecasts.

Kuhn, K. (1999). Conventional analog television—An introduction. *Consumer Electronics Design Education Project.* Retrieved May 28, 2000, from the World Wide Web: http://www.ee.washington.edu/conselec/CE/kuhn/ntsc/95x4.htm.

Lehnert, W. (1998). *Internet 101: A beginner's guide to the Internet and the World Wide Web.* Reading, MA: Addison-Wesley.

Mann, C. (2000). The end of Moore's law? *MIT Technology Review,* May/June. Retrieved May 28, 2000, from the World Wide Web: http://www.techreview.com/articles/may00/mann.htm.

Noble, S. (1999). Nifty high tech tools make the physician's life easier and more productive. *Health Management Technology,* April. Retrieved February 6 from the World Wide Web: http://www.healthmgttech.com/.

PIM. (2000). Darien, CT: Internet.com. Retrieved May 5, 2000, from the World Wide Web: http://www.zd.com/TERM/P/PIM.html.

A primer on the H.323 series standard. (1999). Lexington, KY: Databeam Corporation. Retrieved May 27, 2000, from the World Wide Web: http://gw.databeam.com/h323/h323primer.html.

Rehr, D. (1996). The typewriter. *Popular Mechanics,* August. Retrieved May 30, 2000, from the World Wide Web: http://popularmechanics.com:80/popmech/spec/9608SFACM.html.

Richtel, M. (1998). After falling out of favor, push reinvents itself. *New York Times Technology Supplement,* May 28. Retrieved April 6, 2000, from the World Wide Web: http://www.nytimes.com/yr/mo/day/tech/.

Steele, A. (1999). Computer telephony solution reduces no-shows. *Health Management Technology,* September. Retrieved February 7, 2000, from the World Wide Web: http://216.247.165.30/archives/focus2_0999.html.

Straub, K. (1998). Lives and livelihoods on the line. *Health Management Technology,* September. Retrieved February 6, 2000, from the World Wide Web: http://216.247.165.30/archives/business0998.html.

Zakon, R. (1993-2000). *Hobbes' Internet timeline v5.0.* Reston, VA: The Internet Society. Retrieved May 28, 2000, from the World Wide Web: http://info.isoc.org/guest/zakon/Internet/History/HIT.html

CHAPTER 12

Technology and Distributed Education

SHEILA P. ENGLEBARDT

Learning Objectives

Upon completion of this chapter, the reader will be able to:

1. ***Describe*** the uses of technology in the classroom and in distributed education.
2. ***Match*** the appropriate technology tools to instructional objectives.
3. ***Explain*** the impact of technology on higher education.
4. ***Describe*** the implications of technology on consumer health care education.

Outline

Societal Impetus to Use Technology in Education
Access to Learning
Role of the Teacher
Uses of Technology
Technology in the Classroom
Tools for Teaching With Technology
Online Syllabus
Communication Tools
Technology in Distributed Education
The World Wide Web as an Information Source
Process for Helping Faculty to Adopt Technology as an Educational Strategy
Faculty Development Plan
Quality of Internet-Based Distance Education
Issues of Technology and Education
Faculty Support in Higher Education
Consumer Education

Key Terms

andragogy
asynchronous
chat software
chatware
consumer health care informatics
consumer informatics
distance education
distributed education
Health on the Net Foundation (HDN)
pedagogy
synchronous
teleconferencing

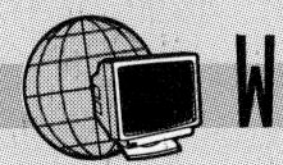

Web Connection

Go to the Web site at http://evolve.elsevier.com/Englebardt/. Here you will find Web links and activities related to technology and distributed education.

If you tell me, I will listen.
If you show me, I will see.
If you let me experience, I will learn.
Lao Tzu (Sixth Century BC)

Changes in the higher-education environment suggest that society is in the midst of a major transformation of educational methods. The transformation is no less dramatic than the change from rhetoric to the alphabet, from papyrus to mass production of paper, or from scribes to the printing press. The innovative application of a variety of technologies to education results from the plethora of available technologies and from a renewed focus on increasing access to higher education via various forms of distance education. In addition, there is a growing emphasis on what is termed "any time, any place" asynchronous educational opportunities. This type of education, often described as flexible delivery, distributed learning, distance education, and online (or Web-based) education, is particularly applicable to health care disciplines, where practitioners with multiple responsibilities require flexibility.

According to John Vaille (2000), digital technologies, in and of themselves, are simply tools unless they are viewed as extensions of human capability. In other words, digital technologies enhance teaching and learning because of the creative imagination of teachers who visualize ways in which technology can enhance teaching and learning processes. In addition, an information-rich learning environment, with changing roles of geographical space and time, enhances learner autonomy, thereby allowing students to be more responsible for their own education. Educators thus have the chance to become more responsive to students' needs for involvement in their own learning (Saba, 2000b). Most educators have decided to be part of the steamroller rather than part of the road (Hale, 2000). A greater number of faculty members are using instructional technologies as part of their teaching repertoires and are seeking effective uses for the growing number of available tools.

Furthermore, changes in the marketplace and the rapid increase in the total body of knowledge are exceeding the ability of people to stay current in their fields. This is especially true in all health care disciplines, where scientific advances have dramatically increased the amount of new knowledge, as well as the application of that knowledge in health care delivery. Estimates are that the volume of life sciences data is doubling every 6 months (IBM Life Sciences, 2000). Therefore health care students and health care practitioners must be lifelong learners. They must avail themselves of a variety of traditional and nontraditional educational offerings across the span of their careers. At the same time, increasing numbers of health care students are often older and have multiple areas of responsibility—family, work, and school. Using technology to provide educational experiences is a solution to acquiring flexible and accessible learning opportunities.

The integration of digital technology into higher education fundamentally changes the way that universities and colleges do business. For example, through the Internet, prospective and current students and faculty members have access to information about institutional policies and procedures, such as registration, program requirements, course and program offerings, and extracurricular activities, in an interactive and immediate way. Students can enroll in programs and courses that are not tied to geographical or time constraints. This widespread phenomenon is reflected in the results of a survey of higher-education members of the National Education Association (NEA). Findings have shown that 1 in 10 higher-education members teaches a distance course and that 90% of NEA members who teach traditional courses work at institutions that either offer or are planning to offer distance courses (NEA, 2000). Both private and public institutions of higher education have invested billions of dollars in distance education (Saba, 2000a). In addition, the Internet, in the form of school Web sites, has become an important and necessary marketing tool for promoting and advertising new and existing courses and programs as well as an effective tool for recruiting new students and faculty.

In addition, access to the Internet has created a new set of student expectations and service priorities. The ease of use, as well as pervasive use, of eMail and Web-based forms has led students to expect rapid responses to their requests for information and immediate feedback from instructors. This ease of communication has changed the work, and increased the workload, of faculty and staff members with both positive and negative consequences. Increased communication facilitates the interchange of ideas and affords faculty the opportunity to clarify and explain course materials and assignments easily and in a timely manner. Student-student and faculty-student interactions are more frequent, thereby creating opportunities for ongoing dialogue and the development of a strong sense of community, leading to collaborative learning experiences. On the other hand, a negative result of the high volume of communications is the large number of messages (often on a 24/7 basis) to which faculty members must respond. The increased number and type of student-faculty interactions has significantly increased faculty workload.

SOCIETAL IMPETUS TO USE TECHNOLOGY IN EDUCATION

In recent years, computers have become ubiquitous in society. In January 2000, nearly 50% of American households were reported to have access to the Internet, with more than 700 new households being connected every hour. In addition, more than half of U.S. classrooms were connected to the Internet compared with less than 3% in 1993 (White House, 2000). Parents purchase learning modules for infants and preschool children; schoolchildren often have access to computer-based learning in elementary, middle, and secondary schools. Many communities have established free access to the Internet in libraries and community centers for those who do not have access at home.

Within 30 years the Internet has grown from a military research network developed to enable the military to survive a nuclear strike (the ARPANET), to the Information Superhighway, and then to the development of Internet2. Just as the railroads of the nineteenth century enabled the Machine Age and revolutionized the society of that time, the Internet has taken us into the Information Age and has profoundly affected our everyday world. There are many examples of the impact of the Information Age. Some people telecommute over the Internet, which allows them to choose where to live on the basis of quality of life rather than on proximity to work. Public schools use the Internet as a vast electronic library, with untold possibilities for students to acquire new information for personal growth and for access to new ideas. Health care providers practice telehealth, using the Internet to consult with colleagues in other geographical locations and provide access to health care in underserved areas. Health care consumers have access to information about diseases, conditions, and medications and often visit their providers with disease- and treatment-specific information in hand and relevant questions about their care. Increasingly, health care providers need to understand **consumer health care informatics** in order to recommend credible health care Web sites to their clients and to use the Web themselves to inform their practice.

As a new generation grows up as accustomed to communicating with a mouse and a keyboard as in person or by telephone, the Internet becomes an increasingly important part of everyday life. A majority of students arrive at institutions of higher education with years of experience using computers and the Internet.

They have high expectations concerning how digital technologies will be used in state-of-the-art teaching at the university level. The number of students entering higher education with sophisticated computer skills grows each year. Some colleges and universities have a computer requirement for incoming freshmen, with some even requiring specific computer configurations and models. Examples with the year of implementation of the requirement are as follows: Wake Forest University, 1995; Georgia Institute of Technology, 1997; Virginia Polytechnic Institute and State University, 1998; and the University of North Carolina at Chapel Hill, 2000. These students and their parents expect faculty members to demonstrate how these expensive required purchases expand and enhance student learning. The need exists to demonstrate the cost/benefit relationship between computers and learning. Faculty members therefore have the additional challenge to develop state-of-the-art computer skills and to demonstrate an understanding of the best pedagogically sound uses of technology to support learning.

The skills needed include the development of Web sites for courses and academic programs, knowledge of the growing and changing numbers and types of technology tools, and an understanding of the fit between each technology tool and pedagogy. Because **pedagogy** usually refers to the education of children, a better term for the learner-focused education on which teaching with technology is based is **andragogy.** Andragogy is a theory about adult education that includes assumptions about the design of learning. These assumptions reflect adults' need to know why they should learn something, learn best by applying new knowledge, approach learning from a problem-solving perspective, and prefer topics that have instant value (Knowles, 1984). In addition, knowledge of learning styles should determine the appropriate use of technology tools while recognizing that all learners do not have similar learning styles.

ACCESS TO LEARNING

It has been predicted that as the children of the baby-boomer generation approach college age, there will not be enough room on traditional campuses for the number of qualified students who apply for admission (Passell, 1997). The National Center for Education Statistics (NCES) has predicted an increase in the number of 18- to 24-year-olds from 25.6 million in 1998 to 30.3 million in 2010. In addition, enrollment in institutions of higher education is expected to increase from 14.6 million in 1998 to 17.5 million by 2010, or 20% (NCES, 2000). With adults changing jobs and careers more often, there is a growing number of adults who are returning to school to pursue new careers. A significant proportion of these adults are interested in careers in health care. In addition, health care professionals are seeking to update their skills and knowledge in existing fields or to move in new career directions within health care.

Advances in technology provide a variety of opportunities for increasing access to higher education by increasing the number of people who seek educational experiences and the number and type of learning experiences. Technology is changing and advancing at a rapid rate; educational technology changes occur in response to these basic technology changes.

Personal computer access has become omnipresent; access exists almost everywhere in our society. Work is in progress to provide access to underserved populations, including people with disabilities. **Asynchronous,** or time-independent, learning opportunities via the Internet open doors for many who cannot attend on-campus or satellite campus classes. Students who have time and place constraints due to family, work, and location issues can enroll in asynchronous courses and programs and complete the required work at their own convenience. Asynchronous learning is typically accomplished via Web-based courses. Therefore access to a computer with Internet capabilities via a modem is the minimum requirement for acquisition of educational resources for people who do not have higher education available in their local environment or who have personal constraints that prevent them from enrolling in face-to-face classes.

In addition to asynchronous Web-based courses, distance learning can occur synchronously (in real time) via videoconference technology. Videoconferencing requires students to be in a specific location at a specific time to attend classes. Thus class scheduling may be similar to campus-based face-to-face offerings; however, cohorts of students in the same class are located at geographically dispersed sites. Videoconferencing enables students to attend class in the geographical location that is most convenient, with the course instructor located at a different site. The H.323 standard provides a foundation for audio, video, and data communications across IP-based networks, including the Internet (DataBeam Corporation, 1997). The H.323 standard, an umbrella recommendation from the International Telecommunications Union, made it possible for real-time desktop videoconferencing to be a reality. As desktop videoconferencing becomes more prevalent with faster and higher bandwidth Internet access, Web-based synchronous educational offerings will increase and synchronous individual conferences (such as advising and counseling sessions) between students and faculty will be facilitated. With the use of desktop video techniques, interactive small-group work among students will be more like face-to-face communication. See Chapters 11 and 17 for additional information about the H.323 standard.

ROLE OF THE TEACHER

The traditional model of the teacher in higher education includes a variety of roles—course designer, lecturer, discussion moderator, and evaluator. This model is often described as the "sage on the stage," where the instructor is considered the content expert who determines what information will be delivered to the students. Students in this model are often passive recipients of the information. Although they are expected to ask for clarification when needed, for the most part they are expected to accept and remember the information presented.

The model of the teacher in the age of technology, on the other hand, is often described as the "guide on the side." In this model, the instructor is a facilitator, and the students take an active role in acquiring, integrating, synthesizing, and analyzing information. Technology can provide the mechanism whereby an interactive learning environment is created in which faculty members and students interact more frequently with each other and with the information-rich Internet environment to learn together. The "guide by the side" model encourages students to take responsibility for identifying their own learning needs, to advance at their own pace, and to better learn to pursue lifelong learning. In addition, students learn to organize material for future retrieval. This new teaching model can be used effectively in the face-to-face classroom, as well as in the distance classroom. The model fits nicely with the principles of adult learning theory.

As computers and the Internet become increasingly prevalent, adult students (those enrolled in academic programs and working professionals who seek to update their knowledge) will need to develop and maintain the skills and abilities needed to use increasingly sophisticated software and hardware. They should be taught how to find and guide themselves through information and helped to become independent, self-directed learners. For additional information concerning technology and learning theory, including adult learning principles, see Chapter 1.

USES OF TECHNOLOGY

Teachers use technology to enhance student learning. When technology is used in education,

Box 12–1 Goals and Objectives for the Learning Experience

1. Technology may be used in the classroom as part of the course content. The following are some examples:
   - Using statistical packages in research and statistics courses as an integral part of the course materials
   - Teaching health care providers how to use U.S. government free databases to guide patient care
   - Using clinical decision support systems to teach approaches to diagnostic decision making in medical schools
2. Technology may be used as an alternative source of learning experiences (e.g., providing students with choices of either attending face-to-face classes or obtaining the same material from the Web or a CD-ROM).
3. Technology may be the prime source of information—such as Web-based courses and videoconferencing.
4. Technology may be used as an adjunct to traditional means of instruction. The preferred method may be for face-to-face classroom activities and Web-based materials to complement each other.

the technology is integrated with the learning experience: the goals and objectives for the learning experience guide how the technology is used (Box 12-1). As indicated in Box 12-1, technology is used when it meets an instructional objective.

TECHNOLOGY IN THE CLASSROOM

The notion of online learning is often interpreted as a form of distance education. However, many people believe that the real power of the Internet in education may be in the enrichment of traditional classroom courses. A face-to-face course experience is supplemented by an online enhancement. Many faculty members use specially designed Web sites and digital communication tools as a routine part of course teaching methods. Enhancements may include electronic syllabi, computer-mediated discussions, course mailing lists (listservs), and Web-based assignments and resources. Educators may access the Internet during an in-class session. The students and faculty access new information, which they question and critique together. Easy-to-use proprietary presentation software, such as Microsoft's PowerPoint and Astound Presentation, have empowered faculty to incorporate technology as a supplement to classroom lectures and to experiment with including audio and video clips in their classroom presentations.

Learning can be enhanced and knowledge retention increased when teachers use colorful, engaging visuals and employ sound and action. Learning is most rapid and retention is highest when multiple senses are involved. In addition, students use presentation software and Web authoring tools to develop classroom presentations. This enables students to learn the skills needed for developing professional presentations in work settings, as well as at professional meetings.

TOOLS FOR TEACHING WITH TECHNOLOGY

The prerequisite for determining which applications are most appropriate for an individual course is the definition of instructional objectives. The marriage of the instructional objective with the appropriate technology tool is critical for effective learning. In addition, higher-order thinking skills, information-seeking skills, and reflection skills are improved when students use interactive applications in their coursework. Comparing multiple ways of teaching and learning encourages educators to examine their goals and the available resources and then to choose the technology that best meets their needs (Levin, 1999).

Online Syllabus

The initial use of technology is often the online syllabus. The electronic syllabus may be a static document that is simply an electronic version of the traditional print syllabus. However, the effective use of electronic media for syllabus design produces a dynamic syllabus. "Dynamic syllabi go beyond online versions of paper syllabi. Instead, they serve as online platforms upon which to stage, manage, and enhance a course and can include electronic resources, instructors' notes, exercises and assignments, course projects, virtual exhibitions, links between course readings and Web resources, rich multimedia resources and students' projects" (Silver, 1998, para. 1).

Issues that must be addressed when planning and developing an electronic syllabus are accessibility, availability, and navigation. Accessibility refers to students' ability to access the syllabus using their usual pathway to the Web. For instance, some Internet service providers (ISPs) use their own proprietary browsers. These browsers may not allow access to all materials on all Web sites. Availability refers to the importance of having needed materials on the course Web site when students need them and updating the materials whenever changes occur. Navigation refers to designing course Web sites that meet students' needs. A well-designed syllabus makes it easy for students to get to the section that they want quickly. In addition, it provides a map that tells students what is available on the site and how to communicate with faculty to request additional information. It is helpful for all courses in an academic program to have similar navigation maps for the same reasons that most books have a table of contents and an index. Ease of use is enhanced if users know how to travel around the site.

Communication Tools

Web-based courses incorporate a variety of communication tools. Communication tools can be asynchronous, with people participating at different times, or **synchronous,** with the interaction between two or more people occurring at (roughly) the same time. Asynchronous communication provides opportunities for students to deal effectively with time and place issues. For example, place-bound students and students who are unable to meet the scheduling requirements of campus-based classes can participate at the time and place that is convenient for them.

The goals for using communication tools are to maximize interactivity among students and between students and faculty, with course materials, as well as with human and informational Web-based resources. Each communication tool serves specific purposes and is therefore chosen to meet specific goals. The following section uses examples to discuss the use of asynchronous tools.

Asynchronous Communication

The most commonly used tool is eMail (electronic mail). Generally, eMail messages between faculty and students are text but may include attachments that are sent in the form of text, graphics, or sound files. The most common objective for using eMail as a teaching tool is to communicate with individuals or small groups of students about issues that are relevant to that student or group and not to the rest of the class. eMail allows students to have easy access to faculty and is useful for brief communications. It is not as useful for lengthy messages and, depending on the ISP, may not be reliable.

A listserv is a mechanism whereby an eMail message is sent to a distribution list (mailing list) automatically. Students must subscribe to a listserv to become members of the list. They can then send eMail to and receive eMail from the list. Subscriptions may be closed to a specific group of people (as in a class listserv) or open for voluntary subscription (as in a professional listserv). Listservs are excellent vehicles for communication among groups of students and faculty in a course. One message is written and distributed to the entire class for such purposes as class announcements, changes in assignments, clarification of assignments, and routine course updates. Generally, both faculty and students can send messages via the course listserv, thereby facilitating communication within the group. Listserv messages should not be used to respond to queries from individual students unless the question and response is pertinent to the entire class.

Electronic discussion forums allow for asynchronous text-based interaction among groups of students. Each topic can be followed as an individual thread with the topical discussion available for review. Also known as discussion boards, bulletin boards, or online conferencing, these applications have several important uses as teaching strategies. Informal discussions (often labeled "student centers," "student lounges," or "discussion cafes") allow for the types of communication that might take place in a campus-based student lounge. Students may ask their classmates clarifying questions about coursework, share personal information or observations, tell jokes, and have other non–course-related discussions. The opportunity for students to share informally builds a sense of community that enables students to get to know one another despite geographical and time separations. These informal electronic discussion forums can function as virtual student lounges performing many of the functions of a traditional student lounge.

Electronic discussion forums are also used as interactive discussion processes for informed discussion of class topics. When used for this purpose, they encourage scholarly discourse about course content. Students, faculty, or invited experts can facilitate these discussions. Because of their format, electronic discussion forums involve public writing exercises. As such, they enhance writing skills and develop expertise in the use of technology. Such discussions may be an integral part of the course assessment process (and be graded), contribute toward a participation grade, or be voluntary. However, overall student participation tends to be higher when participation is part of a graded process. Interactive discussions provide opportunities for students to share ideas, pose questions, and present individual perspectives on the issue at hand. Critical thinking and problem solving can be demonstrated. These discussions may also be used to develop virtual debate sessions and for peer review of student papers. Faculty members can monitor student interactions, pose additional questions, and identify key issues (Figure 12-1).

A key purpose for the use of discussion forums (and other communication tools) is to create a community of learners. Remote learners may feel isolated. Mechanisms that encourage frequent, quality interactions among students, faculty, and other participants in a course are those that provide opportunities for the interchange of ideas, as well as for coaching and mentoring. Distance learners should be able to have personal interactions with faculty and other students just as they would if they were on campus. One example is the concept of virtual office hours. Students are told that at a designated time the faculty member will be available for an online discussion related to questions or problems identified by an individual or by a group of students. Virtual office hours can use discussion forum software or chatware. Using this mechanism, students can drop in to "talk with the faculty member," just as they might stop by an instructor's office on campus.

Synchronous Communication

Chat software (called **chatware**) is used for real-time chat in which the participants alternate typing their comments into a message box. Real-time interactions among distance students can be exciting and informative. However, students who are inexperienced with this type of communication should be adequately prepared for the communication process (Figure 12-2).

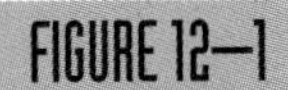
FIGURE 12–1 Example of an Electronic Discussion Forum

Catherine

Excellent example of the complexity of providing for security of information and highlights how we can easily box ourselves in when we make rules and standards that may interfere with our work processes. As I thought about your example of an elevator conversation, I was about to agree wholeheartedly (as I usually do) but then thought about two physicians caring for a critically ill patient who might be responding to a code (or two supervisors covering the house responding to the code) and happen to be in an elevator at the same time. In the interest of time there is the possibility that patient identifiable information may be shared within earshot of others—a breach in security, yes; violation of privacy, yes; violation of confidentiality, yes; typical in the work flow process, yes—so is it wrong? And what should the consequences be?

Donna

Reply

◄◄Previous Message   Next Message ►►

Current Thread Detail:

Security-discussions and solutions	Summey, Meg	02-Oct-2000
Re: Security discussions and soluti...	Bailey, Donna	04-Oct-2000
Re: Security discussions and sol...	Gold, Catherine	05-Oct-2000
Re: Security discussions and ...	Bailey, Donna	06-Oct-2000
Re: Security discussions a...	Dettman, Grace	06-Oct-2000

FIGURE 12–2 Virtual White Board

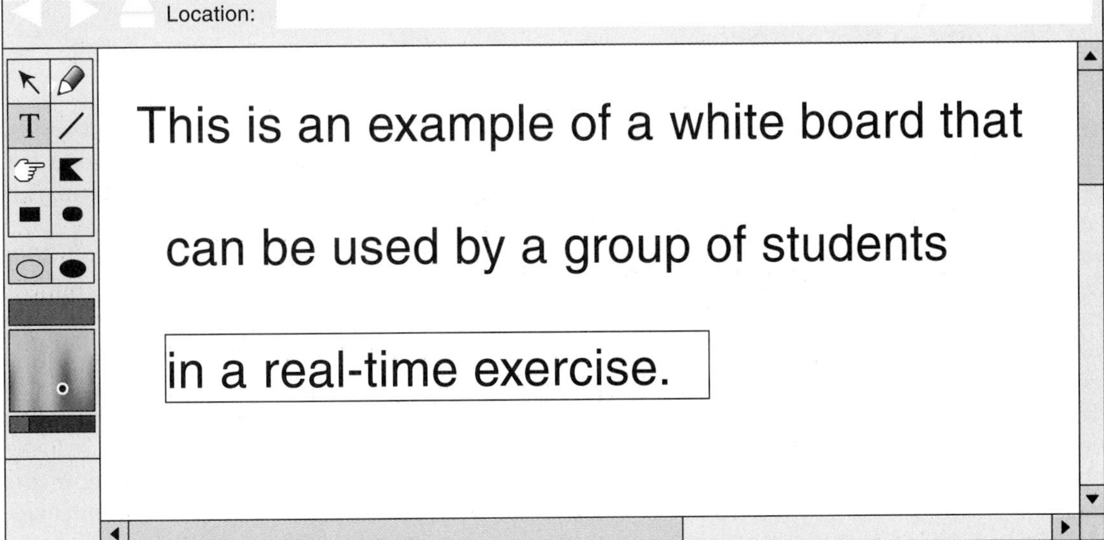

Depending on the software used, results are sent in a scrolling list or in individual boxes for each participant. Although this form of electronic communication is called synchronous, it is important for users to know that there is usually some time lag between comments posted and responses. The time lag is due to speed of typing, as well as electronic transfer of the message. Typographical errors often occur because of the desire to type quickly to maintain the flow of conversation. In addition, if the format is that of a scrolling list, the responses may be displayed in chronological order rather than in logical order. In other words, the person who types more quickly or enters a shorter message will have his or her message viewed first even when the response is not in the appropriate order. Chat may therefore be disjointed and create frustration and fatigue in the participants. Successful synchronous chat occurs in small groups where a group leader directs the interchange among group members and the group has learned to communicate using established protocols.

Future chatware will include audio and video components, making real-time desktop conferencing an exciting part of Web-based educational offerings.

TECHNOLOGY IN DISTRIBUTED EDUCATION

The terms *distributed education* and *distance education* are often used interchangeably. In the broadest sense, **distance education** refers to educational experiences when the instructor and the students are in different geographical locations. Distance education can be accomplished by a variety of methods, including correspondence courses, audiotapes and videotapes, CD-ROMs, broadcast television, and **teleconferencing. Distributed education** denotes a learner-centered environment that uses synchronous and/or asynchronous technologies to supplement traditional courses or deliver distance education.

The development and management of Web-based courses has significant time implications for faculty. Developing and offering any course, traditional or otherwise, involves a number of tasks. Some examples include finding and selecting a textbook or other readings, developing course objectives, outlining the course content, and developing learning units. Developing and offering a Web-based course involves an additional set of tasks. The following list (which is by no means conclusive) is included here to provide an idea of the scope of faculty work involved in teaching a Web-based course. These tasks are in addition to the many tasks required when developing any course:

- Developing Web-based course content
- Locating and integrating links and other Web-based resources into the course
- Updating and maintaining Web pages
- Ensuring currency of content and assignments
- Communicating changes in content and assignments
- Sending periodic reminders of coming deadlines to students
- Receiving and responding to electronic communications
- Grading assignments and recording grades

Web-based courses can be designed using a variety of available tools. Faculty members who are computer buffs may use hypertext markup language (HTML) or a Web authoring application to design a course layout that is individual and unique. This approach requires learning an extensive coding language or a software product, which can be time intensive. Some institutions provide instructional technology support in the form of instructional designers, Web designers, and graphics designers to enable such individualized course development. More often, institutions have adopted one or more course management applications, often called courseware (Blackboard.com's CourseInfo, WebCT) or groupware (Lotus Learning Space), or have outsourced the course development and course management processes to companies that host the courses on their own servers (e.g., Real Education, Eduprise, eCollege). They may also develop partnerships with for-profit entities to market and deliver courses and programs over the Internet to students and organizations in a rapidly growing international marketplace (NextEd).

Course management applications are designed to assist faculty in course development by organizing the materials on a course Web site to enable students and faculty to share and access specific information more easily. Faculty members can administer their courses using built-in controls that allow them to post, update, and remove materials on an as-needed basis. In addition, course statistics are accumulated; electronic grade books are maintained; and online quizzes and surveys can be constructed, administered, and graded. Each application has its own compendium of functions and structures, but most include similar functionality.

Course management applications facilitate interactions between faculty and students and among students. Another term for these applications is courseware. Courseware products include a variety of functions that are available within the shell of the software. Typical provisions are tracking and record keeping, the ability to create groups and mailing lists, and Web forms that enable students and faculty to create individualized quizzes and surveys. The use of intuitive course management software enables educators to produce enhancements to existing face-to-face courses, to develop course materials and learning exercises that decrease the amount of time that students must spend on campuses, or to migrate to totally Web-based courses. Incremental steps toward increased inclusion of digital technology in courses often lead to innovative teaching and learning experiences that are far beyond the original intent.

No matter which course management approach is used, Web-based distributed education usually takes full advantage of the amount of information that is available on the World Wide Web (WWW). This information resource provides opportunities for learning that far exceed historical information resources. Since there is little restriction and oversight of materials that are easily accessed on the Web, learning exercises that use the Web should include modules teaching students how to evaluate Web sites.

THE WORLD WIDE WEB AS AN INFORMATION SOURCE

Health care students and other health care providers who use the WWW as an information resource must know how to evaluate the credibility and usefulness of Web sites for their own and their clients' purposes. Libraries at major universities have taken a leadership role in identifying and providing easily accessible criteria sets for Web site evaluation that can be incorporated into course materials. Health care informatics specialists should be knowledgeable about information retrieval and resources for administrators and clinicians in their work settings.

Web site evaluation criteria typically include such concepts as authority, accuracy, objectivity, currency, and design (Table 12-1). University libraries often include evaluation criteria on their Web sites with suggested processes for using the criteria. Additional information on evaluating Web site information is presented in Chapter 2.

PROCESS FOR HELPING FACULTY TO ADOPT TECHNOLOGY AS AN EDUCATIONAL STRATEGY

Change is difficult for most people under the best of circumstances. Changing teaching strategies is a slow process, especially when technology is part of the equation. There are several ways in which educators might approach the adoption of

Table 12–1 Criteria for Evaluating Web Sites

Criterion	Relevant Questions
Authority	Who is the author? What are the author's qualifications? Who is the publisher/source? What is the author's affiliation?
Accuracy	How reliable and free from errors is the information? For what audience is the information written?
Objectivity	Is the information presented with a recognizable bias?
Currency	How up-to-date is the information? Does the site include the dates on which it was originally posted? Revised?
Coverage	What is covered on the site? How in-depth is the information? Is the depth of coverage congruent with the needs of the expected audience?

Modified from Alexander, J., & Tate, M.A. (1996, revised July 25, 2001). *Evaluating Web resources.* Chester, PA: Widener University. Retrieved August 12, 2001, from the World Wide Web: http://www2.widener.edu/Wolfgram-Memorial-Library/webevaluation/webeval.htm.

technology as part of their teaching methods. Some "early adopters" will take the trial-and-error approach and jump right in. These faculty members are the ones who learn basic HTML so that they can design their own Web pages, sign up for the first training workshops that become available in their work setting, or purchase Web design programs on their own or download shareware from the Web. Early adopters learn best by doing and are willing and able to invest the time and energy to learn on their own. Most faculty members, however, benefit from an incremental approach in which they learn in small bites and apply new skills as they are developed. The process that follows is an example of an incremental approach that requires on-site technical and instructional design support while recognizing that content expertise resides with the faculty member.

Faculty Development Plan

A five-step development plan can be seen in Box 12-2. As technology evolves, new tools become available that will add to those in current use and expand the possibilities for educational innovation. Learning experiences occur in a variety of instructional formats. Some examples of effective learning experiences are small-group projects, discussion groups, real-time activities, and online course materials.

Small-Group Projects

Students are divided into groups of four to seven in which they work collaboratively to complete a single project. Students can determine the communication process that works best for the group. These might be asynchronous or synchronous processes, depending on geographical or time constraints on the members of the group. Some groups will choose to use eMail or a group mailing list, others will post their communications on a discussion forum, and still others will decide to use real-time chat. It is important that the group identify a leader who will keep the group on task, collect the components of the project that each member completes, and compile the final report.

Discussion Groups

The class might be divided into small discussion groups that meet in group-based discussion forums. Each group is assigned a discussion topic. Group members post their comments relative to the assigned subject or reading and then respond to other members' comments. The entire class can discuss some topics in one discussion forum; however, a discussion moderator is needed to keep the discussion flowing and to ensure that all students participate in the discussion. Discussions can receive a participation grade or be vol-

Box 12—2 Faculty Development Plan

1. Take the first bite. Attend a short training workshop, enroll in an online course, initiate a course listserv or discussion forum.
2. Plan the next meal. Examine traditional course materials. Identify the parts of the syllabus to place on the Web, develop a course Web site that includes information that students will think is useful, create a Web-based course calendar, notify students that eMail will be the preferred method of between-class communication.
3. Sit down to eat the meal. Create content modules that can be completed completely online, determine which portions of the course will not require classroom attendance, receive all assignments electronically, return all grades via eMail or an electronic grade book, receive appropriate approval to include online course readings, identify Web resources to assign as learning exercises.
4. Time for dessert. The decision point is now. It is time to decide whether to continue to use the technology to enhance a face-to-face class or to gradually increase the online components so as to migrate to a distance education course.
5. Hungry again! Evaluation at each step of the process will provide input into course revisions, expansions, and enhancements. It is very important to seek student feedback throughout the learning process—to know what works and what doesn't and to pilot revisions. Peer evaluation of course materials by other faculty members provides objective input into subsequent versions of the course.

untary, depending on the instructional objective for the exercise.

Real-Time Activities

Synchronous chat software and white board systems can be used for virtual office hours, student presentations, group evaluation of Web sites, and question-and-answer sessions. Issues related to student schedules and time zone differences must be resolved before scheduling synchronous learning experiences. Decisions about how students who are unable to "attend" synchronous sessions can meet course requirements should be communicated to prospective students before enrollment in the course.

Online Course Materials

There is a growing trend toward including online readings (articles, existing Web sites, and book chapters), lecture notes, and slide presentations in Web-based courses. Lecture notes and slide presentations may be enhanced with accompanying audio tracks or streaming video clips. Decision making regarding the posting of online materials includes a review of intellectual property rules, fair use and copyright regulations, and understanding of organizational policies related to these issues. Consultation with university librarians who have expertise with copyright and intellectual property rules is recommended.

QUALITY OF INTERNET-BASED DISTANCE EDUCATION

The rapid growth of distance education using Internet technology raises issues related to evaluating the quality of teaching and learning using this medium. Benchmarks developed for all types of distance learning have been examined for their

Table 12–2 Benchmarks for Quality in Internet-Based Distance Education

Benchmark Category	Sample Benchmark
Institutional support	The reliability of the technology delivery system is as fail-safe as possible
Course development	Instructional materials are reviewed periodically to ensure that they meet program objectives
Teaching/ learning	Student interaction with faculty and other students is an essential characteristic and is facilitated through a variety of ways, including voice mail and/or eMail
Course structure	Students have access to sufficient library resources that may include a "virtual library" accessible through the World Wide Web
Student support	Students receive information about programs, including admission requirements, tuition and fees, books and supplies, technical and proctoring requirements, and student support services
Faculty support	Technical assistance in course development is available to faculty members, who are encouraged to use it
Evaluation and assessment	The program's educational effectiveness and teaching/learning process is assessed through an evaluation process that uses several methods and applies specific standards

Modified from Institute for Higher Education Policy. (2000). *Quality on the line: Benchmarks for success in Internet-based distance education.* Blackboard.com and National Education Association. Washington, DC: Author.

relevance to Internet-based distance education. Blackboard, Inc., and the NEA were commissioned by the Institute for Higher Education Policy to complete a study related to assessing the quality of online education. In March 2000 the Institute for Higher Education Policy published *Quality on the Line: Benchmarks for Success in Internet-Based Distance Education,* which suggested that for the six institutions studied (universities with Internet-based degree programs), the benchmarks for quality were both important and incorporated into the policies and procedures. The final outcomes are 24 benchmarks organized in seven categories that have been identified as essential to ensure quality in distance education (Institute for Higher Education Policy, 2000). See Table 12-2 for an example of the type of benchmarks in each category.

ISSUES OF TECHNOLOGY AND EDUCATION

Computer- and Internet-based instructional technologies are only tools. Educators and health informatics specialists must learn how these tools can be used to improve the learning environment for students and consumers. Instructional technology is the theory and practice of design, development, utilization, management, and evaluation of processes and resources for learning (Seels & Richey, 1994). It refers to the use of technology to achieve teaching and learning outcomes.

Issues related to the use of technology for educational purposes include the following:

- The need for a variety of faculty supports (technical support, time, incentives and rewards, etc.)
- A fit of technology with the content, audience, and purpose of the educational offering
- Access to appropriate hardware and software by learners and teachers

Faculty Support in Higher Education

Many faculty members acknowledge that they are reluctant to use technology in their teaching (particularly in relation to distance education and Web-based teaching) without receiving appropriate support from their institutions. Support for faculty takes many forms. Issues related to having needed equipment—necessary hardware/software, access to available technical support staff, department and school recognition and valuing attached to electronic educational products; released time to develop materials and learn the skills needed for success in new endeavors; acknowledgment of the effort needed to accomplish required tasks; and intellectual property rights are the issues most often needing resolution.

Valuing of online work as a scholarly endeavor and a respected aspect of promotion and tenure decisions is needed as the movement toward increasing distance education offerings and using technology in campus-based courses grows. Centralized or decentralized technical and instructional design support is needed for faculty training and to convert existing course materials to electronic media. These services may be available in a centralized center or in a specific department or school. Services include training workshops; orientation to Web-based applications; assistance with course design; access to educational research materials, readings, and Web resources about instructional technology; and consultations with peer faculty or instructional designers. Faculty symposia and meetings should be arranged as mechanisms for faculty members to share their experiences and learn from each other.

CONSUMER EDUCATION

The growing trend toward encouraging consumers to be responsible for their own health and the ubiquity of the WWW, with its plethora of health-related information, has changed the way that consumers seek information. Health care organizations, health care professionals, government units, the pharmaceutical industry, and others have invested in the development of health information Web sites that are used by consumers to make decisions about their health care and illness treatment. In 2000 the Pew Charitable Trusts reported that 55% of American adults with Internet access have used the Web to get health or medical information. Seventy percent of these 21 million health seekers reported that the Web information influenced their decisions about how to treat an illness or condition (Pew Charitable Trusts, 2000).

Consumer informatics is a growing subfield within health care informatics. The mission and purpose of the Consumer Informatics working group of the American Medical Informatics Association (AMIA) is "to develop informatics methodologies linked to the evaluation of health status and the optimization of health care and to use informatics to provide clear communication of these issues between provider and client" (AMIA, 2001, para. 1). Consumer health education is just one part of the mission of this group.

It is incumbent on health care professionals (especially informatics practitioners) to evaluate the quality of information on health-oriented Web sites and to recommend Web sites that meet established standards and criteria for electronic resources such as those described in Table 12-1. Several groups are now working to deal with the issues surrounding health information on the Internet. One example is the **Health On the Net Foundation (HON)**, created in 1995. This is a not-for-profit international Swiss organization. Another consumer safeguard is to assess whether health-oriented Web sites subscribe to the HON code—a code of conduct for medical and health Web sites that includes eight principles (HON, 2001). Sites that display the HON code are expected to adhere to the principles. The following are examples of the code principles:

- The site will identify the medical authority who is responsible for the content or acknowledge that the advice comes from a nonmedical source.
- The information is to complement, not replace, the consumer's health care provider.
- Confidentiality of all data shared by consumers will not be shared.

The HON code is a function of the Health on the Net Foundation (a not-for-profit international organization), whose purpose is to guide nonmedical and medical users to useful and reliable online medical and health information.

Other well-respected organizations have developed and maintain sites designed specifically to inform consumers. The following are some examples of such sites (which can be accessed through the Web Connection for this book):

- MEDLINEplus Health Information (National Library of Medicine)
- AARP Health and Wellness (American Association of Retired People)
- AMA Health Insight (American Medical Association)
- Ask NOAH (a cooperative project of the City University of New York, the Metropolitan New York Library Council, the New York Academy of Medicine, and the New York Public Library)
- Healthfinder (Department of Health and Human Services)

The National Library of Medicine (NLM) has had a long-standing interest in ensuring that accurate health care information is available to the public. In 2000 the NLM funded a variety of local and statewide projects related to Health Information for the Public (NLM, 2000). A broad review of these projects in 33 states demonstrates the broad scope of the projects that are meeting the needs of the citizens of these states for accurate health information.

CONCLUSION

As technology becomes an increasing and integral part of the way we live in the twenty-first century, education will change dramatically. According to the final report of the 21st Century Workforce Commission (2000, para. 5), "The current and future health of America's 21st century economy depends directly on how broadly and deeply Americans reach a new level of literacy that includes strong academic skills, thinking, reasoning, teamwork skills and proficiency in using technology." One of the keys to success that is noted in the report is that workers will need to continuously upgrade their skills and knowledge as new technologies emerge. The demand for workers who can apply and use information technology in all industries is increasing.

Demand for health care workers who can transfer computer and information management skills from educational settings to the workplace is increasing as well. A growing number of professional schools in universities and colleges have developed technology infrastructures that enable faculty to use technology effectively in the classroom and at a distance. Students who learn via computers are more likely to transfer technology-oriented skills to the work setting. Thornburg (1995) has suggested that learning via technology not only allows us to do the same thing differently, but it also allows us to do different things. Clearly, as the health care industry embraces administrative, clinical, and reporting technology solutions, educators will need to change to reflect the working environment in which their students will be employed. Technology tools create opportunities for the ongoing development of interdisciplinary learning communities that will enable health care professionals to thrive in the twenty-first century.

The focus must change from one that is instructor-centric to one that is student-centric in order for graduates to learn to think critically, analyze thoughtfully, and take responsibility for meeting their own lifelong learning needs. The opportunity to learn what is needed to maintain continued competencies in a "just in time" and "any time, any place" framework will ensure a health care workforce that is responsive to the needs of society.

The use of technology in higher education is evolving as new tools become available. Student demand for "any time, any place" education is driving the delivery methods. As the use of computers for everyday activities becomes ubiquitous in our society, the demand for their use in traditional classrooms and for online education increases.

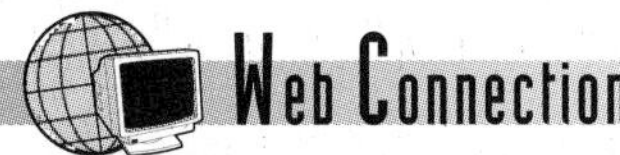

Web Connection

Education has always used processes and technologies to facilitate learning. The dynamic evolution of information and communication technologies is influencing teaching and learning in profound ways. Although promoted as a way to increase access to education, these technologies can be a double-edged sword—access can be enhanced or diminished by factors such as the availability of resources, the quality of the educational product, and the skill of the instructor and the learner. The Web Connection activities for this chapter focus on identifying teaching and learning resources, comparing teaching tools from a variety of authors, and determining the kinds of learning outcomes that can be achieved with current technologies.

discussion questions

1. Discuss three effective ways of using technology to teach in a face-to-face classroom. Explain the impact of this use of technology on student learning.
2. Write three instructional objectives for an undergraduate course in health care informatics. Identify the appropriate technology tool for each instructional objective.
3. Describe the impact of the Internet on higher education in health care.
4. Your employer has asked you, as a health care provider, to develop a handout that includes a process for finding credible health care information on the World Wide Web. Explain how you would design such a handout.

REFERENCES

American Medical Informatics Association. (2001). Consumer Health Informatics Working Group. Retrieved June 25, 2001, from the World Wide Web: http://www.amia.org/working/chi.html.

Brown, M.S. (1997). *Consumer health and medical information on the Internet: Supply and demand.* Retrieved June 22, 2001, from the World Wide Web: http://etrg.findsvp.com/health/mktginfo.html.

DataBeam Corporation. (1997). *A primer on the H.323 series standard.* Retrieved June 20, 2001, from the World Wide Web: http://www.cs.ucl.ac.uk/staff/jon/jip/h323/h323_primer.html#important.

Hale, S. (2000). The last communication revolution. *Good Teacher.* Retrieved June 26, 2001, from the World Wide Web: http://www.theschoolquarterly.com/info_lit_archive/online_ict_learning/00_sh_tlcr.htm.

HON. (2001). *Principles. HON Code of Conduct for medical and health Web sites.* Retrieved June 25, 2001, from the World Wide Web: http://www.hon.ch/HONcode/Conduct.html.

IBM Life Sciences. (2000). *IBM announces $100 million investment in life sciences. News and events.* Retrieved June 22, 2001, from the World Wide Web: http://www-3.ibm.com/solutions/lifesciences/100.html.

Institute for Higher Education Policy. (2000). *Quality on the line: Benchmarks for success in Internet-based distance education.* Blackboard.com and National Education Association. Washington, DC: Author.

Knowles, M. (1984). *Andragogy in action.* San Francisco: Jossey-Bass.

Levin, J. (1999). Multiplicity in learning and teaching: A framework for developing innovative online education. *Journal of Research on Computing in Education, 32*(2), 256-270.

National Center for Education Statistics. (2000). *Projections of education statistics to 2010.* Retrieved June 22, 2001, from the World Wide Web: http://nces.ed.gov/pubs2000/projections.

National Education Association. (2000). *A survey of traditional and distance learning higher education members.* Washington, DC: National Education Association. Retrieved June 22, 2001, from the World Wide Web: http://www.nea.org/he/abouthe/dlstudy.pdf.

National Library of Medicine. (2000). *Health information for the public projects funded by the National Library of Medicine, 2000.* Bethesda, MD: Author. Retrieved June 22, 2001, from the World Wide Web: http://www.nlm.nih.gov/nno/hipprojects.html.

Passell, P. (1997). Long lines outside the best colleges are likely to get longer. Business/Financial Desk. *New York Times,* May 1.

Pew Charitable Trusts. (2000). *Internet and American life.* Retrieved June 22, 2001, from the World Wide Web: http://www.pewinternet.org/reports/toc.asp?Report=26.

Saba, F. (2000a). Why there is no significant difference between face-to-face and distance education. *Distance Education Report, 4*(13), 1.

Saba, F. (2000b). With friends like these? *Distance Education Report, 4*(12), 1-2.

Seels, B.B., & Richey, R.C. (1994). *Instructional technology: The definition and domains of the field.* Washington, DC: Association for Educational Communications and Technology.

Silver, D. (1998). Dynamic syllabi. Technology and Learning. Retrieved June 22, 2001, from the World Wide Web: http://www.georgetown.edu/crossroads/webcourses.html.

Thornburg, D. (1995). *Welcome to the communication age.* Handout based on Education in the Communication Age, Lake Barrington, IL: Thornburg Center. Retrieved June 26, 2001, from the World Wide Web: http://www.tcpd.org/thornburg/handouts/CommunicationAge.pdf.

21st Century Workforce Commission. (2000). *Executive summary. Final report.* Washington, DC: Author. Retrieved June 25, 2001, from the World Wide Web: http://www.workforce21.org/executive_summary.htm.

Vaille, J. *Conversations. The futures channel.* Retrieved May 15, 2000, from the World Wide Web: http://www.thefutureschannel.com/vaille_conversation.htm.

White House. (2000). *Information technology research and development: Information technology for the 21st century* [Presidential Handout]. Retrieved June 21, 2001, from the World Wide Web: http://www.itrd.gov/itrd/it-summary.html.

CHAPTER 13

eHealth Trends and Technologies: The Impact of the Internet on Health Care Providers and Patients

DAVID C. KIBBE

Learning Objectives

Upon completion of this chapter, the reader will be able to:

1. ***Define*** eHealth.
2. ***Describe*** the major trends behind the adoption and use of the World Wide Web for sharing health care information.
3. ***Identify*** the core component technologies of eHealth.
4. ***Discuss*** the advantages of the core components over earlier information technologies.
5. ***Discuss*** the barriers to the adoption of eHealth core components by health care provider organizations.
6. ***Analyze*** the impact of eHealth applications on patients, providers, and payers.
7. ***Discuss*** ethical issues inherent in eHealth.

Outline

Key Terms

ActiveX
application service provider (ASP)
browser
cable modem
common object request broker architecture (CORBA)
digital subscriber line (DSL)
eHealth
extensible markup language (XML)
file transfer protocol (FTP)
graphical interface
Health Insurance Portability and Accountability Act (HIPAA)
Health Level Seven (HL7)
hypertext
hypertext markup language (HTML)
hypertext transfer protocol (HTTP)
Internet
Internet protocol (IP)
intranet
Java

Key Terms—cont'd

simple mail transfer protocol (SMTP)
thin client
transmission control protocol (TCP)
Web server
World Wide Web

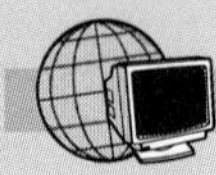

Web Connection

Go to the Web site at http://evolve.elsevier.com/Englebardt/. Here you will find Web links and activities related to eHealth trends and technologies.

It is impossible to predict the ultimate impact of the convergence of the Internet with health care. Most observers agree that it will be very large, even momentous. "The e-health era is nothing less than the digital transformation of the practice of medicine as well as the business side of the health industry" (Coile, 1999, p. 34).

This chapter describes the major technologies and trends that are developing in the arena referred to as **eHealth.** It assesses how eHealth is currently affecting, and may continue to affect, patients and providers in the years to come. The chapter examines the reasons behind the rapid and widespread adoption of eHealth technologies and discusses the health care social and economic context within which eHealth is emerging. A practical application of eHealth technology in a brief case study of Web-based software is presented.

DEFINING eHEALTH

The term *eHealth* is rapidly gaining common usage as a descriptor that encompasses the wide range of health care activities involving the electronic transfer of information. *eHealth* connotes the convenience, low cost, and ready accessibility of health-related information and communication using the **Internet** and associated technologies, such as eMail and the **World Wide Web.** The Internet, in theory, can connect all participants in the health care community, including patients, payers, and providers. eHealth cuts across established intellectual boundaries and has an influence on medicine, public health, and health care informatics (Figure 13-1).

The application of Internet-based technology to health care is a moving target with an uncertain trajectory. Furthermore, eHealth is evolving in the context of the health care industry and the larger society, both of which are undergoing rapid changes at the start of the twenty-first century. Among the most significant of these larger changes are the continued growth of managed care and the aging of American society. It is therefore difficult to predict the dynamic interplay of technology, social change, and economic imperative.

Although they may be difficult and uncertain, the events surrounding the Internet are so important and decisive—both in determining the course of health care delivery and in shaping the development of information technology use by health care professionals—that an attempt to gauge the impact or at least to outline the range of possibilities of eHealth is indicated. The thesis throughout this chapter is that eHealth represents a revolutionary change in the way health care information is accessed and used and there-

FIGURE 13–1 | eHealth Schematic

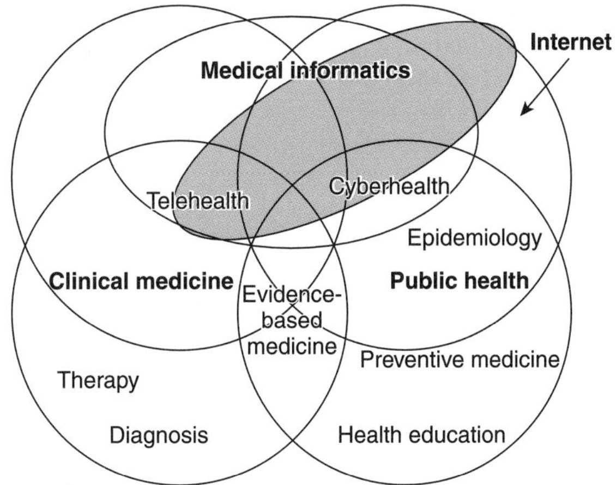

fore poses a fundamental challenge to health care professionals. Health care professionals face a future in which they have much less control over the content and communication channels critical to health care services delivery. This discussion begins with an understanding of how and why the Internet has gained such enormous popularity among the general public and in the wider scope of public affairs and commerce.

INTERNET COMPUTING STANDARDS

In less than a decade the Internet and the World Wide Web have become everyday workplace and household tools, almost as common as the ubiquitous television. This development was made possible by the establishment of rules, or protocols, allowing disparate, geographically separated computers and networks to exchange data, starting in the early 1990s. The **Internet protocol** (IP) and the **transmission control protocol** (TCP) provided the basic tools necessary for Internet connectivity between computers. The **simple mail transfer protocol** (SMTP) made eMail possible. The **file transfer protocol** (FTP) established a standard way to receive, share, and exchange textual information across the Internet. The next great breakthrough of the Internet, the **hypertext transfer protocol** (HTTP), provided a standard way for computers to exchange multimedia information, both text and pictures. Its derivative, **hypertext markup language** (HTML), created the World Wide Web with its dominant feature of hypertext links. This has made **browser** software civilization's most effective communication and information transfer technology. These standards, rules, and protocols are described in greater detail in Chapters 11 and 17.

The widespread adoption of the Internet is due to the combination of user-friendly features embodied in browser software (Internet Explorer, Netscape Navigator, etc.). These features include the standard and intuitive **graphical interface** of the browser software, the easy movement within and between Web documents made possible by **hypertext,** and the low cost of connection—and thus access—to information and applications on the Internet. In turn, these features provide the Internet user with an experience that is different from more traditional modes of processing and communicating information, such as reading, viewing television, or talking on the phone.

The following characteristics of the Internet experience, taken in combination, have driven the behavioral changes at the heart of the new information technology (Evans & Wurster, 1997):

- *Reach* refers to the number of persons exchanging information or who are able to access an information source. Clearly, information published on the World Wide Web attains a reach that is several orders of magnitude higher than a verbal message, even when that message is broadcast on television.
- *Bandwidth* refers to the amount of information that can be exchanged. It is sometimes referred to as the pipe through which data flow. Text requires minimal bandwidth, a still picture requires more, an audio or video signal still more, and so on. Internet-based information sources can deliver their messages across surprisingly diverse bandwidths, considering that for the most part the system consists of two copper wires that form a telephone connection, the electronic equivalent of a soda straw. Higher bandwidth connectivity, for example from cable, satellite dishes, and digital subscriber lines (DSLs), is in huge demand. Three-dimensional imaging, which requires high bandwidth, has become a standard aspect of computer interfaces everywhere, from games to the graphical output of online banking software.
- *Customization* refers to the degree to which the information and its display pertain to or can be adapted by the information seeker. On many Web sites the viewer has the option to turn on or off the graphical content, thus greatly speeding up the delivery of the pages. This is a simple example of customization built into all Internet navigation software. As another example, it has become commonplace for Web **portals** to allow visitors to personalize the configuration of page displays, for example, presenting local weather reports and satellite images each time the user connects to the Internet.
- *Interactivity* refers to the extent to which dialogue, on-demand video and audio, and queries from connected databases are available to the user. Speed of response is a requisite of interactivity. Throughout industry, **intranets** are used largely because they excel in providing swift access to various kinds of data on demand. Chat rooms have become the standard for interactivity online. In summary, the World Wide Web experience combines utility with convenience and both of these with fun. The growth of the Internet has occurred in part because people *seek out* the experience of being informed more directly and interactively than was previously possible; they seek information about issues that matter to them, among the most important being issues involving health and health care. It was reported in one survey that, of active Internet users in 1999, 43% used the Internet for health-related purposes (Forrester Research, 2000, February).

eHEALTH'S EMERGING SECTORS

It is perhaps not surprising that the initial and most visible examples of the Internet's impact on health care have come from the consumer and business domains, rather than from traditional health care providers. Tens of thousands of Web sites have been established, many from commercial for-profit companies offering information on health topics of every kind. This growth includes general and disease-specific Web sites, those devoted to chronic medical conditions, and many that focus on healthy lifestyles and illness prevention. Consumer health sites have become more interactive, offering health information seekers the opportunity to engage in discussions with others as well as with health care professionals and to purchase health-related products. Consumer health sites take advantage of the Internet's broad reach and multimedia delivery to engage large portions of the online population. Health information seekers have in turn contributed significantly to the growth of the use of the Internet.

There are currently at least six broad segments within eHealth that are differentiated by the business models of the companies and sponsoring institutions operating within each sector. These six segments are presented in Box 13-1.

- Content providers broadly represented on the World Wide Web include electronic medical publications and journals, such as *JAMA;* university and other academic Web sites; and disease-specific specialty sites like that of the Alzheimer's Association. Sites are sometimes free to the public and sometimes available through subscription. Content providers often have advertising on their Web pages.
- Health care portals, sometimes called *health care infomediaries,* provide content. They also make available a wide and growing range of information products and services, such as free eMail accounts, expert health care advice, chat rooms for patients with specific conditions, and online financial services. They often are funded by advertising dollars but also rely heavily on networking of services. DrKoop.com, for example, has partnerships with America Online and ABC News, along with the Cleveland Clinic, Dartmouth Medical School, and World Book Encyclopedias. Portals are sometimes judged on how many "eyeballs" they generate (i.e., the numbers of visitors they attract). Well-known health care portals include WebMD.com and Medscape.com.
- eCommerce businesses use the Internet to streamline and automate the purchase of retail health care products such as pharmaceuticals and health supplies. They are among the very few eHealth companies actually earning revenues, and some are making significant profits. Examples include Drugstore.com, PlanetRx.com, and 1 Stop Home Health Care.
- Business-to-business eMarketplaces are rapidly emerging as hospitals, their distributors, and their suppliers go online to contract for and deliver a portion of the huge amounts of money spent on

Box 13–1 Emerging eHealth Market Segments

- Content providers: journals and publications, specialty and disease-specific sites
- Portals: one-stop "infomediaries" for health care consumers
- eCommerce: retail sales sites for health care–related goods and services
- Business-to-business eMarketplaces: provide a link between health care providers and the marketplace
- Connectivity/integrators: making the connections between the players
- Internet applications providers: software applications for administrative and clinical information management that run on the Web

medical supplies, $179 billion in 1999 alone (Forrester Research, 2000, May). Medibuy.com and Neoforma.com exemplify the so-called eProcurement sector of eHealth, using Internet technologies to link hospitals and clinics to the marketplace for medical supplies and equipment.

- Connectivity/integrator companies are attempting to link via the Internet some or all of the major parties to health care transactions, including payers, employers, patients, providers, and physicians. Their business plans involve making administrative transactions more efficient as well as using databases of information for marketing, research, and client support purposes. There is the perception that administrative costs are a disproportionate share of medical expenses and that there are huge potential savings in this sector. Initially these companies have faired well in the stock market. Healtheon, Quintiles Transnational, and ClaimsNet are representative examples from this segment.
- eHealth software application providers are engaged in a completely new model of health care software sales and distribution, known as **application service provider (ASP).** They offer their users the ability to access off-site software programs through a secure connection to the Internet. These programs physically reside off-site on servers in data centers. Unlike traditional stand-alone personal computer (PC) and client server software companies, the business model here includes a role for the ASP as host and security guarantor for health data and information residing on the company's machines. MedicaLogic, Trizetto, Abaton, and Canopy Systems, Inc., are representative examples of eHealth software applications providers.

One thing that is not immediately apparent is that all of these eHealth companies are *interactively* gathering and exchanging data and information from patients, physicians, hospitals, and sometimes even family members. The reach, low cost, connectivity, and personal adaptability of the Internet provide tremendous opportunities for enterprising and imaginative health care professionals and their partners. They are attempting to capitalize on the inefficiencies and inconveniences of the trillion-dollar American health care industry. This activity will most likely result in expected and unexpected consequences for the health care industry and for the public. For example, the interactivity between eHealth and consumers and patients is creating huge new stores of personal health data and information outside of doctors' offices and hospital medical records departments. Most of these data stores are entirely unregulated and unmonitored.

THE SOCIAL AND ECONOMIC CONTEXT FOR eHEALTH

At the same time that eHealth is offering patients and consumers interactive and customizable navigation of health care Web sites, the American health care system is in the throes of change. The focus of attention of most health care providers and administrators during the past few years has not been on using the Internet so much as on meeting the challenges of managed care complexities, the decreased reimbursement for services rendered to Medicare patients imposed by the Balanced Budget Act (BBA) of 1997, and the rapid growth in high-risk populations of elderly and uninsured clients. Several prominent trends have affected the health care industry and eHealth during this period.

- *Aging of the population.* The shifting age distribution indicates that the number of persons aged 65 years or older will double, from 34.7 million in 2000 to 69.4 million in 2030 (U.S. Census Bureau, 1999). Accelerating the impact of the demand and cost for health services will be the soaring number of "old old" (those aged 85 years and above). This group's number is expected to climb from 4.3 million in 2000 to 8.5 million in 2030 (U.S. Census Bureau, 1999). Spillman and Lubitz (2000) estimate that the average cost per person for acute and long-term care from the age of 65 years until death is $164,505 in 1996 dollars.

- *Managed care.* In 1999, 78 million persons, almost 30% of the population, were enrolled in health maintenance organizations (HMOs). Preferred provider organizations (PPOs) have enrolled another 90 million persons in managed care networks (American Association of Health Plans, 1999). The health care industry is becoming a price-competitive sector of the economy as PPOs and HMOs vie with each another to deliver health care services at acceptable premiums. Consolidated and integrated delivery systems are becoming the order of the day. As medical loss ratios—the percentage of health care premiums that plans pay for health care services—rise for HMOs and health insurers, more and more emphasis will be placed on controlling medical and pharmacy costs.
- *New medical technologies.* American consumers have high expectations for medical technology: that it will be available, accessible, and paid for by someone else. New pharmaceuticals increased drug costs at yearly rates of 12% per year during the late 1990s (Levit, 2000). Genomics, the science of targeting drugs and medications based on the knowledge of an individual's specific genetic makeup, is expected to grow enormously and spur the development of many specialized, genetically derived pharmaceuticals. Organ transplants have become nearly routine, and new invasive cardiology treatments are announced regularly.
- *Government payments are changing.* With the Balanced Budget Act of 1997 the government formally abandoned fee-for-service in favor of a fixed-payment financial structure that includes hospital inpatient and outpatient care, laboratory testing, home health, and long-term care. Sharp cuts resulting from the BBA have had an impact on hospitals, skilled nursing facilities, rehabilitation centers, and home care.
- *High administrative costs of paper-based information systems.* Frustration with the complexity and high costs of paper-based information systems used to manage the health insurance industry is reaching a peak. The Health Care Financing Administration (HCFA; now known as the Centers for Medicare & Medicaid Services) estimates that about $250 billion, or nearly 25% of the approximately $1.2 trillion spent on health care, is wasted because of inefficiency that is built into paper-based administrative costs (HCFA, 1999).
- *The health care consumer movement.* There is growing frustration with managed care and with waits and delays, barriers, and lack of choice of health care providers, especially among patients and consumers who receive health care services within HMOs. An Institute of Medicine report (Kohn, Corrigan, & Donaldson, 2000) indicated that medical errors cause as many as 98,000 deaths per year in American hospitals. This report fueled

> the debate about whether managed care reforms have come at the price of decreased quality of care and in some quarters has further eroded public confidence in doctors and hospitals.

eHealth has developed in this context of unprecedented change in the health care industry. The technology of the Internet and its potential benefits are being evaluated by all stakeholders in health care. Quite understandably, eHealth's potential for affecting technical, economic, social, and policy aspects of the health care industry varies according to individuals' perspectives on these issues. For example, consultants for large health care entities such as insurance firms and medical supply companies tend to see the intersection of health care and the Internet as primarily providing a new way of conducting the business of health care, for example, enabling faster and more efficient eCommerce transactions among payers, employers, and providers of care, such as the submission of insurance claims via the Internet or ordering of medical supplies. On the other hand, patient advocacy groups and disease-specific nonprofit foundations see eHealth as having its most profound effect by enhancing the ability of patients and their family members to access information and to use that information to improve the choices they make regarding treatments that affect cost and quality of life. Promoters of health care quality improvement have welcomed the Internet as a source of widespread dissemination of information about the outcomes of care, which patients and corporations may use to help them make choices. Pharmaceutical companies have been quick to grasp the implications of Internet-based applications for facilitating clinical trials, thereby leading to speedier and less costly delivery to market of new drugs and medicines. Public health officials see eHealth developments as capable of permitting earlier and more accurate detection of public health threats, for example, from Internet access to data on the sale of nonprescription drugs and other retail sales analyses that might hint at food or water contamination.

The evolutionary path of health applications on the Internet is unclear. However, the diversity of needs and problems listed and described are certain to drive an increasing number of demonstration projects and commercial implementations that suggest that the Internet is part of the "solution." Thus the impact of eHealth can safely be predicted to be both widespread in society and driven by many, sometimes competing, demands. Notable so far is the relatively quiet voice of the provider relative to the great noise of the consumer and commercial interests in shaping the contours and outlines of eHealth.

THE INTERNET AND HEALTH CARE INFORMATION SYSTEMS

One important impact of eHealth involves how the Internet is used at the level of the health care provider organization, often referred to as health care information systems (HISs). Health care providers have struggled to find effective uses of information technology to manage the challenges presented by client care. Applying information technology in a manner that ensures that the productivity and quality gains are worth the heavy investments in time and money has proved to be a truly daunting organizational task for many during the past 40 years (Kibbe & Bard, 1997).

A high proportion of implementations of information technology in health care organizations have occurred slowly, missed their mark, or failed to achieve the intended benefits. Various reasons have been given for this problem. One reason is the low proportion of budgeted dollars expended for information technology in health care relative to other industries such as banking and retail trade. In 1997 the health care and hospital industry spent 3.91% of its revenue on information systems and technology. In contrast, the financial services and banking industry spent 10.31% of its revenue on information systems

(Gartner Group, 1999). Another reason is the fragmentation typical of most medical communities, where the hospital, doctors, and other provider agencies are all separately owned and operated. Still another cause for the slow pace of information technology adoption in health care organizations is that the there has been a rapid change in information systems technology platforms and infrastructures. As indicated in Table 13-1, in the short time since the end of World War II, the basic technologies for handling data and information in complex organizations such as hospitals have gone through four major shifts from mainframes to intranets and are now entering a fifth major shift involving the Internet. The rapidity of these changes has left many hospitals and their chief information officers (CIOs) struggling to keep up while simultaneously maintaining legacy systems that continue to be useful.

Hospitals and health care organizations including physicians' practices and clinics are just beginning to use Web-based applications for administrative and clinical purposes. During the 1980s and 1990s many HIS vendor companies converted their mainframe and minicomputer-based systems for patient accounting, pharmacy, laboratory, and so forth to client server systems. This transition was costly and complicated. Many hospitals were in the process of making the conversion to locally hosted, on-site client server applications connected via local area networks when Y2K forced them to perform costly analyses and upgrades of their entire electronic environments. At the same time that many health care organizations were completing upgrades, a "better idea" was being introduced and gaining popularity. This "better idea" involves using the Internet and the World Wide Web to replace much of the complexity of client server systems while lowering the cost of enterprise computing. It is know as **thin client** or ASP model computing. An application service provider (ASP) is an organization that hosts software applications on its own servers within its own facilities. Customers access the application via private lines or the Internet. These are also called commercial service providers. In the ASP model of computing the software application is housed on a **Web server,** and the user accesses the application (practice management software, clinical data repository, electronic medical record, etc.) via Web browser software. Using this model of computing a vendor can host one or many software applications from a central geographic location and "rent" access to the software to hospitals, clinics, and doctors' offices.

Table 13–1 Major Shifts in Information Technology Infrastructure From 1950 to the Late 1990s

Decade	Shifts in Information Technology Infrastructure
1950s	Mainframe computers, service model with multiorganizational sharing of applications, tethered "dumb" terminals for users
1960s	Minicomputers, centralized computing and applications within organizations, tethered user terminal
1970s and 1980s	PCs, decentralized users and increasingly decentralized computing and applications hosting on the desktop
1990s	Intranet computing now available, decentralized users, thin client made possible
Late 1990s	Internet widely available, centralized computing and applications hosting, ASP model, "software is a service not a product"

PCs, Personal computers; *ASP,* application service provider.

Generally included in the monthly subscription fees are the operational costs of running and maintaining the hardware and software at the data center.

With truly Web-based software applications, the user needs only minimal computing power on his or her device (hence the term *thin client*) and in fact does not really need any software other than the browser and a connection to the Internet. With Web-based software applications, the health care organization has the option to turn over the capital costs and complexity of maintaining the servers, network administration, and software maintenance to the ASP, thereby lowering the total costs of owning and using the applications. Because the client computers required to run the browser software can be inexpensive network computers without large hard drives and peripheral devices, the cost of these components also decreases. Such systems are easily expandable: new users can be set up and connected anywhere there is a connection to the Internet, at low marginal cost to the institution. In effect, Web-based applications offer a completely new model of information technology access and software distribution that constitutes a way for hospitals and medical practices to outsource some of their information management needs and pay for them on a monthly subscription basis.

The Web's presence and the use of the ASP model are growing at a steady pace and are expected to continue to expand. To meet the demands of the marketplace, older HIS companies, with established customer bases using their client server applications, are Web-enabling their products, or completely rewriting their software in the languages and tools of the Web. These tools include **Java,** HTML, **ActiveX,** and **common object request broker architecture** (CORBA). The process of conversion is expensive and takes a number of years to complete. Experience has proved to HIS buyers that conversions are always difficult and expensive. Vendors do not have a strong economic incentive to recast their products in Web-based versions if they are less profitable for the vendor than their current products. Such conversions can result in "cannibalizing" existing high-margin accounts with less profitable ASP model products. Nonetheless, many companies, among them a large number of start-up companies with venture capital backing, are coming to market with Web-based HIS products. These can be expected to compete with the older client server products, thereby pushing the health care industry toward a higher percentage of Web-based components in hospitals and doctors' clinics.

AN eHEALTH CASE STUDY: DOING COMMUNITY-WIDE CASE MANAGEMENT ON THE WEB

In the practice of case management, case managers coordinate patient care and services in a diversity of settings. They are also responsible for facilitating the administrative and insurance functions between payers and providers. The completion and transmission of forms, messages, and other documents are a high priority for case managers. Two of the major features of ASP model computing are as follows:

- The ready accessibility to users, who need only a browser and an Internet connection to gain access to the software and stored data from any location
- The ease of communications, permitting messages to be transmitted via eMail and from within the Web-based application itself to many parties

So it is natural that one opportunity for using Web-based eHealth applications would be in the field of case management.

Canopy Systems, Inc., in Chapel Hill, North Carolina, has developed a Web-based case management program called Canopy. The program is designed to help case managers become more effective coordinators and advocates for their patients by providing an inexpensive and secure eHealth system. This system links case managers with each other and with providers in communities. Canopy is used by a growing number of hospital case management departments as a navigational tool for screening, coordinating care, and reporting outcomes for patients with complex illnesses and for high-risk patients, as well as for managing care processes across the continuum of care settings.

Canopy is designed to run on the World Wide Web. It is a thin-client application written in Java. All of the software and data are housed in a data center. Case managers and others using the system connect through the Internet (Figure 13-2). Canopy uses multiple layers of security to ensure proper authentication and authorization, organized by user, by site, and by computer. See Chapters 17 and 20 for a discussion of security standards and issues.

Some important features of the security architecture are as follows:

- *User IDs and logins.* When users connect to the site, the server challenges them to supply an identification name (user ID) and password, which are then validated by the application software. The user ID determines the data that the user is authorized to view or edit.
- *Certificates.* Digital certificates, which are almost impossible to forge, allow Canopy to authenticate the computer from which a user is attempting to access the system. Once installed on a user's computer, a certificate provides a unique identifier for that computer. Thus, even if a would-be intruder were to gain access to a legitimate user ID and password, he or she would have to use a certified computer.
- *Encryption.* The stream of data moving into and out of Canopy must not be vulnerable to "eavesdropping" by unauthorized parties. Canopy uses

FIGURE 13–2 | **Canopy and ASP Model Software Application for Case Management**

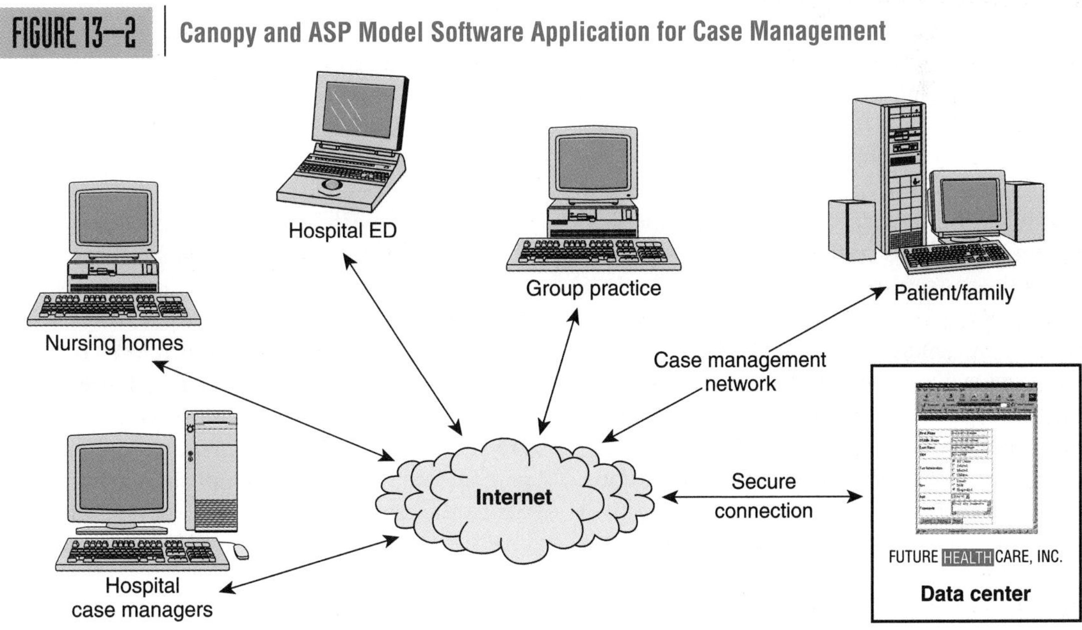

> industry-standard RSA 128-bit public key encryption (an established algorithm for data encryption developed by RSA Security, Inc.) that meets Centers for Medicare & Medicaid Services (formerly known as HCFA) and government standards to ensure that data routed into and out of the server can be read only by legitimate users. If an intruder were to gain access to the data stream, he or she would see only gibberish.

Canopy is used by case managers to screen patients admitted to the hospital in order to identify patients who, because of admitting diagnosis, age, or other comorbid conditions, are likely to benefit from intensive case management. Case managers can accept online referrals from doctors' offices, emergency departments, and community agencies. They can access case management and clinical guidelines on the World Wide Web to help them and their patients evaluate treatment options. They can easily locate and print out patient education materials from credible Web sites. In addition, case managers can immediately access and exchange information with other caregivers and with patients. For example, they can exchange physiological data such as blood pressures and blood glucose readings to make disease management more expedient. Family members who become authorized users use the application to track a loved one's medical progress and stay in contact with the case manager and care team over the Internet. The case manager also gains immediate access to a network of case manager peers around the country. They provide a great source for advice and sharing of professional information. Medication reviews are done online with the aid of Internet-based drug information and drug interaction tools. The case manager can procure and fill medical orders for patients using the eCommerce connections within the application, enabling clients to get medical supplies and services. This same Web-based information system also documents the clinical activities and produces financial and quality of care outcomes reports.

This type of software has created a new set of capabilities for case managers who have been accustomed to using paper-based systems. This has given rise to a new term, *eCase management,* which describes the empowered and connected case manager who is savvy to eHealth.

eHealth applications gain acceptance only if the return on investment (ROI) is worthwhile for the hospitals that purchase and implement the systems. Key to the ROI is the high cost of care and low insurance reimbursement for certain populations of patients. Hospitals recognize that the costs of health care are not evenly distributed. Among patients older than 65 years, just 10% of the population accounts for 70% of the costs in any given year. Whereas persons with chronic medical conditions account for about 69% of hospital admissions, they account for 80% of the total hospital days (Robert Wood Johnson Foundation, 1996). Medicare patients take more than a third of all prescription medicines (U.S. Department of Health and Human Services, 2000). This pattern of uneven distribution and concentration of costs is common among major disease groups. Many hospitals have come to the conclusion that it is in their best economic interest, as well as being congruent with the delivery of quality patient care, to extend the level of case management beyond the four walls of the hospital. Patients with well-managed care are less costly to a health system than those whose care is poorly and inefficiently managed. Improved management leads to fewer complications, fewer days in high-cost facilities, and fewer costly errors that cause costs to mount. To achieve the improvement in management, information systems are needed that increase productivity by case managers and decrease the probability that patients "fall through the cracks" of a fragmented health care system. Web-based systems, such as Canopy, have yet to prove their capabilities but are certainly promising.

BARRIERS AND CHALLENGES TO AND CONCERNS FOR eHEALTH

Expectations for eHealth run high, but for the most part the technology remains to be fully tested and proved in multiple settings and in the complicated environment posed by health care. A barrier to wide-ranging technological change is the vested interests of those who stand to lose by its adoption. Participants in the health care industry have different incentives. They may be on opposite sides of an argument to save money or make processes more efficient if one party's profits are decreased or their jobs are made less valuable. For example, it is widely recognized that physicians and hospitals have potentially opposing incentives in the care of medicare beneficiaries. Doctors are paid on the basis of the numbers of visits they make, and hospitals are reimbursed in one lump sum determined by the diagnosis-related group (DRG). As another example, hospital administrators may see ASP model computing as a means of decreasing overhead and cost of operations. The hospital's CIO may be less enthusiastic because of loss of control over the software application when it and the data are located outside the hospital's information systems department. The health care "system" is actually a highly fragmented pool of resources in any given locale or community. This makes it more difficult for the parties involved to move in unison toward the adoption of new technologies, even those as standardized as the Internet. Ironically the proliferation of start-up eHealth companies selling stand-alone ASP systems may add to the complexity of choice facing the industry as it moves toward adopting the Internet as its communication pipeline.

An important challenge to eHealth concerns the issues of privacy and security. In 2000 the federal government moved slowly but deliberately toward the adoption of national guidelines for privacy and security applied to the electronic transmission and maintenance of patient-identifiable health care information. These guidelines were mandated in the **Health Insurance Portability and Accountability Act (HIPAA)** passed by Congress in 1996. HIPAA guidelines will impose strict new standards for guaranteeing and safeguarding the confidentiality of medical records and insurance information for every party, from a solo practitioner's office to a national insurance company, that participates in eHealth. In the longer term, the HIPAA guidelines are likely to promote the adoption of eHealth by making clear the liability involved in the misuse of health data and by setting the standards for performances that are within those limits. In the short term, the delay and debate surrounding the HIPAA guideline release may give some hospitals and health care institutions reason to move forward cautiously. See Chapters 19 and 20 for a more in-depth discussion of HIPAA, as well as Chapter 17 for a discussion of related HIPAA technical standards.

Two major technological challenges that currently limit the growth of eHealth are bandwidth and the interface problem. Bandwidth, as discussed earlier, refers to the amount of data that can be exchanged per unit of time via a physical conduit (e.g., copper wire, fiberoptic cable, and wireless frequencies). See Chapter 11 for a more in-depth discussion of bandwidth. For the widespread dissemination of eHealth applications to occur, the bandwidth must be high enough to permit large amounts of data to be transferred quickly and reliably. High-speed connection to the Internet, such as through a **digital subscriber line (DSL)** or **cable modem,** although theoretically available in many parts of the country, has been slow to be deployed by the communications and telephone companies that market and install them. Many suburban and rural areas of the country remain dependent on relatively slow, low-bandwidth telephone modem technology for Internet connectivity. In many rural areas no Internet connection is available at all.

The computer interface problem deals with the standards by which computers and their users format data and define the meaning of contained information. Although the Internet has, for all practical purposes, solved the problem of two unconnected computers communicating a message, Internet protocols (IPs) do not deal with the important subtleties of syntax, medical vocabulary, or the meaning of the message itself. For example, if computer data reflecting the vital signs of a group of patients were transferred from a clinic database to a hospital database, the transfer software would require specific tags or labels to identify the packets of data corresponding to the patient's name, medical record number, each vital sign, and so on. The computer at the hospital end can receive the raw data via the Internet; however, the software at the hospital must recognize and interpret the identifying tags in sequence to make any sense from the raw data. Without the data definitions, the raw data are meaningless and unable to be interpreted by the software. An additional aspect of dealing with terminology is the lack of standard terminology within health care. For example, the clinic may define vital signs to include weight and height, along with heart rate, respiratory rate, and temperature, whereas the hospital may only include heart rate, respiratory rate, and temperature.

Standards have been developed for formatting much clinical and administrative health data to permit data transfer to occur automatically, for example, **Health Level Seven (HL7)** standards. However, considerable effort is still required in most institutions to implement interfaces among computer systems that adheres to HL7 standards. There are several versions of HL7 in use, and there is fairly wide latitude of interpretation in the application of these by any given vendor or institution. On the horizon is a powerful new tool, the **extensible markup language (XML)**, which is viewed as the syntax standard for sending and receiving health data. It may prove useful for extracting and standardizing specific data elements in the health care system's existing and largely incompatible information systems (McDonald, 1998). A close cousin to HTML, XML is able, in effect, to read Web-based data content and decide how to route and index the data for multiple users. A complete discussion of these and other health-related technical standards is provided in Chapter 17.

This discussion of the problems involved with bandwidth and interfacing medical information demonstrates the many contingencies that must be dealt with before computers linked by the World Wide Web and Internet will be able to share large amounts of detailed health information easily, securely, and seamlessly.

CONCLUSION

The Internet is arguably the third greatest advance in information technology after the inventions of writing and the moveable type printing press. Significant advances in information technology by decentralizing access to information and knowledge promote revolutionary change. It is too early to call the impact of eHealth revolutionary, but there are increasing signs that the influence of eHealth will affect the very roots of our current health care system.

Removing traditional barriers to information flow within health care creates new opportunities for some and removes or diminishes old privileges for others. eHealth has created a channel for placing very large amounts of health care information at the fingertips of anyone who seeks it. eHealth networks have been created where opinion, knowledge, and health care goods and services are exchanged and relationships are formed between both traditional and nontraditional health care participants. Easy access to health information was previously restricted to the eyes of the professional, mostly in paper format. eHealth creates a new level of access to health care information for both providers and consumers. As this occurs, eHealth shifts the locus of control over health care data and information in the direction of consumers and their partners. Much of what the eHealth consumer does is made possible through retail sales and Internet relationships that are not engineered by the formal health care system. In the eHealth era the shift from a paper-rich environment to an instantaneous electronic environment blurs the traditional divisions of labor and knowledge and therefore changes the power and authority relationship between health care experts and consumers of health care.

Perhaps the most important questions still to be answered about eHealth deal with personal health care data and their appropriate use. With the advent of eHealth, health information of a personal and private nature is stored on Web servers. As the amount of health information proliferates on Web servers located in hospitals, insurance companies, pharmaceutical companies, interactive health portals, and online retailers, so too will grow the possibilities of using the accumulating data for new purposes. These new purposes are certain to raise ethical and moral questions. For example, consider the issue of health insurance discounts for healthy behaviors (e.g., quitting smoking). Health insurance companies may in the future wish to use the new and vast electronic information stores scattered across cyberspace to verify whether an individual has stopped smoking cigarettes and then adjust their premiums accordingly. Is this a fair and ethical use of the data or an intrusion into an individual's privacy? Should online pharmacies be permitted to sell information about customer purchases to online booksellers so that the latter can suggest publications that address specific illnesses and conditions? Should online book sellers be permitted to sell information about the book titles their customers purchase to drug companies so that the latter can suggest new drugs that might be helpful to them or family members? Those kinds of arrangements will be seen as logical and even in the patient's best interest by some but will be vigorously opposed by others who view them as an intrusion into the patient's privacy.

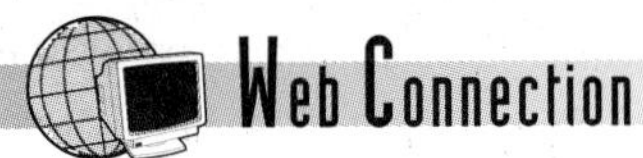

Web Connection

The Internet provides easy access to many kinds of health care information and products. *eHealth* encompasses the wide range of health activities that involve the electronic transfer of information. Convenience, low cost, and accessibility are viewed as benefits of the current and emerging technologies. However, old and new problems are surfacing as we gain experience in using the Internet. Privacy, reasonable access to data and information, and reliability of information are but a few of the issues that informatics professionals are dealing with. The Web Connection activities for this chapter consider the trends and technologies that make up eHealth today. You will explore sites that support eHealth and evaluate their usefulness in health care delivery.

discussion questions

1. Define eHealth. Contrast your definition with the definition of a person who is not involved in the health care industry.
2. Make a list of examples of the ways that you, your friends, and your family members use the Internet and the World Wide Web for health-related purposes. Discuss similarities or differences in these uses of eHealth.
3. Review the privacy policy statement on three different Web sites that provide health information. Explain how these policies do or do not protect the privacy of individuals using the site.
4. Describe the ASP model of computing and explain its advantages and disadvantages.

REFERENCES

American Association of Health Plans. (1999, October). *Enrollment, growth, and accreditation* [Report]. Washington, DC: Author. Retrieved May 15, 2000, from the World Wide Web: http://www.aahp.org/services/government&advocacy/new/enroll.pdf.

Coile, R.C., Jr. (1999, November 2). Keynote address. *Health Internet 2000 conference*. New York.

Evans, P.B., & Wurster, T.S. (1997). Strategy and the new economics of information. *Harvard Business Review, September-October,* 70-82.

Forrester Research. (2000, February). Full-service health sites arise [Report]. Cambridge, MA: Author. Retrieved May 1, 2000, from the World Wide Web: http://www.forrester.com/ER/Research/Report/0,1338,8717,FF.html.

Forrester Research. (2000, May). Hospitals' new supply chain [Report]. Cambridge, MA: Author. Retrieved May 21, 2000, from the World Wide Web: http://www.forrester.com/ER/Research/Report/Interviews/0,1338,9277,FF.html.

Gartner Group. (1999, April). *1998 IT spending and staffing survey results* [Report]. Stamford, CT: Author. Retrieved May 15, 2000, from the World Wide Web: http://gartner.jmu.edu/research/ras/77800/77835/77835.html.

Health Care Financing Administration. (1999). *Fiscal year 1999 annual performance report.* Washington, DC: U.S. Government Printing Office.

Kibbe, D.C., & Bard, M. (1997). Applying clinical informatics to health care improvement: Making progress is more difficult than we thought it would be. *Joint Commission Journal on Quality Improvement, 23*(12), 619-622.

Kohn, L.T., Corrigan, J.M., & Donaldson, M.S. (Eds.). (2000). *To err is human: Building a safer health system.* Washington, DC: National Academy Press.

Levit, K. (2000, January/February). Health spending in 1998: Signals of change. *Health Affairs, 19,* 124-32.

McDonald, C.J., Overhage, J.M., Dexter, P.R., Blevins, L., Meeks-Johnson, J., Suice, J.G., Tucker, M.C., & Schadow, G. (1998). Canopy computing: using the web in clinical practice. *JAMA, 280*(15), 1325-1328.

Robert Wood Johnson Foundation. (1996). *Chronic care in America: A 21st century challenge.* Princeton, NJ: Author.

Spillman, B.C., & Lubitz, J. (2000). The effect of longevity on spending for acute and long-term care. *New England Journal of Medicine, 342*(19), 1409-1415.

U.S. Census Bureau. (1999). *Statistical abstract of the United States.* Washington, DC: U.S. Government Printing Office.

U.S. Department of Health and Human Services. (2000, April). *Report to the President, prescription drug coverage, spending, utilization, and prices.* Washington, DC: U.S. Government Printing Office.

PART FOUR

The Impact of Informatics on the Sociocultural Environment of Health Care

CHAPTER 14

The Impact of Health Care Informatics on the Organization

JACQUELINE DIENEMANN
BARBARA VAN DE CASTLE

Learning Objectives

Upon completion of this chapter, the reader will be able to:

1. ***Describe*** how organization theory and organizational behavior may be used to guide organizational planning.
2. ***Define*** and ***give*** examples of information system characteristics related to the needs of horizontal and vertical integration of health care systems.
3. ***Assess*** the benefits and potential problems for implementing a new information technology application in a health care work environment.
4. ***Describe*** strategies for the successful management of changes in administrative information systems in a health care work environment.
5. ***Describe*** issues and potential solutions related to implementation of a clinical information system using standardized nursing languages.

Outline

Outline—cont'd

Key Terms

cascade effect
coercive pressure
desired health outcomes
evidence-based practice
fluid outsourcing
horizontal integration
loose coupling
middle-range theory
mimetic pressure
normative pressure
open systems
organization science
organization theory
organizational behavior
organizational culture
performance indicators
performance management system
pooled interdependence
reciprocal interdependence
sequential interdependence
vertical integration
virtual organizations

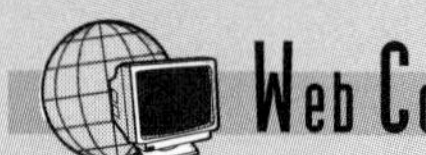

Web Connection

Go to the Web site at http://evolve.elsevier.com/Englebardt/. Here you will find Web links and activities related to the impact of health care informatics on the organization.

Organizations are the structure and process through which health care is delivered to individuals, families, and communities. Communication of information throughout an organization and between the organization and the people it serves is a vital function that often poses barriers to achieving **desired health outcomes** for patients. Analysis shows that health care businesses invest less in technology and technology training to support information flow, accuracy, decision support, storage, and security than do other industries (Newbold, 1998). Yet health care is a service that relies on communication for accurate diagnosis of health problems, description of treatment options, informed consent, effective interventions, and monitoring of responses and effectiveness.

This chapter provides an overview of theories explaining how organizations function and change. These theories are then applied to explain the current impact of health care informatics on health care organizations, as well as the processes that both support and resist incorporation of health care informatics as a tool to support quality services and the success of new strategic initiatives. Managerial and clinical applications are provided as examples of areas where informatics has made an impact. A case study of a health care organization adopting a clinical information system with standardized nursing languages is provided to illustrate the processes of change and organizational impact of innovations in informatics.

RELEVANCE OF THEORIES ABOUT ORGANIZATIONS TO HEALTH CARE INFORMATICS

The discipline of **organization science** has its theoretical roots in psychology, sociology, anthropology, management, and public administration. Research on different types of organizations, such as those that deliver professional services (education, medicine, social work, or nursing), has led to **middle-range theory** development. Middle-range theories are somewhat abstract but include concepts and propositions that are measurable and applicable to practice. Research on different groups within organizations or locations of organizations has also identified middle-range theories about the impact of these variables. From this work, there is now a body of knowledge to explain the impact of informatics on health care organizations and the processes within organizations that support adoption of information technology (IT), as well as those that restrain adoption.

Basic Assumptions of Open Systems Theory

Organization theory focuses on entire organizations rather than on small workgroups or individuals. Theorists seek to explain patterns of activity and the relationships among structure, function, and organizational growth. Many theorists and administrators view organizations as **open systems** with missions and strategic goals. As open systems, organizations respond to environmental demands and changes in resources through the use of technology, policies and procedures, employees, organizational behavior, and task requirements for work. A biological, organic metaphor is used for viewing organizations as organisms. This approach holds two basic assumptions (Dienemann & Navarro, 1998):

1. Organizational growth is necessary for health.
2. Lack of action and response to the environment will lead to organizational decline and eventual death.

Different authors have emphasized different insights provided by open systems theory, including the following:

- Strategic contingency on the impact of changes in the environment
- Resource dependency on the accumulation of power and political impact of control over scarce resources
- Chaos theory on the lack of rationality in response to environmental demands
- Exchange theory on the reciprocity between different sources of power
- The tendency for homeostasis or mutual adjustment to minimize change

Each of these observations offers valuable applications for informatics specialists. Additional information related to systems theory is presented in Chapter 1.

Definitions of Organization Theory and Organizational Behavior

Organization theory seeks to explain why and how organizations change and suggests actions to increase effectiveness when planning change. **Organizational behavior** theories and research, on the other hand, focus on small groups and individuals in organizations. Research from this perspective examines individual and interpersonal work issues, such as career development, job satisfaction,

FIGURE 14–1 Organization Theory and Information Systems

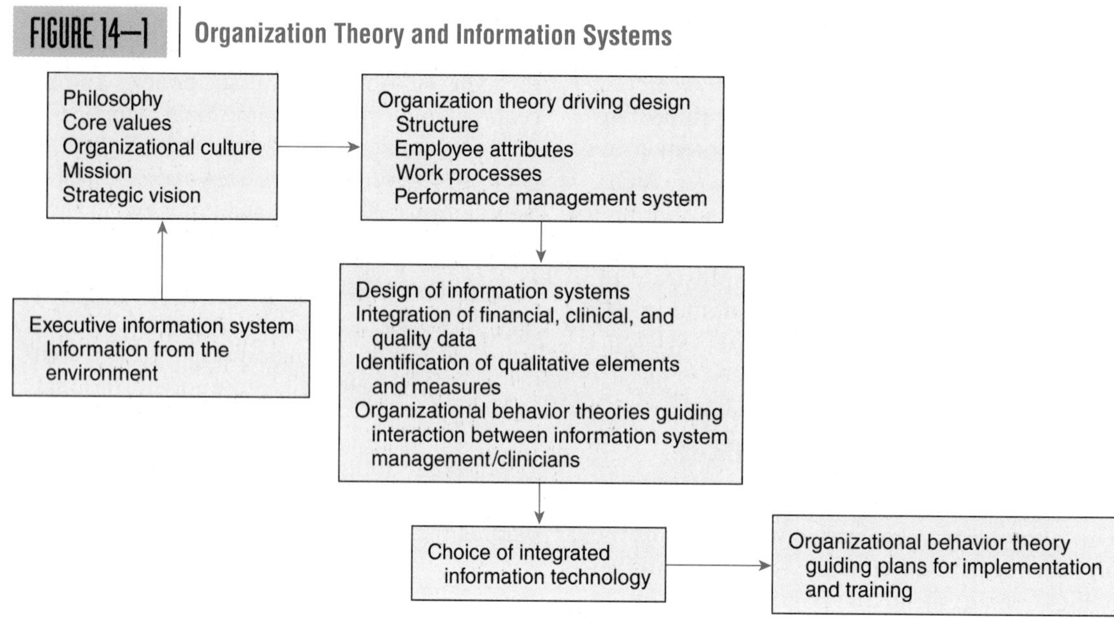

motivation, productivity, group dynamics, work life, ethics, values, and culture. From this perspective, organizational health is based on a balance of autonomy, control, and cooperation among organizational participants. Organizational behavior provides deeper understanding of why, how, and when advances in informatics technology are or are not adopted in a particular organization (Dienemann, 1998). Organization theory and organizational behavior theories have implications for the design and implementation of information systems (Figure 14-1). These implications are discussed throughout this chapter.

INFORMATION NEEDS AND CHALLENGES IN TODAY'S HEALTH CARE ENVIRONMENT

Health Care Informatics as an Environmental Force for Change

Organizations depend on the environment for information on changes relevant to their services, markets, and finances. In the last decade, dramatic shifts in reimbursement mechanisms, costs, competitors, service technology, and population demographics have resulted in an unstable and uncertain health care environment. Advances in IT and the pace of change in the environment have shifted the primary information challenge for executives from access to overload. In response to this challenge, the field of health care informatics developed. It focuses on the information technologies that support patient care decision making by health care practitioners. This focus is evident in informatics clinical practice, education research, and management (Hannah, Ball, & Edwards, 1999). Advances in information applications have created pressure within health care organizations to adopt and use computers to support patient care decision making. For example, information service companies and executive information systems (EISs) that provide summarized and prioritized information to support strategic decision making for groups of providers have emerged.

Virtual Organizations in Health Care

Other environmental forces such as financial risk sharing, a trend toward mergers and acquisitions, and shortages of certain health care personnel have created pressures for health care to become more like other industries. Health care delivery organizations today are likely to be regional, national, or global corporations with a strong emphasis on profitability. They are often referred to as **virtual organizations,** since they are not geographically bound and include various organizational relationships such as consortia, partnerships, strategic limited alliances, mergers, and acquisitions. Characteristics of successful virtual organization systems include a clear mission and vision to unite diverse members; **loose coupling**—a condition where departments in an organization have autonomy and decision-making power at their organizational level; vertical and horizontal integration; **fluid outsourcing**—a situation in which some internal functions are contracted to an external organization while maintaining a core of full-time employees; and integrated information systems. Integrated information systems support feedback of performance data, responsive feedback from the corporate level, and continuous quality and financial improvement (Sebastian, 1999).

Performance Indicators Used by the Mayo Health Care System

The Mayo health care system is a virtual organization that has developed and implemented a **performance management system** using an integrated information system. The **performance indicators** in this system are based on the core business principles derived from a review of the literature and organizational philosophy. These include clinical practice, education, research, mutual respect, continuous improvement, work atmosphere and teamwork, social commitment, and a commitment to sustain the practice financially. Performance measures include customer satisfaction, clinical productivity and efficiency per physician per workday, financial cost per relative value unit of service, internal operations efficiency (average length of stay or waiting time for visits and patient complaints per 1000 patients), employee satisfaction and employee demographics of diversity, and social commitment as shown by community outreach. This is put into a context of external environmental assessment as shown by market share, the board of governor's assessment, and patient characteristics analyzed by geographical area and payer group. Development requires time, commitment, critical thought, new methods of capturing relevant data, and a focus on creating one database to be used for reports to payers, corporate and institutional leaders, staff, and regulators. The development of Mayo's performance management system has been an iterative process that will continue to develop and change over time. For internal use, information gathered from this system is organized into a weekly management report made available through an intranet at the corporate, organizational, and departmental levels. Supplemented by the clinical practice data set, information is also organized into a clinical practice report that is available at the corporate, organizational, and departmental levels and to the clinical practice committee and clinicians at each site (Curtright, Stolp-Smith, & Edell, 1999).

Horizontal and Vertical Integration of Health Care Delivery Systems

Horizontally integrated systems include a group of organizations offering similar services, such as nursing homes, rehabilitation centers, behavioral medicine hospitals, substance abuse programs, or rural hospitals. These include both regional and national chains. To be effective, integrated systems need to achieve economies of scale by using their potential to increase capital funding for acquisition of technology, renovation, and expansion (Charns, 1997). Health care informatics investments are essential to achieve effectiveness. Often, integrated systems standardize IT systems for all agencies within that system. Training, purchasing, allocation of capital, and financial data reporting are centralized. Integrated systems have struggled with decreased revenues from Medicare and Medicaid as a result of cuts caused by the Balanced Budget Act. A key IT challenge facing these organizations is the continuous updating of hardware and software to meet new requirements for timely information on quality improvement, as well as regulatory and accreditation requirements. These organizations are also challenged to take advantage of their **pooled interdependence** in creating increased information sharing, mutual problem solving, and the distribution of positive innovations.

Often accreditation is required by the Centers for Medicare & Medicaid Services (CMS) (formerly known as the Health Care Financing Administration [HCFA]) or state agencies for reimbursement from Medicare or Medicaid. These federal and state agencies work closely with private accrediting bodies to set up databases that can be used to compare the quality of care given by agencies over time. For example, the Joint Commission on Accreditation of Healthcare Organizations' (JCAHO) initiative, ORYX, is developing a process that integrates performance measures into the accreditation process for hospitals and health care networks. Medicare reimbursement is tied to JCAHO accreditation and to participation in the CMS Health Care Quality Improvement Program (HCQIP). Data sets have been developed for specific types of providers, such as home health care. The Outcomes and Assessment Information Set (OASIS) is a data set used by CMS nationally as a condition of participation in the Medicare programs for home health agencies. OASIS is the basis for CMS's Outcome-Based Quality Improvement Program (OBQI). Alternatively, long-term care facilities are required to do patient assessments using the Medicare Minimum Data Set (MDS) and to report changes over time to obtain reimbursement. Managed care organizations providing primary care are accredited by the National Committee on Quality Assurance, which requires them to collect data for the Health Plan and Employer Data and Information Set (HEDIS). CMS requires accreditation and participation in the Quality Improvement System for Managed Care (QISMC) of managed care organizations for reimbursement. Compliance requires that agencies have sophisticated information systems for data entry and retrieval. The cost for manual data entry and compilation is prohibitive (Simpson, 2000).

Vertically integrated systems offer related services within a region, such as health insurance, primary care, laboratory and imaging services, ambulatory surgery or medical day care, hospital care, home health care, rehabilitation care, and nursing home care. In other words, a variety of health care services for an individual may be provided through different parts of one vertically integrated system over time. National and global examples include Kaiser Permanente, the Veterans Administration health care system, and the Mayo health care system. To be effective, vertically integrated systems require clinical coordination of services across member units. The goal is to increase **sequential interdependence** by planning, delivering, monitoring, and adjusting the care of an individual over time, as well as to encourage **reciprocal interdependence** between physicians and member agencies (Charns, 1997). They must also meet the reporting requirements for each provider type included in the system. The integration of data elements, rules for conflicting data, and applications for creating each type of report requires a complex, sophisticated information system. Achievement of their goals for coordinated, efficient care requires extensive relationships with external organizations in the communities served.

Integration of Information Systems in Virtual Organizations

To support integration of clinical information systems for internal and regulatory reporting, the information system must have the capability to (Jacobsen & Hill, 1999):

- Transfer information across settings for each episode of care for one person
- Standardize record keeping
- Monitor quality across settings
- Store data between services
- Provide immediate feedback

Reporting must be organized for frequent and widespread access. Historically, lack of this capability has limited integration and effectiveness. Often the information systems were integrated only at the corporate level, and member organizations operated as independent providers. In addition, the information systems were developed independently and offered sophisticated financial tracking. The information systems between member agencies were incompatible. Thus acquiring software to increase portability and integration of information is the principal goal for information systems within these virtual organizations. Meeting the anticipated demands of the Health Insurance Portability and Accountability Act (HIPAA) in the next decade creates additional pressure for investment in an integrated information system (Waldo, 2000). In addition, international organizations need to acquire software for translations, for internal integration, and for organizational memory systems that support learning and sharing of expertise across the entire virtual organization. Some approaches include extranet capability (i.e., having an intranet that is partially accessible to authorized outsiders) and groupware (software that helps groups of workers attached to a local area network coordinate their activities) (Boudreau et al., 1998).

The implementation, variety, and sophistication of information systems are often unevenly distributed as both horizontally and vertically integrated systems expand through multiple types of relationships. Rather than starting over with a new information system, organizations are investing in IT to link existing systems and add new capabilities. Success is tied to the investment in IT that can operationalize the virtual organization design required by the geographical disbursement of facilities. To move to an integrated IT system for vertically or horizontally integrated health systems will require the organization to make a major investment in needed resources. These resources are needed to create new capabilities for quality monitoring, standardization of terminology and entry requirements, new levels of security, equitable distribution across units, and portability of information for patient mobility, as well as comparisons of similar services. This must be accomplished while maintaining responsiveness to the unique information demands of specialized areas and continuously providing services.

With new hardware, software, and IT changes comes the need for retraining of many people across the organization. For many, it also requires changing the priorities of their work. At the same time, employees are experiencing other changes such as multiple changes of ownership in a short period of time, reorganization of management structure, and reengineering of their work responsibilities and workgroups. Often IT executives planning for system improvement concentrate on hardware and software issues, which are often challenging in themselves, and invest too little time in planning related to motivating people to use the new technology within a fluid, turbulent environment. Implementation plans must include meeting the needs of all workers involved, or employees will sabotage and impede the pace and utilization of the new technology and work processes.

ADVANCES IN HEALTH CARE INFORMATICS IN THE CLINICAL AREA

In addition to the challenges of moving clinical and financial information across geographical locations and types of services, technological advances are creating new opportunities for health care professionals. New services are now being provided, and established ways of doing work have become outmoded.

Telecommunications Applications in Clinical Practice

The most visible advance that most people are aware of is telecommunications applications for health care. The wireless telephone, the facsimile machine, teleconferencing capability, the Internet, and local area networks within health care organizations now make it possible for health care professionals to consult, confer, change orders, and update treatment plans without traveling to the site of the patient encounter. For example, patients may have specially designed telephones or computers to directly measure and transmit assessments of vital signs, chest sounds, or images of wounds from their locations to nurses or physicians. This technology makes it possible to monitor disease or wound management or assess an emergency situation for appropriate care from a distance. Physicians in different countries may now consult on a complex health problem with real-time imaging of the patient, as well as diagnostic data such as an ongoing electrocardiogram reading. Nurse case managers may now participate in multidisciplinary teleconferences with a client and other professionals at distant sites. Patients can make appointments by Internet or obtain answers to their questions concerning their disease or disability via eMail. Other applications include the following (Hannah, Ball, & Edwards, 1999):

- Interinstitutional patient and clinical records and information systems
- Community health information networks for surveillance of infectious diseases, environmental risk factors, and epidemiological analysis
- Health information and education networks and multimedia sources
- Distance learning for both continuing education and degree-granting programs
- Networked research databases and libraries

Telecommunication devices make health care delivery more effective and efficient by reducing the time and effort needed by health care personnel to share information with primary care offices, nursing units, and ancillary services such as pharmacy, radiology, and social work. They also reduce patient and family travel time needed to pick up referrals and managed care authorizations before seeing a specialist. New telecommunications applications are continually being developed and implemented.

Technology Changing the Demand for Inpatient Care

New pharmaceuticals, surgical procedures and devices, and knowledge about disease and disability processes coupled with financial pressures are moving many health care services out of the inpatient, overnight hospital stay and into the office, home, or same-day service mode. This trend, along with advances in telecommunications, is dramatically reducing the demand for inpatient, centralized hospital services and expanding the demand for community-based services. Simultaneously, the pressure to demonstrate effectiveness in reducing costs and increasing desired outcomes is creating new jobs for health care professionals to monitor, measure, manage, and coordinate care for patients across episodes of treatment at multiple sites with multiple providers. These jobs often require computer and telecommunication skills. Another growing area for health care professionals with additional information systems (IS) training is in IT departments. Here their clinical knowledge and technical knowledge of computers and telecommunications provide an ability to work with "both sides." These individuals are effective at problem solving to reduce service gaps and errors, as well as promoting and implementing the use of new applications in a clinical environment.

Responses of Health Care Professionals to Advances in Informatics

New IT applications are both desired and feared by health care personnel with a clinical orientation. Clinicians value individualized care, direct service provision to prolong life, professional autonomy, and a hierarchy of authority. These values may act as barriers to utilization of many IT applications that standardize language and care processes. Health care professionals place a higher value on providing direct services using an individual provider's clinical judgment than on following protocols and documenting observations, services, and outcomes. An assumption is made that "doing the right thing" will result in the right outcome; there is also the belief that documenting desired outcomes is redundant. Clinicians are more motivated to use applications that they perceive as reducing error and transmission time to gateways for services, such as wireless telephone contact between nurses and physicians or facsimile sending of orders between departments or agencies.

Traditional values and practice patterns have created **organizational cultures** (norms, values, and informal standards of behavior that guide behavior in organizations) that conflict with the current trend for **evidence-based practice** to achieve long-term outcomes defined in conjunction with the patient. Evidence-based practice includes the use of interventions and treatments that are research based to support clinical decision making. Payers, researchers, regulators, accreditation agencies, and administrators, seeking to identify the effectiveness of interventions and the quality of patient outcomes, are creating **coercive pressure,** based on power relationships, for clinicians to establish "best practice" standards, develop clinical pathways of recommended interventions, and determine desired outcomes for each clinical condition, disease, and disability. Deviations from these standards and guidelines should be justified with patient data. These groups are also demanding the reduction of costs of care in the final year of a person's life and increased compliance with advanced directives and patients' desires for hospice care (Lundberg, 2000). This conflict with the values and usual practice patterns of health care providers must be addressed to gain their cooperation and collaboration. Signs that leading clinicians are promoting evidence-based practice is shown by the themes of workshops, publications, and "best practice" reports creating **mimetic pressures** for others to follow. In other words, health care professionals are encouraged to practice in ways that imitate standards that have been incorporated into the practice of recognized experts. In time, values will shift to support evidence-based practice creating **normative pressures** for peer acceptance. Normative pressures encourage adoption of behaviors that are accepted by one's group.

Box 14–1 Limitations to Development of Software for Outcomes Measurement

1. Prerequisite of agreement on standards for treatment and desired outcomes across practitioners and settings
2. Clinicians' wariness of technology interfering with practice or lowering productivity
3. Lack of a standardized clinical vocabulary across disciplines and settings

From Simpson, R. (2000). Nursing informatics. *Nursing Administration Quarterly, 24*(2), 87-90.

The speed of these changes will be influenced by the strategies used by payers, researchers, and administrators to introduce and institutionalize evidence-based practice (Scott & Backman, 1990). IT systems are needed to effectively support implementation of evidence-based practice and to convince health care professionals of its value. Limitations to development of software for outcomes measurement are shown in Box 14-1.

The inclusion of patient input for treatment options, advanced directives, and definition of desired outcomes make the algorithms even more complex. Once these algorithms are in place, IT issues of programming, user-friendly software and hardware features, immediate reporting, security of patient information, and faster load time for access can be addressed by the IT industry. In return, health care organizations must decide to invest more in IT systems, hardware for employees, IT maintenance, and IT training (Simpson, 2000).

CHANGES IN PROFESSIONAL PRACTICE DUE TO ADVANCES IN HEALTH CARE INFORMATICS

Access to More Information via the Internet

Advances in health care informatics are increasing clinicians' access to information that is vital to improving their practice. More and more health care organizations are providing Internet access to staff clinicians at the same time that they are creating Web-based policy manuals, formularies, pharmacological protocols, and other internal documents. Clinicians are also using Internet access to obtain information on practice guidelines, continuing education, patient/family educational materials, and even distance learning for academic degrees. Increasingly, integrated health care systems are contracting with multimedia education firms to deliver interactive training simultaneously to multiple sites instead of either sending trainers to sites or having employees travel to central sites (Evans, 2000). This is especially useful when introducing new technology or meeting regulatory requirements for training.

Changes in Time Distribution of Work in Health Care Services

The adoption of other telecommunication devices is discussed earlier. Use of telecommunication technology has changed the time distribution of clinical activity and reduced the time for transmission of information. It has also increased the frequency and timeliness of interaction among staff nurses, allied professionals, and physicians, often resulting in increased collaboration and coordination of care. Simultaneously, it has increased expectations and reduced control of time for nurses and allied professionals carrying cell phones. Their day is now filled with interruptions for real-time communication.

Issues and Solutions When Implementing Physician Order Entry

The electronic health record (EHR), also referred to as the computerized patient record (CPR), is being only partially implemented. The most frequent application now being used is physician order entry (POE), connecting patient care sites with the pharmacy, laboratory, and radiology departments. Adoption of a POE often takes years; for instance, implementation on a pilot unit at Johns Hopkins took 2½ years of planning and an additional 11 months to fully implement. Issues that delayed implementation included the following (Dolan & Kisamore, 1998):

- Development and approval of order sets for frequent configurations of orders specific to high-volume diagnoses on that unit
- State approval for an electronic signature
- Allocation of sufficient personnel hours to task forces
- Alternative paper backup for computer downtime
- Clarification of terminology for the laboratory
- Reduction of the number and complexity of screens for order entry of medications
- Staff acceptance of clinical pathways

Few of these issues could be resolved through technology. Resolution required dealing with the interpersonal barriers relating to the culture of health care that are discussed earlier in this chapter.

Planning for information systems in health care must include an understanding that all problems cannot be anticipated. Therefore senior management must be available at a moment's notice when problems impact patient care delivery. A POE requires ongoing involvement of physicians, staff, and all areas of the information system throughout the adoption process and periodically thereafter as treatment protocols change. Often organizations underestimate the time and commitment of administrators, physicians, other health care professionals, and IS staff that are needed over a period of several years to take any informatics project from planning to adoption throughout an agency. The transition may take several years. Parallel paper and electronic systems, as well as interfaced paper and electronic systems, must be in place to support continuous delivery of services during this time. This duplication of documentation increases time commitments for clinicians. This can dampen their long-term commitment to the project. Once adopted, these systems increase accuracy, eliminate transcription errors, decrease time between order and service, and reduce time needed to track where an order is within the system. However, they do not always reduce the time needed to place an order. This means that the institution may benefit from the automation, but not every staff person will experience the same benefit.

Acceptance of Health Care Informatics by Health Care Professionals

In inpatient and ambulatory care facilities, informatics results in a total change in the work of administrative support personnel, as well as many changes in the workflow of physicians, nurses, and allied health professionals while increasing the need for training in computer and telecommunication skills. Reduction of the transcribing, copying, and distribution work has resulted in a broadening of responsibilities for administrative support personnel. Once an application such as order entry is in place, all professionals need some level of keyboarding skills to interact with most information systems. Technical support for users of the information system during all business hours is essential.

The acceptance by health care professionals has varied from refusal to use the system to pushing for the addition of new applications. For example, some physicians have been so resistant to direct order entry that agencies have hired scribes to provide computer input for physicians' verbal or written documentation, which is then signed off by the physician. Other physicians have been leaders in the design of screens and coordination of rollouts of new applications. In IS environments, nurses and allied health professionals spend less time tracking the status of orders, calling physicians for clarification of orders, or transcribing orders and more time communicating using telecommunication devices and computers.

Access to hardware is an issue on many units. A limited number of workstations or poor geographical distribution of access points can reduce efficiency gains from automation. System downtime and time for reprogramming changes, such as updates in protocols, is an issue in some agencies. Often staff members need retraining and additional information to ensure that they are using the new system appropriately and to communicate changes as problems are addressed and resolved.

Informatics has also provided the communication links to support dispersed services to specialized populations. There has been a rise in health care businesses for specific market niches such as pain management, incontinence management, wellness and fitness management, independent living of the frail elderly, and parish nursing. For these services, telecommunications and computer applications have improved the quality of services and health of the individual patients.

CHANGES IN MANAGEMENT ROLES DUE TO ADVANCES IN HEALTH CARE INFORMATICS

Information Systems Supporting Rapid Response to Change

Today's turbulent health care environment with changing reimbursement mechanisms—along with rapid advances in technology and clinical knowledge—requires rapid response to change through integrated informatics for organizational and system survival. The trend toward larger systems provides the capital and variety of services needed to survive severe cuts in resources and technological obsolescence, and to purchase expensive new technology. Conversely, informatics also supports the localization of decision making. Information systems that support localization of decision making are responsive to changes and needs in specialized service areas. Decentralized decision making creates the need to restructure health care organizations, which have traditionally been hierarchical and bureaucratic. These changes demand a dramatic change in management strategies and skills at all levels.

Leaders' Need for Information Systems Skills

At all levels of management, IT applications are increasingly complex with increased sources of input between levels of management and the environment. More objective data to support decision making is available. Administrators need information about trends throughout all business sectors, not just health care. The challenge for IS design is to create faster, condensed, organized, more accurate feedback that supports decision making without overloading users with information. IT is essential in order for leaders to "read the signposts" and recognize trends in time to envision a plan and respond in an effective manner (Porter-O'Grady, 1998). The administrator may be the leader or deterrent for an organization to successfully adopt new IS technology. Successful adoption is often dependent on the administrator's persistence when problems arise. Martins and Kambil (1999) have found that managers need to be aware that previous experience with adoptions of new IT may lead to overconfidence regarding adoption or to a negative attitude; these responses are independent of the actual issues presented by the new IT change. Successful managers need to be mindful of potential bias caused by untested assumptions.

Critical analysis of sometimes-conflicting information is now a requirement for all administrators working in environments with dispersed power. Even unit or local office managers are being asked to be more accountable for productivity and quality outcomes and cannot rely on "just carrying out orders." Resource dependency theory, an organization theory about political power interactions within organizations, points out that power will accumulate to those who can effectively sort and use information to improve productivity and quality. As IT systems provide more information to managers and clinicians, these persons will be expected to interpret information and act on their analysis to benefit the organization and its customers. Those who use the information well will be rewarded, and those who do not will be sanctioned. In other words, accountability for outcomes is being dispersed throughout the organization; no longer are only executives accountable for the financial, personnel, and quality outcomes of an organization.

Danger of a Cascade Effect When Implementing Changes

Decisions about organizational changes should always include attention to the balance of financial, personnel, and quality factors. Imbalance may create a **cascade effect** where small errors replicate and grow until they destabilize the organization with long-term negative outcomes. One example of a cascade is seen in the reengineering efforts of hospitals that downsized by eliminating most middle management positions, reduced clinical staffing to a theoretical safe minimum, and simultaneously introduced new technical positions. Some organizations did not allow sufficient staffing for training and support of these changes, absorption of existing dysfunctions in the system, or turnover of those who decided not to cope with revolutionary changes. Others made abrupt changes and ignored the slower pace that people need to absorb and collaborate in major changes.

A cascade effect occurred; problems beginning at the pilot stage were ignored and were replicated and multiplied as they reverberated throughout the institutions. Like an error in the beginning of an algebra problem, which results in the wrong outcome even if all of the calculation processes are correct, the agencies could not come to the desired outcome of reduced costs because they did not pay attention to balance in their planning. In these hospitals this led to destablization of nursing and a tarnished image in the nursing community, making recruitment difficult. This destabilization resulted in bed closures and loss of revenue (Kerfoot, 2000). Information specialists should take notice when implementing major changes such as the electronic patient record or a staffing and scheduling system, being mindful of the need to balance financial, quality, and personnel factors and to respond to problems quickly as they arise, to prevent a cascade effect that could occur and take years for organizational recovery.

Box 14–2 Advocacy Responsibilities of Managers

1. Budget to include the staffing time needed for task force and committee work
2. Resources for staff to make informed decisions
3. The power to implement recommendations that originate at the local level
4. Budget to include time for staff to plan, receive training, and implement change on a reasonable learning curve

From Porter-O'Grady, T. (1998). The seven basic rules for successful redesign. In E.C. Hein (Ed.), *Contemporary leadership behavior* (5th ed.). Philadelphia: J.B. Lippincott.

Changing Workgroup Culture

Department managers' work has changed from monitoring to ensure that people follow established policies and procedures to promoting and supporting change and critical thinking for decision making. Leadership has new salience in the managerial role. Having information on using information systems is vital for managers to be effective in their new roles. They are the leaders enabling change to occur that improves services at the point of service. Often this means changing the workgroup culture and establishing new practice patterns. People who become health care professionals share the value of desiring to help patients; this is a unifying theme that many managers have used to motivate changes in practice patterns. For instance, how can information systems be used to maximize the benefit to patients who have a limited length of stay or a limited number of visits as a result of limited insurance coverage? How can information systems be used to provide information on outcomes of patient care? These questions need to be addressed by clinicians in order to improve practice patterns. The manager must encourage decision making about what the workgroup can preserve that supports communication and cohesiveness and what it must discard to better meet the needs of patients. For many clinicians this means learning to use IT. It means getting beyond the initial embarrassment of not being able to do new behaviors well. It also means a reorientation from being concerned only with diagnosis and process to focusing on outcomes. Advocacy responsibilities of managers are shown in Box 14-2.

Short-Term Versus Long-Term Performance Measures

Department managers are often the leaders participating in developing performance measures included in IS reports. IS managers working with administrators and clinicians must be sensitive to the potential use of the data that they organize into information. They must try to include more than financial outcome data. Qualitative information is needed to reflect human tacit wisdom used in decision making. Both long-term trends and immediate objective data are needed for analysis of a broad range of measures such as financial status, adverse events, and personnel turnover. Pfeffer and Veiga (1999) pointed out

Box 14–3 Organizational Changes Needed to Focus on Long-Term Goal Achievement

1. Change the processes for finding and hiring the right clinicians and managers to emphasize enduring attributes, skill sets for critical thinking, and decision making rather than immediate tasks.
2. Develop training programs to prepare workers to do immediate tasks and retrain them as they change.
3. Retain the right people through employment security, comparatively high compensation based on performance by the workgroup, and development of autonomous work teams.

From Pfeffer, J., & Veiga J.F. (1999). Putting people first for organizational success. *The Academy of Management Executive, 13*(2), 37-48.

that organizations that view employees as assets and take a long-term goal achievement approach have substantial financial gains. Yet the focus on long-term goals is counter to American business practices, which usually emphasize short-term return on investment, dependence on quantitative measures, and close, tough supervision. This short-term view treats employees as costs rather than assets.

Administrators must work to change this orientation and increase practices that reflect a commitment to employees and the development of autonomous work teams. This will require dramatic changes in organizational structure and the work of both clinicians and administrators over time. Box 14-3 shows the steps Pfeffer and Veiga (1999) have outlined to accomplish this change.

Widespread IS changes are needed to monitor progress and provide financial and clinical information to the teams so that the work teams are able to make decisions that support the organizational mission and strategic vision. With these changes, many traditional management functions, such as monitoring and adapting work processes, will shift to clinicians. Managers will become system experts, intervening to facilitate change, institutionalize new work processes, and smooth communication. Over time, the gap between managers and clinicians will narrow both in status and salary.

The Paradox of Increased Efficiency

A major change in the work of administrators that is due to the increased efficiencies allowed by integrated IS networks is the paradox of increased efficiency. The new IS processes allow faster communication between and among clinicians and administrators even at distant sites. This has raised expectations for the effective, immediate use of information. Both administrators and clinicians now are expected to do multitasking, or simultaneous processing of multiple sources of information for multiple issues and customers. Gleick (1999) noted that expectations often begin to outstrip human capacity. To deal with this problem, organizations need to devise administrative policies that provide checkpoints ensuring that new information is accurately and effectively being incorporated. These checkpoints slow down expectations and work processes to correspond with the capacity of workers.

CASE STUDY: DESIGN OF A CLINICAL INFORMATION SYSTEM USING STANDARDIZED NURSING LANGUAGES

The ABC Hospital is part of an integrated health care delivery system (IHDS) with services ranging from inpatient acute care to primary care and long-term care. To support the flow of information throughout this vertically integrated system, a decision was made to invest in a clinical information system (CIS) that included interventions by nurses and other allied health personnel in addition to physicians. The leaders of the IHDS recognized that use of a standardized health care language (SHCL) would enable them to add another dimension in comparisons of quality, cost, and provider satisfaction across sites (Johnson, Maas, & Moorhead, 2000).

Goals of Administrators When Planning the Clinical Information System

The administrators set the following goals:

- More effective documentation of assessments, interventions, and outcomes
- Streamlining of charting
- Point-of-service documentation by all disciplines employed
- Detection of steps in patient progress
- Streamlining of report between shifts of nurses

The administrators hoped adoption would lead to more awareness of the various clinicians' impact on patient outcomes and promote job satisfaction. With short lengths of stay, it was hard for health care staff members to see results. With outcomes broken into specific, slight, incremental steps, positive changes could be made visible.

Task Force Choice of Nursing Interventions Classification and Nursing Outcomes Classification

The first step was the formation of a task force to choose the standardized languages to adopt in the CIS. The task force was composed of the bedside clinicians, including the nursing staff, as well as the IS staff. It was decided to limit the review of languages to those approved by the American Nurses Association. The task force selected a modification of the North American Nursing Diagnosis Association (NANDA) taxonomy, Nursing Interventions Classification (NIC), and Nursing Outcomes Classification (NOC) because the terminology was simple, they had been developed jointly, and they had been applied to other CIS applications. Also, the JCAHO had listed the NIC as meeting the requirements for its standard on uniform data (McCloskey & Bulechek, 2000). The task force then held team meetings with other clinical professionals to discover the issues that needed to be addressed by the CIS. They then met with administrators and reviewed policies and standards among all departments to determine what clinical data were needed to support their needs. On the basis of this input, the task force developed a request for proposal (RFP) for vendors to provide the CIS using the SHCLs and meeting the needs of the other professionals and administrators identified from the meetings.

Meanwhile, the task force piloted the use of the NIC and NOC classifications in their current paper charting on a hospital unit to identify any gaps and familiarize staff with the terminology. An expert consultant on these classifications from an affiliated school of nursing was hired to assist in developing the documentation system. The school already used the NIC and NOC classifications in its student care plans, which provided a starting framework. The NIC terms required little change in the format of the progress notes; the outcomes section of the chart needed adjustment to allow for the 5-point rating scale used in the NOC. In instances where care paths were being used, terminology was adapted to use the NANDA, NIC, and NOC taxonomies with outcome scales providing specific measurement. Health care staff members on the pilot unit were then trained in the terminology and given pocket reference tables to use as a resource. Also, a set of tables was laminated and attached to each bedside chart as a resource.

The documentation changes received mixed reactions. The staff members liked having a list for reference but complained that they did not know how to do the outcome ratings. The unit educators used this concern as a chance to provide informal, short in-services for discussions on how to estimate the five levels of ratings for specific outcomes that were often encountered on the unit. Questions also led to providing a copy of the reference books for each taxonomy on the unit for use by the staff.

The chosen vendor then worked with the task force to link the NIC and NOC classifications to the problem lists used by other professional staff members such as respiratory therapists and social workers. There were some issues raised by dietary and respiratory staff members regarding using a "nursing language," but when the terms were examined closely, they were found acceptable. All professional staff members on the pilot unit were then trained in the crosswalk of their old problem list and the NANDA, NIC, and NOC taxonomies. No gaps were found in needed interventions or outcomes, but staff members were encouraged to notify the task force if problems arose in the future. A number of physicians found the list of interventions helpful to their charting, and an in-service was provided for them to incorporate terms they found appropriate.

Screen Development for Ease of Use

The use of a "pick list" for the NIC interventions was chosen as the means to assist documentation using the SNCL. It was thought that a drop-down arrow next to the area for interventions would include the list of all possible interventions. On further thought, it became obvious that the NIC interventions were too numerous to list alphabetically. The decision was made to list only the NIC domains and their class categories. The chosen class brought up a screen with a list of specific interventions in a class; this reduced the search time for an appropriate intervention and allowed professional staff members to visualize all of the interventions in a given class on one screen. This structure of domain, class, and specific intervention was the same process the unit staff had used in the paper charting of NIC interventions and NOC outcomes. The vendor also created a personal library of most-used interventions by individual professionals, which came up when a class was chosen; this both tailored interventions to patient populations served and reduced search time even more.

The vendor then created a report for each patient, listing all of the interventions needed to complete orders and interventions for the next shift. This had been requested by nurses to assist in transferring patients between unit staff members at change of shift. A modified list was added to share planned interventions with nonlicensed personnel working with each patient. A third report for unit managers listed all patients, with the various medical and nursing diagnoses given, and all interventions that were noted for each diagnosis. Outcomes for each intervention were listed, but the rating was not recorded. A fourth report could be generated to look at aggregate interventions and associated outcome ratings.

Lessons Learned

In looking back at the goals originally set, it could be seen that some were met immediately. Others were still in progress. Nurses and other allied health personnel could document diagnoses, interventions, and outcomes at the bedside or a central computer. Clinical staff members found that clicking on preset words increased readability and was faster than narrative reporting. Dietary staff members liked the change-of-shift intervention list and adopted one for their needs. The unit reports were incorporated into weekly status meetings to review issues and to use as a basis for discussion of patient progress. The innovation was evaluated as successful and is now being implemented throughout the hospital. Other member agencies will be included over time.

CONCLUSION

Integration of human factors and technology is necessary to develop optimal technological support for clinical decision making, quality monitoring, cost-efficient care, and strategic visioning in a health care organization. Organization theory acts as a framework for technical experts and managers who are developing and implementing IT to provide this integration. Organization theory can alert technology experts, administrators, and clinicians to issues of culture, interdependence, and change processes, thereby improving the fit between IT systems and those whose work they are designed to support. This leads to wider utilization and faster acceptance.

Web Connection

Health care organizations are dynamic, fluid environments. To remain viable and competitive in a global economy, they must be attentive to the organization, the individual, and the individual's interaction with the organization within a global context. Change theories have traditionally focused on individual or organizational responses to change and innovation. Organizations now realize that attention to only these two dimensions is inadequate to predict the effects of the integration of information technology into the organization. This chapter has provided current perspectives on organizational theory and organization behavior theory. The Web Connection activities explore change as it is presented in various resources and provide opportunities to consider strategies and tools that could be used to understand and assess potential responses to change.

discussion questions

1. Provide an illustration that demonstrates how your health care organization does or does not fit the basic assumptions of open systems theory.
2. Use organization theory to explain the challenges that a health care organization can be expected to experience when additional numbers and types of IT applications are being introduced.
3. Interview a health care professional involved with the introduction of a new telecommunications technology in a health care organization in your area. Determine how the technology was introduced, how long it took before it was fully used as planned, what problems were encountered, and how those problems were solved. What benefits accrued to the organization due to the new technology?
4. What are the sources of data used in your health care organization to measure performance of the department where you are employed? Is the information system used to analyze data on costs, revenues, client satisfaction, and work quality? How is this information shared with staff, and what happens if any measure shows decreased performance?
5. What rating would you give yourself on IT skills on a scale of expert, mastery, competent, or novice? Explain how you defined IT skills and the reason for your ranking.
6. In the case study presented, will the CIS that was designed be able to support achievement of the goals set by the administrators? What do you see as the potential for the system? What do you see as the barriers?

REFERENCES

Boudreau, M., et al. (1998). Going global: Using information technology to advance the competitiveness of the virtual transnational organization. *The Academy of Management Executive, 12*(4), 120-128.

Charns, M.P. (1997). Organization design of integrated delivery systems. *Journal of Healthcare Management, 42*(3), 411-432.

Curtright, J.W., Stolp-Smith, S.C., & Edell, E.S. (2000). Strategic performance management: Development of a performance measurement system at the Mayo Clinic. *Journal of Healthcare Management, 45*(1), 58-67.

Dienemann, J. (1998). Assessing organizations. In J. Dienemann (Ed.), *Nursing administration: Managing patient care* (2nd ed., pp. 267-283). Stamford, CT: Appleton & Lange.

Dienemann, J.A., & Navarro, V.B. (1998). Management and organizational dynamics. In A.P. Harris & W.G. Zitzmann, Jr. (Eds.), *Operating room management* (pp. 1-21). St. Louis: Mosby.

Dolan, C.A., & Kisamore, L. (1998). Cutting the gordian knot: Implementing ordernet in an academic health center. In J. Dienemann (Ed.), *Nursing administration: Managing patient care* (2nd ed., pp. 339-357). Stamford, CT: Appleton & Lange.

Evans, S. (2000). Net-based training goes the distance. *The Washington Post Business Supplement,* May 15, pp. 20-22.

Gleick, J. (1999). *Faster.* New York: Pantheon.

Hannah, K.J., Ball, M.J., & Edwards, M.J.A. (1999). *Introduction to nursing informatics* (2nd ed.). New York: Springer.

Jacobsen, T., & Hill, M. (1999). Achieving information systems support for clinical integration. *Journal of Nursing Administration, 29*(6), 31-39.

Johnson, M., Maas, M., & Moorhead, S. (2000). *Nursing outcomes classification (NOC)* (2nd ed.). St. Louis: Mosby.

Kerfoot, K. (2000). TIQ (technical IQ)—A survival skill for the new millennium. *Nursing Economic$, 18*(1), 29-31.

Lundberg, C.B. (2000). Nursing informatics: Using uniform language in patient care documentation. *Nursing Economic$, 18*(1), 38-39.

Martins, L.L., & Kambil, A. (1999). Looking back and thinking ahead: Effects of prior success on managers' interpretations of new information technologies. *Academy of Management Journal, 42*(6), 652-661.

McCloskey, J.C., & Bulechek, G.M. (2000). *Nursing interventions classification (NIC)* (3rd ed.). St. Louis: Mosby.

Newbold, S.K. (1998). Information systems for managing patient care. In J.A. Dienemann (Ed.), *Nursing administration: Managing patient care* (2nd ed., pp. 323-339). Stamford, CT: Appleton & Lange.

Pfeffer, J., & Veiga J.F. (1999). Putting people first for organizational success. *The Academy of Management Executive, 13*(2), 37-48.

Porter-O'Grady, T. (1998). The seven basic rules for successful redesign. In E.C. Hein (Ed.), *Contemporary leadership behavior* (5th ed.). Philadelphia: J.B. Lippincott.

Scott, W.R., & Backman, E.V. (1990). Institutional theory and the medical care sector. In S.S. Mick (Ed.), *Innovations in health care delivery: Insights for organization theory* (pp. 20-52). San Francisco: Jossey-Bass.

Sebastian, J.G. (1999). Organizational theory and the change process. In J. Lancaster (Ed.), *Nursing issues in leading and managing change* (pp. 91-123). St. Louis: Mosby.

Simpson, R. (2000). Nursing informatics. *Nursing Administration Quarterly, 24*(2), 87-90.

Waldo, B.H. (2000). HIPPA: The new frontier. *Nursing Economic$, 18*(1), 49-50, 31.

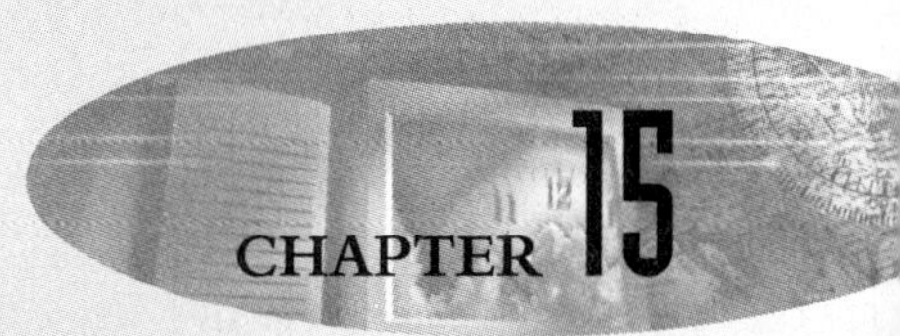

Human-Computer Interaction in Health Care Organizations

NANCY STAGGERS

Learning Objectives

Upon completion of this chapter, the reader will be able to:

1. ***Distinguish*** among the terms *human factors, ergonomics, human-computer interaction,* and *usability.*
2. ***Describe*** the goals of human-computer interaction and its three axioms.
3. ***Identify*** the major components of a model for human-computer interaction in health.
4. ***Compare*** and contrast indicators and methods relevant to usability studies.
5. ***Construct*** a usability test for a health care information application.

Outline

Key Terms

cognitive walk-through
computer-supported cooperative work (CSCW)
contextual inquiry
ergonomics
ethnographic techniques
heuristic evaluations
human factors
human-computer interaction (HCI)
Purdue Usability Testing Questionnaire
push technology
Questionnaire for User Interaction Satisfaction (QUIS)

Key Terms—cont'd

Software Usability Measurement Inventory (SUMI)
task analysis
think aloud
usability
usability assessment
usability questionnaires
user interface (UI)

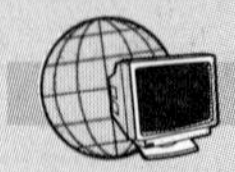

Web Connection

Go to the Web site at http://evolve.elsevier.com/Englebardt/. Here you will find Web links and activities related to human-computer interaction in health care organizations.

Health care informatics specialists are challenged to design, develop, purchase, and implement information systems that are deemed effective and efficient by health users. Concepts about **human-computer interaction (HCI)** can substantially assist informatics specialists in accomplishing this goal. In this chapter, major components of usability and HCI are translated for the health care informatics specialist's needs. The imperative for more usable information systems is delineated with examples of current difficulties. A new health HCI framework is offered for guidance. Usability indicators are outlined, popular methods in usability assessments are offered, and rich examples of usability studies in health settings are presented. At the end of this chapter, health care informatics specialists will be able to evaluate the usability of health care information systems and know how to incorporate HCI concepts into the design, development, or purchase of applications.

HUMAN-COMPUTER INTERACTION

The Problem of Unusable Systems

The ultimate acceptance or rejection of any health care information system by its users is largely dependent on the system's usability (Kushniruk, Patel, & Cimino, 1997). In fact, many authors think that the key barrier to user acceptance of computers is their lack of user friendliness (Ireland et al., 1997; Patel & Kaufman, 1998; Staggers, 1995b), and clinicians often comment that they want systems that are easy to use.

Despite the proliferation of information systems in health care settings, usability issues are a major threat to the success of health care information systems. For example, patients died of radiation overdoses partially because of faulty cursor handling of code in a radiology machine (Leveson & Turner, 1993). According to Salvemini (1998), it is unusual to find a clinical workstation that is successful. Graeber (1997) described a pilot study for a comprehensive, integrated clinical workstation designed to support nurses and physicians during inpatient activities. After an evaluation, the organization decided not to install an integrated workstation for these reasons: the capabilities for user customization were not sufficiently robust, the integration of the system was not sufficient (the communications between ancillary systems such as the laboratory and the new application were inadequate, and the system caused double work), and the presentation of data was poor, especially concerning an overview of the patient's illness, procedures, and medications. The users also evaluated and rejected mobile devices because their screens were too small and the devices were too slow. The organization planned to install a workstation but to begin with only a basic set of functions. The reasons for not installing the initial workstation were usability issues.

In Sweden the installation of a computerized medical records system in primary care increased staff workload by 25% (Nygren, 1997). One of the reasons for this cost impact was the "non-optimal design of HCI functions" (p. 318), which obstructed clinical work. Very recently the U.S. Department of Defense spent 2 years and about a million dollars a day developing its first increment of Composite Health Care System II, an ambulatory application for physicians. When the new application was installed in its first clinic in May 1999, it failed user acceptance testing. The major reasons for failure were because the Web-based application was too slow to support clinical processes and the notes function was considered cumbersome by clinicians. (These are significant usability issues with a negative impact on clinical care.) More important, clinical users were not included in the design and development of the product (Goedert, 2000).

Even without drastic consequences such as deaths and deinstallation of systems, the costs to individuals and organizations for poorly designed systems are substantial. Usability issues can result in decreases in productivity, treatment delays, extreme user frustration, underutilization of applications, errors, the need for extra personnel to install and support cumbersome systems, covert and overt resistance to applications, and the need for substantial funding to redesign and remedy problems. Incorporating HCI concepts into system design, development, and purchase can help defray these organizational and individual costs.

Potential Benefits of Incorporating Human-Computer Interaction Concepts Into Health Care Information Systems

An obvious impact of incorporating HCI concepts, or its subset of usability concepts, into applications relates to patient safety (Salvemini, 1998). Better-designed systems allow for correct data entry, display, and interpretation and contribute to sound clinical decision making, thereby potentially preventing errors. In addition, the use of HCI concepts has a positive influence on the time needed to complete tasks, user disruptions, training time, software rewrites, burden on support staff (Myers, Hollan, & Cruz, 1996), and user frustration. Usability techniques not only allow for identifying user problems with systems but also specifically address *why* users have those problems. Follow-up recommendations can then be made to developers for redesign, especially early in application development. Kushniruk, Patel, and Cimino (1997) have reported that usability can streamline data entry, as well as allow for a tenfold decrease in the average number of reported user problems.

Calculated cost savings due to usability techniques are even more impressive. More than 10 years ago, Karat (1990) reported savings from usability engineering techniques of $41,700 for a small application used by 23,000 marketing personnel and $6,800,000 for a large business application used by 240,000 people. A model constructed from 11 studies estimated that software-created and software-evaluated usability techniques will save a small project $39,000, a medium project $613,000, and a large project $8,200,000 (Nielson & Landauer, 1993). Those projected savings are even higher in today's dollars.

Despite these promising benefits and savings, health informatics specialists have been slow to integrate HCI and usability concepts into computing practices. Medical, nursing, and health informatics educational programs only sporadically offer didactic content about HCI. Yet authors have extolled the need to incorporate usability techniques into the design of health care systems for many years (Orthner, 1996; Staggers, 1991, 1995a; Van Bemmel, 1988). Stating the issue most strongly, Orthner called the interaction between the provider and the computer interface an area in desperate need of attention.

To date, only a few usability initiatives have begun in health care. The Mayo Clinic opened a usability laboratory for health computing in 1997. This was followed by two large clinical application vendors, Shared Medical Systems (SMS) and Cerner, incorporating usability concepts into their applications. Subsequently Cerner purchased SMS. These beginnings are the exception rather than the rule. A health care informatics specialist's goal is to develop and install usable systems. Therefore every informatics specialist and software developer should be knowledgeable about usability techniques.

DEFINITIONS OF TERMS

The term **human factors** is used to describe the general relationship between humans and machines. More specifically, the study of human factors is the scientific study of the interaction between people, machines, and their work environments (Beard & Peterson, 1989). As a broad umbrella term, *human factors* can include topics such as the design of car dashboards to fit human driving activities, how a panel of light switches map or do not map to room configuration, or the intuitiveness of programming a videocassette recorder. Norman (1988) wrote a classic text, *The Psychology of Everyday Things*, about the need for human factors in the design of common objects. The study of human factors includes several subcategories, such as the study of particular machines such as computers. The human factors areas concerned with computers are HCI and ergonomics. HCI is the study of how people design, implement, and use interactive computer systems and how these systems affect individuals, organizations, and society (Myers, Hollan, & Cruz, 1996). HCI blends psychology and/or cognitive science, applied work in computer science (Patel & Kaufman, 1998), sociology, and information science into the design, development, purchase, implementation, and evaluation of computer applications. Essentially, HCI deals with people and computers and the ways that they influence each other (Dix et al., 1998). Box 15-1 lists a sampling of HCI topics.

Ergonomics is intertwined with HCI but focuses on the design and implementation of equipment, tools, and machines in relation to human safety, comfort, and convenience (Loegendoen & Costa, 1994). In Europe the terms *ergonomics* and *HCI* are used interchangeably, whereas in North America the term *ergonomics* is more commonly employed when discussing the physical attributes of equipment used in all work and play activities. For example, ergonomics addresses the optimal design of the handle of a hammer to fit a human hand, the placement of terminals in a patient room, the design of computer chairs to promote comfort and safety, or the design of car dashboards to fit the reach of most people.

Usability is a subset of HCI but only one of its major components. In fact, the term *usability* is at times also used interchangeably with the term *HCI*. More precisely, **usability** addresses specific issues of human performance during computer interactions within a particular context (Rubin, 1994). Usability is multidimensional, including topics such as the following:

- Ease of using an application
- Ease of learning
- Ease of remembering interaction methods
- User satisfaction with system use
- Efficiency of use
- Error-free/error-forgiving interactions
- Seamless fit of an information system to the task(s) at hand

Employing usability techniques means designing or purchasing systems that require a minimum of learning so that users may quickly begin work (Nielson & Landauer, 1993). Ease of use is a general notion that implies many factors from user interface (UI) design to easy naviga-

Box 15–1 A Sampling of Human-Computer Interaction Topics

- The design and use of input and output devices (mouse, trackball, touchscreen, voice-activated applications, printers)
- The impact of user interface (UI) design and its functionality on users' efficiency and effectiveness
- The effectiveness of training
- Tools to design and evaluate UIs
- The design of "help" products
- User documentation
- The relationship between user characteristics and UI design
- Standardization of icons, effective fonts
- Techniques for evaluating the user friendliness of systems
- How to design and evaluate applications or systems that support groups of people, such as eMail
- Principles of effective Web, graphical user interface (GUI), and adaptive interface designs and their impact on users
- The layout of the keyboard
- Navigational aids
- The effective design of virtual work spaces for virtual teams
- Social issues in computing, such as "flaming" in eMail (an emotionally charged, hostile communication using eMail, usually on a listserv)
- Functional allocation of work between humans and computers
- User modeling, such as cognitive analyses of users

tion about the system, visible actions, and/or appropriate language for users within a context. If systems are easy to remember, they will support intermittent usage. Users should find interactions suitable to their purpose, unobtrusive, and facilitative for desired tasks and for indicating overall user satisfaction (Opaluch & Tsao, 1993). The system should be efficient for all levels of users from naïve user to expert by allowing high productivity and shortcuts for adapted uses. The concept of usability implies error trapping to prevent catastrophic errors (Nielson & Landauer, 1993) and the ability to undo actions where and when reasonable.

Goals of Human-Computer Interaction and Usability Concepts

The goals of HCI are to promote acceptance and use of systems by creating better interactive systems and better software, developing new kinds of applications to support specific work (Hartson & Boehm-Davis, 1993), and promoting job optimization with the use of information systems (Howley, 1998). If a system is designed well, the computer interface can effectively disappear, allowing users to focus only on the task at hand. That is, the functionality and design of the application displayed on the computer UI blends seamlessly among users, tasks, system, and environment, providing users immediate benefits when using the system.

The goals of HCI may be expressed in terms of overall effectiveness, efficiency, and satisfaction of users' interactions with information systems (Kushniruk, Patel, & Cimino, 1997; Lin, Choong, & Salvendy, 1997; Nickerson & Landauer, 1997; Preece et al., 1994; Salvemini, 1998). The goals of HCI are further delineated in Figure 15-1.

These are not modest goals. Under the category of effectiveness, the usefulness of an application addresses the fundamental tasks supported by the functions in the application. It

FIGURE 15–1 | Human-Computer Interaction Goals

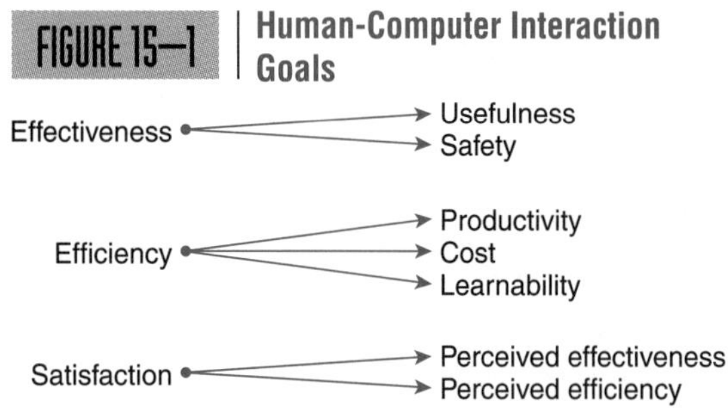

includes the completeness of needed functions within environments and their instantiation as well (i.e., how well the function matches the user's cognitive flow of information, the flow of information among a group of users, and/or the optimal allocation of functions between humans and computers). Nickerson and Landauer (1997) have suggested that assessing a system's social value is a measure of effectiveness.

In life-critical systems, safety of the application is paramount. For example, the accurate transfer of physiological monitoring data to an information system in intensive care units and the accurate display of patient medications in a pharmacy module are critical for patient safety.

The efficiency of systems deals with the expenditures of resources (Lin, Choong, & Salvendy, 1997). Resources include the time, energy, and error rates of users, as well as the costs of the system to the organization in terms of support personnel at the help desk, unused options, and redesign of applications. The learnability of the system is related to productivity, since better-designed systems can take less time to learn; however, learnability is separate from productivity in that learnability is also concerned with the retention of learned material over time.

Users' satisfaction can be expressed as enjoyment or frustration about either the efficiency or the effectiveness of interactions with the system. Users' perceptions about usability and the perceived benefits of using systems are components of satisfaction and can enhance application acceptance and use.

Axioms of Usability

HCI authors agree on three axioms of usability (Hartson & Boehm-Davis, 1993; Rubin, 1994):

1. An early and central focus on users in the design and development of systems
2. An iterative design of applications
3. Empirical usability measures or observations of users and information systems

These original principles have stood the test of time (Gould & Lewis, 1985). The early and central focus on users means understanding users in depth (Rubin, 1994). Direct contact with users in a structured, systematic approach throughout a system's life cycle is needed. In the process of iterative design of a system, users evaluate early prototypes or paper mock-ups of applications to determine their effectiveness. Once a prototype is available, users work with it to determine its effectiveness and efficiency. Identified usability problems are referred back to designers for correction and reevaluation by users in a recurring cycle. Several sequences are usually required to meet basic usability requirements. During usability testing, there is a need for structured observations of users and computers. The data from these observations define the problem areas for redesign, as well as the overall impact of the system on user and organizational productivity and costs.

HCI literature has focused nearly exclusively on the development of software and systems in the past. However, these axioms apply to the selection, purchase, and customization of contemporary systems as well. Off-the-shelf systems require many hours of tailoring to suit an environment; thus an understanding of local users, tasks, and the environment can be critical to selecting an adequate system in the first place and then subsequently customizing the system

FIGURE 15–2 Staggers Health Human-Computer Interaction Framework

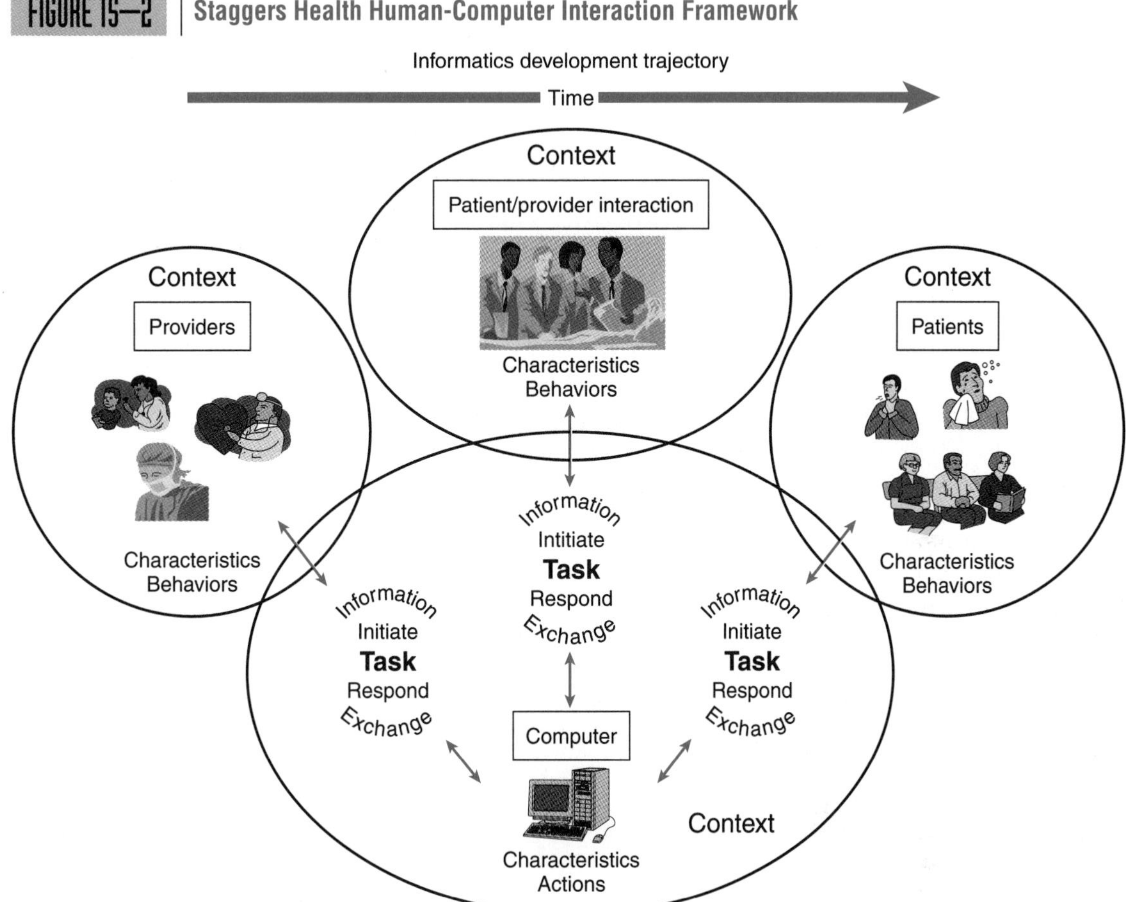

for the environment. Empirical measures can be integrated into selecting and tailoring systems.

A FRAMEWORK FOR HUMAN-COMPUTER INTERACTION IN HEALTH CARE CONTEXTS

HCI goals and axioms are embedded within the major elements of HCI: users, computers, context, tasks, information, interactions, and time. To better understand and study these elements and their relationships, the Staggers Health Human-Computer Interaction Framework was created (Figure 15-2). The framework is useful to help health care informatics specialists remember the components to consider when dealing with HCI. The framework can also help structure usability assessments and evaluate the impact of systems.

The few existing frameworks are inadequate, especially in HCI, because they miss either the context of the interaction in organizations and social settings (Lindgaard, 1992; Mantovani, 1996) or broader concepts such as the design of work or jobs (Beuscart-Zephir et al., 1997). In addition, they do not consider users in group or team situations (Lindgaard, 1992; Mantovani, 1996) or include the time over which the interaction takes place.

The framework in Figure 15-2 builds on work done in the early 1990s to define the dyad of nurse-computer interactions (Staggers & Parks, 1992, 1993). The new framework expands beyond the nurse to the provider or a group of providers, adds a patient or a group of patients, and adds the interaction component among these new elements. In recent years the focus of HCI has changed from attention to a single user interacting with a single computer to how to design systems for groups of users (Lindgaard, 1992; Nickerson & Landauer, 1997; Patel & Kaufman, 1998). Both foci are needed in health care—attention to the dyad of human and computer, as well as attention to groups of users and computers. This new framework allows the focus to be on either a dyad or on groups of users.

As with the previous nurse-computer interaction framework developed by Staggers and Parks (1992), the health HCI framework in Figure 15-2 includes concepts from developmental psychology. These concepts give insight into how to structure elements among nonequivalent members during interactions. Developmental frameworks are limited to human exchanges, yet many concepts are applicable to a human interacting with a nonhuman. Developmental psychologists conceptualize interactions as members interacting in a system of mutual influences and behaving according to respective characteristics. Interactions are embedded in an environment or context. Therefore the outcome of the interaction is different depending on the environment in which the elements interact. The interaction changes across time, and the outcome is dependent on the length of time that the members have been interacting.

Provider-patient-computer interactions allow for managing and communicating information within a health care context. Providers, patients, and computers interact in a system of mutual influences with information as the medium of exchange among them. During this information exchange, provider, patient, and computer behaviors occur relative to their respective characteristics. These interactions occur within a context, even a virtual one, and the interactions develop as they move across time.

The steps in the interaction process are as follows: Humans initiate the process by turning on a computer system and sending information to the computer interface (e.g., requesting a list of patients for today's clinic). From the interface, the information is processed through the computer according to its characteristics; the result of the processed information—the list of patients—is presented back onto the computer interface. Humans observe the information displayed on the interface and process it according to their characteristics (e.g., ensuring that it is the correct list). As the interactive cycle continues, humans behave and computers act. Behaviors include group interactions among humans in a virtual workspace, as well as dyads of providers and patients working with computers.

Patient, Provider, and Computer Behaviors

Behaviors are observable and measurable actions. Behavioral examples are motor movements such as clicking a mouse or speech such as a patient explaining why a Web-based educational application is not as useful as it could be. Behaviors are influenced by the person's respective characteristics but can be impacted by other framework elements as well. These types of characteristics influence the scope of available behaviors. Although people generally initiate interactions, computers may be programmed to independently send information to people using **push technology.** Push technology is a distribution technology in which selected data are automatically delivered to the user's computer or based on preset criteria. This is in contrast to pull technology, in which the user requests something by performing a search or requesting an existing report. For example, push technology can directly feed critical laboratory results to providers' beepers.

User Interface Actions

A **user interface (UI)**, typically a computer screen, allows humans and computers to cooperatively perform tasks. UI actions are the display of data or information on a computer interface or audible responses, such as a beep. UI actions may be a result of a person inputting data into the computer, or they may be a response to a request. Just as human behaviors are related to provider characteristics, computer interface actions are related to computer characteristics, such as their specific programming code. For instance, screen response time (an interface action) is intimately related to the type of microprocessor (a computer characteristic). UI actions might be influenced by other elements of the framework as well. For example, change of shift in acute care contexts may mean that multiple users access the system at the same time, affecting system performance and slowing down UI actions.

Characteristics of Patients, Providers, and Computers

Characteristics are attributes that are measurable but not always observable, such as age. Patients' or providers' acquired knowledge about a particular computer application is considered a characteristic. Characteristics of humans may be attributes such as gender, educational level, computer experience, or cognitive characteristics (such as spatial memory). Computer characteristics, on the other hand, are attributes related to specific hardware and software, such as embedded processing power, programming code, and disk space. Computer characteristics are closely related to computer interface actions but are distinct from them. Programming attributes instruct that data about a certain topic be presented; however, it is the UI that actually allows the data to be visualized. Behaviors, then, are reflective of associated characteristics.

The Task Information Exchange Process

Providers and patients enter data into and retrieve information from a computer to complete a specific task. For example, patients may request information about a diabetes support group from the Internet. An intern and resident may cooperate in completing and signing an order for a radiology request in a clinical information system. Embedded within each specific task is a goal for task completion. The goal may be exploratory or a detailed plan to accomplish a specific action (Kirsh, 1997). Examples of task goals include answering an eMail message from a patient or patients searching the Internet for information about acquired immunodeficiency syndrome (AIDS). Most often, humans specify task goals and communicate these goals by initiating and maintaining the interaction process. Some behaviors and characteristics are outside of the particular task domain. This is because all framework components use only a subset of available behaviors and characteristics during any one task.

Health Context

Interactions are embedded in an environment or context (see Figure 15-2). The context can include a physical or virtual setting (e.g., a rehabilitation unit or a groupware work space for health users in disparate locations), the social or political environment (e.g., corporate structure), individual or corporate cultures, social norms, and physical features (e.g., lighting or noise). The dynamics between humans and computers are defined by these varied contexts. Clearly, the patient-provider-computer interaction that occurs when patients enter their histories online from their home computers is different from the interaction that occurs when they are interviewed in a clinical setting. The context may define interactions more concretely as well. For instance, limited counter space may preclude the use of mice as input devices in an acute care unit.

Informatics Development Trajectory

As may be seen in Figure 15-2, humans and computers progress along a development trajectory over time. Moving along the trajectory, interactions change and mature as new information is incorporated into the interactions. The developmental portion of the framework recognizes the rapid changes that occur in the characteristics of patients, providers, and computers. For example, patients now recognize the power of information on the Internet and can download information they can use to question providers about current treatment modalities. This change in characteristics and the resulting impact on interactions develop over time. As one moves along the informatics development trajectory, new computer characteristics impact the interaction process as well. The introduction of high-speed lines into the homes of users is beginning to change the interaction methods of patients and providers. The future will see a very different level and type of patient-provider interaction.

The match between human behaviors and computer interface actions is important at each stage of the trajectory. In early interactions, less information on screens may be more pleasing to users; however, later in the trajectory, users would rather not have to page through multiple screens to get to information; thus screen density can be increased (Staggers, 1993).

The location of phenomena along the development trajectory is particularly important for usability assessments. For instance, many HCI researchers study users while they interact with systems over an hour's time. This type of assessment necessarily focuses on users' usability problems while learning the system. Another pertinent focus is on usability issues for practiced users that occur later in the development trajectory.

Current Directions in Human-Computer Interaction: Computer-Supported Cooperative Work

Until recently, the focus of HCI was on the interaction of one user with a computer. Thus the methods and guidance for systems are better developed for this dyad than for the complex interactions among groups of users and computers—a new area of focus in HCI. This new and more complex area of HCI is called **computer-supported cooperative work (CSCW)**. CSCW considers people as they act in their normal (work) lives (Mantovani, 1996). CSCW places a strong emphasis on social contexts, norms, and practices, as well as group interactions with computers. Computer support of the task at hand then becomes intertwined with patterns of group behaviors as reflected by social or situational contexts. The optimal allocation of tasks to both humans and computers becomes more of an issue. In fact, some authors suggest that not all work should be supported by computers (Olson et al., 1993). The focus on groups is an important change in direction for HCI because much of the work in business and health settings is completed by teams of people. In health care this change in direction is immediately applicable to the design of applications for health care teams (e.g., supporting patient care completed by the operative team preoperatively, intraoperatively, and postoperatively or the interactions within teams of dental personnel—a dentist, hygienist, and office staff—for scheduling and billing). The framework allows a focus on groups, as in CSCW.

CSCW can be thought of as the study of collaborative science; it is in its infancy (Patel & Kaufman, 1998), far behind the study of the dyad of user and computer (Olson et al., 1993). Olson et al. (1993) noted that all of the same issues in HCI are still prevalent, but now with a twist. In addition to theories and models of users, informatics specialists need to understand conversations, roles, organizational settings, and cultures. Where in the past, HCI focused on psychology and cognitive science to understand the individual, CSCW focuses on sociology and social psychology, as well as communication and management science, to understand group dynamics. Understanding the nature of group work, group processes, and communication processes in both synchronous and asynchronous modes becomes more important. For instance, guidelines for UI displays for online group synchronous interactions have not yet been established. Usability in this area will be a challenge for many years to come.

PERFORMING USABILITY ASSESSMENTS

Even with a global look at an HCI framework to help organize thoughts, usability assessment can seem overwhelming. What exactly is a usability assessment, when is one done, and how does an informatics specialist conduct one? **Usability assessment** is a general term encompassing structured usability testing, as well as other techniques such as task analysis to determine functional requirements. Usability assessments are systematic and structured examinations of the effectiveness, efficiency, or satisfaction of any component(s) or the interactions among the components within the HCI framework. For example, a usability assessment could be done to describe how an emergency dispatch center works, its activities, the cooperation among workers, and how these activities should be supported by information systems. A usability assessment might be conducted to see how a prototype system supports providers' interactions with a patient during an office visit. Another kind of usability test might assess the number of errors users make when they create new patient orders in a clinical information system. Those errors could suggest approaches for redesigning the application to make it more usable. As another example, a usability study might compare an emergency department application with published screen design or usability guidelines.

The range of usability assessments is wide, from modeling the way users' think about health processes in rich, narrative detail to completing formal experiments in laboratory settings that result in quantitative measures of interaction speeds. The type of assessment is dependent on a number of factors, including when the assessment is targeted in the system's life cycle. Usability assessments can be done at any point in the expanded system's life cycle (Thompson, Snyder-Halpern, & Staggers, 1999), from requirements determination and initial design to prototype development, system selection, product customization, or evaluation of the impact of the system during and after installation.

To show how one might accomplish a usability study, some background information is provided. This background includes describing types of usability assessments, outlining usability indicators or measures, discussing usability methods, and listing steps for creating usability studies. Finally, examples of completed usability assessments are presented.

Five Types of Usability Assessments

Usability assessments can be classified into five specific types. These five types include determination of needs and requirements as well as the four types of usability tests described by Rubin (1994):

1. Usability assessment to determine users' needs and requirements
2. Exploratory test
3. Assessment test
4. Validation test
5. Comparison test

Usability Assessment to Determine User Needs and Requirements

The first type of assessment is completed at the beginning of the system's life cycle to elicit users' characteristics, task activities, and interactions among users and tasks in specific environments and/or for particular needs related to the context of interactions. In other words, this is a usability assessment to define functional and technical requirements. This type of assessment answers the following kinds of questions:

- What are basic activities in this context?
- How do users cognitively process information, and what information processing can be supported by technology?
- What special considerations should be made for users in this environment?

Exploratory Test

The first type of usability test, the exploratory test, is conducted early during development after preliminary designs have been determined. Exploratory tests may be performed even before a prototype is developed. The major objective of an exploratory test is to assess the effectiveness of the emerging design concepts, asking questions such as the following (Rubin, 1994):

- Is the basic functionality of value to users?
- Is the navigation around the application intuitive?
- How much computer experience does a user need to use this module?
- Can the application be used without extensive training?

Exploratory tests are rather informal but require extensive interaction between health care informatics specialists and users. This test stresses the usability goal of effectiveness. During the test, users perform common tasks with the UI or step through paper mock-ups of the application. Health care informatics specialists strive to understand *why* users behave as they do with the application rather than how well the application represents a task.

Assessment Test

The second type of usability test, the assessment test, is conducted early or midway into the development of an application after the organization and overall design of the product have been determined (Rubin, 1994). Assessment is a very common type of usability test that evaluates lower-level operations of the application (stressing the efficiency goals of the product) and determines how well the task is presented. Questions during assessment tests might include the following:

- How well can users perform selected tasks?
- Are the terms in the system consistent across modules?
- Are operations displayed in a manner that allows quick detection of critical information?

During an assessment test, users always perform common tasks. The assessment often captures and analyzes quantitative measures of the interaction, such as error rates. Iterative design includes cycles of both exploratory and assessment tests.

Validation Test

The third type of usability test, the validation test, is performed late in the development cycle as the product matures. The purpose of validation is to assess how this product compares with a predetermined standard, benchmark, or performance measure and also to assess how well all of the modules in an application work as an integrated whole (Rubin, 1994). At this point, vendors check the product for major flaws before product release. Questions during this test might include the following:

- Can 80% of the users retrieve a complete blood count (CBC) laboratory result within 60 seconds of interacting with the system?
- Does the product adhere to usability principles? (Principles defined by

Nielson [1994] and Dix et al. [1998] are discussed later in this chapter.)
- Are there "fatal flaws" in the medication administration record?

Validation tests are more highly structured. Specific targets are determined before the test begins, and decisions are made about how each benchmark will be measured. Methods for a validation test can approximate an experimental approach with its concomitant rigor and thoroughness. A validation test is also useful in the system selection process, since decision makers can decide on critical tasks to be supported, develop benchmark standards to measure completion of the tasks, and then assess the degree to which each product under review achieves the standards.

Comparison Test

The fourth type of test, the comparison test, may be conducted at any point in the system's life cycle, from assessing different methods of organizing the design for a product to comparing instantiations of particular tasks in competing products. The major objective of this usability test is to determine which application is easier to use or learn and which design is more effective (complete or accurate, representing a user task) (Rubin, 1994). A side-by-side comparison can be done informally, more systematically with HCI methods, or as a rigorous, classic experiment. Rubin has suggested that better comparison tests are conducted if designs are vastly different from each other.

Health care informatics specialists can use a combination of these usability tests and assessments in conjunction with the usability indicators and methods discussed next.

Usability Indicators

Table 15-1 shows a taxonomy of possible usability measures from which an informatics specialist may choose. Health care informatics specialists can choose among these potential measures of usability depending on the focus of their own usability study. The taxonomy includes measures from three perspectives: users, experts, and organizations. Optimally, informatics specialists choose more than one measure to give depth to a study; however, one indicator may be adequate for some usability assessments.

Sample Methods in Usability Assessments

Usability assessments can use techniques from research, such as experiments, but often rely on other methods unique to HCI and usability assessments. The documentation methods embedded in these techniques overlap at times (e.g., informatics specialists can videotape users during task analysis or during a cognitive walkthrough). A sampling of common HCI methods is presented here with examples of how they are used in HCI work.

Task Analysis

Task analysis is one of the most well known clusters of techniques in HCI. **Task analysis** involves using systematic methods to determine what users are required to do with systems by accounting for behavioral actions between users and computers (Sweeney, Maguire, & Shackel, 1993). More globally, task analysis is used to determine the goals of a new system and the role of information technology in user activities (Nickerson & Landauer, 1997). Using task analysis, informatics specialists typically record user actions in flowcharts and task descriptions. In its purist form, task analysis is the process of learning about and documenting how ordinary users complete actions in a specific context (Hackos & Redish, 1998) and involves interviewing and observing users at their worksites. Informatics specialists may, however, choose to include subject matter experts and developers in these activities (Sweeney, Maguire, & Shackel 1993). Hackos and Redish (1998) have provided a very detailed description of how to perform

Table 15–1 Taxonomy of Usability Indicators

Usability Focus	Usability Indicators
User behaviors (performance)	Task times (speed, reaction times) Percent of tasks completed Number of errors Percent of tasks completed accurately Time, frequency spent in "help" option Number of hits on Web sites Training time Eye movements Frequency of questions to others (e.g., help desk) Facial expressions Range of application usage in actual settings Quality of completed tasks (e.g., quality of decisions) System setup or installation time, complexity Description or modeling of tasks and user behaviors Description of problems when interacting with an application
User behaviors (cognitive)	Description of or system fit with cognitive information processing Retention of application knowledge over time Comprehension of system Fit with workflow
User behaviors (perceptions)	Usability ratings of products Comments during interviews Questionnaires and rating responses
User behaviors (physiological)	Heart rate Electroencephalogram Galvanic skin response Brain-evoked potentials
User behaviors (perceptions about physiological reactions)	Perceptions about anxiety, stress
User behaviors (motivation)	Willingness to use system Enthusiasm
Expert evaluations (performance)	Model predictions for task performance times, learning, ease of understanding
Expert evaluations (conformance)	Level of adherence to guidelines, design criteria, usability principles
Expert evaluation (perception)	Ratings of system, comments
Context (organization)	Economic costs (e.g., calls to help desk about functions) Support staff for application Fit with job design or workflow in departments, organizations, networks of institutions

Modified from Sweeney, M., Maguire, M., & Shackel, B. (1993). Evaluating user-computer interaction: A framework. *International Journal of Man-Machine Studies, 38,* 689-711.

Box 15—2 Sample Presentations of Data Gathered Using Task Analyses

- Profiles of users—brief narrative, visual descriptions, or summaries about the characteristics of users
- Workflow diagrams—models of tasks performed by users or users' cognitive processing
- Task sequences or hierarchies—lists of tasks ordered by sequence or arranged to show interrelationships
- Detailed task descriptions—step-by-step task descriptions in models or outlines
- Task scenarios—narrative, detailed descriptions, from incidents to typical handling of a situation
- Affinity diagrams—bottom-up groupings of facts and issues about users, tasks, and environments to generate design ideas (For example, each issue is placed on a separate piece of paper, and designers then group similar issues into larger categories.)
- Videotape and audiotape highlights—clips that illustrate particular observations about users and tasks in a context

task analysis. The data gathered from task analyses can be presented in a variety of ways, which are listed in Box 15-2.

The informatics specialist selects pertinent methods among those described or other methods, such as photographs, to record user actions. Task analyses are helpful in identifying task completeness, correct sequencing of tasks, accuracy of actions, error recovery, and task allocation between humans and computers. This method can be used throughout the system's life cycle to determine user requirements, to assess the match of a prototype to users' methods of work, or to determine the impact of a system on workflow. An assessment of critical tasks also could be done to assist in system selection and purchase.

Often, task analysis is used early in the system's life cycle. For example, Womack (2000) observed nurses' verbal communication patterns on a busy medical-surgical patient care unit. The observations were recorded in a logbook. She then used affinity diagrams to categorize the activity observations. Affinity diagrams are used to organize large groups of information into meaningful categories. With the transfer of the observed activities onto separate pieces of paper, activities were grouped into categories. With the use of this method, major tasks were identified; nurses could address these verbally and suggest which tasks might be optimally supported by communication technologies in the future. Womack described the perceived difficulties in synchronous communication and the advantages and disadvantages of supporting synchronous communication across disparate geographical locations. Her research provides a detailed description of how nurses communicate to each other during face-to-face interactions in a real world setting.

Task analysis can focus on cognitive processes, observable user actions, or the physical design of a system. For example, informatics specialists can videotape users as they interact with a system, perform specific tasks, and talk about what they are doing. Task analysis may be used in the physical design of a system to determine what users need to see, hear, or manipulate; whether physical space is adequate for projected equipment; and where the potential for error exists (Salvemini, 1998). Informatics specialists may also describe existing systems to help perform a job analysis.

Think-Aloud Protocols or Protocol Analysis

Another common method in HCI is a **think-aloud** technique whereby users talk about what they are doing as they interact with an application. Usually a specific set of tasks is predetermined for inclusion in the study. An evaluator then watches and records actions by one or more of several techniques: videotaping, audiotaping, paper, automatic capture of keystrokes, and/or user and evaluator paper-and-pencil diaries or logs (Dix et al., 1998). The resulting record of actions is called a protocol and is analyzed for common findings; therefore the terms *think aloud* and *protocol analysis* are often used interchangeably.

This method is commonly used in the design, development, or evaluation of applications. Its products allow for a detailed examination of the specified tasks to uncover major effectiveness problems in usability. The analysis of the products of this method can, however, be very time consuming. The ratio of analysis time to observation time can be as high as 10:1. Think-aloud methods can be used in conjunction with other usability methods as discussed in the next section.

Cognitive Walk-Through

The **cognitive walk-through** is a detailed review of a sequence of real or proposed actions to complete a task in a system (Dix et al., 1998) and can be classified as a kind of specialized task analysis (cognitive task analysis) using think-aloud protocols. Users, HCI researchers, and subject matter experts may all be considered as possible reviewers. Reviewers step through the actions and check for potential usability problems, such as in the ease of learning the system through exploration. The following four questions are asked (Dix et al, 1998):

1. Will users be trying to produce whatever effect the action has?
2. Will users be able to notice that the correct action is available?
3. Once users find the correct action on the UI, will they know it is the right action for the effect they want?
4. After the action is taken, will users understand the feedback they get?

These walk-throughs can include recording a think-aloud session with videotaping or creating a structured evaluation method for evaluators to record findings and track problems. The focus is the match between the interface and the cognitive processes of users. Identified problems can help designers address priorities for application changes. This methodical technique can also help informatics specialists better understand user tasks by noting the specified task goals and actions. Cognitive walk-throughs are frequently used early in the system's life cycle and are especially effective for prototyping and initial design sessions. However, they might also be employed as an evaluation technique for established systems to identify usability problems.

Kushniruk and Patel (1995) have outlined a method for coding and analyzing videotapes of physician-computer interactions during cognitive walk-throughs and think-aloud protocols. Their purpose was to describe physicians' cognitive processing of information as they used information systems. The videotapes included rich details about the physical settings and the social context coupled with the physicians' thought processes. The authors interfaced a computer with a videocassette recorder (VCR) to allow researchers to document video frames. Researchers then used the computer to index and search the frames for text notes and time stamps. The text could be searched for key words to determine frequencies of behaviors, problems in interpreting a UI, and/or describing tasks. Kushniruk, Patel, and Cimino (1997) used this method to evaluate how physicians interact with a computer-based patient record as well as to identify UI "hot spots," or major usability problems in systems.

Heuristic Evaluations

Heuristics are rules of thumb. **Heuristic evaluations** are assessments of a product according to accepted guidelines or published usability prin-

Box 15—3 Heuristics Evaluation Criteria

- Organizing principles for systems
  - The purpose of the system
  - The user metaphor
- User locus of control
  - Provide clear exits to applications
  - Provide the user with information on the system status (e.g., "please wait")
- Consistency in terms and interactions
- Supporting a diversity of users
  - Interactions such as menus for novices
  - Shortcuts for experts
- Principle of economy
  - Minimize cognitive workload
  - Minimize user actions to complete a task
- Speak the users' language
- Adequate feedback in system actions
- Minimize errors
  - Provide directions on how to correct errors when made
- Visual appeal
  - Use good Web design, screen design principles
- Measures to assess usability
- Recognition and recall—users should not have to remember information from one option to the next in a system
- Match between the system and the real world

ciples. For example, informatics specialists can use general screen design principles or Web design principles to assess a product. Extensive guidelines are available, such as the classic guidelines by Smith and Mosier (1986) and more recent guidelines by Mayhew (1992). However, these guidelines are hundreds of pages in length. Nielson (1994) has proposed using "discount usability techniques," which are quicker and shorter methods of usability assessments, one of which is heuristic evaluations with a short list of usability principles.

A number of usability heuristics are available to evaluate applications (Dix et al., 1998; Nielson, 1994; Staggers, 1995a). Heuristics include factors such as those mentioned by Staggers (1995b) and Dix et al. (1998), which are listed in Box 15-3.

Heuristics can uncover major usability problems with applications but concentrate more on efficiency usability goals than on effectiveness usability goals. Heuristic methods require reviewers to have knowledge about usability principles.

An example of a heuristic evaluation has been described by Zhang (1999), who compared an electronic medical record with established human factor guidelines. Although Zhang did not specify which guidelines were used, he commented that this particular electronic medical record system increased the cognitive load of users and that the displays could create errors in interpretation.

Usability Questionnaires

Users can interact with applications and then complete structured **usability questionnaires** addressing perceptions of the system's usability. At least three examples of this type of questionnaire are available: the **Questionnaire for User Interaction Satisfaction (QUIS)** (Norman et al., 1998), the **Purdue Usability Testing Questionnaire** (Lin, Choong, & Salvendy, 1997), and the **Software Usability Measurement Inventory (SUMI)** (Kirakowski & Corbett, 1993). The QUIS is a paper-and-pencil or Web-based product that addresses users' perceptions of the system in areas such as overall reaction, terminology, screen layout, learning, system capabilities, and other subscales such as multimedia applications. The instrument underwent psychometric evaluations that demonstrated adequate properties. Also, the QUIS subscales can be selected to fit the usability test at hand. As reported by Staggers and Kobus (2000), nurses took about 10 minutes to complete the QUIS for six of its subscales.

Lin, Choong, and Salvendy (1997) have described a questionnaire for evaluating the usability of a system. After examining UI guidelines and relevant studies, the authors developed a preliminary questionnaire with 100 open-ended questions such as how the data display is or is not consistent with user conventions. This questionnaire appears to be targeted to usability experts rather than actual users, since evaluators would need to have knowledge about usability in order to complete the instrument. Also, reliability and validity assessments of the questionnaire have not been reported.

Little information has been published about the SUMI, including its assessed reliability and validity. The instrument has three components: an overall assessment, a usability profile, and an item consensus analysis. The usability profile examines areas such as efficiency, helpfulness, control, and learnability. The consensus component addresses adherence to well-known design alternatives such as categorical ordering of data in a simple search task.

Ethnographic Techniques

Ethnography is a method borrowed from anthropology and sociology for conducting investigative fieldwork and analysis of people in cultural or social settings. **Ethnographic techniques** are those in which a researcher describes the subject's point of view with a focus on the experience or interactions in social settings rather than on the actions themselves (Dourish & Button, 1998). However, the researcher is an observer and not a participant in the society. Detailed descriptions are generated with an emphasis on social relationships and their impact on work. Ethnographies can be extensive descriptions of users' experiences, from their point of view, in their settings. Because the focus of HCI has shifted to the study of groups cooperating in task completion, this technique has increased importance within CSCW (Dix et al., 1998).

One specialty that finds ethnographic techniques especially useful is sociomethodology, a subspecialty of sociology that focuses on social order and social action. A sociomethodology approach to analysis has enjoyed prominence with the shift in HCI to studying groups because this approach provides rich, ethnographic descriptions of work practices (Dourish & Button, 1998). Dourish and Button have proposed that sociomethodologists can contribute significantly to a system's design and the allocation of functions between technology and people.

An example of an ethnographic approach has been provided by McCarthy et al. (1997), who used these techniques to describe the current conflicting goals in a radiology department. The first goal is to have a complete radiology request form; however, a conflicting goal is that providers are obligated to care for patients even if the form is not properly completed. The authors discussed the implications of these competing goals for the system's design. Mandatory fields will be created for mundane tasks such as the time consumed during the radiology examination, but not for the request to be honored in the first place. Second, an "add comments" field is necessary in the request so that physicians can communicate about the uniqueness of the case, a consideration toward prioritization of completing radiology examinations. Additional information on the use of ethnographic techniques as a research tool is presented in Chapter 16.

Contextual Inquiry

Contextual inquiry is a usability method related to ethnographic techniques that is becoming a popular technique in studying HCI. Compared with ethnographies, it allows quicker determination of rich details of an activity by observing only representative users in actual work settings. With this technique, informatics specialists can understand concrete details of work and its structure and practices that may not be obvious to users. Womack (2000) used this technique to gather data (and develop the affinity diagram to analyze these data) about nurses' synchronous verbal communications cited earlier in this chapter.

Steps in Conducting Usability Assessments

Health care informatics specialists should assemble the framework, types of usability assessments, usability indicators, and methods before actually performing a usability assessment. The process may be divided into five steps.

Step 1: Define the Purpose

A clear purpose will frame the study, allowing informatics specialists to determine the type of assessment and methods needed. Is the purpose to define user requirements for a team of physical therapists in a busy rehabilitation hospital, to select a vendor's system to support all clinical functions in an ambulatory setting, or to evaluate the effectiveness of a newly designed system? Each of these purposes is distinct and points to a need to select different methods for completing the assessment. For example, if the purpose relates to an early question of design, then an exploratory test may be indicated. Specific study questions should then be delineated, such as "What data are needed by nurse practitioners to counsel a new diabetic?"

Step 2: Assess Constraints

Every study has constraints. Constraints include time, user expertise, availability of the software, availability of other equipment such as videocameras, testing laboratories, or users themselves. Constraints may determine portions or nearly all of the assessment techniques. For example, if the interest is in designing an application to support surgeons who perform transplants, the availability of the surgeons for an extensive task analysis may be limited.

Step 3: Use the Human-Computer Interaction Framework to Refine Each Component

Using the major elements of the HCI framework, questions should be asked about each component of the framework that is related to the purpose of the usability assessment. Some questions are as follows: Exactly which users? Which tasks? Exactly what about those tasks are of interest? What information is exchanged during the interaction? What computer characteristics and actions? What setting or context? At which time in the development trajectory? How much practice over time is needed?

Step 4: Emphasize Some Components

Framework components that are of interest should be purposely emphasized, and others that are of little or no interest should be controlled. In more rigorous assessments, assessors will need to ensure that they are measuring only what they want to know. For example, if the purpose is to compare the efficiency (speed) of screen designs between two competitors for an operating room mode, the assessors may need to control for consistency in computer processors, screen size, type of users, and context. However, in other assessments they may purposely emphasize studying a whole team of users in the complexity of their contexts (e.g., they may determine the extent of user requirements in support of a health module to support a youth corrections center).

Step 5: Match Methods to the Purpose, Constraints, and Framework Assessment

The methods selection flows from the previous steps. If the purpose of the study is to understand why users have problems with an installed application to support an emergency department, then a method that allows for rich description should be selected—a cognitive walk-through with protocol analysis, for example. If the purpose is to evaluate the acceptability of a final design, then assessing interaction task times and errors or completing a heuristic evaluation might be more appropriate. Once the method is selected, the assessment team is ready to put all of these pieces into action and conduct the assessment. An example of a rigorous usability test is provided in the following section.

Example of a Comparison Usability Test

The purpose of the comparison usability test conducted by Staggers and Kobus (2000) was to evaluate a text-based UI against a prototype graphical user interface (GUI) for manipulating nursing orders. The authors wanted specific, quantitative data about whether a redesign of a legacy system might have an impact on nurses' performance. The results were to be used by leaders in the organization to decide on a costly change from a legacy text-based system to a more modern UI. The design of the usability test was a formal experiment.

This usability test was one part of a larger study for which the authors had funding. The major constraint in this study was the availability of nurses at the tertiary care center. The tasks and interactions were carefully planned to minimize the amount of time that nurses would be away from clinical care. In addition, all data collection had to be scheduled, coordinated, and completed during a 2-week period before summer vacations and military rotations began.

A nurse-computer interaction framework, similar to the Staggers Health HCI Framework, was used to guide elements in the study. For example, identical computers were used to test both interfaces. The computers were disconnected from the local area network to ensure that system network loads did not affect processing times. Tasks were "real world" nursing orders that any nurse could understand, and the presented tasks were the same for each design. Clinical nurses were the target population for the study; therefore supervisors and nurses in non-clinically related specialties were not included in the study sample. The environment was a computer training room, a quiet room away from patient care. Although testing in a natural setting would be interesting, too many other factors in the setting might affect the results. To understand the pure differences between the UIs, a laboratory setting was chosen. The development trajectory played a significant role in the study because the authors wanted to ensure that users' performance was evaluated when they were well practiced with both interfaces. Otherwise, a short interaction period would only measure how well nurses learned and used a new interface rather than how the interface would behave after users worked with it in daily practice. Therefore 40 tasks for each interface allowed nurses to become practiced with each UI.

The usability test measured the indicators of reaction time (speed), errors, and satisfaction (using the QUIS) for each UI design. Every one of the 98 nurses interacted with both interfaces, but the order in which they were presented was randomized. The findings showed that nurses had significantly faster response times and fewer errors using the GUI when compared with the installed text-based display. The GUI was also rated significantly higher than the text system for nurse satisfaction, and the GUI was significantly easier to learn. The GUI was significantly faster for each type of order and still nearly twice as fast to use after nurses were well practiced in both UIs. Creating orders in the legacy system caused the most errors for nurses. The results were not necessarily anticipated, because nurses used the legacy text system every day and could have had slower speeds with the GUI. These results supported a move to a GUI for moderately complex nursing tasks.

CONCLUSION

In this chapter, reasons why current information systems may not be usable and an explanation of how HCI concepts can help to remedy this situation have been presented. The goal of HCI is to create better information systems and make them useful, safe, satisfying, and efficient to use.

The focus of HCI can be on the interactions of the dyad of user and computer or on cooperative work activities between groups of users and computers. The three axioms of usability are (1) an early and central focus on users in the design and development of systems, (2) iterative design of applications, and (3) empirical usability measures or observations of users and information systems. Major elements of an HCI framework to guide informatics specialists in usability work include patients, providers, computers, context, tasks, information, interactions, and a development trajectory over time. Five usability assessments have been discussed: determining needs and requirements, exploratory tests, assessment tests, validation tests, and comparison tests. Sample methods in usability assessments include task analysis, think-aloud protocols, cognitive walk-throughs, heuristic evaluations, ethnographic techniques, and usability questionnaires. Finally the steps to conduct usability assessments have been discussed. These are as follows: (1) define the purpose; (2) assess constraints; (3) use the HCI framework to refine the study of each component; (4) emphasize or control some framework components; and (5) match methods to the purpose, constraints, and framework assessment. A usability assessment provides an illustration about how informatics specialists can use the concepts in this chapter to conduct a usability assessment.

An example of a health care informatics specialist interested in developing and installing an application to support nurses' assessments of critical care patients at change-of-shift report has been described by Ireland et al. (1997) to determine requirements for a summary screen for an intensive care unit (ICU) information system. The assessment was at the very beginning of the system's life cycle, indicating what authors would emphasize among the framework components: providers in an ICU context in one facility, the task of discovering summary data needed to describe patients' conditions, the interaction of a dyad, and nurses' initial impressions of the summary screen (early in the development trajectory). Their usability goals were to create an efficient, effective, and safe application for frequent system users: the nurses in an ICU.

The driver for usability method selection was not study constraints, but the need for rich detail to determine requirements for the task. The method of task analysis was selected because it would provide the depth of detail needed to describe initial requirements. Initial task observations revealed that ICU nurses should be the target users during this analysis because they were the most frequent potential users of a summary screen in the clinical information system. Interviews with nurses identified that the summary screen should provide data to help nurses get an "awareness" of the patient's overall condition. Data to describe the overall patient condition were obtained via interviews, and then these data were grouped into four categories: cardiovascular (CV), respiratory, fluids, and temperature. These categories were used because nurses' thought processes were organized in this manner.

These requirements and categories were incorporated into the design of a summary screen. Subsequently, an assessment usability test was completed to evaluate whether this one screen provided sufficient information for nurses. A structured questionnaire was used to capture perceptions from 17 ICU nurses about the noninteractive summary screen. The authors asked about the completeness of the data and perceptions about the screen format. The findings gave information about successes and what areas needed to be redesigned; the findings also indicated that required information was readily identifiable, that the information was grouped logically, and that no superfluous information was displayed; however, the findings also indicated that there was some redundancy in the fluid data and that the density of the CV section was too high.

Other types of usability testing could be used as the product is refined. For example, a validation test might measure the product against

Box 15-4 Major Concepts of Human-Computer Interaction

- The purpose of HCI and usability is to promote acceptance and use of systems by creating better interactive systems and better software, and by developing new kinds of applications to support specific work.
- The goals of HCI may be expressed in terms of overall effectiveness, efficiency, and satisfaction of users' interactions with information systems.
- The focus of HCI can be on the interactions of the dyad of user and computer or on cooperative work activities between groups of users and computers (called computer-supported cooperative work [CSCW]).
- The three axioms of usability are an early and central focus on users in the design and development of systems, iterative design of applications, and empirical usability measures or observations of users and information systems.
- The major elements of the Staggers Health HCI Framework are patients, providers, computers, context, tasks, information, interactions, and a development trajectory over time.
- The five types of usability assessments are (1) determining needs and requirements, (2) exploratory tests, (3) assessment tests, (4) validation tests, and (5) comparison tests.
- Sample methods in usability assessments include task analysis, think-aloud protocols, cognitive walk-throughs, heuristic evaluations, and usability questionnaires.
- The steps in conducting usability assessments are as follows: (1) define the purpose; (2) assess constraints; (3) use the HCI framework to refine the study of each component; (4) emphasize or control some framework components; and (5) match methods to the purpose, constraints, and framework assessment results.

predefined standards such as "nurses should be able to detect the four areas of information on the summary screen within 5 seconds of logging on." This example demonstrates how usability concepts are pertinent for designing and installing a useful product.

Major concepts of this chapter are shown in Box 15-4.

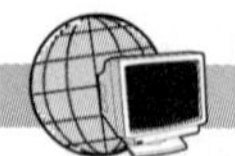

Web Connection

The goal of human-computer interaction is to create information systems and make them useful, safe, satisfying, and efficient to use. This requires attention to people, places, and machines. Clinical information systems, diagnostic technologies, clinicians, and environments of care are examples of areas where human-computer interface concepts of usability are being addressed. The purpose of the Web Connection activities for this chapter is to explore the concepts related to usability that have been introduced in the chapter, such as typical user characteristics, user satisfaction, and system design strategies that are user inclusive. You will evaluate usability of an application using criteria and methods presented in the chapter.

discussion questions

1. How do the terms *human factors, ergonomics, HCI,* and *usability* relate to each other?

2. How might health care informatics specialists use the Staggers Health HCI Framework to conduct a usability assessment to compare two vendors' products?
3. Describe potential advantages and disadvantages of the common usability methods: cognitive walk-through, think-aloud protocols, ethnographics, and questionnaires.
4. Prepare a presentation for your manager explaining why your institution should incorporate HCI concepts into its practices and which concepts are the most important to consider.

REFERENCES

Beard, J.W., & Peterson, T.O. (Eds.). (1989). *A taxonomy for the study of human factors in a management information system (MIS).* Norwood, NJ: Ablex Publishing.

Beuscart-Zephir, M., et al. (1997). Cognitive evaluation: How to assess the usability of information technology in healthcare. *Computer Methods and Programs in Biomedicine, 54,* 19-38.

Dix, A., et al. (1998). *Human-computer interaction.* London: Prentice Hall Europe.

Dourish, P., & Button, G. (1998). On "technomethodology": Foundational relationships between ethnomethodology and system design. *Human-Computer Interaction, 13,* 395-432.

Goedert, J. (2000). Taps for one system, reveille for another. *Health Data Management, 8*(4), 17, 25, 28.

Gould, J.D., & Lewis, C.H. (1985). Designing for usability—Key principles and what designers think. *Communications of the ACM, 28,* 200-311.

Graeber, S. (1997). Application of clinical workstations: Functionality and usability. *Clinical Performance and Quality Healthcare, 5*(2), 71-75.

Hackos, J., & Redish, J. (1998). *User and task analysis for interface design.* New York: John Wiley & Sons.

Hartson, H.R., & Boehm-Davis, D. (1993). User interface development processes and methodologies. *Behaviour and Information Technologies, 12*(2), 98-114.

Howley, K. (1998). Equity, access, and participation in community networks. *Social Science Computer Review, 16*(4), 402-410.

Ireland, R., et al. (1997). Design of a summary screen for an ICU patient data management system. *Medical and Biological Engineering and Computing, 35,* 397-403.

Karat, C. (1990). *Cost-benefit analysis of usability engineering techniques.* Paper presented at the Human Factors Society thirty-fourth annual meeting, Orlando, FL.

Kirakowski, J., & Corbett, M. (1993). SUMI: The software measurement inventory. *British Journal of Educational Technology, 24,* 210-212.

Kirsh, D. (1997). Interactively and multimedia interfaces. *Instructional Science, 25,* 79-96.

Kushniruk, A., & Patel, V. (1995). *Cognitive computer-based video analysis: Its application in assessing the usability of medical systems.* Paper presented at the MEDINFO 95.

Kushniruk, A., Patel, V., & Cimino, J. (1997, October 25-29). Usability testing in medical informatics: Cognitive approaches to evaluation of information and user interfaces. *Conference Proceedings from the American Medical Informatics Association annual symposium* (pp. 218-222). Nashville, TN.

Leveson, N., & Turner, C. (1993). An investigation of the Therac-25 accidents. *IEEE Computing, 26*(7), 18-41.

Lin, H., Choong, Y., & Salvendy, G. (1997). A proposed index of usability: A method for comparing the relative usability of different software systems. *Behaviour and Information Technology, 16*(4/5), 267-278.

Lindgaard, G. (1992). Evaluating user interfaces in context: The ecological value of time-and-motion studies. *Applied Ergonomics, 23*(2), 105-114.

Loegendoen, D., & Costa, D. (1994). *The home office computer handbook.* New York: Windcrest/McGraw-Hill.

Mantovani, G. (1996). Social context in HUCI: A new framework for mental models, cooperation, and communication. *Cognitive Science, 20,* 237-269.

Mayhew, D.J. (1992). *Principles and guidelines in software and user interface design.* Englewood Cliffs, NJ: Prentice Hall.

McCarthy, J., et al. (1997). Accountability of work activity in high-consequence work systems: Human error in context. *International Journal of Human-Computer Studies, 47*(6), 735-766.

Myers, B., Hollan, J., & Cruz, I. (1996). Strategic directions in human-computer interaction. *ACM Computing Surveys, 28*(4), 794-809.

Nickerson, R., & Landauer, T. (1997). *Human-computer interaction: Background and issues* (2nd ed.). Amsterdam: North Holland Elsevier.

Nielson, J. (1993). Interactive user-interface design. *Computer, 26*(11), 32-41.

Nielson, J. (1994). *Heuristic evaluation.* New York: John Wiley & Sons.

Nielson, J., & Landauer, T. (1993). *A mathematical model of the finding of usability problems.* Paper presented at the INTERCHI '93: Human Factors in Computing Systems, Amsterdam, The Netherlands.

Norman, D. (1988). *The psychology of everyday things.* New York: Basic Books.

Norman, K., et al. (1998). *Questionnaire for user interaction satisfaction, version 7.0: Users' guide, questionnaire and related papers.* College Park: University of Maryland.

Nygren, E. (1997). From paper to computer screen: Human information processing and interfaces to patient data. *International Medical Informatics Association, Working Group, 6,* 317-327.

Olson, J., et al. (1993). Computer-supported co-operative work: Research issues for the 90s. *Behaviour and Information Technology, 12*(2), 115-129.

Opaluch, R.E., & Tsao, Y.C. (1993). Ten ways to improve usability engineering—Designing user interfaces for ease of use. *AT&T Technical Journal, 72,* 375-388.

Orthner, H.S. (1996). Series preface. In V.S. Saba & K.A. McCormick (Eds.), *Essentials of computers for nurses.* New York: McGraw-Hill.

Patel, V., & Kaufman, D. (1998). Medical informatics and the science of cognition. *Journal of the American Medical Informatics Association, 5*(6), 493-502.

Preece, J., et al. (1994). *Human computer interaction.* Reading, MA: Addison-Wesley.

Rubin, J. (1994). *Handbook of usability testing: How to plan, design, and conduct effective tests.* New York: John Wiley & Sons.

Salvemini, A. (1998). Improving the human-computer interface: A human factors engineering approach. *M.D. Computing, 15*(5), 311-315.

Smith, S.L., & Mosier, J. (1986). *Guidelines for designing user interface software* (Vol. Report MTR-9420). Bedford, MA: Mitre.

Staggers, N. (1991). Human factors. The missing element in computer technology. *Computers in Nursing, 9*(2), 47-49.

Staggers, N. (1993). The impact of screen density on clinical nurses' computer task performance and subjective screen satisfaction. *International Journal of Man-Machine Studies, 39,* 775-792.

Staggers, N. (1995a). Essential principles for evaluating the usability of clinical information systems. *Computers in Nursing, 9*(2), 47-49.

Staggers, N. (Ed.). (1995b). Usability concepts for the clinical workstation. In M. Ball et al. (Eds.), *Nursing informatics: Where caring and technology meet* (2nd ed.), (pp. 188-199). New York: Springer-Verlag.

Staggers, N., & Kobus, D. (2000). Comparing response time, errors, and satisfaction between text-based and graphical user interfaces during nursing order tasks. *Journal of the American Medical Informatics Association, 7*(2), 164-176.

Staggers, N., & Parks, P.L. (1992). Collaboration between unlikely disciplines in the creation of a conceptual framework for nurse-computer interactions. *Proceedings of the Annual Symposium of Computer Applications in Medical Care,* 661-665.

Staggers, N., & Parks, P.L. (1993). Description and initial applications of the Staggers and Parks Nurse-Computer Interaction Framework. *Computers in Nursing, 11*(6), 282-290.

Sweeney, M., Maguire, M., & Shackel, B. (1993). Evaluating user-computer interaction: A framework. *International Journal of Man-Machine Studies, 38,* 689-711.

Thompson, C.B., Snyder-Halpern, R., & Staggers, N. (1999). Clinical informatics case studies: Analysis, processes, and techniques. *Computers in Nursing, 17*(5), 203-206.

Van Bemmel, J.H. (1998). Medical data, information, and knowledge. *Methods of Information in Medicine, 27,* 109-110.

Womack, D.F. (2000). *Synchronous verbal interaction in acute care nursing.* Master's thesis. Salt Lake City: University of Utah.

Zhang, J. (1999). *How to represent relationship information in electronic medical records: A human factors approach.* Paper presented at the American Medical Informatics Association annual conference, Washington, DC.

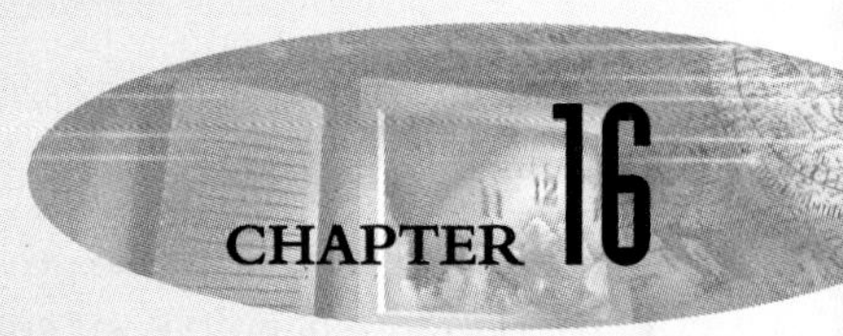

CHAPTER 16

The Implications of Information Technology for Research

JOAN E. THIELE

Learning Objectives

Upon completion of this chapter, the reader will be able to:

1. ***Discuss*** the implications of using information technology to conduct health-related research.
2. ***Explain*** the advantages and disadvantages of using the Internet for health-related research.
3. ***Describe*** how information technology can be used to collect and analyze quantitative and qualitative data.
4. ***Identify*** ethical issues that arise when information technology is applied to the research process in health care.
5. ***Discuss*** informatics research priorities.
6. ***Identify*** informatics-related research resources, including grants and related information.

Outline

Key Terms

CD-ROM
Cumulative Index of Nursing and Allied Health Literature (CINAHL)
Nonnumerical Unstructured Data Indexing, Searching, and Theorizing (QSR NUD*IST)
Statistical Package for the Social Sciences (SPSS)
World Wide Web (WWW)

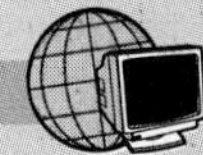

Web Connection

Go to the Web site at http://evolve.elsevier.com/Englebardt/. Here you will find Web links and activities related to the implications of information technology for research.

This chapter discusses the process of using information technology to enhance, support, and conduct research in health care. Ethical issues related to using technology to conduct health care research, as well as issues involved in conducting online research, are discussed. Research topics for health care informatics are identified, as well as sources of information for informatics research. The current state of informatics knowledge and the future of health care information management are briefly addressed.

Early statisticians analyzed their data using quills, bottles of ink, and parchment paper. Described as a "passionate statistician," Florence Nightingale pioneered the use of charts for the presentation of data (McDonald, 1998). These charts were laboriously created by hand. During Nightingale's time, analysis of large data sets was an almost insurmountable task. The difficulties of manually collecting all data and the prohibitive amount of time that was required to perform data analysis severely limited the number and type of research studies that were possible. For example, the first census of the United States population occurred in 1790 and required 18 months just to complete the tally. This census was for the original 13 states, the Southwest Territory (known today as the state of Tennessee), plus the districts of Kentucky, Maine, and Vermont. One hundred years later the census, which is required by the Constitution to be done every 10 years, took close to 10 years to complete. In 1890 the U.S. Census Bureau introduced the Hollerith Punch Card Tabulation Machine and Sorter. The time factor for collection was reduced to 2½ years with the introduction of technology. By comparison, data for the 2000 census were collected and prepared for analysis in 6 months (March to August). These data were analyzed and a report was prepared for the president to be ready December 31, 2000 (U.S. Census Bureau, 2000). This was possible because today's technologies are capable of handling large data sets with incredible speed and accuracy. These technologies have made it possible for all parts of the research process to be accomplished using some form of technology.

Once a research question has been identified, the first step in the research process is a review of the literature. The last step in the research process is to present the research results in the published literature of the discipline. Information technology is now changing both the review process and the publication process, as well as data collection and analysis.

LOCATING RESEARCH INFORMATION

The development of a research study begins with a comprehensive search of the relevant literature. Historically, this review was conducted by manually searching through printed annual volumes of bibliographic databases such as the **Cumulative Index of Nursing and Allied Health Literature (CINAHL)**. This is no longer an accepted or effective method of locating relevant published research. Researchers now begin the review of the literature by accessing multiple bibliographic databases that are stored on automated systems. Electronic bibliographic databases can often be accessed from the researcher's office or home via the Internet. In addition, many medical and health science libraries subscribe to various databases that are available on **CD-ROMs.** These are updated with new versions on a regular basis, often quarterly.

Using subject and/or key words, the researcher can quickly search several databases in a short period of time. Many databases have advanced search features. This can be demonstrated by an example—looking for published research concerning patient education. Advanced search features in automated databases allow scholars to initially use "research" as a search term or selection criterion, then to narrow the search by adding other relevant terms such as "patient education," "literature," or a specific disease name. By combining search terms, the researcher can locate materials that contain the key words "research," "patient education," and "diabetes mellitus." Searches that are organized using relevant terms quickly locate existing pertinent literature. In addition to focusing on key terms in various combinations, electronic searches can be restricted to a specific time frame, such as the last 2 years of articles related to the topics. Careful selection of subject or key words can quickly provide a comprehensive review. Often the assistance of a professional librarian is helpful in selecting the search terms and in learning effective search strategies. A search of several databases may be necessary to produce an exhaustive list of relevant articles for a comprehensive literature review.

Vendors of bibliographic databases provide a number of searching and presentation tools that assist the researcher in locating and reviewing relevant materials. The results of a CINAHL search, for example, would indicate that the search was restricted to particular key words and that specific criteria—such as research and research methodology—were added. In addition, articles that were identified through this search would be displayed in chronological order, with the most recent listed first. Refined capabilities such as the use of key words and search criteria enable the researcher to start a search broadly to determine key words and then to quickly narrow the search to more precise criteria to be addressed in the located materials.

Current databases are constructed so that the researcher can restrict a search to specified years and selected search terms. In fact, linking to MEDLINE (the online corollary to *Index Medicus*) via the **World Wide Web (WWW)** enables the researcher to read the abstracts of selected articles and, in some instances, to obtain full text articles. In addition, the researcher can link to the articles referenced in the selected literature, a possibility not available when using bound volumes of bibliographic citations (Delamothe, 1998). See Chapter 3 for additional detailed information on using online databases to search the literature.

Technology is also changing the way that research results are published in the literature. A growing body of research literature is being disseminated solely by means of the Internet. The last few years have seen a burgeoning of electronic or online journals such as the *British Medical Journal, On-Line Journal of Nursing Issues, Journal of Asynchronous Learning Networks, Journal of Clinical Investigation, Journal of Medical Internet Research, Cardiology Today, Online Journal of Nursing Informatics, Online Journal of Rural Nursing and Health Care,* and *Journal of Community Nursing;* these are just a few of the electronic journals available. (For universal resource locators [URLs], see the Web Connection for this book.) Both peer-reviewed and non–peer-reviewed articles are posted online. The editorial policies and practices of each journal provide information regarding the review procedures for that particular publication.

The ability to publish materials directly on the WWW has changed the mechanisms for peer review. In the traditional approach that is used to produce print journals, peer review and its outcomes are a somewhat private process in which one to three reviewers share their opinions and comments with the editor of the journal. The editor then makes a decision regarding the publication of a submitted manuscript on the basis of the reviews. However, only the editor knows the full scope of the peer critique.

Online publications may invite postpublication review in addition to the traditional prepublication peer review (Bingham, 1998). Both postpublication review and interactive discussions of the published article may be available for reading by the public. Examples of publications that provide full text of articles and reviews of articles include the following: *On-Line Journal of Nursing Issues, Journal of Interactive Media in Education,* and *Australian Electronic Journal of Nursing Education.*

Some electronic journals publish both original articles and reviews or critiques of those articles. The critique addresses strengths and weaknesses of the original article and provides ideas for the conduct of related research or other ways to expand on the original topic.

THE INTERNET AND HEALTH-RELATED RESEARCH

With the exponential growth of the WWW, use of the Internet as a research tool is increasing. The Internet provides a rich resource for identifying pertinent research articles and related materials, as well as a means of collaborating with other researchers worldwide. Concomitant with access to multiple bibliographic databases is the provision of the full text of articles via the Internet. These two capabilities have made the Internet as valuable an information resource as visiting a first-rate library with thousands of journal holdings. Most university libraries have sophisticated Web sites that include access to databases and full text articles for approved users.

In addition to serving as an electronic source of research literature, the ease of use, speed with which data can be obtained, and minimal cost for Internet research are major advantages to using this medium for data collection. Multiple types of descriptive studies, including but not limited to correlation, cross section, and survey research, may be conducted via the Internet (Szabo & Frenkl, 1996).

Quantitative Analysis of Research Data

The simplest and most common format for data collection via the Internet is through structured, closed-response questions. The process of creating an online questionnaire is greatly facilitated by hypertext markup language (HTML), the coding language of the WWW. Once the researcher has decided on the questions to be asked and the response options, a word processor is used to create the form. Questionnaires can be generated with the use of word processing software that includes the ability to convert the entire form to HTML or with the use of a Web creation software program such as Microsoft FrontPage. Using a Web creation application enables the researcher to direct the responses to the questionnaire to a designated text file.

Figure 16-1 displays a portion of an electronic data-collecting form used to obtain patient encounter information in a nurse-managed clinic. These data are analyzed monthly to provide an ongoing productivity report and description of patient demographics about the population served. In this example an online form is completed for each patient seen; the form is electronically transmitted to an informatics specialist who compiles the data. Monthly reports are generated from the electronically stored data.

All electronically generated responses can be automatically accumulated in the designated file and accessed by the researcher for data analysis purposes. Once the participant answers the questions and clicks on the "submit" button, the response is transmitted electronically to the data file designed by the researcher (Lakeman, 1997).

After copying the data file, the researcher can then transfer the data into a comma-delimited file for analysis by a spreadsheet or statistical analysis program. Once the raw data are captured in a file, analysis using predetermined statistical procedures is conducted. Computers are capable of quickly storing and analyzing large volumes of statistical data. See Chapter 3 for additional information about the use of databases.

An example of comma-delimited data from the patient encounter form displayed in Figure 16-1 is shown in Figure 16-2. Once downloaded to a file, the data are then imported to a spreadsheet program for analysis and tabulation of patient care information.

The data shown in Figure 16-2 are more understandable once the file is opened in a spreadsheet or statistical analysis program. Figure 16-3 displays the data in Figure 16-2 after being converted by Microsoft's spreadsheet program, Excel. In this converted format the researcher can

FIGURE 16–1 Example of an Electronic Patient Encounter Form

Today's date

Zip code

New patient? Yes No *Follow-up visit?* Yes *Referral?* Yes

No show? Yes *Walk-in?* Yes

Early intervention patient? Yes

Gender: Male Female *Age (in years)*_________

Insurance? Yes No *If yes, type of insurance:* Private Medicare Medicaid Coupons Other

Marital status: Married Single Divorced *Children:* N/A

Ethnicity: Caucasian Hispanic-Latino African-American American Indian Asian/Pacific Islander Mixed heritage

compute desired calculations and create charts, graphs, and reports. The process for converting the comma-delimited data is exactly the same whether or not the data collection procedure is Web based.

Use of Statistical Packages to Analyze Quantitative Data

The raw materials resulting from research activities are called data. However, data must be converted into a meaningful form to allow for interpretation. The **Statistical Package for the Social Sciences (SPSS)** is an example of a commonly used program for the statistical analysis of quantitative data. In its early days statistical packages were available only to researchers on mainframe, time-sharing computers that required key-punched cards to be submitted for analysis. These packages have evolved to the point where personal computer versions with user-friendly interfaces are in common use. This progression in refinement of the statistical analysis software enables the researcher to perform powerful statistical analyses from the desktop. A wide range of the latest statistical and *post hoc* procedures can be readily calculated from quantitative data using these programs.

Qualitative Analysis of Research Data

Collecting and analyzing qualitative data is a time-consuming and difficult process. This difficulty is caused by two specific problems. First, the richness of qualitative data means that, by its nature, there is a large amount of data. Note, for example, the amount of data that can be contained in a 10-minute videotaped interview. Second, it is difficult to measure qualitative data with precision. For example, using quantitative data collection methods, a researcher might ask a group of subjects if the Internet was used to search for health-related information in the last week. Their yes or no answers can be precisely measured. If these same subjects were asked to explain how they used the information, each subject would use different words, terms, and concepts. Each subject would have a different answer to the question. Whereas the Internet facilitates cost-effective, rapid data collection of large amounts of data from online participants, analysis of those data is a complex process, particularly when qualitative analysis of textual data is the objective. This problem is increased by the amount of data that can accrue when the Internet is used for data collection. In addition, without the verbal and nonverbal cues that are often part of qualitative data collection, there

FIGURE 16–2 Captured Data in a Comma-Delimited Format

"Month","Day","Year","Zip","New_Yes","New_No","Follow_Yes","Referral
_Yes","Referral_Yes1","New_Yes1","WalkinsYes","EarlyIntervPTYes",
"Male","Female","Age","Ins_Yes","Ins_No","Ins_Private","Ins_
Medicare","Ins_Medicaid","Ins_Coupons","Ins_Other","Married",
"Single","Divorced","ChildN/A","Cauc","Hisp-Lat","Afr-Am","Am_Ind",
"Asian","Mixed"
"May","1","2000","99201",,,,,,,,,"2","9",,"2",,,,,,,,,"1","1",,,
,,,"1",,,,,,,,,,"460","","","",,,,,,,,,,,,"2",,,,,,,,,,,"",,"1",
,,"",,"",,,,,,"Submit Query"
"May","1","2000","99212","1",,,"1",,,,,,"2","38",,"2",,,,,,,"2",
,,"1",,,,,,"1,Submit Query"
"May","1","2000","99204",,"2",,,,,,,,"2","33","1",,,,,"1",,,"2",
,,"1",,,,,,"1","","",,,,"1",,,,,,,,,"2",,,,,,,,,,,"1","",,,,,"",,"
",,,,,,"Submit Query"
"May","1","2000","99204",,"2","1",,,,,,,"2","21","1",,,,,,,,"2",
,,"1",,,,,,"1"Submit Query"
"May","1","2000","99201",,"2","1",,,,,,,"2","29",,"2",,,,,,,"2",
,,"1",,,,,,"1"Submit Query"
"May","1","2000","99201","1",,,"1",,,,,,"2","26","1",,,,,"1",,,"
2",,,"1",,,,,,"1
"May","1","2000","99201",,"2","1",,,,,,,"2","21",,"2",,,,,,,"2",
,,"1",,,,,,"1,"Submit Query"
"May","1","2000","99208",,"2","1",,,,,,,"2","17",,"2",,,,,,,"2",
,,"1",,,,,,"1,"Submit Query"
"May","1","2000","99201",,"2",,,,,,,,"2","6","1",,,,,"1",,,,,"1"
,,,,,,"1","1",,,,,,,,,,"034.0","","","",,,,,,,,,,,,"2",,,,,,,,,,
"1","",,,,,"",,"",,,,,,"Submit Query"
"May","1","2000","99201","1",,,,,,,,"1",,"4",,"2",,,,,,,,,"1","1
",,,,,,,,,,,,"1,"Submit Query"

FIGURE 16–3 | **Captured Data Displayed in a Spreadsheet Format**

Month	Day	Year	Zip	New_Yes	New_No	Follow_Yes	Referral_Yes
May	1	2000	99201				
May	1	2000	99212	1			1
May	1	2000	99204		2		
May	1	2000	99204		2	1	
May	1	2000	99201		2	1	
May	1	2000	99201	1			1
May	1	2000	99201		2	1	
May	1	2000	99208		2	1	
May	1	2000	99201		2		
May	1	2000	99201	1			
May	1	2000	99201	1			1
May	2	2000	99206		2		
May	2	2000	99208		2	1	
May	2	2000	99205		2		
May	2	2000	99201		2		
May	2	2000	99201		2		
May	2	2000	99201		2		
May	2	2000	99202		2		
May	2	2000	99205		2		1

are multiple questions regarding the reliability and validity of the data. Using software that is designed to support the analysis of qualitative data helps researchers manage such problems.

Qualitative research software makes it possible to code qualitative data for thematic topics. For example, the data may consist of reports from several patients about their experiences with chronic pain. Each patient's report is contained in a separate document. Each time that anger is expressed, the appropriate part of the document is coded for anger. The software can identify all expressions of anger so that they can be reviewed for common patterns. Software support is most valuable for large numbers of comprehensive reports. This software function can also be used to answer questions regarding the quality and integrity of the data obtained from any source, including the Internet.

One example of qualitative software is **QSR NUD*IST (Nonnumerical Unstructured Data Indexing, Searching, and Theorizing)** (Qualitative Solutions and Research, 1997). QSR NUD*IST provides multiple advantages for the management of textual and multimedia material. As described by the manufacturer, "QSR NUD*IST is a richly featured, highly advanced program for handling qualitative data analysis research projects. It combines rich, editable text and multimedia capabilities to help you bring your data alive" (Qualitative Solutions and Research, 2000). Documents such as transcripts of interviews, field notes, and related articles that have been saved as text files can be analyzed. The challenges of using a software program to analyze qualitative data relate to the restrictions in formatting and the sheer volume of information that may need to be reviewed and coded.

Questions that ask respondents to elaborate on their answers lend themselves to analysis using qualitative, thematic techniques. After saving each narrative response as a single file, the researcher is faced with the question of what to do next. Rather than place notes on cards or on multiple sheets of paper, using a qualitative analysis program enables the researcher to utilize the speed and accuracy of a computer to identify all instances of each selected coding category. Reports can then be generated for each coding category or set of categories. By using concept-modeling techniques, or grouping of statements into related categories, the researcher can organize data in a system of nodes, grouped together in a tree structure with categories and subcategories that are related. Search functions of the software assist the researcher in the exploration process (Tak, Nield, & Becker, 1999).

This software provides the user with a wide range of approaches and techniques that can be used to analyze qualitative data. However, a disadvantage to using software for qualitative analysis is that it requires time to learn to use the software to perform these procedures. An experienced qualitative researcher who is familiar with QSR NUD*IST or another qualitative software application can assist others with learning the efficient use of the software to answer research questions. In addition, analysis of responses to short-answer questions may be completed with a database or spreadsheet program, which the researcher may already know how to use. Before using this type of software it is important for the researcher to determine whether the tree structure itself and its grounded theory basis are consistent with the theoretical underpinnings of the research. Although several software programs are available for qualitative analysis of data, the researcher should consider the advantages and disadvantages of each application and the theoretical basis of the program before data collection and analysis. The computer software only facilitates the mechanics of data handling; the conceptualization of the research question and narrative responses is critical to the accurate interpretation of the outcomes.

ELECTRONIC DISSEMINATION OF RESEARCH RESULTS: SHARING RESULTS WITH OTHERS

Electronic storage of research results fosters information sharing among researchers. Data, text, and other files can be electronically disseminated globally very quickly—often in a matter of seconds. The review of results, sharing of data, and critique of drafts of manuscripts can be accomplished in far less time electronically then with the wait for surface delivery and return of information in a printed format. In fact, although their work would not be classified as a research example, multiple authors in many sites created this book. Materials for review by the editors were transmitted electronically. Feedback, comments, and editing changes were inserted in the manuscripts using the editing functions offered by the word processing package. The authors received the results of the review and recommendations for improvement via the Internet. This same process may be used by researchers at multiple and distant sites who collaborate in research endeavors and in the submission and review of manuscripts and reports denoting their work.

USE OF THE INTERNET FOR RESEARCH

As indicated earlier, the Internet has emerged as a means for conducting research. Three major advantages are (1) speed of data collection, (2) access to large numbers of subjects, and (3) minimal cost. However, the Internet researcher must understand and pay careful attention to the advantages, disadvantages, and ethics of use of this medium for research before beginning Internet-based research.

Advantages of Internet Research

Of the three advantages to Internet research, minimal cost and speed offer the most alluring prospects (Szabo & Frenkl, 1996). From an ethical view, use of the Internet for research removes most doubt as to whether or not the subjects were truly volunteering to participate. Compared with telephone interviews and surveys, Internet subjects can freely log on and offer to participate without any of the agreement being due to the social politeness that telephone interviews may create. Indeed, Web participation in research is a totally volunteer process. Development of hypertext, a standard format that is not dependent on word processors being used by sender and receiver, has facilitated data collection.

With the introduction of HTML and interactive "forms," the Internet became a point-and-click interface for rapid administration of surveys and efficient collection of preformatted data (Houston & Fiore, 1998). Electronic storage and transmission of results enables rapid transfer of the responses into a spreadsheet or statistical analysis program for evaluation of quantitative data. Software capabilities lend themselves to rapid creation of a survey. Distributions of surveys to targeted audiences is facilitated by Usenet newsgroups, mailing lists, and hypertext links from content-related sites. (A listing of sample sites is provided in the Web Connection for this book.) The novelty of Internet research may even be an added incentive to individual respondents, since the WWW has become both an information source and a recreational network (Houston & Fiore, 1988). Electronic data collection via the Internet may be an efficient method of collecting data for pilot studies (Fawcett & Buhle, 1995). As a result, easy access to large numbers of research subjects is provided, with this caveat: researchers beware.

Disadvantages of Internet Research

Before rushing to the computer to interview subjects, one must consider four major disadvantages to Internet research. These disadvantages are as follows:

1. Individuals may easily ignore the criteria for participation. The researcher cannot verify that interested, self-selected, volunteer participants meet the criteria established for subject selection.
2. Individuals may submit false or deceptive answers.
3. Participants may respond to the same set of items multiple times.
4. Participants represent the population unique to the Internet. This population does not match U.S. demographics; therefore, population bias is a factor.

For those desiring international representation among respondents, it is important to know that the United States hosts approximately 63% of all computers connected to the Internet. Many countries have minimal, if any, representation on the Internet (Teese, 1999). Reliability of health assessment data that are computer administered has long been established (Slack & Slack, 1972). Internally consistent responses from WWW-administered health surveys have been demonstrated (Bell & Kahn, 1996). Internet responses offer many advantages over face-to-face interviews; however, the researcher must address the question of whether WWW respondents differ in some systematic manner from respondents in other settings such as clinics or other community settings. The overall question of administering surveys to online participants is one of validity.

The WWW is an open, virtual, public gathering place to which patients may be attracted (Soetikno et al., 1997). Despite the disadvantages of the use of the Internet for research, the easy access to willing participants is a strong motivator to researchers. Ethical use of the Internet for research must be considered.

ETHICS OF ONLINE RESEARCH

The researcher who obtains confidential data or medical information from subjects over the Internet must be keenly aware of security issues. Absolute security of data during transmission from the respondent to the researcher cannot be guaranteed. Several software applications are available to make the transmission and storage of sensitive data as secure as technologically possible. The researcher who uses the Internet for data transmission should consult with computer security specialists and an institutional review board to ensure that the greatest degree of protection of data is provided to potential respondents. Protection must be afforded in accordance with existing regulations related to data collection, handling, and storage. Obviously, researchers who use online resources must be critical readers and exercise caution when evaluating online responses. Several sets of guidelines for the evaluation of online resources have emerged and may be located on the Web (Jacobson & Cohen, 1996).

Guidelines for ethical research have been established by the American Psychological Association (1992). The Internet researcher is bound by the same ethical principles as any other researcher. Therefore the guidelines are the same as for any other method of obtaining data. That is, the researcher is obligated to inform potential subjects of the nature of the research, of the requirements placed on the participant, and about intended uses of data. Informed consent is required, as is the institutional review of the proposed research.

The Internet researcher must also attend to the ethics of data reporting. Because of the inability to verify the demographic data about the online subjects, the researcher must fully and clearly describe the sample, as well as the process for obtaining the sample, and deliberately raise questions about the effect of self-selection of volunteer subjects on the results.

SOURCES OF INFORMATION, SUPPORT, AND ORGANIZATIONS FOR INFORMATICS RESEARCH

In addition to obtaining relevant literature, researchers seek information about grants and funding initiatives on the WWW. Among the "must visit" sites are (1) the National Institutes of Health, (2) the Virginia Henderson On-Line Library at Sigma Theta Tau International Honor Society of Nursing, and (3) the Bureau of Health Professions, Health Resources, and Services Administration. Each of these resources provides a wealth of material regarding research support. Grant announcements, application forms, scientific resources, and lists of funded grants are available through these sources. Multiple databases are available to provide daily updates to online subscribers who wish to be informed of grant opportunities. (See the Web Connection for this book for the URLs of these databases.)

CURRENT RESEARCH IN HEALTH CARE INFORMATICS

As advances in computing technologies continue to enter the health care arena, information management becomes more of a challenge. Issues related to making information management a universally accepted component of health care provide many topics for research. Relevant topics are encompassed as focus areas of a national health information strategy: universal access to health information, greater use of telemedicine and teleeducation, computer-based health records for all health care institutions, continued development of expert decision support systems, and development of standards and issues related to confidentiality and security (American Medical Informatics Association, 1997). Other examples of ongoing research in informatics include models of patient care outcomes, measures of health care quality, consumer informatics, and collaboration projects. Each of these topics presents significant challenges for additional research and development.

CONCLUSION

Information technology has changed all aspects of the research process. Each advance in technology brings new changes. Currently, one of the driving forces changing the process for conducting and disseminating health care research is the Internet. The WWW has opened new vistas for students, researchers, and the general public. The speed with which information can be located makes the WWW an important information access tool for many researchers. Ever-increasing amounts of research-based literature are being made available to Internet users. Many libraries offer gateway services or access to multiple bibliographic search services, providing both abstracts and full text of research articles. In addition, electronic health care and informatics journals are available on the WWW.

Use of the Internet for research purposes is increasing. The low cost of collecting data and the speed with which data can be obtained make the WWW an avenue for conducting exciting new research. However, the reliability and validity of data, as well as the demographic characteristics of the respondents, are serious considerations to be addressed by the researcher when using this approach to data collection. The future will bring further refinement of the WWW as a resource in the preparation of research proposals, in seeking funds to support the research, and as a tool for conducting research.

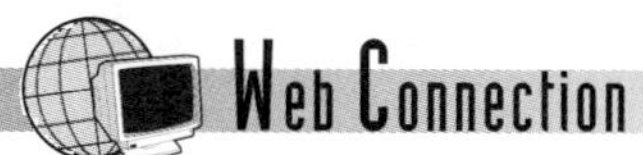

Web Connection

Information technology is a crucial element in an organization's ability to understand the environment of care, the services it provides, the interaction of people with the environment, and the innovations in its processes and technology. Information technology can facilitate the understanding of organizational processes. At the same time, it can be the focus of a research study or process improvement activity on the effectiveness and efficiency of the current methods of collecting organizational data, information, and knowledge. The Web Connection activities for this chapter focus on tools for research processes and resources for conducting Web-based research. You will investigate applications commonly associated with research and explore the emerging area of Web-based research and issues associated with it.

discussion questions

1. How has information technology changed the process and procedures used to conduct health-related research?
2. Describe three major advantages and disadvantages of using the Internet to conduct research.
3. Explain major considerations that the critical reader should consider in reading the results of research conducted via the Internet.
4. Develop a health care informatics–related research question.
5. Identify key areas in health care informatics that need additional research. Explain why you selected these areas, and indicate what kind of research you believe is needed.

REFERENCES

American Medical Informatics Association. (1997). A proposal to improve quality, increase efficiency, and expand access in the U.S. health care system. *Journal of the American Medical Informatics Association, 4,* 340-341. Retrieved September 28, 2000, from the World Wide Web: http://www.amia.org/pubs/pospaper/positio1.htm.

American Psychological Association. (1992). *Ethical principles of psychologists and code of conduct.* Washington, DC: Author. Retrieved May 5, 2000, from the World Wide Web http://www.apa.org/ethics/code.html#materials.

Bell, D.S., & Kahn, C.E. (1996). Health status assessment via the World Wide Web. *Journal of the American Medical Informatics Association, Symposium Supplement,* 338-342.

Bingham, C. (1998). Peer review on the Internet: A better class of conversation. *Lancet, Supplement 1—Guide to the Internet, 351*(9106), 40-46.

Delamothe, T. (1998). The electronic future of scientific articles. *Lancet, Supplement 1—Guide to the Internet, 351*(9106), 5-6.

Fawcett, J., & Buhle, E.L. (1995). Using the Internet for data collection: An innovative electronic strategy. *Computers in Nursing, 13,* 273-279.

Houston, J.D., & Fiore, D.C. (1998). Online medical surveys: Using the Internet as a research tool. *M.D. Computing, 15*(2), 116-120.

Jacobson, T., & Cohen, L. (1996). *Evaluating Internet resources.* University at Albany Library. Retrieved September 30, 2000, from the World Wide Web: http://www.albany.edu/library/internet/evaluate.html.

Lakeman, R. (1997). Using the Internet for data collection in nursing research. *Computers in Nursing, 15*(5), 269-275.

McDonald, L. (1998). Florence Nightingale: Passionate statistician. *Journal of Holistic Nursing, 16*(2), 267-277.

Qualitative Solutions and Research. (1997). *The QSR NUD*IST (version 3.0).* Thousand Oaks, CA: Sage Publications Software.

Qualitative Solutions and Research. (2000). *The QSR NUD*IST computer software.* Thousand Oaks, CA: Sage Publications Software. Retrieved September 29, 2000, from the World Wide Web: http://www.scolari.com.

Slack, W.V., & Slack, C.W. (1972). Patient-computer dialogue. *New England Journal of Medicine, 286,* 1304-1309.

Soetikno, R.M., et al. (1997). Quality-of-life research on the Internet: Feasibility and potential biases in patients with ulcerative colitis. *Journal of the American Medical Informatics Association, 4,* 426-435.

Szabo, A., & Frenkl, R. (1996). Consideration of research on Internet: Guidelines and implications for human movement studies. *Clinical Kinesiology, 50*(3), 58-65.

Tak, S.H., Nield, M., & Becker, H. (1999). Use of a computer software program for qualitative analyses: Part 2. Advantages and disadvantages. *Western Journal of Nursing Research, 3,* 21, 436-439.

Teese, W. (1999). *The Internet index, #24.* Retrieved September 29, 2000, from the World Wide Web: http://new-website.openmarket.com/intindex/99-05.htm.

U.S. Census Bureau. (2000). *Customer services.* Response from Webmaster. Retrieved September 27, 2000, from the World Wide Web: http://www.census.gov/dmd/www/skhome.htm.

PART FIVE

Infrastructure to Support Health Care Informatics

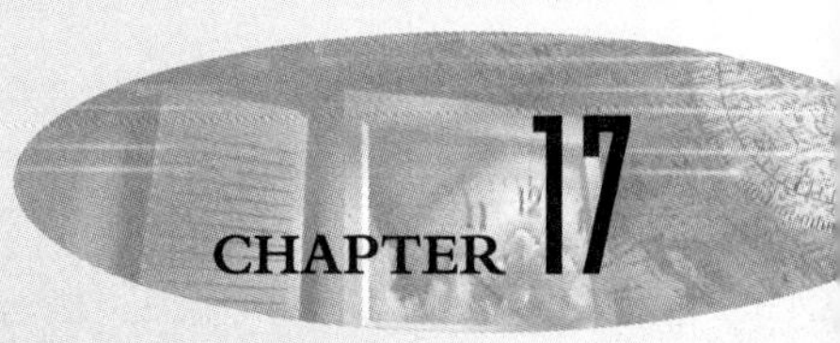

Technical Standards Used in Health Care Informatics

KATHLEEN SMITH

Learning Objectives

Upon completion of this chapter, the reader will be able to:

1. ***Discuss*** the reasons technical health care standards are used.
2. ***Identify*** the major types of technical health care standards.
3. ***List*** the major standards development organizations in the United States and their areas of focus.
4. ***Describe*** the major types of technical standards used in an electronic health record.

Outline

Outline—cont'd

Hypertext Markup Language
Other Web Standards
ActiveX
Telecommunications Standards
Data Interchange Standards Association
Local Area Network
Wide Area Network
Imaging Standards
Infrared Standards
Digital Subscriber Lines
Plain Old Telephone Service

Key Terms

carrier signal
companion standards
electronic commerce
electronic data interchange (EDI)
lexicons
message-bearing signal
multimedia
stand-alone or stovepipe
standard

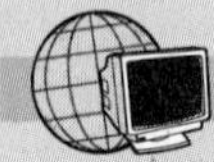

Web Connection

Go to the Web site at http://evolve.elsevier.com/Englebardt/. Here you will find Web links and activities related to technical standards used in health care informatics.

Consider the following. If the electrical industry had not agreed on a **standard** base for a light bulb, you might have to buy a new lamp every time you needed a new light bulb. The standard gauge for railroads is 4 feet 8.5 inches, which is derived from the standard width of a Roman chariot. According to the Old Testament tale about the Tower of Babel, different languages divided mankind so individuals could not communicate with one another. These examples are applicable to a chapter on technical standards because many of the clinical health care informatics applications have not been designed to exchange information easily. In other words, the lack of health care informatics standards has created a "Tower of Babel." This lack of standards is a major barrier to broad implementation of an electronic health record (EHR) and integrated health care delivery systems.

This chapter gives an overview of the major existing and emerging health care information technical standards, as well as the efforts to coordinate, harmonize, and accelerate standards activities. Technical standards are recommended by a number of technical working groups and organizations. In addition, organizations have been established within the United States and internationally to coordinate and standardize data transfer and clinical languages. These organizations, technical standards, and related clinical applications will be explored in this chapter. Technical standards in health care informatics are required for the sharing of data and meaningful information, to develop data warehouses and clinical data repositories, and to contribute to the improved performance of the health care system.

Health care informatics abbreviations used in this chapter are listed alphabetically in Table 17-1. Figure 17-1 shows the technical standards,

Table 17–1 Standards-Related Acronyms Used in Health Care Informatics

Abbreviation	Group
ACR-NEMA	American College of Radiology–National Electrical Manufacturers' Association
ADA	American Dental Association
AHCPR	Agency for Health Care Policy and Research
AHIMA	American Health Information Management Association
ANSI	American National Standards Institute
ANSI HISB	American National Standards Institute Healthcare Informatics Standards Board
ANSI HISPP	American National Standards Institute Healthcare Informatics Standards Planning Panel
ASC X12N	Accredited Standards Committee on Insurance Interchange Standards
ASTM	American Society for Testing and Materials
ASTM E 1029	ASTM Guide for Documentation of Clinical Computer Systems
ASTM E 1238	ASTM Specifications for Transferring Clinical Observations Between Independent Computer Systems
ASTM E 1239	ASTM Guide for Description of Reservation/Registration-Admission, Discharge, Transfer (R-ADT) Systems for Automated Patient Care Information Systems
ASTM E 1284	ASTM Guide for Construction of a Clinical Nomenclature for Support of Electronic Health Records
ASTM E 1381	ASTM Specifications for Low-Level Protocol to Transfer Messages Between Clinical Laboratory Information Instruments and Computer Systems
ASTM E 1384–99e1	Standard Guide for Content and Structure of the Electronic Health Record
ASTM E 1394-97	ASTM Specifications for Transferring Information Between Clinical Instruments and Computer Systems
ASTM E 1460	ASTM Specifications for Defining and Sharing Modular Health Knowledge Bases (Arden Syntax for Medical Logic Modules)
ASTM E 1466	ASTM Specifications for Use of Bar Codes on Specimen Tubes in the Clinical Laboratory
ASTM E 1467	ASTM Specifications for Transferring Digital Neurophysiological Data Between Independent Computer Systems
ASTM E 1633	ASTM Specifications for Coded Values Used in the Computer-Based Patient Record
ASTM E 1712	ASTM Specifications for Representing Clinical Laboratory Test and Analyte Names
ASTM E 1713	ASTM Specifications for Transferring Digital Waveform Data Between Independent Computer Systems
ASTM E 1714	ASTM Guide for Properties of a Universal Healthcare Identifier
ASTM E 1714-95	ASTM Guide for Properties of a Universal Healthcare Identifier
ASTM E 1715	ASTM Practice for an Object-Oriented Model for Registration, Admitting, Discharge, and Transfer Functions in the Computer-Based Patient Record System
ASTM E 1744	ASTM Guide for a View of Emergency Medical Care in the Computerized Patient Record
ASTM E 1769	ASTM Guide for Properties of Electronic Health Records and Record Systems
ASTM E 1869	ASTM Guide for Confidentiality, Privacy, Access, and Data Security Principles for Health Information Including Computer-Based Patient Records
ASTM E 1947	ASTM Specifications for Analytical Data Interchange Protocol for Chromatographic Data
ASTM E 1948	ASTM Guide for Analytical Data Interchange Protocol for Chromatographic Data
ASTM E31	ASTM Subcommittees on Healthcare Informatics
CEFACT	Centre for the Facilitation of Procedures and Practices for Administration, Commerce, and Transport
CEN/TC 215	Comite Europeen de Normalisation, Technical Committee
CMS	Centers for Medicare & Medicaid Services (formerly known as HCFA)
COHR	Computer-Based Oral Health Record
COM	Microsoft's Component Object Model

Continued

Table 17–1 Standards-Related Acronyms Used in Health Care Informatics—cont'd

Abbreviation	Group
CORBA	Common Object Request Broker Architecture
DHHS	Department of Health and Human Services
DISA	Data Interchange Standards Association
DSL	Digital Subscriber Lines
DX DRG	Diagnosis-Related Groups
EDI	Electronic Data Interchange
FDA	Food and Drug Administration
GMN	Gabrieli Medical Nomenclature
HCFA	Health Care Financing Administration (now known as the Centers for Medicare & Medicaid Services [CMS])
HIBCC	Health Industry Business Communications Council
HIN	Health Industry Number
HIPAA	Health Insurance Portability and Accountability Act of 1996
HL7	Health Level Seven
HTML	Hypertext Markup Language
IEEE	Institute of Electrical and Electronic Engineers
IEEE/MEDIX	Institute of Electrical and Electronic Engineers P1157 Medical Data Interchange Standard
IUPAC	International Union of Pure and Applied Chemistry
LAN	Local Area Network
LIC	Labeler Identification Code
LOINC	Logical Observation Identifiers, Names, and Codes
MLM	Medical-Logic Module
MS-HUG	Microsoft Healthcare Users Group, Inc.
NCCLS	National Council for Clinical Laboratory Standards
NCPDP	National Council for Prescription Drug Programs
NDC	National Drug Code
NPF	National Provider File
NPI	National Provider Identifier
OTC	Over the Counter
Pan American EDIFACT	Pan-American Electronic Data Interchange for Administration, Commerce, and Transport Board
POTS	Plain Old Telephone Service
RCS	READ Classification System
SDO	Standards Development Organization
SGML	Standard Generalized Markup Language
SIG VI	Special Interest Group for Visual Information
SSN	Social Security Number
U.S. TAG	U.S. Technical Advisory Groups
UHID	Universal Healthcare Identifier
UN/EDIFACT	United Nations Electronic Data Interchange for Administration, Commerce, and Transport
UPC	Universal Product Code
UPIN	Universal Provider Identifier Number
WAN	Wide Area Network
WEDI	Workgroup for Electronic Data Interchange
XML	Extensible Markup Language

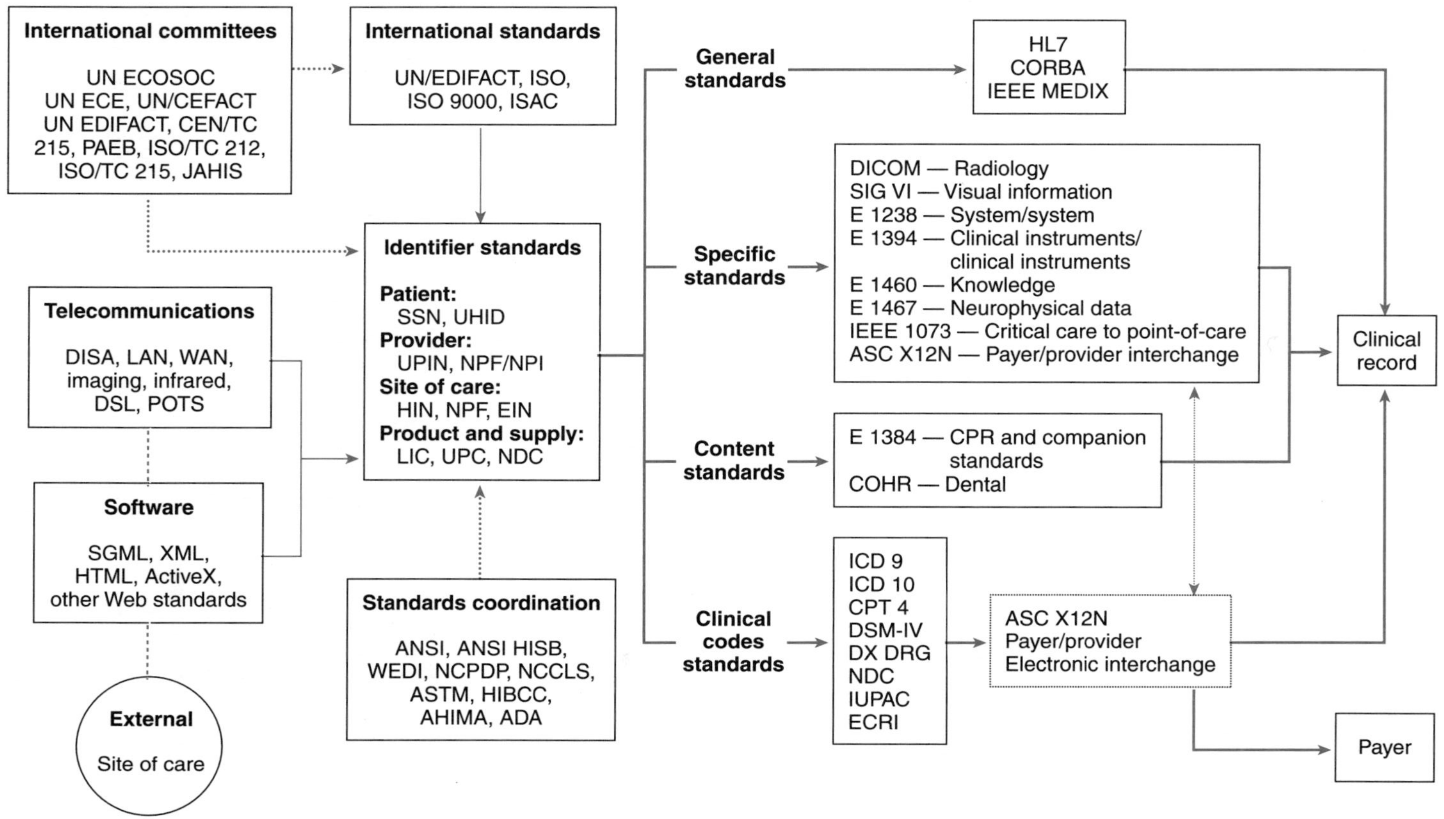

FIGURE 17—1 Technical Standards Used in Health Care Informatics

the standards-setting groups, and the interrelationships between the groups and standards. Each of the standards and standards activities is required to create a clinical or computer-based patient record.

Information systems applications for clinical care evolved during the last 20 to 30 years. Early applications were for a single use; each application was developed as a **stand-alone** system for a specific purpose. Stand-alone systems were called **stovepipe** developments; there was no standardized way to provide continuity of care by sharing patient information across information networks and disparate applications. Today, as additional systems and applications are developed, there is an increasing need to share clinical outcomes measurement and other data. Health care information standards for classifications, guides, practices, and terminology are required to make diverse components work together. Brandt (2000, p. 39) states:

> *In health informatics, a standard defines a commonly agreed-upon manner of collecting, maintaining, or transferring data between computer systems. Until health care providers collect and maintain data in a standard format according to widely accepted definitions, it is nearly impossible to link data from one site to another.*

The use of commonly agreed upon standards makes it possible to share data across systems and to compare data among health care sites.

STANDARDS COORDINATION AND PROMOTION ACTIVITIES

In the United States there are a number of voluntary organizations that coordinate and promote health care information standards. However, there is no national standards-setting group. Some of the standards coordination and promotion activities among voluntary organizations overlap. Some groups are formed to develop standards, and some groups coordinate technical standards in health care informatics. Additionally, some of the professional organizations have special interests in setting standards for a specific application. For example, the American Nurses Association has a process for recognizing standard languages that support the nursing process. In addition a number of companies that develop and market health care informatics applications have joined together to develop voluntary standards. Some of these groups are also involved in standards coordination activities. This section discusses the standards coordination and promotion activities within the United States. Communication-coordinating activities (including data interchange standards) are discussed in the Telecommunications Standards section of this chapter. Communication standards are also discussed in Chapter 11.

Standards-Coordinating Groups

In the United States the groups formed to coordinate the formation of technical health care informatics standards include the American National Standards Institute (ANSI), the Workgroup for Electronic Data Interchange (WEDI), and the National Council for Clinical Laboratory Standards (NCCLS).

American National Standards Institute

ANSI is the administrator and the coordinator promoting and facilitating voluntary consensus standards within the U.S. private sector. ANSI does not develop American National Standards (ANSs); rather it facilitates standards development by establishing consensus among qualified groups. ANSI-accredited developers are committed to supporting the development of national and in many cases international standards, addressing the critical trends of technological innovation, marketplace globalization, and regulatory reform. ANSI promotes the use of U.S. standards internationally, advocates U.S. policy and technical positions in international and regional standards organizations, and encourages the adoption of international standards as national standards where these meet the needs of the user community.

ANSI is the sole U.S. representative of the International Organization for Standardization (ISO) (see discussion of ISO standards later in this chapter). ANSI accredits U.S. Technical Advisory Groups (TAGs), whose primary purpose is to develop and transmit, via ANSI, U.S. positions on activities and ballots to the international technical committee (ANSI, 2000).

ANSI Healthcare Informatics Standards Board

The ANSI Healthcare Informatics Standards Board (HISB) provides an open, public forum for the voluntary coordination of health care informatics standards among U.S. standards development organizations (SDOs). The ANSI HISB works on standards activities for the EHR, coding, terminology, international data exchange, and patient privacy. Members include other SDOs, professional societies, trade associations, medical organizations, corporations, and federal representatives. ANSI HISB deals with coordination of compliance issues in data content development, accreditation of health care security measures, and analysis of the recently compiled administrative and clinical inventories. Every major developer of health care informatics standards in the United States participates in ANSI HISB (Blair, 1996; HISB, 2000; The Latest Word, 1999; Marietti, 1998; Setting up Health Care Services Information Systems, 1999). U.S. standards activities, coordinated under the umbrella of the ANSI HISB committee, are presented in Box 17-1.

ANSI Healthcare Informatics Standards Planning Panel The ANSI Healthcare Informatics Standards Planning Panel (HISPP) was established to perform the function of a standards planning panel in the field of health care informatics. Specifically the planning panel was established to coordinate the work of the standards groups for health care data interchange, health care informatics groups, and other relevant standards groups toward achieving the evolution of a unified set of nonredundant, nonconflicting standards that are compatible with ISO and non-ISO communications environments (Current State of Technology, 1995).

Workgroup for Electronic Data Interchange

The WEDI, formed as a result of the call for health care administrative simplification by the Department of Health and Human Services (DHHS), was incorporated as a formal organization in 1995. WEDI has developed an action plan to promote health care **electronic data interchange (EDI)**, including promotion of EDI standards, architectures, confidentiality, identifiers, health cards, legislation, and publicity (Blair, 1996).

National Council for Clinical Laboratory Standards

The NCCLS is a voluntary consensus SDO that enhances the value of medical testing within the health care community through the development and dissemination of standards, guidelines, and best practices (NCCLS, 1998).

Groups Formed to Develop Standards

The groups formed to develop standards in the United States include the National Council for Prescription Drug Programs (NCPDP), American Society for Testing and Materials (ASTM) Committee E-31 on Health Care Informatics, Health Industry Business Communications Council (HIBCC), and other groups. Each group is composed of individuals, vendors, and other interested parties. They develop and recommend technical standards for applications in health care informatics.

National Council for Prescription Drug Programs

The NCPDP, an ANSI-accredited SDO, recommends the use of a standardized format for electronic communication of claims between pharmacy providers, insurance carriers, third-party administrators, and other responsible parties. This standard addresses the data format and content, the transmission protocol, and other appropriate telecommunication requirements. The standard was developed to accommodate the

Box 17–1 U.S. Standards Activities Coordinated by the ANSI HISB Committee

- American Dental Association (ADA)
- American Society for Testing and Materials (ASTM) E31 Subcommittees on Healthcare Informatics
- Health Industry Business Communication Council (HIBCC)
- Health Level 7 (HL7)
- Institute of Electrical and Electronic Engineers (IEEE)
- National Council for Prescription Drug Programs (NCPDP)
- Accredited Standards Committee on Insurance Interchange Standards (ASC X12N)
- Federal health care informatics standards activities of the following groups:
  - Agency for Health Care Policy and Research
  - Centers for Disease Control and Prevention
  - National Center for Health Statistics
  - Food and Drug Administration
  - Health Care Financing Administration (now known as the Centers for Medicare & Medicaid Services)
  - National Institutes of Health, National Library of Medicine
  - Department of Defense
  - Bureau of Labor Statistics
  - Department of State
  - National Highway Traffic Safety Administration
  - Department of Veterans Affairs
  - Consumer Product Safety Commission
  - Social Security Administration
  - Office of Personnel Management

From Agency for Health Care Policy and Research. (1999). *Health care informatics standards activities of selected federal agencies: A compendium.* Retrieved August 27, 2000, from the World Wide Web: http://www.ahcpr.gov/data/datameet.htm.

eligibility verification process at the point of sale and to provide a consistent format for electronic claims processing. The standard supports the submission and adjudication of third-party prescription drug claims in an online, real-time environment. The standards have been in use since 1985 and now serve almost 90% of the nation's community pharmacies and 70% of the outpatient pharmacies. NCPDP is currently working on standards for adverse drug reactions and utilization review (Blair, 1996; Blair, 1999).

ASTM Committee E-31 on Health Care Informatics

ASTM is one of the largest voluntary standards development groups in the world. Its Committee on Health Care Informatics develops standards for health information and health information systems that are designed to assist vendors, users, and anyone interested in systematizing health information. The current standards address architecture, content, portability, format, privacy, security, and communications. The committee coordinates its efforts with those of other standards developers and is ANSI accredited (Accredited Standards Committee X12, 2000).

Health Industry Business Communications Council

HIBCC is an industry-sponsored, nonprofit SDO. It is a fully accredited member of ANSI. HIBCC's mission is to facilitate electronic commerce by developing appropriate standards for information exchange among health care trading partners, including EDI message formats, bar code labeling data standards, universal numbering systems, and the provision of databases that ensure common identifiers (HIBCC, 1994)

Computer Technology Industry Association and Microsoft Healthcare Users Group, Inc.

The Computing Technology Industry Association (CompTIA) works to develop vendor-neutral eCommerce standards and guidelines. This group helps health care institutions and vendors to simplify practices, reduce expenses, and compete more effectively in an increasingly complex and competitive world. eCommerce standards are increasingly applicable to the health care informatics arena as more and more processes are transmitted electronically to payers and other reporting groups (About CTIA, 2000).

Microsoft Healthcare Users Group, Inc. (MS-HUG), provides a health care industry forum for exchanging ideas, promoting learning, and sharing solutions for information systems using Microsoft technologies. MS-HUG uses this forum to provide industry leadership, drive appropriate standards, and develop associated requirements in support of health care solutions. MS-HUG is not affiliated with Microsoft Corporation. It is an independent, not-for-profit organization catering to the needs of information systems developers and users in the health care industry.

Professional Organizations Supporting the Development of Technical Standards

Several professional organizations within the health care field have working groups interested in developing and recommending technical standards in areas of interest to the group's constituency. Examples of these groups include the American Health Information Management Association (AHIMA) and the American Dental Association (ADA). Other groups are working on issues including standardized languages and other technical issues including privacy, security, and confidentiality. See Chapter 20 for additional information on privacy, security, and confidentiality.

American Health Information Management Association

AHIMA is the professional association that represents health information management professionals who work throughout the health care industry. AHIMA also represents the public by managing, analyzing, and utilizing data vital for patient care, as well as making this information data accessible to health care providers when it is needed most.

American Dental Association

The ADA has formed a task group to initiate the development of technical reports, guidelines, and standards on electronic technologies used in dental practice. Components of the task group include five working groups for clinical information systems. Clinical information systems include all areas of computer-based information technologies, such as digital radiography, digital intraoral video cameras, digital voice-text-image transfer, periodontal probing devices, computer-aided drafting (CAD) and computer-aided machining (CAM), and others. By establishing standards for these modules, the need for several stand-alone systems in the dental office will be eliminated. A Computer-Based Oral Health Record (COHR) concept model has been developed by the Working Group of the Council on Dental Practice (CDP) of the ADA. Standardized messaging formats, vocabulary, and codes for an electronic environment will also be developed for the COHR if they do not exist in current published standards (ADA, 1997).

ESTABLISHING INTERNATIONAL STANDARDS

Internationally at least 140 countries are now developing health care informatics standards. There are many organizations, committees, and subgroups that promote the evolution of health care standards worldwide. This section discusses the international groups developing standards and identifies some of the international technical standards used in health care informatics.

International Standards Committees

The international committees and organizations working on technical standards used in health care informatics include the United Nations Economic and Social Council (ECOSOC), a number of committees and commissions chartered under the ECOSOC, and committees in Latin America and Japan.

United Nations Economic and Social Council

The ECOSOC was established by the General Assembly of the United Nations to promote higher standards of living, full employment, and conditions of economic and social progress and development. Subsidiary bodies in the form of commissions and committees have been formed in economic, social, and related fields (ECOSOC Subsidiary Bodies, 2000).

United Nations Economic Commission of Europe The United Nations Economic Commission of Europe (UN/ECE) is one of the five regional commissions of the United Nations ECOSOC. Its members are from North America, Western Europe, and Eastern Europe, and its headquarters are in Geneva. The primary goal of the UN/ECE is to encourage economic cooperation among the member states, and its focus is on economic analysis, environment and human settlements, statistics, sustainable energy, trade, industry and enterprise development, timber, and transport (UN/ECE, n.d.). To achieve these goals, UN/ECE activities include the development of conventions, regulations and standards, and technical assistance.

United Nations Centre for Trade Facilitation and Electronic Business The United Nations Centre for Trade Facilitation and Electronic Business (UN/CEFACT) is located in the UN/ECE. The mission of UN/CEFACT is to improve the ability of business, trade, and administrative organizations to exchange products and relevant services effectively by improving business and administrative processes, procedures, and information flows (UN/CEFACT, 2000).

Electronic Data Interchange for Administration, Commerce, and Transport The Electronic Data Interchange for Administration, Commerce, and Transport (EDIFACT) Working Group was formed under the auspices of the UN/ECE. The purpose of the UN/EDIFACT Working Group is to maintain the EDIFACT standard, provide the tools and administrative support necessary for the development of EDIFACT, and promote the global use of EDIFACT (EDIFACT, 2000).

Pan American EDIFACT Board The Pan American EDIFACT Board (PAEB) was the official coordinating body of UN/EDIFACT activity in the Pan-American region through 1998. The UN/CEFACT replaced the PAEB and allows coordinating activities on a national basis. As a member country of the UN/ECE, the United States provides its coordination services through the Accredited Standards Committee X12 (ASC X12), which is recognized by the ANSI as the official body to develop EDI standards (Data Interchange Standards Association [DISA], 2000; ASC, 2000).

European Committee for Standards The European Committee for Standards (CEN), also known as the Comite Europeen de Normalisation, Technical Committee (CEN/TC 215), is the international committee for standards in Europe. CEN's mission is to promote voluntary technical harmonization in Europe in conjunction with worldwide bodies and its partners in Europe.

The U.S. TAGs work with the CEN/TC 215 to change the standards-adoption process and industry function in the United States as well as internationally. The ultimate goal of the committee is to adopt a single set of standards. These standards will influence U.S. health care standards development and will have an impact on companies involved in the global market (Blair, 1996).

International Organization for Standardization

The ISO is a worldwide federation of national standards bodies from 140 countries. This nongovernmental organization was established in 1947. The mission of the ISO is to promote the development of standardization and related activities in the world and to develop cooperation in the spheres of intellectual, scientific, technological, and economic activity. The purpose of the ISO is to promote the development of worldwide standardization and related activities (ISO, n.d.a). ANSI was one of the founding members of ISO and is the representative for the United States. ISO includes 223 technical committees that are involved in establishing technical standards (ISO, n.d.b).

ISO Technical Committee 212 The purpose of the ISO Technical Committee 212 (ISO/TC 212) is to provide a focus for coordination of international standardization in the clinical laboratory-testing field. ANSI, as the U.S. member of ISO, is listed as the Secretariat of ISO/TC 212. The scope of ISO/TC 212 is standardization and guidance in the field of laboratory medicine and in vitro diagnostic test systems (NCCLS, 1998).

ISO Technical Committee 215 Health Informatics Chartered in February 1998, ISO Technical Committee 215 (ISO/TC 215) is establishing a system of liaison with other standards-setting organizations to negotiate overlapping issues and coordinate content. See Box 17-2 for a list of the ISO Technical Committee 215 working groups.

Box 17–2 The ISO TC 215 Working Groups

- WG 1: Health records and modeling coordination
- WG 2: Messaging and communications
- WG 3: Health concept representation
- WG 4: Security
- WG 5: Health cards

From Chute, C.G. (1999). ISO TC 215: What the health world needs now. *MD Computing, 16*(3), 21-22.

Japanese Association of Healthcare Information Systems Industry

The Japanese Association of Healthcare Information Systems Industry (JAHIS) was established for the following purposes:

- Contributing to the development of the health care information systems industry
- Improving the health, medical treatment, and welfare of the nation
- Making technological improvements
- Ensuring quality and safety
- Promoting the standardization of health care information systems

It also plans to promote international cooperation in the fields of health, medical treatment, and welfare (Blair, 1996). JAHIS works with other international groups, including ASTM, to develop and promote standardization of health care informatics.

International Standards

The international committees and working groups strive to develop and adopt international standards in health care and EDI. Some of the international technical standards applicable to health care informatics include UN/EDIFACT, ISO, ISO 9000, and Image Store and Carry (ISAC).

United Nations Electronic Data Interchange for Administration, Commerce, and Transport

In 1986 the UN/ECE launched UN/EDIFACT, a single international standard for EDI flexible enough to meet the needs of governments and private enterprise worldwide. UN/EDIFACT eliminates manual copying and entering of data and provides for common, paperless documentation and a single "language," which speeds up international trade transactions and cuts costs.

UN/EDIFACT contains a set of standards, directories, and guidelines for the electronic interchange of structured data, and in particular the data related to trade in goods or services between independent computerized information systems. Recommended within the framework of the United Nations, the rules are approved and published by the UN/ECE in the United Nations Trade Data Interchange Directory (UNTDID) and are maintained under agreed procedures. UN/EDIFACT is widely used in Europe and in several Latin American countries. In addition, UN/EDIFACT has developed message format standards that support interactive eligibility/information and inquiry (Blair, 1996; Blair, 1999).

International Standards Reference Model

The purpose of the International Standards Reference Model of Open Systems (commonly called the open systems model, open systems interconnection [OSI] model, or ISO model) is to provide a common basis for the coordination of standards development for systems interconnection. The reference model contains seven layers, and with the exception of the application layer, each layer provides services to support the layer above it. Box 17-3 lists the seven ISO layers.

The Institute of Electrical and Electronic Engineers P1157 Medical Data Interchange Standard (IEEE/MEDIX) and Health Level Seven (HL7) (see discussion of IEEE/MEDIX and HL7 later in this chapter) have recognized and built upon the ISO/OSI framework. ANSI HISPP has stated as one of its objectives the encouragement of U.S. health care standards compatibility with ISO/OSI. The ISO activities related to information technology take place within the Joint Technical Committee (JTC) 1 (Blair, 1999; Blair, 1996).

Box 17–3 The Physical Layers of the ISO Module

- Layer 7: Application—The end user view or exchange of information
- Layer 6: Presentation—The conversion of code and data reformatting
- Layer 5: Session—The coordination interaction between two processors
- Layer 4: Transport—The end-to-end data integrity and quality of service
- Layer 3: Network—The switching and routing network
- Layer 2: Data link—The transmission of a unit of data
- Layer 1: Physical—The hardware transmission of a bitstream

From Vargo, J., & Hunt, R. (1996). *Telecommunications in business strategy and application* (pp. 152-154). Boston: Irwin McGraw-Hill.
The upper three layers (application, presentation, and session) deal with information activities associated with host applications. The lower three layers (network, data link, and physical) are concerned with the mechanisms of the communication network. The transport layer forms a bridge between the two groups and is relative to both host and network services.

ISO 9000

ISO 9000 is a set of five universal standards for a quality assurance system that is accepted around the world. Currently 129 countries have adopted ISO 9000 as a national standard. Purchase of a product or service from a company registered to the appropriate ISO 9000 standard provides assurances for the quality of the product. ISO 9000 registration is rapidly becoming a requirement for any company that does business in Europe. Many industrial companies require registration by their own suppliers. There is a growing trend toward universal acceptance of ISO 9000 as an international standard (ISO Easy, 2000; ISO 9000, 2000).

Image Store and Carry

A Japanese consortium that includes Sony, Toshiba, and Canon has implemented a videodiskbased patient record system called ISAC. This standard provides structures for storing patients' demographic data, all kinds of medical images, electrocardiograms, laboratory data, and clinical information. ISAC includes both the ASTM E1238 (ASTM Specifications for Transferring Clinical Observations Between Independent Computer Systems) and Digital Imaging and Communications in Medicine (DICOM) standards (Blair, 1996).

The remainder of this chapter discusses the standards and supporting standards used in the United States to develop and maintain an EHR or computer-based patient record.

IDENTIFIER STANDARDS

Health care identifier standards are needed to uniquely specify each patient, provider, site of care, and product in an electronic format. A number of groups are working on various aspects of identifier standards including the ASTM, DHHS, Food and Drug Administration (FDA), Centers for Medicare & Medicaid Services (CMS), and HIBCC. To date there is no universal acceptance and/or satisfaction with the existing standards. Controversy continues among the various groups and agencies about identifier standards used in the United States and internationally (Appavu, 1999; Paul, 1998). See Figure 17-1 for the identifier standards discussed in this section.

In 1996 Congress passed the Health Insurance Portability and Accountability Act (HIPAA), which includes provisions to address the need for a standard national provider identifier, national employer identifier, national health care provider identifier, and other standards, including a national individual identifier, that would lead to administrative simplification. HIPAA mandates the use of these standards in the following electronic transactions (HCFA, 1999b):

- Health claims
- Health encounter information
- Health claims attachments
- Health plan enrollments and disenrollments
- Health plan eligibility
- Health care payment and remittance advice
- Health plan premium payments
- First report of injury
- Health claim status
- Referral certification and authorization

The Notice of Proposed Rule Making (NPRM) by the DHHS contains the administrative simplification regulations specified by the HIPAA. The standards were required to be implemented within 2 years of the effective date of the final rule (see Chapters 19 and 20 for additional information on HIPAA).

Patient Identifiers

The proposal for a National Individual Identifier through HIPAA is on hold until other security and privacy standards are in place. Opinion about an individual identifier is deeply divided in the United States. Adequate security and privacy measures are needed before the individual's health information is identified. Individuals have various identifying numbers assigned by different health plans and health providers. Currently there is no way to cross-reference this information to provide a lifetime history for an individual. Duplicate medical record numbers have plagued the health care industry for a variety of reasons, including name changes, misspelled names, use of nicknames, and use of aliases (HIPPA, 2000b).

Social Security Number

In the United States the social security number (SSN) has been considered as a potential patient identifier. Critics point out that the SSN is not an ideal identifier because not everyone has an SSN, several individuals may use the same SSN, and the SSN is so widely used for other purposes that it presents an exposure to violations of confidentiality. The SSN is not used outside the United States, and nonresident and illegal aliens do not have SSNs assigned. There is also a concern that the use of the SSN for a patient identifier may link credit and financial information to health information.

Universal Health Care Identifier

ASTM Committees E 1714-95 are developing guidelines and properties for a universal health care identifier (UHID). The criteria necessary for a UHID include an alphanumeric or numeric identifier scheme; a mechanism to identify information; an index; a mechanism to encrypt the identification; and the technology infrastructure to search, identify, match, and encrypt the information (ASTM, 1999).

Provider Identifiers

Currently each health plan assigns identifying numbers to health care providers including individuals, groups, or organizations. If a provider does business with multiple plans, he or she will have multiple identifiers. At this time, provider identifiers created by different U.S. federal agencies include the Universal Provider Identifier Number (UPIN) and the National Provider Identifier (NPI) or National Provider File (NPF).

Universal Provider Identifier Number

The HCFA (now known as CMS) created the UPIN to identify physicians and others who provide primary care to Medicare patients. Health care providers who do not treat Medicare patients may not have UPINs.

National Provider Identifier

Although there has been no universal agreement on a single standard for identifying providers, HIPAA requires the Secretary of the DHHS to adopt standards for unique health identifiers for each individual, employer, health plan, and health care provider. HIPAA also requires that the adopted standards specify for what purpose unique health identifiers may be used (HCFA, 1999a; HIPAA, 2000a). The DHHS has proposed use of an eight-digit alphanumeric NPI to uniquely identify all providers. As a part of HIPAA, the NPRM was published by the DHHS in May 1998. The final rule was published as part of the *Federal Register* on August 17, 2000, to become effective on October 16, 2000. The standard will be implemented within 2 years of the effective date of the final rule. Provider identification is an important issue in health care to identify providers for eligibility certification requirements, utilization review, claims reimbursement, and a means to reduce the costs of health care. In designing the NPI the DHHS considered the following criteria:

- Need to improve the efficiency and effectiveness of the health care system
- Ability of the NPI to be comprehensive and meet the needs of the health data standards user community
- Need to be consistent and uniform with HIPAA and other private and public sector health standards in providing for privacy and confidentiality
- Ability to incorporate flexibility and adapt easily to changes (HIPAA, 2000a)

Site-of-Care Identifiers

Two site-of-care identifier systems are currently in wide use. One is the Health Industry Number (HIN), issued by the HIBCC. The HIN is an identifier for health care facilities, practitioners, and retail pharmacies. It was created as a universal identification number to be used in all electronic communications and is widely used in both the private and public sectors for EDI transmissions. CMS has also defined the provider of service identifiers for Medicare usage. Both the CMS's provider of service identifier and the UPIN identifier will be replaced by CMS's NPF for Medicare Usage (HIN System, n.d.).

The HIPAA rule proposes both a standard for a national employer identifier and requirements for the use of the identifier by health plans, health care clearinghouses, and health care providers. These groups would use the identifier, among other uses, in connection with certain electronic health care transactions. For example, this requirement will enable employers to identify themselves in electronic transactions when they enroll or disenroll employees in their health plan or when they make premium payments to health plans. The DHHS consulted with several standard-setting organizations, including the National Uniform Billing Committee, the National Uniform Claim Committee, WEDI, and the ADA, to identify that no standard has been developed, adopted, or modified by a standard-setting organization to meet the requirements of HIPAA. The DHHS has proposed use of the Employer Identification Number (EIN) to meet HIPAA requirements. The EIN (the taxpayer identifying number for employers) is assigned by the Internal Revenue Service (IRS), Department of the Treasury.

Product and Supply Labeling Identifiers

To transmit business information electronically, trading partners must be able to identify quickly and efficiently the three most common elements in every transaction: the buyer, the seller, and the item. A bar code system provides the unique identifiers that allow this to occur. The bar code uses a series of patterns representing letters and numbers that produce a machine-readable code representing any kind of data. The data are read by an optical scanner and can be transmitted through EDI for payment purposes, printed on paper, or transmitted to an electronic record. See Box 17-4 for a listing of the product and supply labeling identifiers (Bar Code Labeling Standard, n.d.).

Box 17–4 Product and Supply Labeling Identifiers

- Labeler Identification Code (LIC)
- Health Industry Bar Code Standard (HIBC)
  - Supplier Labeling Standard
  - Provider Application Standard
- Health Industry Number (HIN)
- Universal Product Number (UPN)
- Universal Product Code (UPC)
- National Drug Code (NDC)

Labeler Identification Code

The Labeler Identification Code (LIC) identifies the manufacturer or distributor of a product or supply and is issued by the HIBCC. The LIC is used both with and without bar codes for products and supplies distributed within a health care facility. The LIC database provides identifiers that are key elements in EDI transaction messages. These globally unique identifiers are used for health care products, transplant organs, specimens, x-ray images, and procedures (Labeler Identification, n.d.).

Health Industry Bar Code

The Health Industry Bar Code (HIBC) Standard is composed of the Supplier Labeling Standard and the HIBC Provider Applications Standard. The HIBCC created this standard in an effort to reduce labor costs and human error. The Supplier Labeling Standard and the Provider Application Standard are ANSI approved (Bar Code Labeling Standard, n.d.).

Supplier Labeling Standard The Supplier Labeling Standard details the data structures and bar code types that are acceptable for the labeling of health care products. It identifies the labeler, the product code, and the unit of measure for each product. First approved in 1984, these standards recognized the need of the medical manufacturing industry to encode product identification using alphanumeric symbols.

Provider Application The Provider Application Standard is used for patient bar codes, specimen bar codes, intravenous admixture bar codes, and medical record/x-ray bar codes. The data structure carries information describing what the data are and where they are located. The identification must be specific enough to describe "where" the patient identity came from, that is, the patient wristband or the patient chart.

Health Industry Number

The HIN is assigned by HIBCC to every health care provider facility in the United States and was designed to be used for electronic communications. The HIN is the electronic "address" on the information superhighway; it is currently used by hospitals, nursing homes, buying groups, pharmacies, manufacturers, and distributors. It is widely used in the public and private sectors for EDI transactions. HIN databases identify customers by "facility address." The databases are composed of three separate files including the facility database, the prescriber database, and the animal health database (HIN System, n.d.).

Universal Product Number

The Universal Product Number (UPN) is based on the Supplier Labeling Standard. The UPN was developed to identify medical/surgical products in the supply chain and to facilitate product distribution. In 1995 the Department of Defense (DOD) adopted the UPN standard for all medical/surgical products sold to military hospitals. Subsequently, manufacturers of such products applied bar codes. The UPN was extended to other health care industries and to most countries in Europe, Latin America, Australia, and Canada (Mosher, 1996; Longe, 1999).

Universal Product Code

The Universal Product Code (UPC) is maintained by the Uniform Code Council and is typically used to label products that are sold in retail settings. Grocery retailers and manufacturers adopted the UPC in early 1970. Since that time it has been adopted for most retail products. The UPC is a 12-digit product identifier consisting of a 6-digit manufacturer identification number, a 5-digit item number, and a calculated check digit.

National Drug Code

The National Drug Code (NDC) was originally established by the FDA as an essential part of an out-of-hospital drug reimbursement program under Medicare. The NDC serves as a universal product identifier for human drugs. The current edition of the *National Drug Code Directory* is limited to prescription drugs and a few selected over-the-counter (OTC) products (HIBCC, 1994; Blair, 1996).

Once the patient, provider, site-of-care, and supply or product are uniquely identified, the electronic format of a clinical record can be transferred (communicated) from one site to another, or from one software application to another. The first set of technical standards, the General Communication Standards, is identified in Figure 17-1.

GENERAL COMMUNICATIONS (MESSAGE FORMAT) STANDARDS

These communication message standards are used for most electronic message transactions in health care and have been generally accepted both by users and by vendors. These standards are in various stages of development, but they are generally more mature than those in most of the other topic areas (Blair, 1996; Blair, 1999).

Health Level Seven

HL7 is one of several ANSI-accredited SDOs operating in the health care arena. HL7 develops specifications that allow different health care software applications to communicate with each other; the most widely used specification is a messaging standard that enables disparate health care applications to exchange key sets of clinical and administrative data. Like all ANSI-accredited SDOs, HL7 adheres to a strict and well-defined set of operating procedures that ensures consensus, openness, and balance of interest. There are 14 technical committees and 14 special interest working groups within HL7. The technical committees are directly responsible for the content of the standards. Special interest groups serve as a test bed for exploring new areas that may need coverage in HL7's published standards (Health Level Seven, n.d.; Williams, 1997).

The term *HL7* indicates that the message is an application or level seven message. *Level seven* refers to the highest level of the ISO's communications model for OSI—the application level. (See Box 17-3 for a description of the physical layers of the ISO module.) The application level addresses the definition of the data to be exchanged, the timing of the interchange, and the communication of certain errors to the application. The seventh level supports such functions as security checks, participant identification, availability checks, exchange mechanism negotiations, and most importantly, data exchange structuring (Health Level Seven, n.d.).

The format of HL7 messages conforms to HL7-specific encoding rules. The beginning of a segment is delimited by its three-letter code, such as MSH (the message header) or PID (patient identification); the vertical bar separates segments. The MSH segment accompanies every HL7 message, communicating information such as the version of the HL7 standard being used, the type of message being sent, and the encoding characters used for field and segment separators. Each segment is terminated with a carriage return; there is no special termination character to mark the end of the message. HL7 version 2.4 was approved by ANSI in October 2000. HL7 version 3.0, which is scheduled to be published and distributed to the HL7 membership near the end of 2001 (Health Level Seven, n.d.), will offer a defined method of structuring and designing messages so there is less room for interpretation by software vendors. The standard will use component technology and extensible markup language (XML) to achieve more interoperability between information systems. Version 3.0 will enable the transfer of structured content over the Internet. Another feature of version 3.0 will be the ability to cross-reference diagnostic codes from multiple clinical vocabularies (Chin, 1999). Plans are for version 3.0 to be published and ANSI approval obtained by winter 2002 (Health Level Seven, n.d.).

The most widely used HL7 specification, the Application Protocol for Electronic Data Exchange in Healthcare Environments, is a messaging standard that enables disparate health care applications to exchange data. In its simplest form, the standard provides the layout of messages that are exchanged between two or more applications. The developers of the HL7 Standard realized that real-world events, called trigger events, cause the need for information to be exchanged between two or more systems. For example, when a patient is admitted to an inpatient facility, the finance department needs to open an account for the patient. Using the HL7 Standard, information such as the patient's demographics and next-of-kin data that are collected by an Admissions, Discharge, and Transfer (ADT) system at the time of an inpatient admission are electronically transmitted to a financial system and used to establish an account for the newly admitted patient. Using the HL7 standard to exchange data between systems saves time and money by eliminating the need to rekey data into multiple systems and/or to develop custom interfaces that would otherwise enable two systems to exchange data (Health Level Seven, n.d.).

Common Object Request Broker Architecture

The member companies of the Object Management Group (OMG) produce and maintain a suite of specifications that support distributed, heterogeneous software development. One of these standards sets is referred to as CORBA (common object request broker architecture). OMG's CORBA consortium develops object-oriented interoperability standards. The standards support an open architecture and infrastructure that computer applications use to work together over networks. Using the standard protocol, a CORBA-based program on almost any computer, operating system, programming language, and network can interoperate with a CORBA-based program on almost any other computer, operating system, programming language, and network. CORBA is vendor-neutral middleware.

CORBA has authenticity as the ISO standard 14750. The CORBA Component Model (CCM) aims to improve adaptability and simplify the task of writing distributed applications. CORBA supports many types of hardware platforms, operating systems, programming languages, and network architectures and was designed to eliminate language barriers. CORBA MED uses existing health care content standards such as HL7, Unified Medical Language System (UMLS), and CEN TC 251. Its design is based on ISO standard translations for common middleware technologies including DICOM, Java, CORBA, and XML. CORBA MED includes standards for the following:

- Person Identification Service (PIDS) to enable master patient indexes
- Terminology Query Service (TQS) for access and translation between coded information in public and private terminologies
- Clinical Observation Access Service (COAS) to integrate clinical information in a distributed enterprise
- Healthcare Resource Access Decision (RAD) for application-level security policies

CORBA and CORBA MED are integral parts of the U.S. government Computer-Based Patient Record (G-CPR) framework (Marietti, 1998, 1999).

Institute of Electrical and Electronic Engineers P1157 Medical Data Interchange Standard

One of the standards for the exchange of data between hospital computer systems was developed by the Institute of Electrical and Electronic Engineers (IEEE) P1157 Medical Data Interchange Standard (MEDIX). Based on the ISO standards, MEDIX is working on a framework model to guide the development and evolution of a compatible set of standards. This activity has been carried forward as a joint working group under ANSI HISPP's Message Standards Developers Subcommittee (MSDS). IEEE is recognized as an accredited organization by ANSI (Blair, 1996).

Although general communications standards can be used for many electronic messages, each independent system or application also has a unique set of standards. See Figure 17-1 for a listing of the specific health care communication standards discussed in this chapter.

SPECIFIC COMMUNICATIONS STANDARDS

Many SDOs produce standards (sometimes called *specifications* or *protocols*) for a particular health care domain such as pharmacy, medical devices, imaging, or insurance (claims processing) transactions. This section discusses some of the more common specific communications standards used in health care.

Digital Imaging and Communications in Medicine

DICOM is the industry standard for transferral of radiological images and other medical information between computers. Developed by the American College of Radiology–National Electrical Manufacturers' Association (ACR-NEMA), DICOM defines the message formats and communications standards for diagnostic and therapeutic images. Most radiology Picture Archiving and Communications Systems (PACS) vendors support DICOM. DICOM permits the transfer of messages and images made by multiple vendors and located at one site or many sites to communicate across an open-system network. As a result, medical images can be captured and communicated more quickly, physicians can make diagnoses sooner, and treatment decisions can be made in a more timely manner (Blair, 1996; DICOM, 1997).

ASTM Communication Standards

ASTM E 1238 Standard Specification for Transferring Clinical Observations Between Independent Computer Systems

E 1238 was developed by ASTM Subcommittee E31.13 Clinical Laboratory Information Management. It enables any two systems to establish a link for communicating text to send results or request information in a standard and interpretable form. This standard is used by most of the commercial laboratory vendors in the United States to transmit laboratory results. It has also been incorporated into the Japanese (ISAC) standard. HL7 has incorporated E 1238 as a subset within its laboratory results message format (Blair, 1996; Wilhelm, 2000; Computer-Based Patient Record Institute, 1995). In addition to the ASTM E 1238 Standard, there are a number of guides developed by the ASTM subcommittees (Box 17-5). These guides offer directions without recommending a definite course of action. The purpose of these guides is to offer a consensus of viewpoints and increase the awareness of the user concerning available techniques (Wilhelm, 2000).

ASTM E 1394-97 Standard Specification for Transferring Information Between Clinical Instruments and Computer Systems

This standard covers the two-way digital transmission of remote requests and results between clinical instruments and computer systems. It is intended to document the common conventions required for the interchange of clinical results and patient data between clinical instruments and a computer system (ASTM, 1999b, 2000b). The clinical laboratory instruments are those that measure one or more parameters from one or more patient samples. Examples of automated instruments that measure many parameters from many patient samples include chemistry analyzers, hematology analyzers, and electrolyte analyzers. Typically the computer system will be a Laboratory Information Management System (LIMS) (ASTM, 2000b).

ASTM E 1460 Specification for Defining and Sharing Modular Health Knowledge Bases (Arden Syntax)

This specification covers the sharing of computerized health knowledge bases among personnel, information systems, and institutions. The Arden Syntax for knowledge representation is a balloted and internationally deployed standard that was created with the goal of allowing users to create and share pieces of medical knowledge in a form that can be used by computer systems. Because of a confluence of complementary activities within other standards groups, the Arden Syntax has come under the HL7 umbrella and is now maintained within the Clinical Decision Support Technical Committee of HL7 (Health Level Seven, n.d.; ASTM, 1999).

The Arden Syntax was developed primarily to address the need for "data-driven" decision support, which means that logic rules are invoked as a result of changes to patient data in a clinical system. The objective is to enable sharing of medical knowledge by providing a standard language for clinical decision rules. Clinical decision rules are encoded as medical-logic modules (MLMs). Each MLM also contains management information to help maintain a knowledge base of MLMs and links to other sources of knowledge. MLMs are commonly used to represent alerts and reminders in clinical-information systems. In May 1999, ANSI approved the Arden

Box 17–5 Guidelines for Clinical Laboratory Systems

These guidelines, developed by ASTM subcommittees, provide additional information pertaining to clinical laboratory information systems. A guideline is a compendium of information that does not recommend a specific course of action.

E 792 Standard Guide for Selection of a Clinical Laboratory Information Management System
This guide covers the selection, purchase, use, enhancement, and updating of computer technology supplied by a vendor as a complete system in the clinical laboratory.

E 1029 Standard Guide for Documentation of Clinical Laboratory Computer Systems
The documentation includes how users interact with and operate the system, training documentation, and reference documentation such as a terminal operator's guide.

E 1246 Standard Practice for Reporting Reliability of Clinical Laboratory Computer Systems
This practice describes a system for collecting data, maintaining records, and reporting on the reliability of operating clinical laboratory computer systems.

E 1381 Standard Specification for the Low-Level Protocol to Transfer Messages Between Clinical Laboratory Instruments and Computer Systems
This specification describes the electronic transmission of digital information between clinical laboratory instruments and computer systems.

E 1466 Standard Specification for the Use of Bar Codes on Specimen Tubes in the Clinical Laboratory
This specification stipulates the way bar-coded sample identification labels are applied to clinical specimen containers. Information technology is used to document the form, placement, and content of bar code labels on specimen tubes that are used on clinical laboratory analyzers. It enables laboratory information system vendors to produce reliable bar-coded symbols that are readable by any complying clinical laboratory analyzer vendor.

E 1639 Standard Guide for Functional Requirements of Clinical Laboratory Information Management Systems
This guide covers the capabilities needed for a logical structure of a Clinical Laboratory Information Management System (CLIMS). It is written so that both the vendors and developers of CLIMS and laboratory managers have a common understanding of the requirements and logical structure of a laboratory data system.

E 1712 Standard Specification for Representing Clinical Laboratory Test and Analyte Names
This specification covers the construction of elected laboratory procedure and analyte names because data concerning clinical laboratory procedures must identify these procedures in a common fashion if such data are to be transferred between databases or to be recognized in lookups or searches.

Syntax Standard Version 2.0 for Medical Logic Systems (Clinical Context Management, 1999; Broverman, 1999).

ASTM E 1467 Specification for Transferring Digital Neurophysiological Data Between Independent Computer Systems

This standard defines codes and structures needed to transmit electrophysiological signals and results produced by electroencephalograms (EEGs) and electromyograms (EMGs). The methods for encoding waveforms used in this standard would be suitable for encoding other tests involving waveforms such as electrocardiograms (ECGs), vascular/intracranial pressure monitoring, or gastrointestinal motility studies. It is similar in structure to the ASTM E 1238 for sending information from system to system and the HL7 formats. This standard is being adopted by all of the manufacturers of EEG systems (Blair, 1996; Blair, 1999; ASTM, 1999b).

Although the following standard is used for a specific purpose, it is shown in Figure 17-1 as the link between the transmission of the clinical codes and the payer of the test or procedure.

Accredited Standards Committee X12

The Accredited Standards Committee (ASC) X12, composed of cross-industry representation, delivers electronic data interchange (EDI) standards that interact with a multitude of eCommerce technologies and serves as a primary source for integrating electronic applications. The main objective of ASC X12 is to develop standards to facilitate electronic interchange relating to such business transactions as order placement and processing, shipping and receiving, invoicing, payment, cash application, insurance transactions, and others associated with the provision of products and services. The aim of ASC X12 is to structure standards so those computer programs can translate data to and from internal formats without extensive reprogramming. ASC X12 includes several subcommittees including ASC X12N, the subcommittee focused on standards related to insurance. Insurance is defined as including all products and services functionally equivalent to insurance, such as government health care programs like Medicare and Medicaid. All Medicare carriers and intermediaries have implemented ASC X12N standards for claims. Many other payers have followed HCFA's (now CMS) lead and implemented the standard as well (Blair, 1999; What Is ASC X12?, n.d.).

IEEE Medical Information Bus 1073 Standard for Medical Device Communications

The IEEE promotes the engineering process of electrical and information technologies and sciences. The scope of the Medical Information Bus (MIB) is to provide open systems applications. A Bus is a channel or path for transferring data or power from one of many sources to one or more destinations. The IEEE MIB Standard 1073 defines the linkages of medical instrumentation (e.g., critical care instruments) to point-of-care information systems. It addresses the needs of patient-connected bedside medical devices. The standard is designed for use by devices that are run by microcontrollers and microprocessors and have limited processing bandwidth available for communications. The MIB Standard is complementary to the HL7 Standard. Device data can be comprehensively and accurately captured with MIB and stored in an HL7-based data repository. The MIB defines a complete seven-layer communications stack for devices in acute care settings. The layering allows a plug-and-play interoperability between various devices. The lower layers of the IEEE standard cover the connections of patient monitors and infusion pumps. The lower layers are like a telephone line that carries the message to its destination in a reliable manner (IEEE, 1999; Blair, 1996).

Special Interest Group for Visual Information

The Special Interest Group for Visual Information (SIG VI) is a consortium of more than 20 clinical information systems vendors and pioneering end-user organizations. The group, formerly know as the Clinical Context Object Workgroup (CCOW), joined HL7 in 1998 (CCOW, 1998). The SIG VI publishes standards for the visual integration of cooperative interaction among independently authored health care applications at the point of use. The standard emphasizes applications with graphical user interfaces operating together on a personal computer or workstation. In July 2001 the Clinical Context Management (CCM) specifications (version 1.3) were approved as an ANSI standard. CCM supports specific plug-and-play capabilities based on component-based technology. The patient link capability maps patient identifiers across multiple applications and points all applications that are patient-link enabled to the same patient. The specification includes a high-level architecture that is technology neutral and maps to specific target technologies such as ActiveX (ANSI Approves Data Integration Standard, 2001).

The general and specific standards are aimed at the current legacy systems used in clinical applications. The content standards and guides are presented as ongoing work to create a true EHR, or computer-based patient record. See Figure 17-1 for the standards discussed in this section.

CONTENT AND STRUCTURE STANDARDS

Work in this area is primarily directed both at developing standards for the design of the EHR and on the Computer-Based Oral Health Record (COHR) (Blair, 1999). The guides offer direction based on agreement of viewpoints, but they do not establish a standard practice for users to follow.

ASTM E 1384–99e1 Standard Guide for Content and Structure of the Electronic Health Record

This guide covers all types of health care services, including those given in acute care hospitals, nursing homes, skilled nursing facilities, home health care, specialty care environments, and ambulatory care. The guide applies to both short-term contacts (e.g., emergency departments and emergency medical service units) and long-term contacts (primary care physicians with long-term patients). The purposes of the guide are as follows:

- Identify the content and logical structure of an EHR
- Define the relationship of data coming from diverse source systems
- Provide a common vocabulary, perspective, and references for those developing, purchasing, and implementing CPR systems
- Describe ways that logical data structures might be accessed or displayed
- Relate the logical structure of the EHR to the essential documentation currently used in the health care delivery system in the United States

The guide is divided into four parts:

- Part 1 identifies all of the information carried in the traditional patient record (doctor's progress notes, nurses' notes, ECG reports, etc.)
- Part 2 presents the operational principles of a computer-based patient record, including privacy and security
- Part 3 describes a common data model for an EHR
- Part 4 discusses the minimum data elements that should be contained in an EHR (descriptions of the longitudinal health record are included in this section)

The ASTM E 1384-99e1 (EHR guide) has been selected as the foundation EHR content requirement in the information services plans for several health care systems, including the Group Health Cooperative of Puget Sound, and as a component in the EHR plans of the Veterans Affairs (VA) Administration (ASTM, 1999, 2000a). Within the broad, general guidelines for an EHR, a group of guides and standards called **companion standards** address components of the EHR. See Box 17-6 for a listing of these companion standards and guides for the EHR, including the following:

- Guides for the description of reservation/registration, admission, discharge, and transfer (R-ADT) activities of patients in a health care institution (E 1239)
- The coded values recommended for use in an EHR (E 1633)

Box 17–6 Companion Standards for the Computer-Based Patient Record

ASTM E 1239-94 Standard Guide for Description of Reservation/Registration-Admission, Discharge, Transfer (R-ADT) Systems for Automated Patient Care Information Systems
This guide identifies the minimum information needed for the R-ADT functions. These R-ADT functions are used in an ambulatory care system or a hospital system. It is intended to assist in the application of information technology to the processes of patient registration and inpatient admission in health care institutions and the use of registration data in establishing the demographic segment of the automated patient care record (ASTM, 1999).

ASTM E 1284-97 Standard Guide for Construction of a Clinical Nomenclature for Support of Electronic Health Records
This guide covers the clinical terms used in everyday clinical communications. It is intended to list the concepts for a clinical nomenclature that is designed to support electronic health care records. The purpose of the guide is to describe the needed requirements for a nomenclature dedicated to clinical use and a way to maintain nationwide compatibility among electronic health records (ASTM, 1999).

ASTM E 1633-96 Standard Specification for Coded Values Used in the Computer-Based Patient Record
This specification covers the identification of the **lexicons** to be used for the data elements identified in Appendix X1 of Guide E 1384 (ASTM, 1999).

ASTM E 1715-99 Standard Practice for an Object-Oriented Model for Registration, Admitting, Discharge, and Transfer (RADT) Functions in the Computer-Based Patient Record System
This practice amplifies and complements other guides and standards by detailing the objects that make up the RADT functional domain of the primary record of care. This is the first model used to create a common library of objects and their attributes as applied to the health care domain. The object-oriented modeling domain is influential in all patient record and ancillary system functions, including messaging functions used in telecommunications. For example, it is applicable to clinical laboratory information management systems, pharmacy information management systems, and radiology, or other image management and information management systems. The object

Continued

Box 17–6 Companion Standards for the Computer-Based Patient Record—cont'd

model terminology is used to be compatible with other national and international standards for health care data and information systems engineering or telecommunications standards applied to health care data or systems. This practice is intended for those familiar with modeling concepts, system design, and implementation. It is not intended for the general computer user or as an initial introduction to the concepts.

ASTM E 1744-98 Standard Guide for a View of Emergency Medical Care in the Computerized Patient Record
This guide covers the identification of the information that is necessary to document emergency medical care in a computerized patient record that is part of a paperless patient record system. The intent of a paperless patient record system will be to improve efficiency and cost-effectiveness. It is intended to amplify guides E 1239, E 1384, and E 1715.

ASTM E 1769-95 Standard Guide for Properties of Electronic Health Records and Record Systems
This guide covers the current understanding of the requirements for the electronic health record (EHR), which is using currently available technology to document clinical activities and related information generated during the care of an individual (ASTM, 1999). The criteria and characteristics for an EHR include:

- A description of the data input and source identification
- A description of the longitudinal health record
- A description of the accessibility and reliability of the EHR
- The security of the EHR
- A description of the inference engine to create, use, and maintain rules to support the EHR
- A description of mechanisms to optimize practitioners' practices, including decision support tools, access to knowledge databases, outcome information, cost information, and quality assurance information

- E 1715 (Object-Oriented Model for the EHR)
- E 1744 (Guide for Emergency Medical Care in the EHR)

Computer-Based Oral Health Record

In the future the COHR will replace paper charts and enable better care delivery in the process. The COHR will contain all information that is now stored in hard copy records. Because this information can include text, numbers, drawings, models, images, or video, it is represented on the computer in multimedia format. **Multimedia** simply means that a record is stored in more than one medium such as text, audio, graphics, animated graphics, and full-motion video. COHRs enable mechanisms that are useful to tracking the oral health of individuals, practice populations, and communities in ways that the paper record cannot (Temple University, 1996).

The next section of technical standards contains the clinical data representation codes. See Figure 17-1 for a listing of the standards in this section. These clinical data codes are also discussed in Chapter 18 with other standardized languages. They are discussed in this chapter in terms of technical standards and coding schemes used to transmit the data in an electronic format.

Box 17–7 A Sample Coding Scheme for ICD-9

Angina (attack) (cardiac) (chest) (effort) (heart) (pectoris) (syndrome) (vasomotor) 413.9

Appendicitis 541
with perforation, peritonitis (generalized), or rupture 540.0
with peritoneal abscess 540.1
  peritoneal abscess 540.1
  acute (catarrhal) (fulminating) (gangrenous) (inflammatory) (obstructive) (retrocecal) (suppurative) 540.9
  with perforation, peritonitis, or rupture 540.0
  with peritoneal abscess 540.1
  peritoneal abscess 540.1

CLINICAL DATA REPRESENTATION (CODES)

Clinical data representation codes are widely used to document diagnoses and procedures. There are more than 150 known coding systems developed by different organizations with different focuses. The discussion of clinical codes in this section is centered on the technical standards and coding schemes used to transmit the data in an electronic format.

International Classification of Diseases, 9th Revision

The World Health Organization (WHO) *International Classification of Diseases, 9th Revision* (ICD-9), codes are primarily used in the United States to facilitate billing and other medical claims. These codes are accepted worldwide. In the United States, HCFA (now CMS) and the National Center for Health Statistics (NCHS) have supported the development of a clinical modification of the ICD codes (ICD-9-CM). An example of the ICD-9-CM coding scheme is shown in Box 17-7.

International Statistical Classification of Diseases and Related Health Problems, 10th Revision

The WHO has been developing the *International Classification of Diseases and Related Health Problems, 10th Revision* (ICD-10), which is currently used in several countries. CMS (formerly HCFA) has formed a voluntary technical panel to assist with the development of the ICD-10. However, CMS projects that it will be a few more years before ICD-10 will be available for use within the United States. Payers require the use of ICD-9-CM codes for reimbursement purposes. However, ICD-9 lacks clinical specificity and therefore has limited value for clinical and research purposes (Blair, 1996).

Current Procedural Terminology, 4th Edition

Current Procedural Terminology (CPT) codes are maintained by the American Medical Association (AMA) and are widely used in the United States for reimbursement and utilization review purposes. The CPT-4 is the fourth edition of these codes and descriptions. The codes are derived from medical specialty nomenclatures and are updated annually (Blair, 1996). For example, a procedure to measure pulmonary function before and after bronchodilation would be coded as follows: 94060 PRE and POST BD spirometry before and after a bronchodilator (or before and after exercise).

Systematized Nomenclature of Medicine

The Systematized Nomenclature of Medicine (SNOMED) is maintained by the College of American Pathologists (CAP). "SNOMED's design is based on the premise that a detailed and specific nomenclature is essential to accurately reflect, in computer readable format, the complexity and diversity of information found in a patient record" (CAP, 2000; SNOMED, n.d.).

It has a multiaxial (11 fields) coding structure that gives it greater clinical specificity than the ICD and CPT codes, and it has considerable value for clinical purposes. The CAP has begun to coordinate SNOMED development with the message standards organizations HL7 and ACR-NEMA (Clinical Vocabulary, 1999; www.snomed.org). See Chapter 18 for a description of the relational database and structured languages used in SNOMED-RT.

Diagnostic and Statistical Manual of Mental Disorders

The *Diagnostic and Statistical Manual of Mental Disorders* (DSM) is now in its fourth edition (DSM-IV). The American Psychiatric Association (APA) maintains this code structure. It sets forth a standard set of codes and descriptions for use in diagnoses, prescriptions, research, education, and administration for psychiatric and mental disorders (Blair, 1996; Hinckley, 1997). For example, the DSM-IV classification for "Dementia of the Alzheimer's Type, With Late Onset, Uncomplicated" has a numerical value of 290. "Dementia of the Alzheimer's Type, With Early Onset, With Delusions" is coded 290.12.

Diagnosis-Related Groups

Diagnosis-related groups (DRGs) classify hospital stays in terms of what was wrong with (major diagnosis) and what was done for (resources used) a patient. DRGs are maintained by CMS (formerly HCFA). They are derivatives of ICD-9-CM codes and are used to facilitate reimbursement and case-mix analysis. In the United States, the basic sets of DRG codes are those defined by CMS (formerly HCFA) for adult Medicare billing. For other patient types and payers such as Medicaid, commercial payers for neonate claims, and worker's compensation, DRG Groupers (CMS DRG Assignment software) and additional DRG codes are used (Blair, 1996).

National Drug Codes

The National Drug Codes (NDCs) are maintained by the FDA and are required for reimbursement by Medicare, Medicaid, and most commercial insurance companies. The NDCs serve as a universal product identifier for drugs used in human beings. The current edition of the NDC directory is limited to prescription drugs and a few selected over-the-counter products. Each drug product is assigned a unique 10-digit, 3-segment number. This number identifies the labeler/vendor, product, and trade package size (Blair, 1996; USFDA, 2000).

International Union of Pure and Applied Chemistry

The International Union of Pure and Applied Chemistry (IUPAC) is a voluntary nongovernmental, nonprofit organization that unites chemists from all over the world. It is recognized as the world authority on chemical nomenclature, terminology, and standardized methods for measurement, atomic weights, and many other critically evaluated data. The standardization of weights, measures, names, and symbols is essential to the smooth development and growth of international trade and commerce (IUPAC, 2000).

Emergency Care Research Institute Medical Equipment Codes

The Emergency Care Research Institute (ECRI) is an independent, nonprofit institution that provides the health care community, both nationally and internationally, with information about the safe and efficacious use of medical technology. The Health Devices Sourcebook, a directory file produced by ECRI, contains current address and marketing information on U.S. and Canadian manufacturers and distributors of more than 4500 classes of medical devices. The database uses ECRI's internationally endorsed Universal Medical Device Nomenclature System (UMDNS) and International Medical Device Codes (IMDC) for product classification. An online thesaurus is available as an aid in locating broader, narrower, and related product names.

The file contains three types of records: product (device) records, manufacturer records, and service records. International coverage of companies is also provided. The UMDNS is intended for classifying medical devices for purposes of indexing, storing, and retrieving device-related information (e.g., inventory control and adverse incident tracking). The UMDNS terms as well as the corresponding five-digit codes are widely incorporated into publications, databases, medical information systems, hazard-alerting systems, and other software used by government agencies, health care systems, and facilities worldwide (National Committee on Health and Vital Statistics, 2000).

STANDARDS FOR SOFTWARE APPLICATIONS

To transmit the identifier, general, specific, and content standards and clinical codes, a variety of software applications are required. In recent years there has been more interest in the use of Web technologies in health care. Web-related standards play a major role in distance education and telehealth. These standards are used to transfer information and data through the World Wide Web (WWW). They are important for use in health care informatics with applications that are developed to use the Web for transferring information from remote computers, such as in physicians' offices, to a hospital information system. Additional information concerning this group of standards is also presented in Chapter 11.

Standard Generalized Markup Language

Standard Generalized Markup Language (SGML) is an ISO standard that establishes rules for identifying elements within a text document. Once identified, or "tagged," the elements can be further interpreted by other markup languages such as hypertext markup language (HTML), standard markup language (SML), and dynamic hypertext markup language (DHTML). SGML promises to offer solutions for managing text-based information because it is a standard that is explicitly designed to provide mechanisms for encoding the contents of a virtually endless array of documents, from the very simple to the very complex (The Latest Word, 1999; Williams, 1997; Lincoln, Essin, Anderson, & Hare, 1994).

Extensible Markup Language

XML is a subset of the SGML defined in ISO Standard 8879:1986. It is designed to make it easy to interchange structured documents over the Internet. XML describes the content in terms of the data that are being described. XML files always clearly mark where the start and end of each of the logical parts (elements) of an interchanged document occur. XML restricts the use of SGML constructs to ensure that fallback options are available when access to certain components of the document are not currently possible over the Internet. It also defines how Internet uniform resource locators (URLs) can be used to identify component parts of XML data streams. By defining the role of each element of text in a formal model, known as a document type definition (DTD), users of XML can check that each component of document occurs in a valid place within the interchanged data stream. An XML DTD allows computers to check, for example, that users do not accidentally enter a third-level heading without first having entered a second-level heading, something that cannot be checked using HTML.

However, unlike SGML, XML does not require the presence of a DTD. If no DTD is available, either because all or part of it is not accessible over the Internet or because the user failed to create it, an XML system can assign a default definition for undeclared components of the markup. XML allows users to do the following (Anderson & Colin, 2000; An Introduction to the Extensible Markup Language, 1997):

- Bring multiple files together to form compound documents

- Identify where illustrations are to be incorporated into text files and the format used to encode each illustration
- Provide processing control information to supporting programs, such as document validators and browsers
- Add editorial comments to a file

Hypertext Markup Language

HTML is the authoring language used to create documents on the WWW. HTML is similar to SGML, although it is not a strict subset. HTML defines the structure and layout of a Web document by using a variety of tags and attributes. It is a collection of platform-independent styles (indicated by markup tags) that define the various components of a WWW document and how the content is displayed (HTML, 2000; Anderson & Colin, 2000).

Other Web Standards

The network interface device (NID) functions as an Internet access device and supports applications executed from browser-style commands in a Web-based environment. The NID, also referred to as a *thin client,* relies on Java and ActiveX programming technologies to compress data and application information so that applications and documents can be easily accessed and retrieved over a high-speed network. The data and application are transferred and downloaded to the NID flash memory via Java applets or ActiveX components. Java/ActiveX technologies compress the application and data structures for high-speed transport to the desktop. The NID supports the major Internet, WWW, and mail protocols for a robust application and communications environment (Gilreath, 1997).

ActiveX

ActiveX is grounded in Microsoft's Component Object Model (COM). Although COM is not accredited by an independent standards organization, it is so widely available that it is fast becoming a de facto standard. A number of applications support ActiveX/COM. MS-HUG is the health care task force group working on the development of these standards. The first reference for implementation was 1997. In addition to software required to carry the information, a mechanism is required to transmit the information. Telecommunication is the science or technology of communicating by telephone, telegraph, or computer. See Figure 17-1 for the telecommunications standards discussed in this section.

TELECOMMUNICATIONS STANDARDS

These standards are used to communicate information and **electronic commerce.** Electronic commerce is the exchange of business data among small and large businesses.

Data Interchange Standards Association

DISA is the foremost association for electronic commerce. DISA offers the world's leading conference on electronic commerce and provides a variety of seminars on various types of communications standards. DISA publishes implementation guides and the X12 standards and hosts standards-setting and networking forums. Representing eCommerce professionals from around the world, DISA's affiliation with electronic commerce user groups, the ASC X12 and many others facilitates an interchange of eCommerce topics for the global market. In an effort to facilitate emerging Internet technologies of U.S. and international eCommerce environments, the DISA committee is working on the next generation of EDI (DISA, 2000).

Local Area Network

A local area network (LAN) is a computer network that spans a relatively small area. Most LANs are confined to a single building or group of buildings connecting workstations and personal computers. Each node (individual computer) in a LAN has its own central processing unit (CPU) with which it executes programs, but it is also able to access data and devices anywhere on the LAN. This means that many users can share expensive devices, such as laser printers, as well as data. Users can also use the LAN to communicate with each other by sending eMail or engaging in chat sessions. The most common LAN for personal computers is an Ethernet. LANs are capable of transmitting data at very fast rates, much faster than data can be transmitted over a telephone line; however, the distances are limited, and there is also a limit on the number of computers that can be attached to a single LAN (Local-area network, 1998).

Wide Area Network

A system of LANs connected to other LANs over any distance via telephone lines and radio waves is called a wide area network (WAN). A WAN is a computer network that spans a relatively large geographical area. Computers connected to a WAN are often connected through public networks, such as the telephone system. They can also be connected through leased lines or satellites. The largest WAN in existence is the Internet (Wide-area network, 1997).

Imaging Standards

Imaging standards are used to transfer medical or other images such as pictures via computer systems. There are five types of standards relevant to medical imaging (Introduction to Medical Image Communication Standards, n.d.):

- Specific medical image communication standards (e.g., DICOM, MEDICOM)
- General imaging standards (e.g., IPI)
- Compression standards (e.g., JPEG, JBIG)
- Other medical imaging standards (e.g., IS&C, Interfile); these have been implemented but are not widely available
- General communications standards; these are of use in, or closely associated with, medical imaging

Infrared Standards

The Infrared Data Association (IrDA) is a group of device manufacturers that developed a standard for transmitting data via infrared light waves. Increasingly computers and other devices (such as printers) come with IrDA ports. This enables transfer of data from one device to another without cables. IrDA ports support roughly the same transmission rates as traditional parallel ports. The only restrictions on their use are that the two devices must be within a few feet of each other and there must be a clear line of sight between them. As health care informatics applications develop handheld devices, the transfer of data using infrared technology is increasing (HTML, 2000; IrDA, 1996).

Digital Subscriber Lines

Digital subscriber lines (DSLs) refer to all types of digital subscriber lines. DSL technologies use sophisticated modulation schemes to pack data onto copper wires. Modulation takes a **message-bearing signal** and superimposes it upon a **carrier signal** for transmission. DSLs are sometimes referred to as last-mile technologies because they are used only for connections from a telephone switching station to a home or office, not between switching stations. xDSL is similar to an Integrated Services Digital Network (ISDN) inasmuch as both operate over existing copper telephone lines (plain old telephone service [POTS]) and both require short runs to a central telephone office (usually less than 20,000 feet). However, xDSL offers much higher speeds—up to 32 million bits per second (mbps) for downstream traffic, and from 32 kilobits per second (kbps) to more than 1 mbps for upstream traffic (POTS, 1998; xDSL, 2000).

Plain Old Telephone Service

POTS refers to the standard telephone service that most homes use. In contrast, telephone services based on high-speed digital communications lines, such as ISDN and Fiber Distributed Data Interface (FDDI), are not POTS. The main distinctions between POTS and non-POTS services are speed and bandwidth. POTS is generally restricted to about 52 kbps (52,000 bits/second). The POTS network is also called the public switched telephone network (PSTN) (POTS, 1998). Additional information on these standards can be found in Chapter 11.

CONCLUSION

The first electronic health care applications were developed for niche or stand-alone applications in financial and/or billing departments. Early applications used mainframe computers to hold and manage the volume of data collected. As other applications were developed, the need to transmit data between applications and systems developed. In recent years the computer environment has moved to a distributed environment operating on personal computers.

The health care industry in the United States has grown and changed as a result of technological and health care innovations, the rules of business, marketplace globalization, corporate mergers, and efforts to obtain larger market shares. The result is an increased need for information sharing and decision support to manage complex health care environments. In the current health care informatics arena, a number of technical standards and committees are supporting the development of standards necessary for information sharing and decision support. In addition to work by a variety of U.S. committees, a number of international committees are striving to design and develop technical standards for health care delivery. Although each of these committees is diligently working on technical standards, the lack of a single national standardizing body in the United States and the lack of mandated standards have slowed the development of integrated health care computing in this country. The move to a global market is also slowed by the lack of standards.

The standards required to transmit electronic health data for the HIPAA of 1996 have accelerated the development of electronic data interchange standards. Suppliers of electronic health care applications are striving to meet the disparate requirements to link and transmit data between applications and systems. However, the expense of changing software applications to meet multiple standards and operate on multiple platforms increases the cost of the software applications. The decision to adopt a particular standard is often time-consuming and difficult when these decisions depend on fragmented national standards for privacy, security, and confidentiality, as well as fragmented technical infrastructure standards that are required to transmit data across systems. The lack of national and international health care informatics standards is a major barrier to the implementation of an EHR. Until information is collected and maintained in a common format, it will be impossible to create a true lifetime EHR.

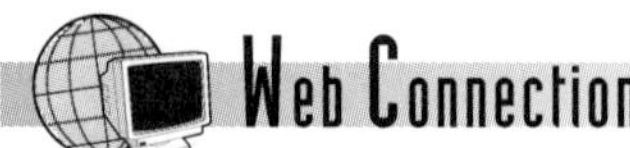

Web Connection

The use of commonly agreed upon standards is bringing the health care industry closer to integrated information systems that allow easy data exchange and knowledge discovery in data sets. Technical standards focus on the processing and management aspects of information such as production, use, and archiving. The Web Connection activities examine the standards and organizations introduced in the chapter to provide an understanding of the complexity of the infrastructure behind information use, management, and archiving in health care. You will visit Web sites that describe the positions, foci, and practice areas affected by work on technical standards.

discussion questions

1. Why are technical health care standards needed and how are they used?
2. Identify three major types of technical health care standards. What is the purpose of each type of standard?
3. What is the purpose of SDOs in the United States? Identify the key SDOs and include a description of the organizations and the type of standards developed by each organization.
4. Discuss the major types of technical standards used in an EHR. Which organization is responsible for each standard? What is the interrelation among the standards?

REFERENCES

About Computing Technology Industry Association. (2000). Oakbrook, IL: Author. Retrieved October 25, 2000, from the World Wide Web: http://www.comptia.org/aboutus/index/htm.

Accredited Standards Committee (ASC) X12. (2000). *Health care task*. Washington, DC: American National Standards Institute. Retrieved May 25, 2000, from the World Wide Web: http://aspe.hhs.gov/admnsimp/hisbinv2.htm.

Agency for Health Care Policy and Research. (1999). *Health care informatics standards activities of selected federal agencies: A compendium.* Washington, DC: Author. Retrieved August 27, 2000, from the World Wide Web: http://www.ahcpr.gov/data/datameet.htm.

American Dental Association for Accredited Standards Committee MD156. (1997). Chicago, IL: Author. Retrieved May 23, 2000, from the World Wide Web: http://www.va.gov/publ/standard/health/ADA.htm.

American National Standards Institute. (2000). *An introduction to ANSI American National Standards Institute.* Washington, DC: Author. Retrieved May 27, 2000, from the World Wide Web: http://web.ansi.org/public/ansi_info/ansi_iso.html.

American Society for Testing and Materials. (1999a). ASTM E 1714-95 standard guide for properties of a Universal Healthcare Identifier (UHID). *Annual Book of ASTM Standards* (Vol. 14.01, Healthcare Informatics: Computerized Systems and Chemical and Material Information). West Conshohocken, PA: Author.

American Society for Testing and Materials. (1999b). *Annual Book of ASTM Standards* (Vol. 14.01, Healthcare Informatics: Computerized Systems and Chemical and Material Information). West Conshohocken, PA: Author.

American Society for Testing and Materials. (2000a). *E1384-99e1 standard guide for content and structure of the electronic health record (EHR).* West Conshohocken, PA: Author. Retrieved May 27, 2000, from the World Wide Web: http://www.astm.org/cgi-bin/SoftCart.exe/DATABASE.CART/PAGES/E1384.htm?L+mystore+eenj9364+959410877.

American Society for Testing and Materials. (2000b). *E1394-97 standard specification for transferring information between clinical instruments and computer systems.* West Conshohocken, PA: Author. Retrieved October 17, 2000, from the World Wide Web: http://astm.micronexx.com/DATABASE.CART/PAGES/E1394.htm.

Anderson, M., & Colin, J. (2000). XML—Helping exchange data on the Internet. *Internet Health Care Magazine, March/April,* 87-88.

ANSI approves data integration standard. (2001). *Health Data Management.* Retrieved August 26, 2001, from the World Wide Web: http://www.healthdatamanagement.com/HDMSearchResultsDetails.cfm?DID=8455.

Appavu, S. (1999). Unique patient identifiers—What are the options? *Journal of AHIMA,* October, 50-57. Retrieved May 18, 2000, from the World Wide Web: http://www.ahima.org/journal/features/feature.9910.2.html.

Bar Code Labeling Standard. (n.d.). Retrieved October 20, 2000, from the World Wide Web: http://www.hibcc.org/auto.htm.

Blair, J.M. (1996). *An overview of healthcare information standards.* Retrieved May 18, 2000, from the World Wide Web: http://www.cpri.org/resource/index.html.

Blair, J.M. (1999). *Setting up healthcare services information systems: A guide for requirements analysis, application specification, and procurement* (CD-ROM, Section F, Standards p. 6). Washington, DC: Pan American Health Organization.

Brandt, M.D. (2000). Health informatics standards: A user's guide. *Journal of AHIMA,* April, 39-43. Retrieved May 18, 2000, from the World Wide Web: http://www.ahima.org/journal/features/feature.0004.1.html.

Broverman, C.A. (1999, Summer). Standards for clinical decision support systems. *Journal of the Healthcare Information and Management Systems Society.* Retrieved April 10, 2000, from the World Wide Web: http://www.himss.org/himss-nbin/loadframes?/jhim.side.nav.html?membersl/members/secure/journal/14-1/14-1.index.html.

Chin, T.L. (1999). New HL7 standard strives to achieve plug-and-play. *Health Data Management, 7*(2), 136-138, 140, 142, 144.

Chute, C.G. (1999). ISO TC 215: What the health world needs now. *MD Computing, 16*(3), 21-22.

Clinical context management specifications becomes a new ANSI national standard. (1999). *HIMSS News, 10*(12), 8.

The Clinical Context Object Workgroup: Its standard and methods. (1998). Retrieved May 25, 2000, from the World Wide Web: http://www.hl7.org/special/Committees/ccow_sigvi.htm.

Clinical vocabulary hits high gear. (1999). *Healthcare Informatics, 16*(2), 30.

College of American Pathologists. (2000). *About SNOMED.* Retrieved July 10, 2001, from the World Wide Web: http://www.snomed.org/.

Computer-Based Patient Record Institute. (1995). *Description of the Computer-Based Patient Record (CPR) and Computer-Based Patient Record System.* Retrieved June 6, 2000, from the World Wide Web: http://www.cpri.org/resource/index.html.

Current State of Technology. (1995). *Electronic network solutions for rising healthcare costs.* Retrieved October 25, 2000, from the World Wide Web: http://www.njit.edu/njIT/Publications/Reports/HINT/CHAPTER3.htm.

Data Interchange Standards Association (DISA). (2000). Alexandria, VA: Author. Retrieved May 27, 2000, from the World Wide Web: http://www.disa.org/aboutdisa.htm.

Data Interchange Standards Association. (2000). *Pan American EDIFACT Board (PAEB).* Alexandria, VA: Author. Retrieved May 21, 2000, from the World Wide Web: http://www.disa.org/paeb.

DICOM: The value and importance of an imaging standard. (1997). Oak Brook, IL: Author. Retrieved June 3, 2000, from the World Wide Web: http://www.rsna.org/REG/practiceres/dicom/index.html.

Economic and Social Council Subsidiary Bodies. (2000). New York: United Nations. Retrieved October 27, 2000, from the World Wide Web: http://www.un.org/esa/coordination/ecosoc/subsidiary.htm.

EDIFACT. (2000). UN/EDIFACT Working Group Organisation. New York: United Nations. Retrieved October 27, 2000, from the World Wide Web: http://www.edifact-wg.org.

Gilreath, H. (1997, March). The thin client: Let the feast begin. *Healthcare Informatics.* Retrieved April 10, 2000, from the World Wide Web: http://www.healthcareinformatics.com/issues/1997/03_97/cover.htm.

Health Care Financing Administration. (1999a). *National provider identifier frequently asked questions.* Washington, DC: Author. Retrieved October 13, 2000, from the World Wide Web: http://www.hcfa.gov/stats/npi/faq3%2D99.htm.

Health Care Financing Administration. (1999b). *The national provider identifier (NPFI).* Washington, DC: Author. Retrieved May 21, 2000, from the World Wide Web: http://www.hcfa.gov/stats/npi/overview.htm#hipaa.

Health Industry Business Communications Council. (1994). *Standards for bar coding.* Retrieved February 28, 2000, from the World Wide Web: http://www.hibcc.org/barcodel.htm.

Health Industry Number (HIN) System. (n.d.). Retrieved October 20, 2000, from the World Wide Web: http://www.hibcc.org/hin.htm.

Healthcare Informatics Standards Board (HISB). (2000). Washington, DC: American National Standards Institute. Retrieved August 26, 2000, from the World Wide Web: http://www.ansi.org/rooms/room_41/default.htm.

Hinckley, N. (1997). The cure for interoperability headaches? *ADVANCE for Health Information Executives, 1*(5), 27-29. Retrieved June 5, 2000, from the World Wide Web: http://www.appi.org/dsm.html.

HIPAA. (2000a). *NPI standards.* Phoenix Health Systems: Gaithersburg, MD. Retrieved October 28, 2000, from the World Wide Web: http://www.HIPAAdvisory.com/regs/natstandardhcprovidid/npistandard.htm.

HIPAA. (2000b). *Unique identifier.* Phoenix Health Systems: Gaithersburg, MD. Retrieved October 28, 2000, from the World Wide Web: http://www.hipaadvisory.com/action/faqs/FAQ_Identifiers.htm.

Health Level Seven. (n.d.). *HL7 standards.* Ann Arbor, MI: Author. Retrieved May 29, 2000, from the World Wide Web: http://www.hl7.org.

HTML. (2000). Retrieved May 28, 2000, from the World Wide Web: http://webopedia.internet.com/TERM/H/HTML.html.

Infrared Data Association. (1996). Retrieved May 28, 2000, from the World Wide Web: http://webopedia.internet.com/TERM/I/IrDA.html.

Institute of Electrical and Electronic Engineers. (1999, August). *The relationship between IEEE 1073 and HL7.* Retrieved June 2, 2000, from the World Wide Web: http://www.manta.ieee.org/groups/mib/articles/hl7&mib.pdf.

International Organization for Standardization. (n.d.a). *Introduction: What is ISO?* Retrieved July 3, 2001, from the World Wide Web: http://www.iso.ch/iso/en/aboutiso/introduction/whatisISO.html.

International Organization for Standardization. (n.d.b). *Standards development: List of technical committees.* Retrieved July 3, 2001, from the World Wide Web: http://www.iso.ch/iso/en/stdsdevelopment/tc/tclist/TechnicalCommitteeList.TechnicalCommitteeList.

International Union of Pure and Applied Chemistry. (2000). *About IUPAC.* Retrieved September, 12, 2000, from the World Wide Web: http://www.iupac.org/general/about.htm.

An introduction to the extensible markup language (XML). (1997). Retrieved May 27, 2000, from the World Wide Web: http://www.personal.u-net.com/~sgml/xmlintro.htm.

Introduction to medical image communication standards. (n.d.). Retrieved May 27, 2000, from the World Wide Web: http://www.standards.nhsia.nhs.uk/spg/step/stepdocs/H223-2.htm.

ISO Easy. (2000). *What are ISO 9000 and ISO 9001? International standards for quality assurance.* Middletown, NJ: Author. Retrieved April 11, 2000, from the World Wide Web: http://www.isoeasy.org.

ISO 9000 translated into plain English. (2000). Retrieved April 11, 2000, from the World Wide Web: http://connect.ab.ca/~praxiom/.

Labeler Identification. (n.d.). Retrieved October 20, 2000, from the World Wide Web: http://www.hibcc.org/auto.htm.

The latest word (1999). *Healthcare Informatics, 16*(1), 57-58, 60-62, 64-67.

Lincoln, T.L., Essin, D.J., Anderson, R., & Hare W.H. (1994). *The introduction of a new document processing paradigm into health care computing: A CAIT Whitepaper.* Santa Monica, CA: Rand Corp. Retrieved February 10, 2000, from the World Wide Web: http://www.mcis.duke.edu.

Local-area network. (1998). Retrieved May 25, 2000, from the World Wide Web: http://webopedia.internet.com/TERM/l/local_area_network_LAN.html.

Longe, K.M. (1999). *UPN bar code labeling: A guide for implementation in healthcare.* Retrieved October 13, 2000, from the World Wide Web: http://upnTOC.htm.

Marietti, C. (1998). ActiveX vs. CORBA. *Healthcare Informatics, 15*(11). Retrieved April 10, 2000, from the World Wide Web: http://www.healthcare-informatics.com/issues/1998/11_98/activex.htm.

Marietti, C. (1999). Middle managers. *Healthcare Informatics, 16*(10), 28.

Mosher, W.M. (1996). *Bar code standards: For medical products, more work is needed.* Retrieved October 13, 2000, from the World Wide Web: http://www.devicelink.com/mddi/archive/96/09/005.html.

National Committee on Health and Vital Statistics. (2000). *Report to the secretary on uniform standards for patient medical records.* Retrieved August 26, 2000, from the World Wide Web: http://www.ncvhs.hhs.gov/.

National Council Clinical Laboratory Systems. (1998). Retrieved May 23, 2000, from the World Wide Web: http://www.nccls.org/.

Paul, L. (1998). Public outcry over patient IDs. *Healthcare Informatics, 15*(9), 17.

POTS. (1998). Retrieved May 25, 2000, from the World Wide Web: http://www.webopedia.com/TERM/P/POTS.html.

Temple University. (1996). *Temple University School of Dentistry Session summary—The Computer-Based Oral Health Record.* Philadelphia: Author. Retrieved May 27, 2000, from the World Wide Web: http://www.temple.edu/dentistry/di/curric/di96/cohr.htm.

United Nations Centre for Trade Facilitation and Electronic Business. (2000). *Knowledge of UN/CEFACT.* Geneva, Switzerland: United Nations Economic Commission for Europe. Retrieved October 27, 2000, from the World Wide Web: http://www.unc\ece.org/cefact/knowledge.htm.

United Nations Directories for Electronic Data Interchange for Administration, Commerce and Transport. (1995). Geneva, Switzerland: United Nations Economic Commission for Europe. Retrieved October 26, 2000, from the World Wide Web: http://www.unece.org/trade/untdid/.

United Nations Economic Commission of Europe. *The UN/ECE in a nutshell.* (n.d.). Retrieved March 25, 2001, from the World Wide Web: http://www.unece.org/oes/eceintro.htm.

U.S. Food and Drug Administration. (2000). *The national drug code directory.* Washington, DC: Author. Retrieved August 26, 2000, from the World Wide Web: http://www.fda.gov/cder/ndc/.

Vargo, J., & Hunt, R. (1996). *Telecommunications in business strategy and application* (pp. 152-154). Boston: Irwin McGraw-Hill.

What Is ASC X12? (n.d.). Retrieved October 20, 2000, from the World Wide Web: http://www.x12.org/x12org/about/index.html?whatis.html.

Wide-area network. (1997). Retrieved May 26, 2000, from the World Wide Web: http://webopedia.internet.com/TERM/w/wide_area_network_WAN.html.

Wilhelm, R. (2000). Know your types of standards. *ASTM Standardization News, 28*(10), 22-23.

Williams, J.P. (1997). *Healthcare informatics standards: An electronic health record developer's perspective.* Retrieved May 19, 2000, from the World Wide Web: http://www.hytime.org/ihc97/papers/williams.html.

xDSL. (2000). Retrieved August 28, 2000, from the World Wide Web: http://webopedia.internet.com/TERM/x/xDSL.html.

CHAPTER 18

Professional Health Care Informatics Standards

CAROL J. BICKFORD

Learning Objectives

Upon completion of the chapter, the reader will be able to:

1. ***Describe*** three characteristics of a health care profession.
2. ***Identify*** three groups of health care professionals and explain how each might implement professional standards.
3. ***Differentiate*** between the internal and external regulatory activities and the standards affecting a specific health care profession.
4. ***Discuss*** the various organizing frameworks that health care professionals use during their work.
5. ***Identify*** at least one standardized language or code set for each phase of health care delivery that can describe the associated activities.
6. ***Discuss*** how the National Guidelines Clearinghouse supports quality in health care.
7. ***Describe*** two health care evaluation programs and how they use standards to measure quality of care.

Outline

Key Terms

ASTM Committee E31
credentialing
Health Plan Employer Data and Information Set (HEDIS)
Logical Observation Identifiers Names and Codes (LOINC)
medical logic modules (MLMs)
National Practitioner Databank–Healthcare Integrity Protection Database (NPD-HIPD)
Nursing Management Minimum Data Set (NMMDS)
NURSYS

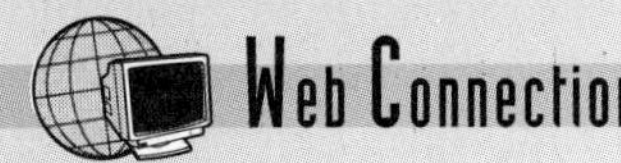

Go to the Web site at http://evolve.elsevier.com/Englebardt/. Here you will find Web links and activities related to professional health care informatics standards.

Every health care system involves people engaged in their roles as clinicians, administrators, educators, researchers, and finally, consumers, who are identified as patients when they have some health problem, injury, or disease. Each professional interacts with others within the health care system and uses other health care resources to complete activities whose purpose is to accomplish specific health goals or targeted outcomes. All of these initiatives, including the patient-clinician encounter can be depicted by the concept of complexity.

The richly detailed data and information about individuals and their characteristics, activities, and relationships within the context of the health care setting compose a portion of the content that informatics professionals address and information systems capture, process, store, and communicate. Many external environmental influences affect the health care system and its internal informatics environment. This chapter explores the relationship and impact of various professional standards on health care information systems.

THE PEOPLE WITHIN A HEALTH CARE SYSTEM

Many types of individuals and groups can be identified within a health care system. Because this chapter addresses professional standards in health care, this discussion about people is limited in focus to health care consumers and health care professionals.

Health Care Consumers

The health care delivery system is evolving from an illness treatment model to a system that includes health promotion activities and a focus on maintaining wellness. At times, these changes seem to be moving at the rate of a slow-moving glacier. Therefore health care consumers continue to be identified as patients, regardless of the care setting, in professional literature, languages, health care system models, databases, and information systems that collect and process data and report information about health care consumers and health care resources.

Labeling all health care consumers as patients is complicated by the current definition of the word *patient. Patient* may refer to a single individual, an unborn child, a group of individuals constituting a family, a group of individuals referenced as a community, a group of individuals considered to be a population, or an aggregate of communities (also known as a population). These apparent inconsistencies and incompatibilities in the use of *patient* demand constant scrutiny by vigilant informatics professionals to ensure the construction and implementation of correct identification strategies and information structures. The application of appropriate standards, data definitions, and algorithms is critical to ensure the assignment and maintenance of unique patient identifiers. The informatics professional must consult with applicable health care professionals to facilitate correct decision making in naming and labeling individuals as patients or health care consumers.

Health Care Professionals

Although the health care industry includes the use of increasing numbers of technology and computer applications and instruments, it remains labor intensive, relying on many people to provide care, support, and administrative services. Titles of health care professionals and their assignments and professional activities vary depending on their assumed professional roles in various work settings. Health professionals tend to be part of a very mobile workforce, often moving from location to location in their daily activities. Professionals need unique identifiers, just as do the health care consumers they serve, as tracking mechanisms to link them to decisions, outcomes, and resource utilization. Using recognized standards to create uniform identification processes and naming conventions that use a set of rules for item names, architecture, and the user interface assists in creating high-quality data and information.

Health care system workers may be categorized as professionals or nonprofessionals. The professionals claim membership in a profession that has the following characteristics (Wilson & Neuhauser, 1982):

- A defined body of scientific knowledge and certain required technical skills
- A code of ethics
- A national or regional professional association
- Formal education and examination required for membership in the profession
- Certification or licensure required for membership in the profession

Another characteristic is that members of the profession demonstrate expertise in decision making in their area and practice with a degree of authority.

The professional is educated through undergraduate and graduate academic programs that include content structured to prepare the professional to pass certification or licensure examinations that test for required knowledge and skills. During professional development experiences, the professional-in-training most often learns about the mandate for professionals to conduct themselves in accordance with a specific code of ethics and may be introduced to the importance of the national professional association. The individual may also learn about the value and necessity of becoming an active member of one or more specialty professional organizations, such as pediatric nursing, ophthalmology, oral surgery, neurology, internal medicine, health care informatics, or nursing informatics. Professionals appreciate their own roles and their contributions toward the development of professional standards.

Code of Ethics

One characteristic of a profession is the presence of a code of ethics. A code of ethics provides the public with a list of principles and values that are foundational to the profession and that are embraced by those who practice the profession. The professional association serves as the developer and custodian of the code and undertakes periodic reviews and revisions of that code. Those wishing to learn about a profession and its accountability statement can begin by reviewing its code of ethics. For example, the following professional organizations have posted their professional code of ethics statements on their public Web sites:

- American Association of Pastoral Counselors (AAPC)
- American Dental Association (ADA)
- American Dietetic Association (ADA)
- American Health Information Management Association (AHIMA)
- American Medical Association (AMA)
- American Nurses Association (ANA)
- American Pharmaceutical Association (APhA)
- American Physical Therapy Association (APTA)
- American Psychological Association (APA)
- Association for Computing Machinery (ACM)
- Institute of Electrical and Electronics Engineers, Inc. (IEEE)
- International Association of Medical Laboratory Technologists (IAMLT)
- Medical Library Association (MLA)
- National Association of Social Workers (NASW)
- Software Engineering Coordinating Committee (SWECC)

For almost every one of these organizations, access to and use of information are key aspects of the code of ethics.

Abdelhak, Grostick, Hanken, and Jacobs (2001) discuss the integration into practice of several tenets from the American Health Information Management Association's (AHIMA) Code of Ethics. This code mandates that the health information management professional respect the rights and dignity of all individuals. The AHIMA Code of Ethics also highlights the professional's responsibility to promote and protect the confidentiality of primary and secondary health records and health information. By the nature of their role, health care informatics professionals often gain knowledge of privileged corporate and operational information, which should be kept confidential and secure. Similarly, other codes of ethics for health care professionals include language mandating protection of patient privacy and patient information confidentiality by all its members. These responsibilities may not be recognized or shared by other individuals or professionals not associated with health care and may result in professional conflict.

Professional organizations often incorporate content from their code of ethics in their other publications. For example, the American Nurses Association (ANA) references the *Code of Ethics for Nurses* (ANA, 2001) in the *Scope and Standards of Nursing Informatics Practice* (2001) and the earlier version of that code in the second edition of the *Standards of Clinical Nursing Practice* (ANA, 1998), *Scope and Standards of Public Health Nursing Practice* (ANA, 1999), *Scope and Standards of Psychiatric–Mental Health Nursing Practice* (ANA, 2000), *Standards of Practice for Nursing Informatics* (ANA, 1995), and other nursing specialty scope and standards documents. Although health care professionals may not consciously consider using codes of ethics in their daily work or informatics activities, they have integrated key content from the appropriate code of ethics into all aspects of their professional conduct and decision making.

Regulations, Statutes, and Credentials

Although a health care profession monitors and regulates its own practice and the practice of its professionals, there are also external controls on the profession. External controls may include state legislation in the form of statutes and regulations that establish professional practice acts and licensure requirements. Health care professionals must comply with these rules to obtain and maintain current licenses to practice. Failure to do so incurs certain penalties. This control process is meant to assure the public that the professional has specific competencies and has met the minimal qualifications to provide professional services. In addition, external controls may include federal rules and laws governing reimbursement and prescriptive authority for health care clinicians. Often these regulations include specific coding and reporting requirements that need to be considered in the development and implementation of information systems.

Because health care employers are often mandated to verify that their professional employees have valid, current professional licenses, credentialing processes are established. In addition, **credentialing** usually involves confirmation of educational preparation, experience, employment history, and level of prescriptive authority.

Maintenance of licensing and credentialing information is now supported by electronic databases, which may or may not be accessible to the public. Health care consumers and professionals are finding that more and more states have posted licensee information about health care professionals on government Internet sites as part of initiatives to increase access to public records. There is increased interest in including disciplinary actions in these public records. Members of the various professions have also expressed concern when these information displays include personal residence addresses and current telephone numbers.

Although electronic databases may begin as stand-alone proprietary entities, new reporting

Table 18–1 NURSYS Content and Definitions

Content	Definition
Personal information	A nurse's identity and specified residential/mailing addresses
License description information	Information about an individual's nursing license
Education information	Information about an individual's education relative to nursing and a specific license
Disciplinary action information	Information about disciplinary actions taken against and reported for an individual
Verification request and fee tracking information	Information about the tracking of the receipt of verification requests and associated fee payments from an individual and the licensing member board's verification review process
Historical information	Any changes to the types of data mentioned above will cause the original information to be kept as history
Source information	Source of each piece of data is tracked so that appropriate security measures can be enforced

From National Council of State Boards of Nursing. (1999). Frequently asked questions about NURSYS. Retrieved November 15, 2000, from the World Wide Web: http://www.ncsbn.org.

requirements require linkages among databases. Examples of professional databases are **NURSYS,** a central repository of nurse license information throughout the United States and its territories, created by the National Council of State Boards of Nursing (NCSBN); the American Medical Association's (AMA's) Masterfile, a comprehensive and accurate source of physician information, with profiles of more than 700,000 physicians; and Health carePro Connect, established by the AMA in 2000 to provide an accurate and comprehensive information source about physicians and other health care professionals. These databases contain data and information that must be reported to the National Practitioner Data Bank, which is maintained by the U.S. Department of Health and Human Services, Health Resources and Services Administration, Bureau of Health Professions. See Table 18-1 for examples of information contained in the NURSYS database, with a definition of each content element.

Professional Standards

Professions often elect to define additional specific standards that reflect an even greater commitment to the public. This voluntary professional self-monitoring process may even prevent imposition of legislative and regulatory constraints.

In this instance, professional standards are authoritative statements that provide direction for practice and describe the profession's responsibilities for which it is accountable to the public. Professional standards include measurable criteria and provide a framework for evaluation (ANA, 1998). If the profession has established specialty and subspecialty groups, each of these may have specialty standards of practice that build on the general, overarching professional standards but also reflect the uniqueness of the specialty. For example, the nursing profession has standards of practice for nursing informatics that build on the profession's standards of clinical practice but also describe practice and professional performance for nurses engaged in the specialty of nursing informatics practice (ANA, 2001).

Groups of Health Care Professionals

Although physicians and registered nurses are the most often named health care professionals, other professionals who are integral to the health care system should also be represented in standards development and other health care informatics discussions. Laboratory technologists, dietitians, pharmacists, physical and occupational therapists, and registered health information administrators (RHIAs), formerly known as registered record administrators (RRAs), participate in the life cycle of health care information systems. Social workers and chaplains are seldom consulted, although they access and document patient information. Dentists, audiologists, epidemiologists, and public health officers practice primarily in ambulatory care settings and have somewhat different health care information requirements. Other support and administrative services professionals include medical librarians, professional development educators, health services administrators, and accountants, as well as human resources, quality improvement, information management, and facilities and operations management professionals. Veterinarians and researchers are other groups of health care professionals who have unique data, information, and knowledge management needs. Such a cosmopolitan constituency, with diverse data and information needs and knowledge work activities, demands similar diversity in its supporting information systems.

Frameworks for Information Management and Knowledge Work

Most health care professionals rarely, if ever, recognize and appreciate that they are always doing information management and knowledge work. Their role models and educational systems prepare them for their responsibilities and work as clinicians, administrators, educators, and researchers. However, the perspective of information and knowledge creation, use, and dissemination has not been a historical focus.

The clinician invests heavily in data and information retrieval activities and knowledge work to make evidence-based patient care decisions. The administrator seeks answers and crafts plans on the basis of available information resources and projections. Educators and researchers use clinical and other health care information in their work. Both educators and researchers have assimilated and, sometimes unknowingly, integrated professional standards into their decision-making framework and problem-solving strategies.

Health care professionals focus their attention on health care delivery events. The clinician is concerned about actually providing direct patient care activities, whereas the administrator focuses on the enterprise, surrounding environment, resources, quality issues, and business processes to support direct patient care delivery. The researcher may examine specific health care clinical events and outcomes or related nonclinical activities, products, services, or other concepts or entities. The educator is a specialist in providing academic, professional development, or patient education activities, or any combination of these or other educational activities.

Significant record-keeping functions are integral to the work of all health care professionals. In the past, record-keeping activities primarily focused on creating paper-based, handwritten documentation, often in the form of patient charts, personal notes, logbooks, laboratory notebooks, reports, presentations, and correspondence. The introduction of automated instrumentation and information systems has not always reduced the professional's record-keeping responsibilities or burden. Automated media may produce faster, more legible, and more accessible content, but past practices of installing multiple systems without the development of an integrated information management strategy have resulted in significant redundant data entry activities, causing many complaints from health care professionals.

Health care events reflect the continuum of the life span from the prenatal to postmortem state. These events occur in very diverse delivery settings and may or may not involve the actual or virtual presence of patients or clinicians. Health care events are best described as scenarios of complex information—stories rich in details—and are always iterative with multiple feedback loops and recurrent decision-making and processing activities that integrate text; images; waveforms; and audio, video, analog, and digital components. This diversity begs for the application of standards for input, processing, and output phases. However, the challenges of such complexity suggest that standards development and implementation may be daunting.

The scientific method serves as an organizing framework for health care professionals and consists of assessment, diagnosis, planning, expected outcomes, implementation, and evaluation phases when the framework is used for patient care activities. The presentations of written and verbal data and information about patient care most often reflect these categories. Weed (1993) introduced an alternative information management technique for decision making using subjective, objective, assessment, plan, implementation, and evaluation headings for clinical record keeping. Because these category labels are frequently missing in clinical documentation, those interested in identifying and following a plan of care or evaluating the outcomes of care cannot easily do so. Individuals unfamiliar with health care structures, operations, processes, traditions, and languages can find the documentation unfathomable, even when it is legible.

THE CONTENT WITHIN HEALTH CARE

People involved in health care delivery must communicate about their activities with others within and outside of the health care system. The substance of clinicians' thoughts, concepts, communications, messages, images, and recordings constitutes the communication content. Although clinicians have traditionally used free text and natural language formats in their documentation activities, ongoing standardization efforts to create effective communication, reporting, and analysis have gained increased importance as managed care and evidence-based practice requirements demand data evaluation and changes in care delivery practices. Comparisons across units, departments, agencies, facilities, and enterprises at the regional, state, national, and international levels require the use of standardized terms and definitions to ensure data integrity and appropriate computations that accurately describe health care delivery activities.

Health care clinicians are usually educated in professional schools that focus on clinical activities and the associated necessary recordkeeping processes rather than on the financial or reimbursement elements of care. Consequently, early standardization efforts began as mechanisms to establish codes representing descriptions of real-world observations, or the actual health care services provided. This approach has evolved to one that is driven primarily by financial or reimbursement pressures and issues, with supporting documentation deemed necessary for reimbursement. Another perspective is that accurate clinical descriptions should be the focus for data definition and collection, with financial elements captured transparently in the background.

Standards of the American Society for Testing and Materials

The American Society for Testing and Materials (ASTM), organized in 1898, has grown into one of the largest voluntary standards systems in the world. The ASTM defines a standard as a document that has been developed and established within the consensus principles of the society and then meets the approval requirements of ASTM procedures and regulations (ASTM, 2001). **ASTM Committee E31** has responsibility for health care informatics standards. The majority of its work is completed by volunteers involved in many subcommittees' initiatives. The consensus process incorporates multidisciplinary participation by individuals within health care, vendor representatives, consumers, and other interested parties to craft draft standards, complete the ballots to be distributed for standards approval, and prepare the final standards for publication.

The current ASTM standards address the following:

- Confidentiality
- Security
- Documentation in the clinical laboratory
- Properties of the universal health care identifier
- Electronic authentication of health care information
- Content and structure of the electronic health record
- User authentication and authorization
- Training of persons who have access to health information
- Other aspects of health care information creation, processing, storage, and communication

As the need for new standards becomes apparent, existing or new subcommittees begin to formulate the new standards. Standards are being prepared for the format of transcribed health information and for the content of Web-based personal health records. Unfortunately, many health care and informatics professionals do not know about these existing and proposed health care informatics standards and therefore do not integrate them into procurement of systems, operational settings, and practice. See Chapter 17 for additional information on ASTM and other technical groups as well as for a review of applicable technical standards.

Standardized Languages

One way to organize discussion of the diverse standardized language initiatives is to identify the language that supports each portion of the health care delivery process: diagnosis, interventions, outcomes, and evaluation. Another strategy is to examine the languages that have been developed or used by each profession. Alternatively, discussion could focus on the primary functions of languages to support clinical or administrative activities. The problem-solving strategy is inherent in all clinical practice activities and has served as the impetus for most of the language development work; therefore the following discussion uses the problem-solving framework.

Diagnosis

In the United States the diagnosis component of medical practice is most often represented by the *International Classification of Diseases, 9th Revision, Clinical Modification* (ICD-9-CM). The World Health Organization developed the ICD as a classification system of groups of related disease entities and procedures to facilitate statistical reporting. The ICD-9-CM, modified by the National Center for Health Statistics from the World Health Organization's ICD-9, provides a way to classify morbidity data for indexing medical records, medical case reviews, and ambulatory and other medical care programs (National Center for Health Statistics, 2000).

The *International Statistical Classification of Diseases and Related Health Problems, 10th Revision* (ICD-10), is the latest version of the series that began in 1893 as the Bertillon Classification or International List of Causes of Death (World Health Organization [WHO], 1999). This updated classification extends beyond diseases and injuries, with conditions grouped in a way that was thought to be most suitable for general epidemiological purposes and the evaluation of health care. The ICD-10 is in use in other nations but has not yet been incorporated into the reporting requirements of the Centers for Medicare

& Medicaid Services (CMS) (formerly known as the Health Care Financing Administration [HCFA]), the leading government agency requiring submission of coded data for reimbursement of Medicare claims.

The World Health Organization's ICIDH-2: International Classification of Functioning Disability and Health (WHO, 2000) provides a complementary classification system to permit an even richer description. While the National Center for Health Statistics is a collaborating center of the WHO, ICIDH-2 is less well known in the United States. The ICIDH-2 systematically groups functional states associated with health conditions (i.e., disease, disorder, injury or trauma, or other health-related state) in an effort to provide a unified and standard language and framework for the description of human functioning and disability as an important component of health. This classification covers any disturbance in terms of "functional states" associated with health conditions at body, individual, and society levels. The three dimensions of body functions and structure, activities at the individual level, and participation in society describe the functioning and disability terms.

The dental profession found the ICD inadequate in specificity for its purposes and has developed the *Current Dental Terminology,* 3rd edition (CDT-3). Similarly, the American Psychological Association (APA) created the *Diagnostic and Statistical Manual of Mental Disorders* (DSM-IV) to assist in appropriately describing psychiatric–mental health diagnoses. The DSM-IV serves as a source of diagnostic information for clinical practice, research, and education and serves as a language to communicate diagnostic information among colleagues, hospital administrative bodies, journals, government agencies, insurance companies, and others (APA, 2000).

During the early 1980s, the nursing profession began to develop new research-based diagnostic codes that represent another approach to defining and describing patient problems. The North American Nursing Diagnosis Association (NANDA) maintains this diagnosis coding system and has developed a multiaxial system for the new version, Taxonomy II (NANDA, 1999). The Omaha System, Home Health Care Classification (HHCC), Patient Care Data Set, and Perioperative Nursing Data Set also include diagnostic terms that have been uniquely defined and coded for each system.

Implementation or Intervention

The implementation component of the health care event may be represented by the Alternative Billing Codes (ABC). ABCs are intended for use by health plans, health clearinghouses, and health care providers for processing electronic claims requiring a code for an alternative medicine procedure, service, or supply. ABCs were developed by Alternative Link, Inc., as a classification system designed to relay state-by-state information to map procedural codes to categories of practitioners who are allowed to do specific procedures. Services provided by acupuncture, chiropractic, holistic medicine, homeopathy, massage therapy, midwifery, naturopathy, osteopathy, and nursing are included. Currently this classification system contains about 800 nursing procedures gathered from the Nursing Interventions Classification (NIC), Omaha System, HHCC, and a new terminology system, the Sexual Assault Nurse Examiner (SANE), as well as those procedures done by other nonphysician providers. The system solidifies communication to payers and claims processors with content that presents billable information about the procedures used to treat patients and delineates time, setting, and difficulty parameters (Alternative Link, 2001).

Similarly, terms in the AMA's fourth edition of *Current Procedural Terminology* (CPT) (AMA, 2000) can represent the implementation phase of the health care event. The descriptive terms and identifying codes in the CPT are used to report medical services and procedures, thereby supporting administrative claims processing and the development of guidelines for medical care review. Early editions of the CPT codebook contained primarily surgical procedures, with limited sections for medicine, radiology, and laboratory procedures. Although all sections have been expanded to facilitate reimbursement of claims for physicians, some physician specialty and subspecialty societies have joined nonphysician health care professionals in calling for major CPT revisions to incorporate many more interventions to more accurately reflect the reality of care delivery activities. The AMA has established a strategy to develop CPT-5 over the next few years (AMA, 2000).

Although the NIC system describes activities most commonly performed by registered nurses (McCloskey & Bulechek, 2000), other nonphysician health care professionals have found that many of the terms apply equally well for their patient populations and work settings. The Omaha System, HHCC, Patient Care Data Set, and Perioperative Nursing Data Set also include codes for interventions that are uniquely structured for each language system. The American Dental Association has integrated procedure codes within CDT-3.

Outcomes or Goals

Outcomes codes that are uniquely structured for each system are described in the Nursing Outcomes Classification (NOC) system (Johnson, Maas, & Moorhead, 2000), Omaha System, HHCC, and Perioperative Nursing Data Set. The Patient Care Data Set identifies the results of care interventions as goals, rather than outcomes. These varied representations of the outcomes or goals provide choices but also create challenges for the user and information system developer and programmer.

The Outcome and Assessment Information Set (OASIS) was developed to provide a group of data elements that represent core elements for a comprehensive assessment of an adult home care patient. These data will provide the basis for measuring patient outcomes for outcome-based quality improvement initiatives for Medicare, permit patient assessment and care planning for individual adult patients, and support agency-level case mix reports of patient characteristics, such as demographics, health, or functional status when care began (HCFA, n.d.a).

Evaluation

Evaluation in health care can be supported either with integrated language systems containing assessment, diagnosis, planning, outcomes, and interventions capabilities or with individual languages that address only one or two components but have the ability to link with other languages. In nursing, for example, the Omaha System, HHCC, Perioperative Nursing Data Set, and Patient Care Data Set support evaluation activities.

The International Council of Nurses (ICN) has undertaken a major initiative to develop an international nursing language, the International Classification for Nursing Practice (ICNP). At the time this chapter was written, the Beta Version was available on the Internet. Earlier versions have evolved into a multiaxial structure used to describe the phenomena, outcomes, and actions of concern to nursing.

In addition to the Nursing Minimum Data Set (NMDS) described in Chapter 10, the nursing profession has developed the **Nursing Management Minimum Data Set (NMMDS)** to describe the health care and nursing environment associated with the diagnosis, intervention, and outcome segments from the administrative, management, and resource management perspectives. The NMMDS is composed of 17 data elements organized into three categories: environment, nurse resources, and financial resources. The focus is on the nursing delivery unit/service/center of excellence level and numerous constructed variables; in addition, data aggregation is supported.

As demonstrated here nursing professionals have developed many standard languages using terms that overlap and conflict. In 1999 several nursing language developers participated in the first of a series of meetings, the Vanderbilt Nursing Languages Summit, to identify the language issues that can be resolved and to plan appropriate activities to attempt to converge the irreconcilable differences toward a closer agreement and toward potential consolidation in the future. The Vanderbilt Nursing Languages Summit in June 2000 expanded the work of the 1999 summit to include an international perspective with a focus on proposing specific nursing language initiatives in the international standards environment. Consequently, the ICN, the organization consisting of national nursing associations and which represents all of the world's nurses, has partnered with the International Medical Informatics Association's (IMIA's) Nursing Informatics Special Interest Group to prepare a series of nursing language proposals for presentation to the International Organization for Standardization (ISO).

Other Languages

The Read Codes were invented and developed by Dr. James Read in 1982 as a computer-based system for general practice physicians. In 1990, the United Kingdom's National Health Service (NHS) bought the Read Codes; made them an NHS standard; expanded the codes to cover all areas of clinical practice, nursing, physiotherapy, and health visiting; and commissioned the Clinical Terms Projects to collect all relevant terms from specialists in each field. The collected terms became the Read Version 3 (a national thesaurus of clinical terms) in 1995 (NHS, n.d.). Although the Read Codes are not presently used in the United States, SNOMED Clinical Terms (SNOMED CT), which is currently under development, will include these terms.

SNOMED, the Systematized Nomenclature of Medicine, is a comprehensive, multiaxial, controlled terminology created for the indexing of the entire medical record. Population-based outcomes analysis, cost-effectiveness studies, and practice guidelines are supported with the SNOMED-coded vocabulary, which is organized in a hierarchical, systematized structure. Development work has begun to combine the current SNOMED terms and Read Codes into the SNOMED Clinical Terms, or SNOMED CT—targeted for release in 2001. The new work combines the robust strength of SNOMED RT (SNOMED Reference Terminology) in specialty medicine, including pathology, and the richness of Clinical Terms Version 3 (also known as Read Codes V3) for primary care.

The **Logical Observation Identifiers Names and Codes (LOINC)** database provides a standard set of universal names and codes that identifies individual laboratory results (e.g., hemoglobin, serum sodium concentration), clinical observations (e.g., vital signs, hemodynamics, intake/output, diastolic blood pressure, and other clinical observations), and diagnostic study observations (e.g., cardiovascular PR interval, cardiac echo left ventricular diameter, and chest x-ray impression). The LOINC database currently contains about 29,000 observational terms. Nearly 20,000 of these observational terms relate to laboratory testing. It includes chemistry, toxicology, serology, microbiology, and selected clinical variables. This database includes fields for each of the six parts of its name. These six parts include the component (e.g., hemoglobin), the property measured (e.g., enzyme activity), the timing (e.g., 24-hour urine), the type of sample (e.g., blood), the scale (e.g., ordinal), and the method used to produce results. The database also contains International Union of Pure and Applied Chemistry (IUPAC/IFCC) codes and ASTM codes, as well as related words, synonyms, and comments. The related words, synonyms, and comments are included to facilitate searches for individual laboratory test and clinical observation results. Although developed by the Regenstreif Institute for Health Care as a proprietary system, the LOINC database is incorporated into the Unified Medical Language System (UMLS), is being adopted by information systems vendors, and is now available for free public use on the Internet (Regenstreif Institute for Health Care, n.d.).

The UMLS began as a National Library of Medicine (NLM) research and development project in 1986 to develop systems to help health professionals and researchers retrieve and integrate electronic biomedical information from a variety of sources (NLM, 2000). The project included development of three "knowledge sources": the Metathesaurus, Lexicon, and Semantic Network. The Metathesaurus now provides a uniform, integrated distribution format linking the many different names for the same concepts from about 60 biomedical vocabularies and classifications. The Lexicon contains syntactic information for many terms, component words, and English words, including verbs that do not appear in the Metathesaurus. The Semantic Network contains information about the types or categories (e.g., "disease or syndrome," "virus") to which all concepts have been assigned and includes the permissible relationships among these types (e.g., "virus" causes "disease or syndrome"). This long-term initiative, funded with public dollars, has been instrumental in establishing a standardized mechanism to access health care literature. This foundational language work has also been instrumental in facilitating development of other federal databases, such as the National Guidelines Clearinghouse maintained by the Agency for Healthcare Research and Quality (AHRQ), and the Cancer Trials supported by the National Cancer Institute, as well as other public and private database activities.

The initiation of the U.S. Human Genome Project in 1990 was expected to be a 15-year effort coordinated by the U.S. Department of Energy and the National Institutes of Health. However, rapid technological advances have accelerated the expected completion date to 2003. The goals of the Human Genome Project are to (Human Genome Program, 2001):

- Identify all of the 100,000 genes in human DNA
- Determine the sequences of the 3 billion chemical base pairs that make up human DNA
- Store this information in databases
- Develop tools for data analysis
- Transfer related technologies to the private sector
- Address the ethical, legal, and social issues (ELSIs) that may arise from the project

The resultant avalanches of data are challenging researchers and language experts as they struggle to organize the findings within gigantic databases using standardized naming conventions and rules. Informatics professionals are now beginning to engage in discussions to identify the resulting significant information management and professional practice and standards challenges that are associated with this new health care technology.

American Nurses Association Recognition Programs

In the early 1990s the American Nurses Association (ANA) established specific criteria for nursing languages as part of its new nursing languages recognition program. Recent changes in ANA recognition criteria reflect the increasing sophistication of the language development process. See Box 18-1 for the recognition criteria. By January 2000, 12 nursing languages had received ANA recognition. (Contact information for these languages is available through the Web Connection of this book.)

In 1997 the ANA launched the Nursing Information and Data Set Evaluation Center (NIDSEC), a unique and complementary evaluation program focusing on the recognition of information systems vendors and their products that support nursing by integrating at least one ANA-recognized nursing language into those products. Again, the evolving industry has mandated the recent revision of the recognition criteria. These standards have been valuable resources for nurse and health care administrators during system selection and implementation activities. Similarly, vendors have used the standards during product development work.

Box 18–1 American Nurses Association Recognition Criteria for Languages for Nursing

I. Criteria
   A. Core criteria for ANA recognition of nursing data sets, classification systems, and nomenclatures; documentation supports evidence of:
      1. Support of nursing practice by providing clinically useful terminology (e.g., nursing diagnoses, nursing interventions) and rationale for development
      2. A level of development beyond an application, adaptation, or synthesis of currently recognized ANA vocabulary/classification schemes or presents an explicit rationale for seeking recognition for synthesis, application, or adaptation of existing schemes
      3. Clear and unambiguous concepts
      4. Documented testing of reliability, validity, and utility in practice
      5. A systematic method of development
      6. A named entity responsible for a formal process of documenting evolving development and maintenance, including tracking of deleted concepts/terms and version control
      7. A coding scheme that provides a unique identifier for each concept
   B. Additional recognition criteria for specific systems:
      1. *Data set:* Must meet all core criteria *plus:*
         a. Identify pertinent data elements as the variables of interest to whom and within what context
         b. Define the set of possible values for each variable
      2. *Classification system:* Must meet all core criteria plus:
         a. Provide a clear description of a defined structure or architecture with explicit principles of division
      3. *Nomenclature:* Must meet all core criteria *plus:*
         a. Contain terms that can be combined to represent more complex concepts
         b. Include a classification structure that supports multiple parents and multiple children as relevant
         c. Include preestablished rules for combining the concepts/terms

From American Nurses Association Committee on Nursing Practice Information Infrastructure. (2001). *ANA recognition criteria for languages for nursing.* Washington, DC: American Nurses Association. Printed with permission of the American Nurses Association.

Decision Support and Rule Making

To counter deficiencies in the current health care delivery systems and to promote increased quality of health care, the Agency for Health Care Policy and Research (AHCPR) established a research program in the early 1990s to develop clinical practice guidelines. Recent funding directives and operational mandates resulted in the agency's name change to the Agency for Healthcare Research and Quality and included the establishment of the National Guidelines Clearinghouse (NGC). The AHRQ is the lead agency charged with supporting research designed to improve the quality of health care, reduce its cost, and broaden access to essential services.

The AHRQ has established criteria for the evaluation of submitted guidelines for inclusion in the NGC. A clinical practice guideline must

Box 18—2 Criteria Necessary for Inclusion in the National Guidelines Clearinghouse

1. The clinical practice guideline contains systematically developed statements that include recommendations, strategies, or information that assists physicians and/or other health care practitioners and patients to make decisions about appropriate health care for specific clinical circumstances.
2. The clinical practice guideline was produced under the auspices of medical specialty associations; relevant professional societies; public or private organizations; government agencies at the federal, state, or local level; or health care organizations or plans. A clinical practice guideline developed and issued by an individual not officially sponsored or supported by one of the above types of organizations does not meet the inclusion criteria for NGC.
3. Corroborating documentation can be produced and verified that a systematic literature search and review of existing scientific evidence published in peer-reviewed journals was performed during the guideline development. A guideline is not excluded from NGC if corroborating documentation can be produced and verified detailing specific gaps in scientific evidence for some of the guideline's recommendations.
4. The guideline is in English language, current, and the most recent version produced. Documented evidence can be produced or verified that the guideline was developed, reviewed, or revised within the last 5 years.

From National Guidelines Clearinghouse. (2000). Retrieved from the World Wide Web: http://www.guideline.gov.

meet all of the criteria shown in Box 18-2 to be included in the NGC.

The guidelines must be reviewed at least every 5 years with subsequent implications for informatics professionals. Because clinicians use the guidelines for decision making in the health care delivery setting, for the development and implementation of plans of care, and for evaluation of the processes of decision making and health care delivery, exquisite tracking of the previously and currently available versions of the guidelines becomes an integral concern to clinicians and informatics professionals. The information system must accommodate timely installation of new guidelines with associated new rules and links; at the same time, past versions and relationships must be retained for legal, risk, and clinical practice evaluation reviews and for research initiatives.

The Arden Syntax for **medical logic modules (MLMs)** is a language for encoding medical knowledge. It was developed primarily to address the need for data-driven decision support, invoking logic rules in response to patient data changes. In 1992 the ASTM adopted and integrated the Arden Syntax Version 1.0 into document E1460 under subcommittee E31.15 Health Knowledge Representation. Sponsorship of this standard was moved to Health Level Seven (HL7) in 1998, with its maintenance now overseen by the Clinical Decision Support and Arden Syntax Technical Committee of HL7. HL7 and American National Standards Institute (ANSI) formally adopted Arden Syntax Version 2.0 in August 1999. Each MLM contains sufficient logic to make a single medical decision and has been used to generate clinical alerts, interpretations, diagnoses, screening for clinical research, quality assurance functions, and administrative support (CPMC, n.d.).

As part of the federal government's Internet activities to increase information access for improved decision making and informed consent, the NLM maintains a hyperlinked listing of online resources in its list of organizations. Now health care consumers and their clinicians are supported in their decision-making activities by having access to Web-based and printed resources available from MEDLINEplus. MEDLINEplus is the National Library of Medicine's Web site for consumer health information. One of the resources in MEDLINEplus is MEDLINE. MEDLINE is the National Library of Medicine's database of references to more than 11 million articles published in 4300 biomedical journals (NLM, 2000). This increasing demand for and reliance on Internet-based educational and decision support materials creates new technical, fiscal, legal, ethical, and social concerns and challenges for the clinical and informatics communities.

THE CONTEXT OF THE HEALTH CARE SYSTEM

Previous sections of this chapter have highlighted some of the standards associated with the person and the content components of health care. The complexity is even greater when discussing how informatics professionals can use standards within the context component of health care. In the past, less attention has been paid to the environment, organizational setting, and "systems" aspects except when the emphasis focused on reduction of resource expenditures, recruitment of needed human resources, and the bottom line. However, the recent Institute of Medicine's report, *To Err Is Human: Building a Safer Health System* (2000) has served as a catalyst to heighten public and legislative interest in the environmental context and to define how informatics can make a difference in the context of doing more with less while maintaining the same quality of care.

Reporting About Quality of Care

In an effort to monitor the quality of services delivered by health care practitioners, providers, and suppliers, the U.S. Department of Health and Human Services, Health Resources and Services Administration, Bureau of Health Professions, was charged to establish the **National Practitioner Databank-Healthcare Integrity Protection Database (NPD-HIPD)**. This restricted-access database permits summaries to be compiled of adverse action reports, including licensure and other adjudicated actions as well as civil judgment or criminal conviction. Registered entities began reporting in November 1999. Queries are authorized for hospitals, other health care entities, state licensing boards, and professional societies.

The **Health Plan Employer Data and Information Set (HEDIS)** is a set of standardized performance measures designed to ensure that purchasers and consumers of health care have the information they need to reliably compare the performance of managed health care plans. HEDIS 3.0 was developed by the National Committee for Quality Assurance (NCQA) in conjunction with public and private purchasers, health plans, researchers, and consumer advocates. The performance measures in the HEDIS are related to significant public health issues such as cancer, heart disease, smoking, asthma, and diabetes. The HEDIS also includes a standardized survey of consumers' experiences to evaluate plan performance in areas such as customer service, access to care, and claims possessing. The HEDIS is sponsored, supported, and maintained by the NCQA (HCFA, n.d.b).

Accreditation

URAC (also known as the American Accreditation HealthCare/Commission) is a not-for-profit entity that establishes accreditation standards for managed care organizations, including utilization review, networks, credentialing, and workers' compensation managed care. The URAC conducts on-site reviews as part of its determination of eligibility for accreditation and provides each of its proposed standards for public comment during the development phase (URAC, n.d.). Both the NCQA and the URAC evaluation criteria include review processes to examine the applicant organization's mechanisms for ensuring that appropriate, competent clinicians provide quality health care to all clients.

The Joint Commission on Accreditation of Healthcare Organizations (JCAHO) has a well-established and extensive accreditation program for many types of health care organizations that is based on triennial site surveys with a focus on site survey evaluation activities (JCAHO, 2000). The JCAHO standards cover requirements for the people, content, and context components of the health care delivery system. Information management standards are integral to every self-review and accreditation survey, with expected continuous compliance during nonsurvey periods.

ORYX is the name of the Joint Commission's initiative to integrate performance measures into the accreditation process. The JCAHO is implementing ORYX, a continuous monitoring program using core measurement data to review an accredited organization's performance between site surveys. The long-range goal of the ORYX initiative is to establish a data-driven, continuous survey and accreditation process to complement the JCAHO standards-based assessment. The five initial core measurement areas for hospitals are as follows (JCAHO, 2000):

1. Acute myocardial infarction (including coronary artery disease)
2. Heart failure
3. Pneumonia
4. Surgical procedures and complications
5. Pregnancy and related conditions (including newborn and maternal care)

Professional education and academic programs also are subject to accreditation mandates. Federal funding for health profession education programs may be contingent on the current status of educational program accreditation. The individual health care professional is also affected by the accreditation status of the educational program because initial professional licensing prerequisites usually include graduation from an accredited professional education program. As an example, nursing education programs may be accredited by the National League for Nursing (NLN) or the American Association of Colleges of Nursing (AACN) after a review of the program's compliance with standards applied during the application, self-assessment, and site survey processes. Additional information on accreditation in health care informatics can be found in Chapter 19.

Electronic Mail and Electronic Information

Once relegated to the office and scientific communities, electronic mail (eMail) has become an integral communication technology in health care services delivery. Some would argue that the consumer population has led health care professionals in the use of electronic technology to communicate via eMail and to search for health care information and services. The unregulated and unstructured burgeoning cyber-environment fosters the invasion of personal, corporate, and organizational privacy and often permits breaches of confidentiality and security. The ASTM and other recognized standards bodies continue to develop standards to address information system deficiencies in this area. Various industry groups also are developing self-regulatory activities to prevent further governmental involvement and control in relation to confidentiality and security.

To begin promoting dialogue about the development of standards and guidelines for the use of eMail in health care, the American Medical Informatics Association published a set of guidelines for the use of clinic-patient eMail in 1998 (Kane & Sands, 1998). More recently, the Association of Records Managers and Administrators

International (ARMA International, 2000) released its publication, *Guideline for Managing E-mail.* To date, no health care standards body has undertaken the development of consensus standards for eMail, leaving both consumers and health care professionals at risk as they use this communication strategy.

CONCLUSION

The health care delivery system in the United States includes significant numbers of individualized, noncollaborative activities associated with providing care and attempting to manage the necessary resources for care delivery. Some professional standards initiatives are beginning to demonstrate a gradual evolution from independent to collaborative environments to successfully address the significantly complex data and information management issues inherent in the health care system. Health care informatics professionals continue to be leaders in identifying issues and then raising clarifying questions about the people, content, and contexts that need attention, discussion, and resolution for the implementation of professional standards. Armed with an understanding and appreciation of the multitude of professional issues affecting clinicians, administrators, educators, and researchers in the health care environment, health care informatics professionals can provide the environment, context, and content to support health care consumers and professionals in their decision making and quest for high-quality health care.

Web Connection

This chapter discusses the standards for professional and nonprofessional staff. Organizations must manage and develop processes according to these standards to achieve their goals and objectives safely, efficiently, and effectively. Additionally, organizations are accredited and certified by agencies to ensure that care meets acceptable standards. The Web Connection activities for this chapter focus on professional standards and the organizations that develop and maintain these standards and review organizational compliance. You will be able to identify several organizations that are closely involved in standards for informatics professionals.

discussion questions

1. What is the impact of professional standards on the development of health care information systems? Give examples to demonstrate this impact.
2. Explain the health care information management issues that surround the description of professional practice.
3. Describe how professional standards affect a facility's strategic plan for information management.
4. Describe acceptable solution alternatives when disparate information-reporting requirements and data definitions occur.
5. Which standards development activities should receive priority when clinicians, administrators, educators, and researchers join information management professions in standards initiatives? Consider the inherent limitations on time, money, and human resources in a health care facility or organization.

REFERENCES

Abdelhak, M., Grostick, S., Hanken, M.A., & Jacobs, E. (Eds.). (2001). *Health information: Management of a strategic resource* (2nd ed.). Philadelphia: W.B. Saunders.

Alternative Link, Inc. (2001). *ABC-codes.* Las Cruces, NM: Author. Retrieved from the World Wide Web: http://www.alternativelink.com.

American Medical Association. (2000). Chicago: Author. Retrieved from the World Wide Web: http://www.ama-assn.org/ama/pub/category/3113.html.

American Nurses Association. (2001). *Code of ethics for nurses.* Washington, DC: Author.

American Nurses Association. (2001). *Scope and standards of nursing informatics practice.* Washington, DC: Author.

American Nurses Association. (1997). *NIDSEC: Standards and scoring guidelines.* Washington, DC: Author.

American Nurses Association. (1998). *Standards of clinical nursing practice* (2nd ed.). Washington, DC: Author.

American Nurses Association. (1999). *Scope and standards of public health nursing practice.* Washington, DC: Author.

American Nurses Association. (2000). *Scope and standards of psychiatric–mental health nursing practice.* Washington, DC: Author

American Nurses Association. (2001). *Scope of practice of nursing informatics and standards for the informatics nurse specialist.* Washington, DC: Author.

American Psychological Association. (2000). Retrieved from the World Wide Web: http://www.psych.org/clin_res/dsm_iv.html.

American Society for Testing and Materials. (2001). *Annual book of ASTM standards 2000.* West Conshohocken, PA: Author.

ARMA International. (2000). *Guideline for managing e-mail.* Prairie Village, KS: Author.

CPMC. (n.d.). Retrieved from the World Wide Web: http://www.cpmc.columbia.edu/arden.

Health Care Financing Administration. (n.d.a). Retrieved from the World Wide Web: http://www.hcfa.gov/medicaid/oasis/hhoview.htm.

Health Care Financing Administration. (n.d.b). Retrieved from the World Wide Web: http://www.hcfa.gov/stats/hedis.htm.

Human Genome Program. (2001). *Human Genome Project information.* Washington, DC: U.S. Department of Energy. Retrieved from the World Wide Web: http://www.ornl.gov/hgmis/.

Institute of Medicine: Committee on Quality of Health Care in America. (2000). In L.T. Kohn, J.M. Corrigan, & M.S. Donaldson (Eds.), *To err is human: Building a safer health system.* Washington, DC: National Academy Press.

Johnson, M., Maas, M., & Moorhead, S. (2000). *Nursing outcomes classification (NOC)* (2nd ed.). St. Louis: Mosby.

Joint Commission on Accreditation of Healthcare Organizations. (2000). *2000 automated comprehensive accreditation manual for hospitals* (CD-ROM). Oakbrook Terrace, IL: Author.

Joint Commission on Accreditation of Healthcare Organizations. (2000). Retrieved from the World Wide Web: http://www.jcaho.org/standards_frm.html.

Kane, B., & Sands, D.Z., for the AMIA Internet Working Group, Task Force on Guidelines for the Use of Clinic-Patient Electronic Mail. (1998). Guidelines for the clinical use of electronic mail with patients. *Journal of the American Medical Informatics Association, 5*(1), 104-111.

McCloskey, J.C., & Bulechek, G.M. (2000). *Nursing interventions classification (NIC).* (3rd ed.). St. Louis: Mosby.

National Center for Health Statistics. (2000). Retrieved from the World Wide Web: http://www.cdc.gov/nchs/icd9.htm.

National Health Service of the United Kingdom. (n.d.). Retrieved from the World Wide Web: http://www.cams.co.uk/faq.htm#446011520.

National Library of Medicine. (2000). Retrieved from the World Wide Web: http://www.nlm.nih.gov/research/umls.

National Library of Medicine. (2000). Retrieved from the World Wide Web: http://www.nlm.nih.gov/medlineplus/organizations.html.

North American Nursing Diagnosis Association. (1999). *NANDA nursing diagnoses: Definitions and classification 1999-2000.* Philadelphia: Author.

Regenstreif Institute for Health Care. (n.d.). Retrieved from the World Wide Web: http://www.regenstrief.org/loinc/loinc.htm.

URAC/American Accreditation Healthcare Commission. (n.d.). Retrieved from the World Wide Web: http://www.urac.org/about.htm.

Weed, L.L. (1993). Medical records that guide and teach. *MD Computing, 10*(2),100-114.

Wilson, F.A., & Neuhauser, D. (1982). *Health services in the United States*. Cambridge, MA: Ballinger Publishing.

World Health Organization. (1999). Retrieved from the World Wide Web: http://www.who.int/whosis/icd10/descript.htm.

World Health Organization. (2000). Retrieved from the World Wide Web: http://www.who.int/icidh/intro.htm.

CHAPTER 19

The Implications of Accreditation and Governmental Regulations for Health Care Informatics

DONNA W. BAILEY
KAY S. LYTLE

Learning Objectives

Upon completion of this chapter, the reader will be able to:

1. ***Describe*** how accreditation standards influence information management systems in health care organizations.
2. ***Analyze*** how governmental regulations influence health care information technologies.
3. ***Explain*** the role of the informatics professional in the health care setting in relation to accreditation and governmental regulations.

Outline

Key Terms

accreditation
certification
code sets
governmental regulation
regulation
transaction standards
unique identifiers

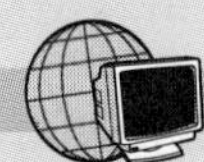

Web Connection

Go to the Web site at http://evolve.elsevier.com/Englebardt/. Here you will find Web links and activities related to the implications of accreditation and governmental regulations for health care informatics.

Accreditation, certification, and regulatory requirements play a major role in determining the infrastructure that supports health care informatics. Accurate, timely, and accessible data and information are required for organizations to understand and improve their processes and quality of services. Understanding health care delivery processes and improving these processes produce additional data to be analyzed and folded back into organizational quality improvement, resource management, and evaluation of the organization's strategic plan. The underpinnings of accreditation and regulatory requirements are often embedded in internal organizational improvement or quality assurance efforts. Accreditation and regulatory influence is part of a structure that begins with internal quality improvement efforts. When these quality processes are viewed as a continuum, it is easy to see how institutional data, information, and knowledge are critical components of quality improvement. Furthermore, the processing and management of data, information, and knowledge is essential to assessing compliance with internal performance standards and external requirements. There are two sides of the coin for informatics professionals. On one side of the coin, they are charged with creating, implementing, maintaining, and evaluating effective information management processes. On the other side, they must interact and communicate effectively with the users of the information management processes. Informatics professionals must ensure that these users have the necessary knowledge and skill to work with and within those information management processes.

Performance assessment begins with internal continuous quality improvement (CQI) or total quality management (TQM) efforts. These efforts are followed by solicitation of external accreditation or certification to independently validate an organization's or individual's performance. The same data, information, and knowledge are used in both the internal and external quality improvement processes.

There is a continuum of compliance with standards that assumes that organizations will manage their processes in such a way that they achieve compliance with quality standards in their day-to-day operations. If compliance does not occur, then governmental regulators may intervene to mandate a particular level of compliance. Accreditation and certification represent self-regulation within an industry or profession. Failure to self-regulate and/or improve processes can result in governmental regulation. **Governmental regulation** includes legislated laws, rules, and regulations that mandate compliance or conformance to a particular set of performance processes, standards, or outcomes. This chapter explores the major accreditation and certification organizations and standards, as well as the governmental regulations that are of primary concern to health care informatics professionals.

ACCREDITATION AND CERTIFICATION

Accreditation is a process by which a health care entity is given official or formal authorization, approval, or recognition for its practice (Merriam-Webster, 2000). It generally requires an external review of performance by knowledgeable reviewers against a set of accepted standards. **Certification** is a written statement indicating that an individual has met a particular set of standards or requirements. According to the American Nurses Association (ANA), "Certification is a process by which an individual licensed to practice a profession is attested to have met certain predetermined standards specified by that profession for specialty practice. Its purpose is to ensure various publics that an individual has mastered a body of knowledge and acquired skills and abilities in a particular specialty" (ANA, n.d.a).

Each of these processes uses data and information to assess compliance with the accreditation or certification standards. The key element of both processes is the evaluation of performance against a standard. This is the concept of interest to informatics professionals. They are concerned not only with the data and information that are used to complete the work of the organization or individual, but also with how the data and information are used to evaluate the performance of the organization or individual. The terms *accreditation* and *certification* are common to the United States. These terms are often used interchangeably in discussions of compliance with external standards; however, more appropriately, accreditation refers to organizations and certification refers to individuals.

In the United States there are several organizations that offer accreditation and certification services related to health care informatics. This chapter provides an overview of these organizations, their standards, and the role of the informatics professional in relation to accreditation and certification. The primary agency that accredits health care organizations is the Joint Commission on Accreditation of Healthcare Organizations. This organization includes in its standards a comprehensive list of information management standards.

Joint Commission on Accreditation of Healthcare Organizations

As the primary accrediting body for health care organizations, the Joint Commission on Accreditation of Healthcare Organizations (JCAHO) evaluates and accredits more than 195,000 health care organizations in the United States. A variety of health care agencies are reviewed by the JCAHO, such as hospitals, health care networks, managed care organizations, and health care organizations that provide home care, long-term care, behavioral health care, laboratory services, and ambulatory care services. The mission of the JCAHO is to continuously improve the safety and quality of care provided to the public through the provision of health care accreditation and related services that support performance improvement in health care organizations (JCAHO, 2000a). This mission translates into policies and procedures that health care organizations use to assess and improve their performance. These policies and procedures are based on the organizations' own internal standards, as well as on the standards set forth by the JCAHO.

The JCAHO accreditation process is designed around three functional areas: patient-focused functions, organizational functions, and structure-related functions (JCAHO, 2000a). Patient-focused functions describe functions that are necessary in the direct provision of patient care. They include assessment of patients, care of the patient (planning care, anesthesia care, medication use, nutrition care, operative and special treatments), education, and the continuum of care, as well as patients' rights and organizational ethics. Organizational functions deal with the functions that support patient care. These include improving organizational performance; leadership; management of the environment of care; management of human resources; management of information; and surveillance, prevention, and control of infection. Structure-related functions deal with structures that are closely involved in the management and delivery of patient care. These include, for example, the governance and management of medical and nursing staff.

The information management standards specifically address how information is managed within the organization. Although the information management function resides within the organizational function section of the JCAHO standards, the information management function encompasses all of the other functional areas, since the management and processing of information is essential to effective performance of all those functions. The information management standards are reviewed from an organization-wide perspective and encompass a wide variety of information processes. A brief outline of the ten information management standards is provided in Table 19-1.

At the most basic level, the JCAHO standards address both the definitions of data and

Table 19–1 Joint Commission on Accreditation of Healthcare Organizations Information Management Standards

Focus	Standard Number	Standard
Information management planning	IM.1	Information management processes are planned and designed to meet the health care organization's internal and external information needs.
	IM.2	The information management function provides for information confidentiality, security, and integrity.
	IM.3	When feasible, uniform data definitions and methods for capturing data are in place.
	IM.4	Decision makers and other individuals in the organization who generate, collect, and analyze data and information are educated and trained in the principles of information management.
	IM.5	The transmission of data and information is timely and accurate.
	IM.6	The information management function enables the combination of data and information, makes information from one system (clinical and/or organizational) available to another, provides reports, clarifies and interprets data and information, and enables linkages of patient care and non–patient care data and information over time among the organization's departments and provider resources for all care settings.
Patient-specific data and information	IM.7	The information management function provides for the definition, capture, analysis, transformation, transmission, and reporting of individual patient-specific data and information related to the process(es) and/or of the outcome(s) of the patient's care.
Aggregate data and information	IM.8	The information management function provides for the definition, capture, analysis, transformation, transmission, and reporting of data and information that can be aggregated to support managerial decisions and operations, performance improvement activities, and patient care.
Knowledge-based information	IM.9	The management of knowledge-based information (also known as "literature") provides for the identification, organization, retrieval, analysis, delivery, and reporting of clinical and managerial journal literature, reference information, and research data for use in designing, managing, and improving patient-specific and organizational processes.
Comparative data and information	IM.10	The information management function provides for the definition, capture, analysis, transformation, transmission, and reporting and/or use of comparative performance data and information, the comparability of which is based on national and state guidelines for data set parity and connectivity.

From Joint Commission on Accreditation of Healthcare Organizations. (2000). *2000 hospital accreditation standards.* Oakbrook Terrace, IL: Author.

information and the information management processes. Standards require that the movement of information within the organization, among organizational units, and external to the organization should be carefully planned and monitored to meet the health care organization's internal and external information needs. Informatics professionals who are familiar with the development and structure of databases are required to perform these functions. They need to develop strategies that connect a variety of vocabularies and classifications, such as the *International Classification of Diseases, 9th Revision, Clinical Modification* (ICD-9-CM); *Current Procedural Terminology, 4th Edition* (CPT-4); and the *Code on Dental Procedures and Nomenclature* (CDT). On the hardware side, most health care organizations have a vast array of older and newer information systems that sometimes do not communicate well with one another. This creates problems that interfere with the quality of data. These problems include delays in the transmission of data, conflicts in data definitions, and inaccessibility of data when systems are down and unavailable for accessing the needed data.

The JCAHO information management standards address issues of confidentiality, security, and integrity (JCAHO, 2000a). In health care, confidentiality, security, and integrity of information are mission-critical processes that require exquisite planning, design, and implementation. Confidentiality refers to those actions taken to protect data and information by allowing access only to persons who have a need or reason to access the data and information and who have permission to access it. Security includes the processes that organizations implement to protect information and information systems from damage. Integrity refers to the accuracy, consistency, and completeness of the data. Quality indicators such as timeliness of information transmission, availability, accessibility, consistency, and accuracy provide barometers of process performance. These indicators also point out the unique nature of health care information in that data and information that are unavailable or inaccurate potentially jeopardize people's lives (Kohn, Corrigan, & Donaldson, 1999).

Aggregate patient-specific and organizational data and information are necessary to evaluate patient and organizational outcomes respectively. Aggregate data and information are data and information that have been combined and standardized. Aggregating data and information requires uniform data definitions. The JCAHO information management standards speak to the process of defining, capturing, analyzing, transforming, transmitting, and reporting patient-specific and organizational data and information. These evaluation processes generate their own sets of data and information that must be analyzed and managed. Evaluation activities based on sound information management processes ultimately inform patient care, organizational strategic plans, and local, state, and, regional health policy.

Data and information that are transformed into knowledge are deemed essential by the JCAHO for designing, managing, and improving patient and organizational processes. Reference libraries and databases are examples of knowledge-based information sources. The ability to compare data and information is the basis for a major JCAHO project, ORYX. The ORYX initiative is designed to link the accreditation process to outcomes and other performance measures (Kreider & Haselton, 1997). ORYX is not an acronym. It is the name given to this effort that is aimed at providing a data-driven performance evaluation process that is continuous and outcomes based. ORYX can be used to benchmark processes and outcomes (JCAHO, 2000b). Evidence-based practice with the focus on outcomes evaluation depends on data and information that can be systematically compared across settings, providers, and patient populations.

The focus of the JCAHO is on improving organizational performance through the use of processes for managing data, information, and knowledge. The information management standards set the stage for organizations to improve processes, thereby ensuring, first, that the right thing is done and, second, that the right thing is done well. Today, the JCAHO is not alone in the quest to ensure quality and safe care. A number of other organizations have joined this commission in the accreditation process.

Other Accreditation Organizations

Health care accreditation has become more widespread and now includes a variety of agencies that focus on specific areas of health care delivery. The National Committee for Quality Assurance (NCQA) is a private, not-for-profit organization that assesses and reports on the performance and quality of care provided by managed care organizations (NCQA, n.d.b). Like the JCAHO, the NCQA assesses the quality of key systems and processes. Data and information are systematically collected, analyzed, and evaluated to demonstrate quality organizational performance. The management and processing of data, information, and knowledge is used to achieve the mission of providing "information that enables purchasers and consumers of managed health care to distinguish among plans based on quality, thereby allowing them to make more informed health care purchasing decisions" (NCQA, n.d.b). The survey process includes an overall assessment of how the organization is organized and managed, as well as a comparison with performance standards. The Health Plan Employer Data and Information Set (HEDIS) provides performance standards related to significant public health issues (such as cancer, heart disease, smoking, asthma, and diabetes) and is intended to provide a reliable, standardized set of performance measures that allows for more informed decision making by employers selecting managed care plans. The HEDIS data set and measures are a part of the NCQA accreditation process (NCQA, n.d.a). For the informatics professional, knowledge of the standards and required data sets is essential to manage the accreditation process. Working in partnership with organizational teams, the informatics professional provides technical support, as well as information processing and management strategies, to facilitate the accreditation process.

In addition to the JCAHO and NCQA, other examples of accrediting bodies and their focus are provided in Table 19-2.

Table 19–2 Examples of Accreditation and Certification Agencies

Agency	Focus
American Osteopathic Association (AOA)	Osteopathic hospitals
College of American Pathologists (CAP)	Laboratories
Commission on Accreditation in Physical Therapy Education Programs (CAPTE)	Physical therapy education programs
Commission on Accreditation of Rehabilitation Facilities (CARF)	Rehabilitation facilities
Community Health Accreditation Program (CHAP)	Home health agencies
Joint Commission on Accreditation of Healthcare Organizations (JCAHO)	Hospitals, non–hospital based psychiatric and substance abuse centers, home care organizations, ambulatory care organizations, long-term care organizations, and organization-based laboratory and pathology services
National Committee on Quality Assurance (NCQA)	Managed care organizations

Accreditation in health care is not limited to health care organizations and their specific populations or services. Institutions offering educational programs also participate in the process of accreditation. Accreditation in this setting ensures that the educational program is designed to produce quality practitioners. Examples of accrediting agencies concerned with the preparation of health care providers are the Commission on Accreditation of Allied Health Education Programs, the National League for Nursing, the American Medical Association, and the American Nurses Credentialing Center. Educational accreditation agencies impact informatics in two ways. First, they can include educational standards concerning computer, information, and informatics literacy. Second, increasingly these agencies are including standards related to the use of technology in education. For example, many of these organizations have standards related to the use of distance education.

Other programs exist to evaluate health care organizations against standards in particular areas of performance. Although not accrediting bodies in the sense of agencies like the JCAHO, they provide the organization and public with an external evaluation of organizational performance. Examples of this type of recognition program include the American Nurses Credentialing Center (ANCC) Magnet Nursing Services Recognition Program and the International Organization for Standardization (ISO 9000). The ANCC Magnet Nursing Services Recognition Program was established in 1993 to recognize acute care and general care facilities, long-term care facilities, rehabilitation services, and psychiatric nursing services that demonstrate excellence in nursing services, have a professional practice environment, and encourage professional development of nursing staff (ANCC, n.d.).

The ISO 9000 is published by the International Organization for Standardization (ISO, 1998). The intent of the ISO standards is to promote international standards for quality assurance across all industries. Their focus is on generic standards that can be used across a broad range of manufacturing and service industries, including health care. Both the ANCC and the ISO reviews include an evaluation of the organization against standards related to the quality of the services provided.

Professional organizations can also influence informatics practice by impacting vendor requirements. For example, the ANA established the Nursing Information and Data Set Evaluation Center (NIDSEC). The intent of this center is to develop and distribute standards for information systems that will represent nursing practice (ANA, n.d.c).

Part of the mission of the NIDSEC is to evaluate information systems against these standards with the intent to recognize those systems that support the documentation of nursing care in computerized patient records (ANA, 1997).

Professional organizations also impact informatics standards through the development of certification processes. For example, another way that the ANA influences nursing informatics practice is through the ANCC informatics certification process. This process provides recognition that the recipient of certification has demonstrated knowledge specific to the practice of informatics (ANA, n.d.b).

As these organizations demonstrate, the processing and management of information is essential to ensuring that health care organizations and professionals adhere to standards of practice and care that are safe and effective. Data, information, and knowledge describe care processes and their effectiveness and efficiency in the provision of care. Staff members with informatics knowledge, experience, and expertise are an imperative component in facilitating an organization's successful meeting of accreditation standards by ensuring continuing improvement in the quality of care offered.

Role of the Informatics Professional

The informatics professional plays a critical role in the accreditation process. As a result, the informatics practitioner must be knowledgeable about the agencies, the accreditation processes, and the standards. Informatics-related standards typically focus on information management and planning, different types of data/information (patient-specific versus organizational), and comparative processes that allow benchmarking among organizations. Many informatics practitioners participate in the development of both internal and external standards. Often they are involved in developing the systems needed to meet these internal and external standards. For example, an informatics specialist might develop information systems that monitor and trend data and information related to medication errors or falls. The system then forms the basis for assessing the organization's compliance with standards of patient care.

Finally, informatics professionals are intimately involved in the implementation of standards across the organization in terms of both the information processes and their outcomes. One example is the development or acquisition of databases that provide data and information about clinical processes and also provide data that can be correlated with financial data to assess cost outcomes. A cardiac care database is one example that may be used to monitor clinical outcomes, as well as cost relationships. As standards are developed, they are often a result of rules and regulations required by government agencies. Often embedded in many of the standards are rules and regulations that are required by government agencies.

GOVERNMENTAL REGULATION

A **regulation** is a rule issued by governmental authorities that has the force of a law. Regulations can be issued at the federal, state, or local level. Most regulations are aimed at issues of quality, utilization, and cost of care (Ray, Cofer, & Coburn, 1996). The primary U.S. federal agency that has issued regulations related to health-related information systems is the U.S. Department of Health and Human Services. However, other federal agencies are also involved in issuing regulations that impact health care information systems. For example, the Occupational Health and Safety Administration has issued regulations related to ergonomics.

U.S. Department of Health and Human Services

The U.S. Department of Health and Human Services (DHHS) is the branch of federal government primarily responsible for the regulatory programs for the health care industry (USDHHS, 2000g). The DHHS is responsible for oversight and implementation of the Health Insurance Portability and Accountability Act (HIPAA) of 1996, the Food and Drug Administration (FDA), and the Centers for Medicare & Medicaid Services (CMS) (formerly the Health Care Financing Administration [HCFA]). This law and these two agencies have recently issued several regulations that directly affect health care information systems.

Health Insurance Portability and Accountability Act

The Health Insurance Portability and Accountability Act (HIPAA) passed in 1996 amended the Public Health Service Act (PHS Act), the Employee Retirement Income Security Act of 1974 (ERISA), and the Internal Revenue Code of 1986 (HCFA, n.d.a). It has five purposes:

1. To improve portability and continuity of health insurance coverage in the group and individual markets
2. To combat waste, fraud, and abuse in health insurance and health care delivery
3. To promote the use of medical savings accounts
4. To improve access to long-term care services and coverage
5. To simplify the administration of health insurance and for other purposes

The purpose of the section of the law dealing with simplifying the administration of health insurance is to improve the Medicare program under title XVIII of the Social Security Act, the Medicaid program under title XIX of the Social Security Act, and the efficiency and effectiveness of the health care system by encouraging the development of a health care information system by establishing standards and requirements for electronic transmission of certain health information (USDHHS, 1996).

To achieve these purposes, HIPAA includes a series of "administrative simplification" (AS) provisions that required the DHHS to adopt national standards for electronic health care transactions. These provisions call for the establishment of standards related to the electronic data interchange (EDI) of certain administrative and financial transactions while protecting the security and privacy of the transmitted information (USDHHS, 2000h). Current security and privacy protections are not universally applied. Practices are unregulated, and privacy laws vary widely from state to state. AS standards apply to providers, plans, and clearinghouses (agencies that process claims). Civil and criminal penalties exist for noncompliance, with fines up to $250,000 and imprisonment up to 10 years.

AS includes standards for transactions and code sets, unique identifiers, security and electronic signature, and privacy and confidentiality. Table 19-3 lists the AS standards and time lines (USDHHS, 2000i). Each standard is initially issued by the DHHS in the *Federal Register* as a "notice of proposed rule making" (NPRM). There is a public comment period, and later the final rules are published. The rules are effective within 60 days of publication, and compliance is usually required within 24 months of the final rule effective date. Small health plans have 36 months for compliance. The DHHS defines a small health plan in accordance with the Small Business Association definition of annual receipts with a maximum of $5 million (USDHHS, 2000f). The DHHS adjusted the time lines for expected final publication and on March 20, 2000, removed expected dates for all standards except those for transactions and code sets. The DHHS has reported delays related to the large number of comments received. For example, the standards for transactions and code sets received 17,000 comments.

HIPAA Administrative Simplification Transactions Standards and Code Sets The standards for electronic transactions and code sets are the only standards available to date in final rule status. The DHHS estimates that 400 formats are currently in use for electronic claims processing (USDHHS, 2000f). The final rules mandate standards for transactions and code sets. Table 19-4 lists the mandated transactions. The **transactions standards** for data transactions include health

Table 19–3 HIPAA Administrative Simplification Standards and Time Lines*

HIPAA Standard	Date Published for Public Comment (NPRM)	Final Publication	Required Compliance Date
Transactions and Code Sets	5/7/98	8/17/00	10/16/02†
National Provider Identifier	5/7/98		
National Employer Identifier	6/16/98		
Security	8/12/98		
Privacy	11/3/99	12/28/00	4/14/03
National Health Plan Identifier	Not published		
Claims Attachments	Not published		
Enforcement	Not published		
National Individual Identifier	On hold pending privacy legislation or regulation		

Data from U.S. Department of Health and Human Services. (2000). *Tentative schedule for publication of HIPAA administrative simplification regulations.* Retrieved July 11, 2001, from the World Wide Web: http://aspe.os.dhhs.gov/admnsimp/pubsched.htm.
NPRM, Notice of proposed rule making.
*Small health plans have 12 additional months to comply—8/16/03.
†The initial final dates for the standards have typically changed before truly becoming final dates.

Table 19–4 HIPAA-Mandated Transaction Standards

Transaction	Standard
Patient plan eligibility (inquiry and response)	ANSI ASC X12N 270 and 271
Claims status reports (request and response)	ANSI ASC X12N 276 and 277
Referral certification and authorization	ANSI ASC X12N 278
Plan premium payments	ANSI ASC X12N 820
Enrollment and disenrollment in health plan	ANSI ASC X12N 834
Payment and remittance advice	ANSI ASC X12N 835
Claims: dental, professional, and institutional	ANSI ASC X12N 837
Retail drug claims	NCPDP Telecommunications Standard Format Version 5.1 or NCPDP Batch Standard Version 1.0
Claims attachments	Pending separate NPRM and final regulations: ANSI ASC X12N 275

claims and equivalent encounter information, enrollment and disenrollment in a health plan, eligibility for a health plan, health care payment and remittance advice, health plan premium payments, health claim status, referral certification and authorization, and coordination of benefits (USDHHS, 2000b). The transaction standards mandate using the standard format developed by the American National Standards Institute's Accredited Standards Committee X12N subcommittee, version 4010, for all transactions except retail pharmacy. The National Council for Prescriptive Drug Programs (NCPDP) standard was chosen for retail pharmacy because it is already in widespread use (USDHHS, 2000b). Code sets are required under the HIPAA for data elements in the transaction standards. A **code set** is used to encode data elements such as terms, medical concepts, diagnosis codes, or procedure codes (USDHHS, 2000a). Table 19-5 lists the mandated code sets (USDHHS, 2000f). Additional information on codes and technical standards can be found in Chapter 17.

Implementation of the transactions and code sets may result in a boom for claims clearinghouses as one method of compliance with defined standards for provider and payer organizations that do not already use the defined code sets (Briggs, 2000). A survey of 65 clearinghouses indicates that 57% have at least one of the nine ANSI ASC X12N standards already and a few have met all nine standards (Briggs, 2000). The final standards define designated standard maintenance organizations (DSMOs). These are listed in Box 19-1 (USDHHS, 2000e). DSMOs are responsible for maintaining the standards for health care transactions adopted under HIPAA requirements, including evaluation of requests for standard changes. The DHHS estimates that implementations of the transactions and code sets will cost the industry $7 billion over 10 years and produce net savings of $29.9 billion over the same time period (USDHHS, 2000f). Average costs to large health plans are estimated at $1 million, costs to 100-plus bed hospitals at $250,000, and costs to individual providers at $1500.

HIPAA Administrative Simplification Unique Identifiers **Unique identifiers** are a standardized method to recognize entities within a specified group. These remain unchanged and are usually in the form of an alphanumeric code of a specified length (USDHHS, 1998c). HIPAA require-

Table 19–5 HIPAA–Mandated Code Sets

Data Elements	Code Set and Agency/Organization Responsible for Maintenance
Conditions	
Diseases Injuries Impairments Other health-related problems and their manifestations Causes of injury, disease, impairment, or other health problems	*International Classification of Diseases, 9th Revision, Clinical Modification* (ICD-9-CM), Volumes 1 and 2 maintained by the USDHHS
Inpatient hospital diseases, injuries, and impairments	
Prevention Diagnosis Treatment Management	*International Classification of Diseases, 9th Revision, Clinical Modification* (ICD-9-CM), Volume 3 maintained by the USDHHS
Drugs and biologics	National Drug Codes (NDC) maintained by the USDHHS
Dental services	The Code on Dental Procedures and Nomenclature (CDT) maintained by the American Dental Association (ADA)
Physicians' services Physical and occupational therapy services Radiological procedures Clinical laboratory tests Other medical diagnostic procedures Hearing and vision services Transportation services, including ambulance	The combination of the Health Care Financing Administration (HCFA) Common Procedure Coding System (HCPCS Level II) and the Current Procedural Terminology (CPT-4); USDHHS maintains HCPCS and the American Medical Association (AMA) maintains CPT-4
Medical supplies Orthotic and prosthetic devices Durable medical equipment	HCFA Common Procedure Coding System (HCPCS) Level II maintained by USDHHS

Data from U.S. Department of Health and Human Services. (2000). Health insurance reform: Standards for electronic transactions. *Federal Register, 65*(160), 50312-50372. Retrieved October 12, 2000, from the World Wide Web: http://aspe.os.dhhs.gov/admnsimp/final/txfinal.pdf.
USDHHS, U.S. Department of Health and Human Services.

ments include unique identifiers for providers, employers, health plans, and individuals. Current practice is for health plans to assign identification numbers to providers of services. As a result, providers who work with multiple health plans have multiple identification numbers (USDHHS, 2000c). The national provider identifier (NPI) will give each provider a unique number that will be used by all health plans. Providers will include all providers of services, such as physicians, nurse practitioners, hospitals, laboratories, nursing homes, pharmacies, and medical supply companies. The proposed standard for providers in the NPRM was an eight-character alphanumeric identifier. The DHHS received many comments recommending a 10-character numeric identifier with a check digit to detect keying errors (USDHHS, 2000c). The projected 5-year costs for implementation are $5.8 billion with a net savings of $1.5 billion

Box 19–1 U.S. Department of Health and Human Services–Designated Standard Maintenance Organizations

1. Accredited Standards Committee X12 (ASC X12)
2. Dental Content Committee of the American Dental Association
3. Health Level Seven (HL7)
4. National Council for Prescription Drug Programs (NCPDP)
5. National Uniform Billing Committee (NUBC)
6. National Uniform Claim Committee (NUCC)

From U.S. Department of Health and Human Services. (2000). Health insurance reform: Announcement of designated standard maintenance organizations. *Federal Register, 65*(160), 50373. Retrieved October 12, 2000, from the World Wide Web: http://aspe.os.dhhs.gov/admnsimp/final/dsmofr.pdf.

(USDHHS, 1998c). As of July 2001, the final standards for the NPI had not been published.

The national employer identifier is proposed for identifying employers as sponsors of health insurance on electronic transactions (USDHHS, 1998b). The DHHS is proposing the use of the taxpayer identification number that is currently assigned by the Internal Revenue Service as the employer identification number (EIN). The taxpayer identification number is nine digits with the first two digits separated by a hyphen (e.g., *00-0000000*). The tax identification number is proposed because most if not all employers already have an assigned number (USDHHS, 1998a). As of July 2001, the final EIN standards had not been published. No standard has been proposed for health plans or individuals, and both are still awaiting NPRMs by the DHHS.

HIPAA Administrative Simplification Security and Electronic Signature Standards Security and electronic signature standards are designed to protect the confidentiality, integrity, and availability of individual health information while allowing appropriate use by providers, plans, and clearinghouses (USDHHS, 2000d). The security standards apply to health data stored electronically or transmitted over a network. The proposed security standards include standards for administrative procedures, physical safeguards for data, technical security services, and technical security mechanisms (USDHHS, 1998d). The first three categories are designed to guard data integrity, confidentiality, and availability. The fourth category, technical security mechanisms, is to prevent unauthorized access.

Administrative procedures are documented procedures to manage the selection and execution of security measures and the conduct of personnel (USDHHS, 1998d). Proposed administrative procedures include certification, chain-of-trust agreements, contingency plans, formal mechanisms for processing records, information access control, internal audits, personnel security, security configuration management, security incident procedures, security management processes, termination procedures, and training. Physical safeguards protect computer hardware and buildings. Proposed physical safeguards include assigned security responsibility, media controls, physical access controls, policy or guidelines on workstation use, workstation security, and security awareness training. Technical security services are processes to protect, control, and monitor access. Proposed technical security services include access controls, audit controls, authorization controls, data authentication, and entity authentication. Technical security mechanisms are processes designed to protect data from unauthorized access as they are transmitted over a network. Proposed technical security mechanisms include integrity controls, message authentication, and either access controls or encryption. If a network is being used, the required technical security mechanisms include alarm, audit trail, entity authentication, and event reporting.

Electronic signature is the act of applying a signature to a document by electronic means. Applying a signature to a document accomplishes authentication, nonrepudiation, and assent (Michael, 2000). Authentication means that the signature identifies the source of a document. Nonrepudiation means that the person signing the document cannot later deny signature or approval of contents. Assent means that the parties approve of the terms or contents of the document. The proposed HIPAA standard for electronic signature is a digital signature with three required features: message integrity, nonrepudiation, and user authentication (USDHHS, 1998d). The DHHS defines a digital signature as "an electronic signature based on cryptographic methods of originator authentication, computed by using a set of rules and a set of parameters so that the identity of the signer and the integrity of the data can be verified" (USDHHS, 1998d, p. 43269). The electronic signature standard applies when HIPAA-specified transactions require the use of an electronic signature. As of July 2001, none of the transaction standards required an electronic signature.

Security standards will detail how data are stored and transmitted, and although the regulations may not specify a given technology or solution except for encryption, they may be specific enough to limit available choices (Hilts, 2000). Using technology alone does not mean that organizations are in compliance with the regulations (Gillespie, 2000). Technologies are typically used to support and reinforce efforts. Compliance with the regulations will require specific institutional policies and procedures.

HIPAA Administrative Simplification Privacy Standards Privacy is a means of protecting health information so that it is not used or disclosed except as authorized by the individual (USDHHS, 1999). The proposed HIPAA regulations would allow disclosure of health information for treatment; payment; or health care operations such as quality assurance, utilization review, or credentialing (Phoenix Health Systems, 2000). Any other disclosure of health information would require individual authorization. Privacy and confidentiality include consumer controls and protections for health records created or stored electronically, including the paper printouts of electronic documents. There are severe civil and criminal penalties for noncompliance (USDHHS, 1999). Providers, plans, or clearinghouses must maintain audit trails of information disclosure, including the paper printouts (Phoenix Health Systems, 2000). In addition to providers, plans, and clearinghouses, the privacy regulations would also apply to any business partner contracts between organizations (Christiansen, 2000). A business partner contract binds the business partner to the same privacy requirements as the provider, health plan, or clearinghouse.

Security standards also apply to data that are collected for research purposes. The standards require that data be stripped of all identifiers so that techniques cannot be used to reidentify the individuals. The DHHS has proposed a list of 19 identifiers for removal, such as name, address, telephone number, birth date, relative's name, and employer's name (USDHHS, 1999). The estimated costs for implementation are $3.8 billion over 5 years. The data privacy rule is the most controversial rule in the regulations. This may not be published on schedule because of the heavy volume of comments and the need to make rules dovetail with the security standards. The proposed privacy standards received 150,000 comments, whereas other proposed HIPAA standards had only 2000 or fewer comment (White House, 2000).

One common misconception about the HIPAA standards is that implementation is primarily an information systems issue (Walker & Spencer, 2000). The HIPAA standards affect a variety of business processes, procedures, and operations. The DHHS estimates that 80% to 90% of HIPAA implementation is administrative and that the remainder is technical (Amatayakul, 2000). The DHHS estimates that the costs of implementing the HIPAA standards will rival and perhaps exceed the cost of fixing the Y2K problem, whereas other analysts estimate that implementing the HIPAA standards will cost providers anywhere from $10 to $43 billion (Kirchheimer, 2000). HIPAA implementation requires large-scale planning and changes in information systems and business processes much like the work that was done for the Y2K problem (Tabar, 2000).

An interdisciplinary approach is recommended, since operational changes will cut across the organization (Amatayakul, 2000). One unique strategy is the statewide HIPAA compliance effort begun by the North Carolina Healthcare Information and Communication Alliance (NCHICA) (Scott, 2000). NCHICA members include provider organizations, health plans, research organizations, state government agencies, state professional associations, and business partners. More than 100 individuals representing 50 NCHICA member organizations are working on five HIPAA-related task forces. It is likely that the success of the implementation of the HIPAA regulations will by necessity require this kind of multiorganizational approach because of the complexity of information processing and management of health care.

The DHHS, in addition to providing oversight for HIPAA compliance, is the reporting structure for the Food and Drug Administration.

Food and Drug Administration

The Center for Devices and Radiological Health (CDRH) of the Food and Drug Administration (FDA) develops and implements a national program to protect the public health related to medical devices (FDA, n.d.). The regulations were established in the Medical Device Amendments to the Federal Food, Drug, and Cosmetic (FFD&C) Act enacted in 1976. The FFD&C Act was most recently amended by the FDA Modernization Act of 1997. Health care information systems are regulated by this agency as medical devices if they are part of instruments, machines, or other related articles intended for use in the diagnosis of disease or other conditions.

Medical devices are classified into one of three groups on the basis of the level of control necessary to ensure safety (FDA, n.d.). Class I requires general controls; class II requires general controls and special controls; and class III requires general controls, special controls, and premarket approval. Class I devices present minimal potential for harm to the user and require manufacturing in accordance with "good manufacturing practices." Class II devices require special controls. Special controls may include special labeling requirements, guidance documents, mandatory performance standards, and postmarket surveillance. Class III devices are typically items that support or sustain human life. A 510(k) submission or premarketing submission to demonstrate device safety is required for specified class II and class III devices. A 510(k) review of a device is made to determine whether it is substantially equivalent to a device already legally marketed in the United States (FDA, 2001). The required practices, audit trails, and system checks are intended to improve quality and system integrity. When information systems that interface with physiological monitoring devices are being purchased, FDA approval for these systems will most likely be required.

Centers for Medicare & Medicaid Services

The Centers for Medicare & Medicaid Services (CMS) (formerly HCFA), established in 1966, is responsible for the rules and regulations that govern the Medicare program (HCFA, n.d.b). To be eligible for Medicare and Medicaid reimbursement, providers must demonstrate compliance with the "conditions of participation" (COP) (Social Security Administration, n.d.b). Compliance certification is the responsibility of states; however, Title XVIII of the

Medicare act specifies that facilities accredited by the JCAHO or American Osteopathic Association (AOA) are deemed compliant (Social Security Administration, n.d.a). COP revisions are published in the *Federal Register.*

The Outcomes and Assessment Information Set (OASIS) is a core group of data elements that include items of a comprehensive assessment for an adult home care patient and form the basis for measuring patient outcomes for purposes of outcome-based quality improvement (OBQI) (HCFA, 2000). OASIS data are a key component of the revised COP for Medicare-certified home health agencies. Also identified are data submission standards that home health agencies must follow in their submission of required OASIS data to the state.

The CMS also uses the Minimum Data Set (MDS) as the means of collecting specific data on the long-term care patient. The first version of the MDS was used in 1990. The data elements included resident background, activities of daily living, cognition, physical functioning, health problems, psychological status, and a body systems review (Fletcher, 1997). Each state must specify a resident assessment instrument (RAI) for use by all long-term care facilities to assess and plan for a resident's care (HCFA, 1998). The minimum requirement for the state RAI is the CMS's MDS. The idea behind the MDS was to standardize data elements related to the care that was provided to long-term care patients, as well as provide a means to consistently evaluate the quality of care provided.

The proposed HIPAA standards, the FDA guidelines for medical devices, and the CMS guidelines for Medicare and Medicaid demonstrate the impact of governmental regulations on the complexity of health care information systems and information management. To ensure that health care institutions maintain compliance with the regulations, it is essential for health care informatics specialists to stay abreast of the changes in these types of regulations.

Other Regulatory Agencies and Regulations

Other regulatory agencies and regulations of interest to the informatics professional include the Occupational Safety and Health Administration and the Consumer Internet Privacy Enhancement Act.

Occupational Safety and Health Administration

The Occupational Safety and Health Administration (OSHA), an agency of the U.S. Department of Labor, was formed after Congress passed the Occupational Safety and Health Act in 1970 (OSHA, 1998). OSHA published the proposed rules and regulations for an ergonomics program in the *Federal Register* on November 23, 1999. The proposal underwent a public comment period and public hearings. The proposed rules pertained to work-related musculoskeletal disorders (MSDs). MSDs include carpal tunnel syndrome and tendinitis. Risk factors for MSDs include repetitive motions, awkward postures, and static postures. The OSHA proposal identified a full ergonomics program with six elements of management: leadership and employee participation, hazard information and reporting, job hazard analysis and control, training, MSD management, and program evaluation (OSHA, n.d.).

Professional organizations varied in their response and support of the proposed OSHA ergonomic standards. The ANA supported the OSHA ergonomic standards. The American Health Care Association did not support the proposed standards because it believed the requirements would have a significant and negative financial impact on long-term care facilities. The American Hospital Association and the American Society for Healthcare Human Resources Administration also believed that the costs for implementation were underestimated (Trossman, 2000). Much of the controversy that surrounded the ergonomics rules concerned the additional costs that businesses would incur. In March 2001, President Bush signed into law S.J. Res. 6, a measure that repealed the proposed regulations dealing with ergonomics (U.S. Government, 2001).

Ergonomic principles are important in the design and implementation of computer workstations. As a result of these rules, the informatics professional must consider the environmental dimension of user information processing and management. Ergonomically designed workstations and furniture are only now being developed as people experience the long-term effects of sustained nonneutral body positions. It appears that the effects of poor body mechanics related to these postures accumulate over time and possibly interact with other factors, making it difficult to pinpoint an exact point of injury (Steering Committee for the Workshop on Work-Related Musculoskeletal Injuries, 1998). The potential for user injury and subsequent cost to the organization requires that the informatics professional broaden the traditional life cycle of an information system to include the user environment from the physical dimension. A discussion of ergonomics and other aspects of human-computer interaction is included in Chapter 15.

Consumer Internet Privacy Enhancement Act

In its research report titled *The Online Health Care Revolution: How Americans Take Better Care of Themselves,* the Pew Internet Project of the Pew Research Center identified fear of privacy violations as one of the major fears of individuals seeking health information on the Internet (Pew Internet Project, 2000). The Consumer Internet Privacy Enhancement Act was introduced in the U.S. Senate on July 26, 2000 (S. 2928). The bill was designed to protect the privacy of individuals using the Internet. With this bill, Web sites may not collect personally identifiable information unless the consumer is notified and has the ability to limit marketing use and third-party disclosure. The Web site notice must include the identity of the Web site operator and any involved third parties, a list of information collected, a description of how the information is used, any requirements to provide information in order to use the Web site, and steps taken to protect the security of the information. The bill was referred to the Senate Committee on Commerce, Science, and Transportation. Although there is some agreement that such legislation is needed, compromise will be required. Congress is likely to continue to focus on privacy issues. Although this specific bill may not become a law, as consumers become more aware of the implications of providing information about themselves to organizations, they will demand higher levels of accountability and appropriate protection of their privacy.

Implications for Informatics Professionals

The OSHA-proposed ergonomic standards and the proposed Consumer Internet Privacy Enhancement Act provide examples of how regulations and legislation are important to the informatics professional. The standards, rules, and regulations will change over time. The importance of the health care informatics specialist staying current and understanding the implications of government laws and regulations cannot be overemphasized.

This chapter has focused on national laws and regulations. State and local level regulations can also have an impact on health care informatics practice. Keeping abreast of regulatory changes contributes to the complexity of challenges facing the informatics professional. Balancing system knowledge, organizational knowledge, and the changing regulatory environment across all levels often seems like building a house of cards that can come crashing down at any moment.

Unlike accreditation and certification, regulations tend to be a moving target for the informatics professional, especially in the early days of their interpretation. Implementation and integration of standards and regulatory requirements into clinical information systems is dependent on the interpretation of the rules and regulations.

Sometimes the "interpretation" requires interpretation. The informatics professional is dependent on keen project management skills to avoid making costly mistakes by failing to plan, in his or her particular setting, for required regulations and rules. Networking people by nature, savvy informatics professionals interact regularly with peers and industry leaders to be sure that their approach in their organization is a sound one.

CASE EXAMPLE

A case example from Women's Hospital illustrates the importance of accreditation and regulation in the selection and installation of an obstetrical information management system. Throughout the system's life cycle, there are many opportunities for the informatics professional to apply knowledge of accreditation and regulation.

Women's Hospital (Women's) is a 150-bed facility that is part of the Special Health Care System. The leadership at Women's is planning the purchase of an obstetrical information management system. The system will be used in the 30-bed labor and delivery unit, the 20-bed antepartum unit, and the 30-bed postpartum unit. Currently the hospital delivers about 3200 newborns per year. The physician practice groups include attending physicians, residents, and medical students, along with private-practice groups of obstetricians and family practitioners. Providers also include midwives in both private practice and academic service.

Initial project objectives have been outlined. These include increased compliance with the JCAHO standards regarding clinician documentation, medication use, and continuity of care. Defined requirements include components related to fetal monitoring and fetal monitoring strip archiving. These requirements necessitate compliance with FDA regulations. Mechanisms for appropriate dispensing and management of medications are a key aspect of the cost management goals.

Infant morbidity and mortality rates are high in this area. Women's hopes to lower these rates by ensuring continuity of care during the prenatal and postpartum period. Continuity of care is necessary to decrease the costs related to prematurity. Prematurity is a common cause for lengthy newborn hospital stays at Women's. The administrators believe that having a common information system across departments will enhance continuity of care because data and information would be accessible, available, and complete.

Aware of the problems that changes in information systems create for the clinician, the informatics professional involves key end users in the process of developing system objectives. End user involvement provides another resource for understanding the accreditation and regulatory standards and their impact on practice within the framework of the current information system and the proposed system. An added benefit of clinician involvement is having knowledgeable people at the point of care who can convey to other staff members why certain project decisions were made on the basis of standards, rules, and regulations.

As requests for proposal are developed, the organization includes statements regarding the need to comply with JCAHO standards and FDA requirements. During product demonstrations, the informatics professional evaluates whether the system meets the identified standards and regulations. Once a purchase decision is made, contractual language is developed to specifically target compliance with accreditation standards and regulatory requirements. During the selection phase, comparisons of current process capabilities form the basis for later evaluation. The informatics professional is involved in the ongoing data collection and analysis of continuous process improvement projects that were drivers of the decision to select an information system solution.

Implementation planning identifies needs for customization to meet organizational priority items. In this phase the project manager and team consistently refer back to the business plan and to how the system will facilitate maintaining compliance with regulations and accrediting requirements. Staying current with the changing regulatory and accrediting requirements as the implementation progresses allows for system adaptation and is less of a burden on the staff in terms of learning new requirements. Using the system implementation as a way to reinforce regulatory and accrediting requirements also provides just-in-time review and reinforcement so that the staff can more easily make the connections between the old way of doing business and the new way of working through the standards and regulations.

Ongoing system evaluation includes maintaining compliance as standards and regulations change. The informatics professional applies knowledge of the appropriate accreditation standards and regulatory requirements throughout the system's life cycle. Integrating the requirements into the new system, as well as into the process improvement plans, provides for a smooth transition and more systematic analysis of whether the information solution achieved the outcomes it was designed to meet.

CONCLUSION

Health care informatics professionals who understand the processes necessary for effective and efficient management of data, information, and knowledge are required for the organization to meet accreditation and regulation requirements. Effective and efficient management of data, information, and knowledge places a health care organization on solid ground to successfully complete the accreditation processes and meet regulatory requirements. Coupled with the need to understand data, information, and knowledge management, the informatics professional is required to be knowledgeable of the rules, regulations, and standards of the different accrediting and regulatory agencies. Ideally, compliance with accreditation and regulatory requirements demonstrates that the organization is strategically positioned to be competitive in the health care arena. Effective information and knowledge management related to accreditation and regulation places the organization in a much better position to meet internal and external standards more efficiently and effectively.

Web Connection

The introduction of or change in an organization's information and communication technologies is highly influenced by accreditation and governmental regulations. The primary element in both processes is evaluation of performance against a standard. Informatics professionals facilitate the interpretation of standards and regulations and assist the organization to achieve and maintain compliance with them. The Web Connection activities for this chapter introduce the organizations that deal with accreditation and regulation. Using the regulations mandated by the Health Insurance Portability and Accountability Act, you will examine different perspectives to be considered in achieving compliance with these regulations.

discussion questions

1. Discuss how effective and efficient data, information, and knowledge management is required to successfully meet accreditation and regulation requirements.
2. Using examples, explain the impact of accreditation, certification, and governmental regulations on the life cycle of a health care information system.
3. Describe the purpose of the accreditation process and the role of the informatics professional in the process.

4. List the sources of governmental regulation in health care and explain how the informatics professional facilitates regulatory compliance.
5. Discuss the HIPAA regulations and their significance to health care information management policies and procedures.

REFERENCES

Amatayakul, M. (2000). HIPAA 2000 conference report: HIPAA is heating up. *MD Computing, 17*(4), 15-17.

American Health Care Association. (2000). *OSHA's proposed ergonomic standard: A groundless regulation.* Retrieved October 12, 2000, from the World Wide Web: http://www.ahca.org/brief/ISS-Ergo.htm.

American Hospital Association. (2000). *Letters to the hill.* Retrieved October 12, 2000, from the World Wide Web: http://www.aha.org/ar/ergonomics600.html.

American Nurses Association. (1997). *Nursing information and data set evaluation center: Standards and scoring guidelines.* Washington, DC: American Nurses Publishing.

American Nurses Association. (n.d.a). *Fact sheet on ANCC certification program.* Washington, DC: American Nurses Publishing. Retrieved October 19, 2000, from the World Wide Web: http://www.ana.org/ancc/fsancc.htm.

American Nurses Association. (n.d.b). *Informatics nurse certification.* Washington DC: American Nurses Publishing. Retrieved October 22, 2000, from the World Wide Web: http://www.nursingworld.org/ancc/certify/catalogs/2000/cbt/infonurs.htm.

American Nurses Association. (n.d.c). *What is NIDSEC?* Washington, DC: American Nurses Publishing. Retrieved October 15, 2000, from the World Wide Web: http://www.ana.org/nidsec/index.htm.

American Nurses Credentialing Center. (n.d.). *Magnet nursing services recognition program.* Washington, DC: American Nurses Publishing. Retrieved October 12, 2000, from the World Wide Web: http://www.ana.org/ancc/magnet.htm.

Briggs, B. (2000). Early HIPAA feast for clearinghouses? *Health Data Management, 8*(8), 76-78, 80.

Christiansen, J. (2000). Tips for negotiating HIPAA contract requirements: Business partners and chain of trust agreements. *IT Health Care Strategist, 2*(5), 6-7.

Consumer Internet Privacy Enhancement Act, S. 2928, 106th Cong., 2D Sess. (2000). Retrieved October 12, 2000, from the World Wide Web: http://frwebgate.access.gpo.gov/cgi-bin/getdoc.cgi?dbname=106_cong_bills&docid=f:s2928is.txt.pdf.

Fletcher, D.M. (1997). Outcome assessment information set (OASIS) for home care. *Journal of the American Health Information Management Association, 68.* Retrieved October 4, 2000, from the World Wide Web: http://www.ahima.org/journal/working.smart/97.09.html.

Food and Drug Administration. (2001). *What is premarket notification?* [Premarket Notification]. Rockville, MD: Author. Retrieved June 26, 2001, from the World Wide Web: http://www.fda.gov/cdrh/devadvice/314.html#link_1.

Food and Drug Administration. (n.d.). *Center for Devices and Radiologic Health.* Washington, DC: Author. Retrieved October 12, 2000, from the World Wide Web: http://www.fda.gov/cdrh/index.html.

Gillespie, G. (2000). How will CIOs protect data to comply with HIPAA? *Health Data Management, 8*(8), 41, 43, 46, 48, 50-52.

Health Care Financing Administration. (1998). *Specification of HCFA's MDS/RAI and effective dates.* Washington, DC: Author. Retrieved October 12, 2000, from the World Wide Web: http://www.hcfa.gov/medicaid/mds20/mdsdates.htm.

Health Care Financing Administration. (2000). *OASIS overview.* Washington, DC: Author. Retrieved October 12, 2000, from the World Wide Web: http://hcfa.hhs.gov/medicaid/oasis/hhoview.htm.

Health Care Financing Administration. (n.d.a). *HIPAA insurance reform.* Washington, DC: Author. Retrieved October 12, 2000, from the World Wide Web: http://hcfa.hhs.gov/medicaid/HIPAA/topics/more.asp [no longer available].

Health Care Financing Administration. (n.d.b). *Welcome to HCFA.* Washington, DC: Author. Retrieved October 12, 2000, from the World Wide Web: http://www.hcfa.gov.

Hilts, M. (2000). Authentication in HIPAA. *Health Management Technology, 21*(7), 38.

International Organization for Standardization. (1998). *Selection and use of ISO 9000.* Geneva: Switzerland: Author. Retrieved October 12, 2000, from the World Wide Web: http://www.iso.ch/9000e/selusee.pdf.

Joint Commission on Accreditation of Healthcare Organizations. (2000a). *2000 hospital accreditation standards.* Oakbrook Terrace, IL: Author.

Joint Commission on Accreditation of Healthcare Organizations. (2000b). ORYX: *The next evolution in accreditation.* Oakbrook Terrace, IL: Author. Retrieved October 12, 2000, from the World Wide Web: http://wwwb.jcaho.org/perfmeas/oryx_qa.html.

Kirchheimer, B. (2000). Report predicts huge HIPAA price tag. *Modern Healthcare.* Retrieved October 12, 2000, from the World Wide Web: http://www.modernhealthcare.com/currentissue/pastpost.php3?refid=5985.

Kohn, L.T., Corrigan, J.M., & Donaldson, M.S. (1999). *To err is human: Building a safer health system.* Washington, DC: National Academy Press.

Kreider, N.A., & Haselton, B.J. (1997). *The systems challenge: Getting the clinical information you need to support patient care.* Chicago: American Hospital Association.

Merriam-Webster. (2000). *Merriam-Webster WWW dictionary.* Springfield, MA: Author. Retrieved March 9, 2000, from the World Wide Web: http://www.m-w.com/.

Michael, E.L. (2000). Electronic signature legislation. *Ubiquity.* Retrieved October 12, 2000, from the World Wide Web: http://www.acm.org/ubiquity/views/e_michael_1.html.

National Committee for Quality Assurance. (n.d.a). *Health plan employers data and information set.* Retrieved October 12, 2000, from the World Wide Web: http://www.ncqa.org/Pages/Programs/HEDIS/index.htm.

National Committee for Quality Assurance. (n.d.b). *National Committee for Quality Assurance: An overview.* Retrieved October 12, 2000, from the World Wide Web: http://www.ncqa.org/Pages/about/overview3.htm.

Occupational Safety and Health Administration. (1998). *OSHA strategic plan.* Washington, DC: Author. Retrieved October 12, 2000, from the World Wide Web: http://www.osha.gov/oshinfo/strategic/pg1.html#intro.

Occupational Safety and Health Administration. (n.d.). *How does this standard apply to me?* Washington, DC: Author. Retrieved October 12, 2000, from the World Wide Web: http://www.osha-slc.gov/ergonomics-standard/preamble/IV_905-910-APPLY.html.

Pew Internet Project. (2000). *The online health care revolution: How Americans take better care of themselves. Pew Internet and American Life. Pew Internet Project.* Washington, DC: Pew Research Center. Retrieved from the World Wide Web: http://www.pewinternet.org/reports/toc.asp?Report=26.

Phoenix Health Systems. (2000). HIPAAfaq: Privacy. *HIPAAdvisory.* Retrieved October 12, 2000, from the World Wide Web: http://www.hipaadvisory.com/action/faqs/FAQ_Privacy.htm.

Ray, M.N., Cofer, J., & Coburn, V.R. (1996). Health care systems. In M. Abdelhak, S. Grostick, M.A. Hanken, & E. Jacobs (Eds.), *Health information: Management of a strategic resource.* Philadelphia: W.B. Saunders.

Scott, L. (2000). Coordinating compliance. *Modern Healthcare,* October 2. Retrieved October 12, 2000, from the World Wide Web: http://www.modernhealthcare.com/article.php3?refid=59.

Social Security Administration. (n.d.a). *Social Security Act, Title XVIII Health Insurance for the Aged and Disabled: Effect of accreditation.* Washington, DC: Author. Retrieved October 12, 2000, from the World Wide Web: http://www.ssa.gov/OP_Home/ssact/title18/1865.htm.

Social Security Administration. (n.d.b). *Social Security Act, Title XVIII Health Insurance for the Aged and Disabled: Use of state agencies to determine compliance by providers of service with conditions of participation.* Washington, DC: Author. Retrieved October 12, 2000, from the World Wide Web: http://www.ssa.gov/OP_Home/ssact/title18/1864.htm.

Steering Committee for the Workshop on Work-Related Musculoskeletal Injuries: The Research Base, Committee on Human Factors, & Commission on Behavioral and Social Science and Education. (1998). *Work-related musculoskeletal disorders: A review of the evidence.* Washington, DC: National Academy Press.

Tabar, P. (2000). CIOs speak out. *Healthcare Informatics Online,* April. Retrieved October 12, 2000, from the World Wide Web: http://www.healthcare-informatics.com/issues/2000/04_00/hipaa.htm.

Trossman, S. (2000). Moving violations: Working to prevent on-the-job injuries. *The American Nurse, 32*(5), 1, 12-14.

U.S. Department of Health and Human Services. (1996). *Health Insurance Portability and Accountability Act.* Washington, DC: Author. Retrieved from the World Wide Web: http://aspe.hhs.gov/admnsimp/pl104191.htm#261.

U.S. Department of Health and Human Services. (1998a). *Frequently asked questions about the national standard employer identifier (EIN).* Washington, DC: Author. Retrieved October 12, 2000, from the World Wide Web: http://aspe.os.dhhs.gov/admnsimp/faqemp.htm.

U.S. Department of Health and Human Services. (1998b). Health insurance reform: Standard employer identifier. *Federal Register, 63*(115), 32784-32798. Retrieved October 12, 2000, from the World Wide Web: http://aspe.os.dhhs.gov/admnsimp/nprm/empnprm.pdf.

U.S. Department of Health and Human Services. (1998c). National standard health care provider identifier. *Federal Register, 63*(88), 25320-25357. Retrieved October 12, 2000, from the World Wide Web: http://aspe.os.dhhs.gov/admnsimp/nprm/npinprm.pdf.

U.S. Department of Health and Human Services. (1998d). Security and electronic signature standards. *Federal Register, 63*(155), 43241-43280. Retrieved October 12, 2000, from the World Wide Web: http://aspe.os.dhhs.gov/admnsimp/nprm/secnprm.pdf.

U.S. Department of Health and Human Services. (1999). Standards for privacy of individually identifiable health information: Proposed rule. *Federal Register, 64*(212), 59918-60065. Retrieved October 12, 2000, from the World Wide Web: http://aspe.os.dhhs.gov/admnsimp/nprm/pvcnprm.pdf.

U.S. Department of Health and Human Services. (2000a). *Frequently asked questions about code set standards adopted under HIPAA.* Washington, DC: Author. Retrieved October 12, 2000, from the World Wide Web: http://aspe.os.dhhs.gov/admnsimp/.

U.S. Department of Health and Human Services. (2000b). *Frequently asked questions about electronic transaction standards adopted under HIPAA.* Washington, DC: Author. Retrieved October 12, 2000, from the World Wide Web: http://aspe.os.dhhs.gov/admnsimp/faqtx.htm.

U.S. Department of Health and Human Services. (2000c). *Frequently asked questions about the national provider identifier (NPI).* Washington, DC: Author. Retrieved October 12, 2000, from the World Wide Web: http://aspe.os.dhhs.gov/admnsimp/faqnpi.htm.

U.S. Department of Health and Human Services. (2000d). *Frequently asked questions about security and electronic signature standards.* Washington, DC: Author. Retrieved October 12, 2000, from the World Wide Web: http://aspe.os.dhhs.gov/admnsimp/faqsec.htm.

U.S. Department of Health and Human Services. (2000e). Health insurance reform: Announcement of designated standard maintenance organizations. *Federal Register, 65*(160), 50373. Retrieved October 12, 2000, from the World Wide Web: http://aspe.os.dhhs.gov/admnsimp/final/dsmofr.pdf.

U.S. Department of Health and Human Services. (2000f). Health insurance reform: Standards for electronic transactions. *Federal Register, 65*(160), 50312-50372. Retrieved October 12, 2000, from the World Wide Web: http://aspe.os.dhhs.gov/admnsimp/final/txfinal.pdf.

U.S. Department of Health and Human Services. (2000g). *HHS: What we do.* Washington, DC: Author. Retrieved October 12, 2000, from the World Wide Web: http://www.hhs.gov/about/profile.html.

U.S. Department of Health and Human Services. (2000h). *Other frequently asked questions about administrative simplification.* Washington, DC: Author. Retrieved October 12, 2000, from the World Wide Web: http://aspe.os.dhhs.gov/admnsimp/faq-othq.htm.

U.S. Department of Health and Human Services. (2000i). *Tentative schedule for publication of HIPAA administrative simplification regulations.* Washington, DC: Author. Retrieved October 12, 2000, from the World Wide Web: http://aspe.os.dhhs.gov/admnsimp/pubsched.htm.

U.S. Government. (2001). S.J. Res. 6. Retrieved from the World Wide Web: http://www.whitehouse.gov/news/releases/2001/03/20010321.html.

Walker, J. & Spencer, J. (2000). Ten deadly sins. *Health Management Technology, 21*(7), 10.

White House seeks to distort privacy rules and rush them out this year. (2000). *Inside Healthcare Computing, 10*(21), 1-3.

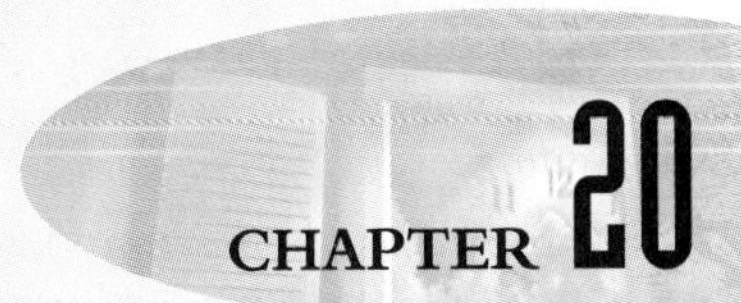

CHAPTER 20

Protection of Health Care Information

DONNA W. BAILEY
W. HOLT ANDERSON

Learning Objectives

Upon completion of this chapter, the reader will be able to:

1. ***Identify*** the essential dimensions of performance involved in protecting health care information.
2. ***Explain*** the differences among privacy, confidentiality, and security.
3. ***Illustrate*** the complexity of protecting health care information using the virtual health record.
4. ***Outline*** the legal and policy implications for protection of health information.
5. ***Identify*** elected practices currently used to protect patient information and discuss the issues associated with their use.

Outline

Dimensions of Performance
- *Access*
- *Integrity*
- *Availability*

Transition From Paper to a Virtual Health Record
- *New Methods of Linking Records*
- *Privacy, Confidentiality, and Security in the Virtual World*

Legal and Policy Implications
- *Legal Protection*
- *Ownership and Control of Health Information*
- *DNA Matching*
- *Health Insurance Portability and Accountability Act: A Federal Initiative*
- *Reengineering Health Care for Compliance*

Key Terms

access
administrative simplification
authentication
availability
confidentiality
digital certificates
eHealth
health information
Health Insurance Portability and Accountability Act (HIPAA)
integrity
privacy
Public Key–Encryption Infrastructure (PKI)
security
virtual health record

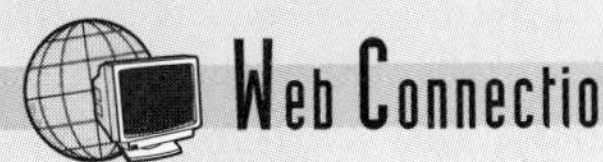

Web Connection

Go to the Web site at http://evolve.elsevier.com/Englebardt/. Here you will find Web links and activities related to the protection of health care information.

Modern information and communications technologies present both opportunities and challenges to providing high-quality, efficient health care. Just a few decades ago, the landscape of health care services consisted primarily of the family practitioner and the corner pharmacy using simple paper records to provide care for generations of a family. Today's complex world is made up of health plans, managed care options, specialists, and pharmacies that are increasingly using the Internet and electronic records to create a new health care economic model called **eHealth.** Information generated in this new landscape is receiving heightened attention. The technologies are fundamentally different from paper-based records and communications in several ways. Differences include the ease of access, the potential for loss of integrity, and issues related to storage and future availability. In this transition from paper-based, traditional methods of communicating to almost instantaneous exchange of information, the management of health care information based on well-understood and articulated public policy and commonly accepted technical standards has lagged (Dick, Steen, & Detmer, 1997).

Protection of health care information is a complex endeavor requiring that the informatics professional be aware of more than the obvious issues related to protecting current personal information. Information and communications technologies will change, innovate, and become outdated. To facilitate efficient access to reliable data and information, professionals must also have an eye on the future, as well as the past.

Informatics professionals are key players in the development of technologies and processes within their organizations, in all levels of government, and in the information and communication systems industries. They are well aware of the dimensions of performance necessary to protect personal and organizational health information.

Health information has been defined as:

> *. . . any information, whether oral or recorded in any form or medium that is created or received by a health care provider, health plan, public health authority, employer, life insurer, school or university, or health care clearinghouse; and related to the past, present, or future physical or mental health or condition of an individual, the provision of health care to an individual, or the past, present, or future payment for the provision of health care to an individual. (U.S. Department of Health and Human Services, 1998, p. 43264)*

This definition highlights the multifaceted nature of health care information protection by including the multiple producers, intermediaries, and users of health care information. Key aspects of the information protection function of the health care informatics specialist are management and facilitation of information in terms of who has access to data and information; when access occurs; how access is obtained; and how data and information are used, transformed, and made available for future review and transformation. The health care informatics specialist's role in ensuring the protection of health care information focuses on several dimensions of performance.

DIMENSIONS OF PERFORMANCE

The dimensions of performance that are necessary to protect health care information include access, integrity, and availability. Within these focal areas are key concepts that are used to describe information protection.

Access

The first dimension of performance is access. **Access** refers to the ability to obtain data and information for specific purposes and by specific users. This dimension of performance is the most commonly thought of when protecting health care information and is highly interrelated to the dimensions of integrity and availability. The terms *privacy, confidentiality,* and *security* are used to describe aspects of access. There are a multitude of definitions for each of these terms

(Committee on Maintaining Privacy and Security in Health Care Applications of the National Information Infrastructure, 1997; Joint Commission on Accreditation of Healthcare Organizations, 1999; Strum, 1998). In this chapter the definitions provided by the Institute of Medicine study—For the Record: Protecting Electronic Health Information—are used:

> ***Privacy*** *refers to an individual's desire to limit disclosure of personal information.* ***Confidentiality*** *is a condition in which information is shared or released in a controlled manner.* ***Security*** *refers to measures that organizations implement to protect information and systems, including efforts to ensure the integrity and availability of that information and the information systems used to access it. (Committee on Maintaining Privacy and Security in Health Care Applications of the National Information Infrastructure, 1997, p. 1)*

Access issues are not new to the health care setting. Traditional patient records and verbal communications are also susceptible to inappropriate or accidental access. Every institution has policies and procedures aimed at protecting individually identifiable data and information. Some of these policies meet the requirements of accrediting bodies. Increasingly, there are federally legislated laws and regulations aimed at protecting health information. Some examples include the Freedom of Information Act, the Privacy Act of 1974, regulations on confidentiality of alcohol and drug abuse records, and most recently, the Health Insurance Portability and Accountability Act (HIPAA) of 1996. In addition, there are many state laws to protect health information; however, these laws form a patchwork of protections that are increasingly complicated and difficult to administer because of the increasingly global nature of health care (Dennis, 2000).

With the advent of the Internet and the ability to easily transmit information rapidly and to large numbers of individuals, these rules and regulations seek to impose severe consequences for violating privacy, breaching confidentiality, or failing to provide adequate security measures for health information. Closely related to access is the integrity of health information.

Integrity

Integrity of health information is concerned with ensuring the completeness and accuracy of data and information, as well as the protection of data and information from processes that would invalidate them (Collen, 1995). Completeness of records is dependent on the careful construction of templates and processes required to capture and represent desired data and information. Increasingly, a team approach to the development of languages is necessary so that the language used by one provider does not invalidate the entries, analyses, and decision-making processes of other providers. The need to create common languages is, in part, driven by the need to ensure that the data and information that are available to providers are easily understood by all users. Consistent and commonly used coding processes facilitate the integrity of data and information. The consistency of coding is essential as software is developed to interface with the myriad sources of health care data and information. The potential for data to be altered or lost in the transmission between programs is related to the ability of the software to recognize and accept the data.

Another threat to data integrity is the accidental entry of incorrect data or information into the record. Transcription errors are common. One of the highly touted reasons for implementing a clinical information system is to provide clinicians with the ability to easily enter their own data and information into the record, thereby decreasing transcription errors. At the same time that clinical information and communications technologies are proliferating, there is an increase in interfaced medical information devices that stream data into records independent of the provider. Ensuring that these data are accurate and consistent with the clinical picture of the patient adds additional information protection processes to an already-complicated picture of information security.

More sinister is the intentional reading, alteration, or tampering with data and information that occurs through inappropriate or unauthorized access. The increased number of users requiring access to health information has led to the difficult process of ensuring that the right users are accessing the information for the right reasons (Committee on Maintaining Privacy and Security in Health Care Applications of the National Information Infrastructure, 1997). Unfortunately, for a variety of reasons, some authorized users intentionally provide confidential information to others. Less commonly considered by the average information user is the disruption caused by the increasing number of computer viruses and worms. A computer virus is software that infects a computer by burying its code within an existing program. The effect of a virus can vary from a simple irritation such as message that pops up on the screen to a major loss of software or data. A worm is a destructive program that replicates itself throughout disk and memory and uses up the computer's resources. A worm can cause a computer to operate so slowly that it is not useable (TechEncyclopedia, 2001). These programs disrupt systems and can cause loss of data or alterations in data that may go unnoticed (Collen, 1995). Because health information is increasingly seen as a resource that spans the "cradle to the grave" for an individual, the potential for unnoticed alterations and data loss may seriously affect the validity and reliability of this resource.

Availability

Each individual's data and information serve as the basis for individual and aggregate health decisions. Therefore it is important to ensure that the information is available when needed. **Availability** refers to the ability of information users to easily access data and information appropriate to their authorization level when needed. In the short term, this requires systems that protect data and information through a variety of security measures, including access controls, personnel security, training, organizational policies and procedures, and network/workstation controls (Dennis, 2000). The ability to access the information should not be hampered by cumbersome processes that are complex and slow. Every practitioner can relate to waiting for the delivery of an old chart from the medical records department, only to find that the material in the chart folder is either incomplete or unavailable.

In the long term, storage capabilities and media life expectancies form the basis for ensuring that data and information are reliably and readily available. Archival systems that consider that individual records may span over a century are necessary (McCall & Mix, 1995). Storage strategies that take into consideration access, natural disasters such as fire or flooding, and innovations in the technology are necessary. An example of an innovation that has gone by the wayside is the obsolescence of media such as microfilm and microfiche. Records that were recorded on microfiche as recently as the late 1980s can be difficult if not impossible to read today because of a lack of microfiche readers.

Whether the health care system is ready for innovations in information and communications technologies to enhance information availability and access is not the question. Rather, the question is how to best move forward and keep pace with technological innovations in the area of information protection.

TRANSITION FROM PAPER TO A VIRTUAL HEALTH RECORD

With the dispersal of information across multiple care settings, the gathering and presentation of individual health information at the point of care becomes critical to providing high-quality treatment and to avoiding medical mishaps (Kohn, Corrigan, & Donaldson, 2000). Administrative functions that have become more complicated are as follows: filing electronic claims, coordination of benefits among multiple insurers, and verification of eligibility at the time of care.

The use of computers in health care first appeared in the administrative and research arenas and has evolved slowly to include health records that were traditionally kept in paper form (Collen, 1995). With the increasing mobility of the population, the change in health plans, and the use of specialists and pharmacy benefit managers, an individual's health record may exist in a dozen or more different locations. Slightly more than a decade ago, a family physician treated patients in a small-practice office and the patient's complete paper record was kept in a file cabinet or a central file room. The dispersed functions and records in today's health care world (e.g., pharmacy, laboratory, specialty practice, home care, urgent and emergency care) make the caregiver's job much more difficult.

In one of the first collective efforts in the nation, the major health associations and societies in North Carolina* have joined forces to create a vision of "paperless, person-centered health records by 2010" and have achieved organizational approval to establish this as one of their goals. Included in this group are the North Carolina Nurses Association, the North Carolina Medical Society, the North Carolina Health Information Management Association, the North Carolina Hospital Association, the North Carolina Association of Pharmacists, the North Carolina Association of Local Health Directors, and the North Carolina Health Care Facilities Association. Central to this effort has been the definition of the health record in 2010 as "a *virtual digital record* of an individual's health information and all episodes of care. This record is *maintained by multiple providers* and shared when necessary for care of that individual (as allowed by patient consent and/or law)."

Two of the main benefits of achieving this vision are expected to be the improvement of care and the reduction of medical errors that occur when decisions are based on incomplete or missing information. Computers and communications networks can provide the ability to link dispersed records into one **virtual health record.** The other major benefit will be the reduction of administrative costs that are due to the inefficiencies of paper-based processes and the related storage, retrieval, and management costs.

New Methods of Linking Records

The linking of records raises concerns from consumers who perceive that concentrating their information in one location or database invites accidental disclosure or unauthorized access. Frequent news stories about computer "hackers" breaking into and interrupting computer systems heighten the public's suspicion of the security of systems that contain their private health information. There are instances where the inappropriate disclosure or use of health information may lead to discrimination in employment or insurability (Health Privacy Project, 2000).

New technological approaches provide the ability to assemble information, through the linking of records from disparate databases, to allow for targeting information for health care, marketing, or other purposes. It has been demonstrated that matching a limited number of demographic factors such as age, zip code, and sex with publicly available relational databases can lead to the identification of individuals with a high degree of certainty. This technique is extremely useful in health care, where the data accumulated over years in separate databases are combined to create a longitudinal view of a patient and all episodes of care. In the past, exact matches had to occur in the spelling of names, addresses, Social Security numbers, age,

*The Standing Advisory Committee to the Board of Directors of the North Carolina Healthcare Information and Communications Alliance, Inc. (NCHICA), a 501(c)(3) nonprofit organization, is the organizer and proponent of this effort.

telephone numbers, etc., before records could be combined. Now, probabilistic matching allows decisions to be made on the basis of choices culled from a large data set. Advances in data mining and knowledge discovery in large data sets are providing practitioners and organizations with information for evidence-based practice and continuous process improvement. Additional information about data mining and knowledge discovery can be found in Chapter 5. Balancing privacy with the need to improve and innovate is a tough balancing act for the informatics professional and health care provider or organization.

Privacy, Confidentiality, and Security in the Virtual World

As has been demonstrated, the concepts of privacy, confidentiality, and security may be confusing, and the terms are often used interchangeably. An individual with a certain medical condition possesses information that is private only so long as it is not conveyed to another party. In the past it was assumed that when private information was conveyed in confidence to another party for the purpose of obtaining medical treatment or insurance, that information would be held in confidence by the other party and would be used only for the purposes for which it was given. To protect the privacy of the individual and the confidentiality of the information and to keep the information from unintentionally being available to others who do not have the right to access it, the involved party needs to use security mechanisms, policies, and practices.

At the same time that the use of computers and electronic communications has increased, the public has become more aware of and sensitive to the potential for inappropriate and malicious use of private information. Concerns about confidentiality and security of personally identifiable health information in electronic form have grown as public awareness of this issue has increased.

Organizations that deal with health information must take strong measures to engender the trust of their patients/clients/customers. Physicians and nurses are reporting a reluctance of patients to share personal data when they perceive that the information will be entered into a computer. Providers of services to the public are discovering a heightened interest by their clients in the protection of their privacy to the greatest extent possible. One strategy that clients use without realizing the consequences for themselves and the practitioner is the withholding of information (Alderman & Kennedy, 1995; Dennis, 2000). There is no doubt that many consumers would change providers if there were any suspicions about the trustworthiness of an enterprise or its personnel. In addition to suffering the loss of valuable relationships, breaches of trust can expose an organization and its staff to potential civil and even criminal penalties.

Physicians and nurses are familiar with the portion of the Hippocratic oath that stipulates "that whatsoever you shall see or hear of the lives of men or women which is not fitting to be spoken, you will keep inviolably secret."* Others such as marketing, research, and consulting organizations that are in contact with health information are not bound by a code of ethics or by clear legal direction. This is changing as a result of new federal policy and state laws that will require greater protection of identifiable health information (American Health Information Management Association, 1999).

LEGAL AND POLICY IMPLICATIONS

Protecting health care information has always been a key issue in the legal arena. The potential for individual and organizational damage because of a violation of privacy and breach of confidentiality has heightened the need for secu-

*Hippocratic oath. (2000). *Microsoft Encarta Online Encyclopedia:* http://encarta.msn.com © 1997-2000 Microsoft Corporation. All rights reserved.

rity and, along with physical and procedural measures, the perceived need for strong consequences when confidentiality is breached. Although some measures have addressed privacy issues over the years, today there are a number of additional solutions, regulations, and rules being promulgated. This section discusses the Health Insurance Portability and Accountability Act (HIPAA) of 1996 and the implications of this act for protecting health care information.

Legal Protection

Legal protection to ensure the confidentiality of electronic health information traditionally has been the responsibility of state governments. Laws that reflect individual state needs and that have been created over time have resulted in inconsistencies among states and even within the statutes of a single state. The resulting national legal framework created uneven coverage and protection of health information and resulted in substantial uncertainty and confusion when health information needs to be conveyed across state or national boundaries. Federal preemptive legislation could standardize the requirements and provide consistency, but states are unwilling to cede their responsibility when the resulting protections may be less than what currently exists. Efforts to harmonize and standardize the laws in this area continue but are not easy tasks. Once this problem has been solved within the United States, consideration must be given to laws in other countries in which U.S. multinational companies exist and where health information must cross international boundaries. Laws that specify how the protection or security must be implemented (e.g., 128-bit encryption for transmission over the Internet) rather than relying on the general principles of appropriate and inappropriate uses of information inevitably will fail to keep pace with the continuing and rapid advances in technology. The most obvious example of a general principle would be that health information gathered for a specific purpose (such as treatment or payment) should not be used for any other purpose without the explicit permission of the patient or as permitted by law.

Ownership and Control of Health Information

The traditional viewpoint of health information held that the physician or hospital "owned" the medical records of its patients and that patients generally had the right to a copy of their records. The emergence of the informed consumer has challenged this premise with the idea that patients should "own" their records. Emerging in the area of policy between these two ideas is the concept that the physician or institution that collected and recorded the information about a patient owns the medium on which the information is recorded and is responsible for maintaining the integrity and confidentiality of that record. At the same time, the individual has the right to control the use of his or her private health information (through consent or authorization). There are exceptions to the rules requiring consent before disclosure or use of the information. These exceptions are primarily in the area of public health surveillance (e.g., for tracking communicable diseases) and for certain health research purposes, such as epidemiological studies requiring large populations that are conducted under the close supervision of institutional review boards whose role is to protect the identities and privacy of the individuals whose records are being used.

DNA Matching

As the mapping of the human genome progresses, there will be increased emphasis on the protection of individual privacy and public concern over the collection of identifying information in linked databases that might be accessed and used for purposes such as marketing and public safety surveillance without adequate oversight. The Human Genome Project will provide tools to look specifically at generations of a specific family and to predict future health conditions accurately. This may be desirable from a health surveillance point of view, but there has been limited discussion in this area, and very little public policy has been developed. The use of DNA information is certain to be a major topic of debate over the next decade as the power of this technology becomes more apparent.

Health Insurance Portability and Accountability Act: A Federal Initiative

The **administrative simplification** provisions of the **Health Insurance Portability and Accountability Act (HIPAA)** of 1996 (P.L. 104-191) were passed to provide standards and a regulatory framework to assist the health care industry in overcoming the multiplicity of proprietary solutions developed by scores of vendors to support the collection, storage, access, transmission, and use of health information in electronic form. The regulations mandate standards for electronic administrative transactions (e.g., claims, referrals, eligibility, enrollment, payment); codes for medical procedures, diagnosis, devices, drugs, and so forth (e.g., CPT, ICD, NDC, HCPCS); and unique identifiers (for providers, health plans, employers, and potentially for individuals) for precise linking of records, security, and privacy.

Data and Network Security

The HIPAA regulations mandate certain security considerations "to protect data integrity, confidentiality, and availability" for data in electronic form. These include physical protection of devices and media and may be as simple as locks on critical doors or as complicated as requiring biometric authentication of individuals for access to certain records, with audit trails and monitoring to ensure accountability of individuals.

The difficulty of linking policies and technology increases markedly as one moves from a single enterprise approach, to the linking of a limited number of enterprises, and finally to the secure networking of the entire health care community that is required to achieve the virtual digital health record. The HealthKey Project is a consortium of five nonprofit organizations from the states of Massachusetts, Minnesota, North Carolina, Utah, and Washington.* These organizations have joined forces to develop a "technology roadmap" that demonstrates the complexities of such a system-wide approach. Many large health systems may already be using many of the technologies involved, but smaller practices are most likely using very few of these. Smaller practices tend to be constrained by the lack of human and capital resources. The consortium has focused on a number of clinical applications whose usefulness and security can be enhanced through the use of technology. **Public Key–Encryption Infrastructure (PKI)** technology is thought to be a promising technology for high-value or high-vulnerability applications where strong authentication of the individual or institution is desired. However, most experts agree that PKI implementation in the health care arena is moving slowly and is creating other informatics issues, such as the management of public and private keys (Committee on Maintaining Privacy and Security in Health Care Applications of the National Information Infrastructure, 1997).

Patient Consent and Authorization

Although the federal government is issuing regulations covering the "appropriate" use of information, there continues to be differences of opinion among consumers, health researchers, pharmaceutical manufacturers, health plans, and public health regarding what is appropriate use. To frame this debate, some consumer advocates

*The five state organizations participating in the HealthKey Project are the Massachusetts Health Data Consortium (MHDC), the Minnesota Health Data Institute (MHDI), the North Carolina Healthcare Information and Communications Alliance (NCHICA), the Utah Health Information Network (UHIN), and the Washington Foundation for Health Care Quality (FHCQ).

believe that explicit consent must be given for any use of identifiable health information, even sharing among health professionals for treatment of that patient, whereas commercial interests believe that any information they can gather about individuals will enable them to develop and target the marketing of products to meet specific consumer needs. Between these opposing extremes are public health and health research practitioners, who depend on insights gained from the analysis of large health-related data sets to protect the public from contagious diseases or to develop new drugs or methods for treating disease. These types of activities become extremely difficult to carry out if individual consent has to be obtained, because of the difficulty of locating the individuals many years after the original treatment was administered. This debate falls into the area of privacy and the appropriate use of information, but it also affects concerns about protection and security of information. Individuals are more likely to allow their personal health information to be used to improve the health of the general public if they are confident that their personal privacy is protected from unauthorized use and that the systems containing their personally identifiable information are secured from unauthorized access.

To emphasize and enforce this point, the HIPAA regulations mandate that health care providers obtain patient consent before sharing their information for treatment, payment, and health care procedures. Furthermore, explicit patient authorization is required for all other disclosures of information, with several exceptions made for public health and research purposes that are carried out under strict guidelines. These requirements are aimed at offering the individual some control over how his or her information may be accessed and used, thereby creating an environment where health care information can be viewed as a critical resource for the individual, the provider, and the organization. In other words, the responsibility and accountability for the accessibility, integrity, and availability of a complete health record could potentially be shared by all parties involved rather than by just the organization and the provider.

With the HIPAA regulations, patients are gaining new rights, such as the right to see and have a copy of their health record, to request an amendment of the record when they disagree with the record, and to receive a record of disclosures of their health information outside of treatment or payment purposes. Additional information about HIPAA is found in Chapter 19.

Reengineering Health Care for Compliance

A very high degree of protection for health information will be required in an electronic world where remote access to the virtual health record via the Internet will be commonplace. Innovative technology vendors will be relied on to provide solutions that enable and facilitate remote access without placing additional time-consuming or expensive requirements on caregivers. Technical solutions have been estimated to be only 30% of that which will be required to ensure security of health information. The bulk of the required resources will be related to the creation, monitoring, and enforcement of internal policies and processes and the requisite training required. Very few organizations are self-sufficient in the handling of equipment or databases containing health information; therefore many organizations outsource analytical and administrative processes (such as transcription) to third parties. The HIPAA regulations require the custodians of health information to have contractual agreement with their business associates to protect the information to the same degree as the original party. In addition to civil monetary penalties for violation of the regulations, criminal fines and imprisonment may be applied to particularly egregious privacy violations, such as obtaining health information under false pretenses or for the sale of such information for profit, personal gain, or malicious intent.

Incentives for Change

Avoiding civil or criminal liability and negative public reaction to inappropriate disclosure of or access to sensitive and confidential health information will be the primary drivers for change. Prudent risk management and regulation will require protecting the integrity of the information and its availability at the time when it may be required for treatment of a patient. Organizations will need to reengineer the way they do business and rethink the way they use information as a key operational resource (Shortell & Kaluzny, 1994).

Physical and Contractual Precautions

Beyond solutions such as placing physical and electronic locks on equipment and time-out features on workstations, care will need to be taken when replacing or disposing of computers and media. Disks may need to be physically broken or melted to avoid the recovery of data previously thought to have been erased. Access to systems, networks, and data by third-party vendors for service or other authorized purposes presents a threat to security that generally is not recognized. Business associate contracts and agreements should be carefully constructed and reviewed periodically for coverage of responsibilities in this area. Providers and health plans routinely outsource contract for services such as transcriptions and quality assessments that require access to individually identifiable patient data without necessarily auditing the third party's policies and procedures. Privacy laws may not forgive a lack of due diligence on the part of a custodian of health information, and a closer monitoring of business associates or third-party certification may become common practice.

Internal Processes and Policies

In addition to technical and physical solutions for protecting electronic information, the majority of resources necessarily will be focused on internal processes and procedures regarding the way information is handled. Current policies need to be reviewed and revised or augmented because they may have been written for the paper world and may not address electronic means of collecting, storing, accessing, or sharing health information. Personnel training, monitoring, and disciplinary actions for breaches of policy must be documented to prove due diligence in the event that legal action is brought against the custodian of health information. This shift in providing heightened protection of personal health information will require a cultural shift that can be achieved only through continuous training and support from executive management levels.

Remote Access

Authentication is used to prove the identity of individuals who are accessing health data over a network. This requires strong technical means that allow audit and review of all accesses of the data and make the denial of access by a valid and authorized user of the information extremely difficult. Public Key–Encryption Infrastructure (PKI), or rendering the health information unintelligible without special codes combined with **digital certificates** or the electronic equivalent of an individual's signature and personal seal, is a means of positively identifying an individual, sealing a message, and providing secret coding of the data through encryption as the information moves across networks. Digital signatures are increasingly being recognized as the electronic equivalent of the pen-and-ink signature on paper documents and are legally binding in most cases. The terms *electronic signature* and *digital signature* are often used interchangeably. Electronic signature refers to the application of a signature to a document by electronic means and accomplishes authentication, nonrepudiation, and assent. Simply put, an electronic signature identifies the source of the document (authentication), ensures that the person signing the document cannot deny the document (nonrepudiation), and verifies that the parties approve of the term/contents (assent). The U.S. Department of Health and Human Services (DHHS) defines a digital signature as "an electronic signature based on cryptographic methods of originator authentication, computed by using a set of parameters so that the identity of the data can be verified" (USDHHS, 1998, p. 43269). A digital signature as defined by the DHHS is a type of electronic signature.

The emerging field of biometric identification through fingerprint recognition, retinal or facial scanning, and voice recognition may provide a significantly higher level of personal identification than has previously been available. Combinations of PKI and biometric technologies will provide organizations with a high degree of confidence that only authorized individuals are able to view an individual's health record. Unauthorized sharing of passwords and electronic accounts will be much more difficult when combined with biometrics. In any case, sharing of one's own personal identification to allow another individual access to health information may result in severe penalties, including termination in appropriate circumstances, and may be cause for criminal prosecution.

Cost of Compliance

Most health record professionals recognize that the costs of increased security methods and systems are necessary to protect the private information of their patients and clients. It makes good business sense to take all reasonable and appropriate steps because of the potential liability and loss of business if the confidentiality or privacy of this information is compromised. Certainly, as the public is made aware of the measures taken to protect health care information, public confidence in institutions should increase. On the other hand, there are sure to be highly publicized instances where organizations skimp on resources and health information is inappropriately exposed, thereby not only creating significant damage to that institution but also eroding the image of all health care organizations. HIPAA compliance requires that providers and health plans take reasonable and appropriate steps to protect health information; this requirement makes it essential for each organization to undertake a risk management evaluation within the context of its own business environment and base its compliance plan and action accordingly. There is no effective measure or means to project the cost of compliance, since the paths taken by each institution will be determined by individual circumstances.

CONCLUSION

Protecting health care information covers two important constituencies in the health care arena. First and foremost are the patients and clients, who rightly have an expectation that information about them will be managed appropriately. Second, organizations cannot afford the potential damage that breaches of patient confidentiality or organizational confidentiality might incur. The challenge for the health care informatics profession is to be knowledgeable of the vulnerabilities and to develop strategic plans for information management and protection that provide appropriate access, secure the integrity of the data and information, and ensure efficient availability processes.

The mobility of the population, an increasing reliance on health care specialists, and a variety of purchasing choices will further diffuse an individual's health record into many settings. The provision of high-quality care demands that critical portions of the health record be available to the health care professional at the time that care decisions are made. Electronic health records that may be assembled from disparate locations in a secure and certain manner will require the increasing use of technology to quickly locate a record, provide proper authentication to the remote source, and effect secure transmission of the record to the target location. Future advances in computing and communications will continue to outstrip our ability to anticipate and develop public policy. Procedural and technological solutions will be needed to counter security threats to systems and the confidentiality of information contained therein. New computing capabilities have given rise to data mining and direct/targeted marketing from information previously thought to have been stripped of identifiers. More powerful computing capability will break encryption algorithms previously thought impregnable. Multinational companies need to exchange information with health care organizations across state and national political boundaries with differing rules and standards that make protection of the data very difficult. Just from these few challenges alone, there appears to be no end in sight for the need to continually upgrade and enhance every organization's security policies, procedures, technical methods, and training to meet the legal, ethical, and moral responsibilities of protecting a patient's identifiable health information from inappropriate or unauthorized access.

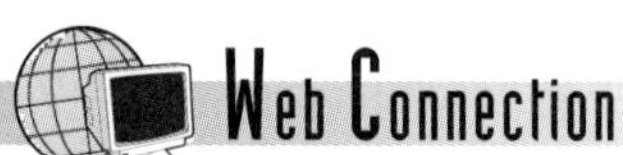

Web Connection

Protection of health care information is a complex endeavor. Privacy, confidentiality, and security are not new concepts to health care. Health care providers work hard to ensure the confidentiality of personal information, but the paper-based information world has not been as secure as desired. Many argue that automation of the clinical record enhances security of personal information; however, the integration of information technologies into health care settings has increased the amount of available and potentially accessible information. Exploring the concepts of privacy, confidentiality, and security, these Web Connection activities will facilitate your understanding of the complexity of protecting health care information. You will learn the different perspectives of this issue and identify how the Health Insurance Portability and Accountability Act is shaping the health care industry's approach to making health care information secure.

discussion questions

1. Describe the differences among the concepts of privacy, confidentiality, and security.
2. Name four methods for ensuring physical security of health information.
3. What is a virtual health record?
4. How are medical records handled differently today from in 1950?
5. Why does individually identifiable health information need protection?
6. What key areas of public policy will continue to be debated as electronic technology and electronic health records increasingly become an integral part of health care delivery and administration?

REFERENCES

Alderman, E., & Kennedy, C. (1995). *The right to privacy.* New York: Alfred A. Knopf.

American Health Information Management Association. (1999). *Confidentiality of medical records: A situational analysis and AHIMA's position.* Retrieved May 1, 1999, from the World Wide Web: http://www.ahima.org/infocenter/current/white.paper.html.

Collen, M.F. (1995). *A history of medical informatics in the United States: 1950-1990.* Indianapolis: American Medical Informatics Association.

Committee on Maintaining Privacy and Security in Health Care Applications of the National Information Infrastructure. (1997). *For the record: Protecting electronic health information.* Retrieved May 12, 1998, from the World Wide Web: http://www.nap.edu/readingroom/books/for/.

Dennis, J.C. (2000). *Privacy and confidentiality of health information.* San Francisco: Jossey-Bass.

Dick, R.S., Steen, E.B., & Detmer, D.E. (1997). *The computer-based patient record.* Washington, DC: National Academy Press.

Health Privacy Project. (2000). *Medical privacy stories*. Retrieved May 1, 1999, from the World Wide Web: http://www.healthprivacy.org/usr_doc/43842%2Epdf.

Joint Commission on Accreditation of Healthcare Organizations. (1999). *Joint Commission on Accreditation of Healthcare Organizations*. Retrieved April 17, 2000, from the World Wide Web: http://www.jcaho.org/.

Kohn, L.T., Corrigan, J.M., & Donaldson, M.S. (2000). *To err is human: Building a safer health system*. Washington, DC: National Academy Press.

McCall, N., & Mix, L.A. (1995). *Designing archival programs to advance knowledge in the health fields*. Baltimore: Johns Hopkins University Press.

Shortell, S.M., & Kaluzny, A.D. (1994). *Health care management: Organization design and behavior* (3rd ed.). (Series in Health Services.) New York: Delmar.

Strum, P. (1998). *Privacy: The debate in the United States since 1945*. Fort Worth: Harcourt Brace College Publishers.

TechEncyclopedia. (2001). *TechWeb: The business technology network*. Point Pleasant, PA: Computer Language Company. Retrieved June 27, 2001, from the World Wide Web: http://www.techweb.com/encyclopedia/defineterm?term=worm.

U.S. Department of Health and Human Services. (1998). Security and electronic signature standards. *Federal Register, 63*(155), 43241-43280. Retrieved October 12, 2000, from the World Wide Web: http://aspe.os.dhhs.gov/admnsimp/nprm/secnprm.pdf.

PART SIX

Yesterday, Today, and Tomorrow

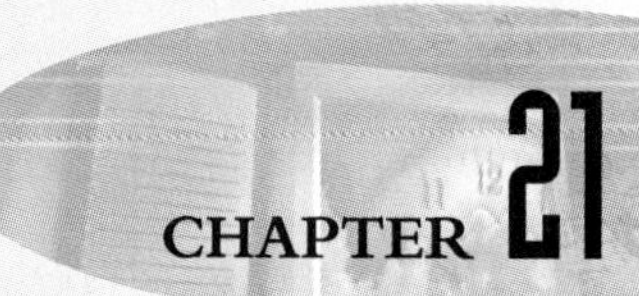

The History of Health Care Informatics

KAY M. SACKETT
WILLIAM SCOTT ERDLEY

Learning Objectives

Upon completion of this chapter, the reader will be able to:

1. ***Describe*** the evolution of the term *health care informatics.*
2. ***Describe*** the history of health care computing internationally and in the United States.
3. ***Describe*** the evolution of health care informatics internationally and in the United States.
4. ***Analyze*** the paradigm shift (a change from one way of thinking to another) that is occurring with the advancement of health care informatics worldwide.

Outline

History and Development of Computing and Informatics in Health Care
- *Pre-1800s*
- *1800 to 1900*
- *1900 to 1950*
- *1950s*
- *1960s*
- *1970s*
- *1980s*
- *1990s*

Historical Development of Educational Programs in Health Care Informatics

Key Terms

bioengineering
data
first-generation computer
health care informatics
informatics
information
knowledge
medical informatics
minicomputers
nomenclature
number crunching
nursing informatics
relational databases
second-generation computer
stakeholders
standardized languages
stored program concept
systems approach
transistors
wisdom
working partnerships

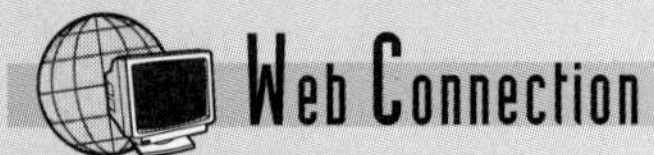

Go to the Web site at http://evolve.elsevier.com/Englebardt/. Here you will find Web links and activities related to the history of health care informatics.

This chapter examines the history of health care computing and informatics, exploring its development in both the United States and international arenas. The first generations of computers were analog devices that focused on military communication and tabulation for cryptography—missile launch, guidance, and space exploration. The initial focus was on the development of computer hardware. Expansion to include computer applications for business administration and accounting tasks followed. The subsequent invention of **transistors**—solid state semiconductors—resulted in the second generation of computers. These computers were digital devices that were both smaller and faster than analog computers. Silicon chips that were smaller and more powerful than transistors eventually replaced transistors and advanced the process of miniaturization of computing equipment.

As computer technology evolved, so did the terminology to describe various applications and theoretical perspectives. Blum's seminal work (1986) on the history of clinical computing describes the intersection of biology and engineering to form bioengineering. Blum (1986) also delineated the concepts of **data, information,** and **knowledge** and their relationship to the management of information and technology in medicine. Over time, the Russian term *informatika* evolved into the French *informatique* and subsequently into the English **informatics** (Box 21-1). The designation of informatics as a profession's specialty was identified through the placement of the profession's name in front of the term, such as *medical informatics, nursing informatics,* or *dental informatics.* The term *nursing informatics* was probably first used and defined by Scholes and Barber (1980) in their address to the MEDINFO conference that year in Tokyo. Mandil used the term *health care informatics* in 1987.

Graves and Corcoran (1989) used the data, information, and knowledge concepts defined by Blum to define nursing informatics. Nelson and Joos (1889) as well as others (Slawson, Shaughnessy, & Bennett, 1994) added a fourth concept, **wisdom.** Turley (1996) proposed a conceptual framework of **nursing informatics** that integrated information science, cognitive science, and computer science within the realm of nursing science. In general, this theoretical and semantic progression mirrored the evolution of the integration of computers in health care.

Table 21-1 demonstrates how the use of the concepts of data, information, knowledge, and wisdom has evolved since the 1950s. The decades are provided to give a general overview of the increasing use of these concepts. The symbol before the decade indicates the flexibility of these time periods. The evolution begins with the recognition of these terms as distinct concepts. For example, in the past the terms *data* and *information* have been used interchangeably by many. Today most people recognize that these terms represent different concepts. Once a term has been identified as representing a distinct concept, it is possible for that concept to be used in activities such as thinking, experimentation, and research. In health care this research and experi-

Box 21–1 Translations of the Terms *Informatics* and *Medical Informatics*

Informatika: Defined in 1966 by Russian scientist A.I. Mikhailov as "the discipline of science which investigates the structures and properties (not specific context) of scientific information, as well as the regularities of scientific activity, its theory, history, methodology and organization" (Collen, 1995, p. 39).
Informatik, informatikki, informatsii, informatsiya: Terms also used by Mikhailov.
Informatique: French term for informatics.
Informatics: The scientific discipline that studies the structure and general properties of scientific information and the laws of all processes of scientific communication.
Informatyki medyczinei: Polish term first used in 1972 about informatics in health care.
Medicine et informatique: French term for medical informatics.
Medicinski informatike: Serbo-Croatian term for medical informatics.
Medical informatics: Defined by Collen (1995) to be "the application of computers, communications and information technology, and systems to all fields of medicine—to medical care, medical education and medical research" (p. 41).

Table 21–1 Evolution of Data, Information, Knowledge, and Wisdom

	~1950	~1960	~1970	~1980	~1990	~2000
Wisdom application					Concept	Research
Knowledge application	Concept	Concept	Research	Prototype	Mature	
Information application	Concept	Research	Prototype	Mature	Refined	
Data application	Research	Prototype	Mature	Refined		

Data from Blum, B. (1986). *Clinical information systems.* New York: Springer-Verlag; Blum, B., & Duncan, K. (1990). *A history of medical informatics.* New York: ACM Press; Nelson, R., & Joos, I. (1989). On language in nursing: From data to wisdom. *PLN Visions,* Fall, p. 6; Joos, I., et al. (1992). *Computers in small bytes—The computer workbook* (2nd ed.). New York: National League of Nursing Press; and Slawson, D., Shaughnessy, A., & Bennett, J. (1994). Becoming a medical information master: Feeling good about *not* knowing everything. *Journal of Family Practice, 38*(5), 505-513.

mentation resulted in the development of prototype health care information systems. For example, the period from the "mid 1960s to the mid 1970s was primarily characterized by accomplishments in the processing of medical data" (Blum, 1986, p. 36). The initial systems were for the most part stand-alone systems. As these prototype and stand-alone systems matured, they became the basis for a major industry. Many of these stand-alone systems are now being integrated with one another and refined as they change the health care delivery system.

In the United States, health care administrators and providers each required unique information, from health care information technology, to facilitate their work. Health care providers needed information to guide the management of patient health while administrators focused on resource management such as the allocation, control, and analysis of human and financial resources. Health care providers demanded quick access to information and unlimited access to facilities, services, and resources. Administrators also required information systems that increased the efficiency of operations and decreased costs. To further complicate the situation, health care informatics was characterized by the development of proprietary applications and a lack of standards. The intersection of these and other stakeholder groups was affected by the change in the U.S. health care system from a fee-for-service to a capitated, managed care environment.

The international community was affected by these same groups of stakeholders. However, additional factors also complicated and complemented the international community's adoption of health care information technology. International health care informatics was characterized by the building of partnerships among stakeholders on several continents and by the preliminary adoption of standardized nomenclature. These stakeholders included members from Europe, Africa, Eastern Europe, Russia, Asia, Australia, and South America.

HISTORY AND DEVELOPMENT OF COMPUTING AND INFORMATICS IN HEALTH CARE

Pre-1800s

Communication and tabulation were necessary ingredients for the exchange of information and for mathematical computations in all early societies. Examples of ancient methods of communication included speech, cave art, the use of Oriental characters for writing, and hieroglyphics. Ancient tabulation devices included shells, rocks, and pieces of bone that were added or subtracted to create a sum. The Chinese abacus was created around 5000 BC for purposes of counting.

Early human communication was also influenced by migration, wars, and communication among tribes. Passage from the Dark Ages into the Renaissance period heralded a myriad of changes that positively altered communication and tabulation. Blum (1986) has described some counting devices that were created during the mid-1600s, such as the Rabdologia, or Napier's Bones, and Pascal's Arithmetic Engine. Napier's Bones, named for John Napier, were numbered white rods that when laid side by side allowed a person to multiply numbers. Pascal's Arithmetic Engine was a gear-and-wheel device that was able to subtract and add numbers. The movement of people and ideas from the Old World to the New World also influenced the development of computation and tabulation devices and provided the foundation for preliminary work on rudimentary computers.

1800 to 1900

International Developments

The latter part of the 1800s witnessed the development of Babbage's Difference Engine in England. The Difference Engine was composed of rods, wheels, and gears and was designed to automate geometric functions. Ada Byron, the Countess of Lovelace, who worked with Charles Babbage, is considered the first woman programmer (Blum, 1986; Hannah, Ball, & Edwards, 1999).

Another important invention that impacted the intersection of computers and health care was the development of a standardized language. Peter Roget, an English philologist, scientist, and physician is credited with creating the first standardized **nomenclature** for the English language. He created *Roget's Thesaurus of English Words and Phrases* based on synonyms in 1852. American inventions such as the telephone, typewriter, electricity, and locomotion were soon adopted in Europe. These winds of change coincided with the beginning of the twentieth century and laid the groundwork for computer development in the next century.

Developments in the United States

Medicine and computing began to overlap and be interrelated in the United States in the late 1800s. John Billing Shaw, a physician considered by many to be the first person to integrate medicine and computational devices, accepted the task of conducting the U.S. census of 1880. This task led Shaw to discussions with Herman Hollerith, an engineer. Hollerith had a way to automate the tedious task of compiling data from the census through the use of a card-punching machine. The 1890 census employed over 50 of Hollerith's machines. This automation was subsequently powered by electricity. Because of Shaw's involvement and his use of a tabulation device, the 1890 census automation is thought to be the starting point of medical informatics in the United States (Collen, 1995).

Hollerith founded the Tabulating Machines Company in 1896. Thomas Watson, Sr., joined the company in 1914 and after rising through the ranks, eventually purchased the company. In 1924 Watson changed the company's name to its current name, International Business Machines (IBM) (Collen, 1995; Saba & McCormick, 1986). Another significant event that occurred during this period was Alexander Graham Bell's invention of the telephone in 1876. The telephone provided the infrastructure that would eventually support computer connectivity.

1900 to 1950

The period of 1900 to 1950 was filled with national and international strife, including World War I, World War II, the armed conflict in Korea, the Cold War, and the spread of Communism. These events hastened the development of computational devices that communicated and tabulated information over vast distances. However, it was in the late 1930s and early 1940s that the push for computational services and devices was actualized. It would be these devices, developed to battle distant enemies, maintain demographic population data in Germany, and take lives, that would ultimately evolve into lifesaving tools for health care professionals.

International Developments

In 1938 Konrad Zuse of Germany created the ZI computer, and during World War II he created the Z2 and Z3 machines. The completion of Z4 was interrupted by the end of the war. As electromechanical relay machines, these are referred to as being among the first **second-generation computers** (University of St Andrews, Scotland: School of Mathematics and Statistics, 1999).

The Colossus computer was designed by Alan M. Turing and built by M.H.A. Neuman at the University of Manchester, England, in 1941. The Colossus, a room-sized computer, was used to decipher coded transmissions of the Germans and the Japanese. This invention marked the first time a computational device effectively combined communication and tabulation to facilitate information management. During these early years the British, Germans, and Russians continued to develop digital computers and applications for military use, as well as for data processing functions.

Developments in the United States

The initial reason for developing electronic computational devices was to calculate missile flight paths. Before the existence of these computational devices, a large amount of manpower was necessary to perform these calculations. The realization that machines could perform the calculations revolutionized the world. Even though these machines were used toward the end of World War II, their impact on the world continues. The Mark I (1943 to 1944) was the result of a project led by Howard Aiken of Harvard and IBM that led to the first electromechanical computational device (Saba & McCormick, 1986). The Mark I was controlled by prepunched paper tape, was based on the decimal system, and used relays and wheels to calculate flight paths (Collen, 1995).

In 1945 John von Neumann, a researcher at Princeton, developed the idea of storing programs and data in the actual computer. This development diminished the need to enter data and also reduced the rewiring of circuits and changing of tubes previously required to run each program. This application, known as the **stored program concept,** necessitated a switch from a base 10 to a binary framework (Saba & McCormick, 1986).

John W. Mauchly and J. Presper Eckhert completed the Electrical Numerical Integrator Computer (ENIAC) in 1946 at the University of Pennsylvania. Its function was to tabulate the immense tables used for ballistic path calculations. It had no moving parts, weighed over 30 tons, and contained over 19,000 vacuum tubes (Payne & Brown, 1975; Saba & McCormick, 1986). Later in the 1940s, Mauchly and Eckert used von Neumann's stored program idea to develop the Universal Automatic Computer (UNIVAC), which was able to handle both numeric and alphabetic data. The UNIVAC I, used for the 1950 census data, had 5000 vacuum tubes. The vacuum tubes created considerable heat and required that the computer be placed in an air-conditioned room (Collen, 1995; Saba, 1986).

It was around this time that An Wang (founder of Wang Laboratories) patented the idea of magnetic core memory. This storage mode was faster, lighter, and produced less heat than tubes. In addition, magnetic core memory was able to retain data and programs after the power was turned off (Collen, 1995). The Whirlwind digital computer at MIT (1953) was the first computer to employ this type of memory.

1950s

International Developments

International developments in health care and technology were limited during this period. As noted earlier, the term **bioengineering,** a combination of the application of biology and engineering, was used to describe the application of electronic digital computers in medicine (Blum & Duncan, 1990). With limited functionality, computers in health care were used for their financial and data processing capabilities. However, the use of computers to influence health care practices was the next step in the evolution of this technology.

Developments in the United States

One of the earliest computers used for medical research was the IBM 704. For its time, this computer was extremely advanced, using magnetic core memory, FORTRAN programming, and a cathode ray tube (CRT) monitor (Collen, 1995). This system was in the vanguard of change for computational devices. Until this time, computers were primarily tubes and wires, unwieldy to work with and prone to failure. With the advent of transistors in 1958, computational machines could be programmed with comparative ease. A natural transition from building computer hardware to the creation and use of increasingly sophisticated software applications was begun. The software to be developed over the next several decades would focus on managing data, information, and knowledge.

The establishment of the Joint Commission on Accreditation in Healthcare (JCAH), the forerunner of the Joint Commission on Accreditation of Healthcare Organizations, in 1951 was an important variable that compelled the need for accurate documentation by health care providers. The JCAH increased the requirements for documentation and recording of patient-related activities in the hospital. For example JCAH required that the hospital demonstrate a relationship between patient needs and staff allocations. The need to document and monitor nursing activities as they related to staffing allocations added to the impetus for computer usage and suggested what software would be needed. This type of mathematical calculation was a repetitious, tedious task and ideal for the computer (Saba & McCormick, 1986).

Until this time, computational devices were primarily used for **number crunching** (the performance of considerable mathematical calculations by a computer), whether ballistic calculations or census tabulations. According to Collen (1995), Robert Ledley was the first to employ a computer for health purposes. Ledley used computer applications at the National Bureau of Standards to study dental projects. Farley and Clark (1954) reported on a simulation modeling of learning that employed computers. In general, however, reports of computer utilization in health care were not published until the mid-1950s.

1960s

International Developments

Brandejs (1976), Elioutina and Tarasov (1995), Hannah, Ball, and Edwards (1999), and Hogarth (1997) have highlighted significant accomplishments that occurred in the emerging field of informatics during the 1960s. The International Federation for Information Processing (IFIP) was formed in 1960. In the late 1960s, exploratory work began in Moscow, Novosibirsk, Kemerovo, Novokuznetsk, St. Petersburg, and other Russian cities on the use of information systems in health care. The first hospital information system made up of patient administrative services, laboratory services, and x-ray services using visual display units was implemented in the United Kingdom in 1967 at the London Hospital. In 1966 the Council of Hospital Operation Rationalization (SJURA) in Sweden began investigating the use of computerized databases in hospitals.

Developments in the United States

Transistor use in computers marked the end of **first-generation computers** and the beginning of the second generation. Jack Kilby and Robert Noyce worked independently but, almost at the same time, discovered that transistors could function as their own circuit boards, thus greatly diminishing the size and power requirements of computers (Collen, 1995). The discovery that transistors greatly increased computational power moved computers from academia to the business world. These types of computers came to be called **minicomputers.** Noyce and his colleagues also developed the first integrated silicon chip, thus making it possible to miniaturize electronic components, which eventually led to the use of very large scale integration chips in the late 1960s (Collen, 1995). These integrated circuits demarcated second-generation computers (Blum, 1986; Saba & McCormick, 1986). Noyce founded Intel in the late 1960s, which is now the world's leading manufacturer of computational chips. Intel was involved in the production of these and other chips (e.g., random access memory [RAM] chips).

In the health care arena, computer use at this time was limited to nondigital machines for electrocardiograms (ECGs) and electroencephalograms (EEGs) (Payne & Brown, 1975). In the 1950s and 1960s, ECG signals provided one of the first areas for using computers in health care. Hubert Pipberger, in the late 1960s used the analog-to-digital converter—a device that converts an analog signal to a digital signal to represent the same information—that was invented at the National Bureau of Standards to enable digital computers to monitor and analyze ECG signals (Rautaharju, 1999).

In 1962, Wesley Clark and Charles Molnar of the Massachusetts Institute of Technology (MIT) developed a specific laboratory computer called the LINC (Collen, 1995). PLATO, developed in the late 1960s, was one of the first computer-based education programs. During this decade, legislation also began to have an impact on the development of informatics. The Social Security Act amendments that established Medicare and Medicaid were passed in 1965. The subsequent need to maintain health care records, resulting from these amendments, lent strong additional impetus to the development of informatics in the United States.

To keep up with the ever-increasing volume of biomedical literature included in the *Index Medicus* bibliography, the National Library of Medicine committed to computerization in the early 1960s. A computerized literature retrieval system, known as MEDLARS, became totally operational in 1964. It performed thousands of searches before online searching capabilities and databases, such as MEDLINE, became available in 1971 (National Library of Medicine, 1999).

Several independently developed information systems for health care emerged in the United States during this decade. The Technicon Medical Information System (TMIS) started in 1965, was a collaborative project between Lockheed Systems and the El Camino Hospital in El Camino, California. This system took a modular approach to the development of a medical information system. Continuing the integration of the computer and its software applications into health care, the first module implemented 2 years after development began was the financial module. In 1971 Technicon purchased the system outright from Lockheed (Collen, 1995).

The Problem Oriented Medical Record (POMR) and Problem Oriented Medical Information Systems (PROMIS) were also introduced in the 1960s. These applications, based on the research method, attempted to standardize the organization of medical information in a patient's chart. Concurrently, Kaiser Permanente in California, Massachusetts General Hospital in Boston, the National Bureau of Standards in Washington, D.C., and Estrin Brain Research Institute in Boston all received institutional and financial support to experiment and develop individual medical information systems.

The *CO*mputer-*ST*ored *A*mbulatory *R*ecord (COSTAR) was developed and implemented in the late 1960s at the Harvard Community Health Plan. It used the Massachusetts General Hospital Utility Multiprogramming System (MUMPS) as its programming language, in addition to using its own vocabulary. COSTAR was designed to meet both clinical and financial needs of health care practices outside of the traditional hospital by (Barnett et al., 1989):

- Facilitating patient care
- Providing a more efficient billing system
- Enhancing day-to-day care of a practice group
- Assisting administrative and ancillary data processing requests
- Facilitating report generation, both standard and specific
- Increasing ease of quality assurance processes

The initial development of the Health Evaluation Through Logical Processing (HELP) system began at the LDS Hospital in Salt Lake City, Utah, in the late 1950s and early 1960s. The HELP system was a clinical program that supported medical decision making to assist both physicians and nurses with their decision-making processes. The system was able to assist with decision making through the inclusion of preset conditions that indicated decision points in a patient's illness. The decision process used multiple data entries, including data from manual entries, laboratory results, and/or prior decisions made by the system for a similar situation. The health care professional could also practice decision making using dummy data. The coding system used by the HELP system for patient discharge was the Systematized Nomenclature of Pathology (SNOP), which at that time had four axes and approximately 10,000 codes. The HELP system was one of the first software applications for critical care clinicians (Warner, Olmstead, & Rutherford, 1971).

1970s

International Developments

Boutros (1993), Brandejs (1976), Collen (1995), Elioutina and Tarasov (1995), Hannah, Ball, and Edwards (1999), and Mandil et al. (1993) have described a shift in health care informatics in the

1970s from a focus on the use of computer hardware to a focus on the use of computer applications to manage medical, nursing, and health information. In Canada and the United Kingdom, several computerized information systems were implemented in nursing practice. At King's College Hospital in London, computerized nursing care plans were implemented. Ninewells Hospital in Dundee, Scotland, implemented a real-time system for nursing documentation. York Central Hospital in Richmond Hills, Ontario, implemented a computerized patient care system. At the same time as these systems were being implemented, the Canadian health care system began introducing computerized medical information records and health care databases into the offices of family practice physicians (Hannah, Ball, & Edwards, 1999).

In 1974 the first MEDINFO Conference was held by the International Federation for Information Processing (IFIP). The Fourth Technical Committee (TC-4) of the IFIP later became the International Medical Informatics Association (IMIA). Illustrative of the interest in informatics in general and the burgeoning interest in the area of medical informatics, 3 years later the MEDINFO 77 hosted 199 papers, 146 of which were international papers.

During 1975 the Union of Soviet Socialists Republics (USSR) Council of Ministers supported the formation of automated regional computer informatization management centers governed by the Health Ministry (Elioutina & Tarasov, 1995). Countries in Africa also launched initiatives that furthered the adoption of information management systems. In 1978 the Egyptian Ministry of Health initiated a pilot project to develop its national health information system. The use of microcomputers at the subministerial level in selected areas was intended to improve management functions and enable coordination and support of public health programs (Boutros, 1993).

In another part of the world, a significant event occurred that was to further shape the use and spread of computerization and informatics in medicine, nursing, and health care. This event, sponsored by the World Health Organization, was the Alma-Ata Conference of 1978. At this conference the participants unanimously voted to adopt a resolution that primary health care services become globally available (Health for All) by the year 2000. Also included in this resolution was a document that described the use of health care information systems worldwide (Boutros, 1993; Mandil et al., 1993).

Developments in the United States

In the United States the development of hospital information systems saw the addition of care management and cost control functions. The silicon chip, with its miniaturization of transistors and electronic switches, was developed in the United States and increased the access and availability of computers and technology for everyone.

Collen (1970) published his seminal work on medical information systems. In it, he listed general requirements to which any medical information system should adhere. Included was this definition of a medical information system—electronic data processing (computer) and communication equipment for online processing of medical data with real-time output. His general requirements incorporated the following:

- Continuous data capture (laboratory values, ECG, etc.)
- Provision for data on demand by physicians
- A data repository for research purposes
- The ability to meet any legal requirements

The medical information system was to be the data repository for any patient treated at a hospital. This article was one of the earliest articulations in support of an electronic patient record as a prerequisite for construction of a data repository. At about the same time as Collen published his work, Edgar Codd explored **relational databases** in his book *Relational Model for Large*

Shared Data Banks (Haux, Knaup, & Schmucker, 1999). The ability to manipulate relational databases within medical information systems to explore patterns and variances among and between patient populations was to have a profound impact on future health care systems.

During the 1970s various attempts at hospital information systems began to appear at Charlotte Memorial Hospital in Charlotte, North Carolina, as well as at the Institute of Rehabilitation and Research in Houston, Texas. Other systems of note were Technicon Medical Information System (TMIS) at El Camino Hospital in El Camino, California (a continuation of work from the mid-1960s), and PROMIS at the Medical Center Hospital in Burlington, Vermont (Collen, 1995). The Patient Care System (PCS), developed at Duke University Medical Center, Durham, North Carolina, was a customizable, general-purpose software base with the primary focus of nurse staffing needs. This system was used to organize and transform staffing data into a usable and manageable form for administrative purposes.

Weed further refined PROMIS in the late 1970s. PROMIS used a computer system to organize the medical record. The premise of PROMIS was the efficient and systematic organization of data to deal with patient problems. The data, arranged or categorized in the computer, would allow the physician to focus on the patient and the diagnosis of the patient's problem. The Problem Oriented Medical Record (POMR), the basis of PROMIS, also allowed for auditing of medical problems and examination of any sort of discontinuity of patient care. With PROMIS, these audits, as well as systematic analysis of patient care, could be facilitated. This in turn would assist with the overall provision of patient care by the physician (Weed, 1968).

McDonald (1976) articulated the perspective that computers were necessary to help the physician with handling the vast amounts of information necessary for practice. Physician error was attributed to information overload, and McDonald ascribed much of this to basic, repetitive tasks, such as the reordering of medications, ordering of tests, and other similar repetitive tasks that could be done by computers. However, protocols were needed to direct these computerized repetitive tasks. A system developed with this focus was implemented at the Regenstrief Institute in Indianapolis, Indiana. The computer was used as a reminder tool and not specifically for decision making. The reminders were to gather more data, order a particular diagnostic test, or change/alter a therapeutic regimen (McDonald, 1976). This type of system was one of the first to show the practicality of using computers in health care and eventually led to the inclusion of reminders in applications developed by vendors today.

Yet another system, created by Shortliffe and Buchanan (1975), was a computer software application called MYCIN, one of the first expert systems developed for diagnosing medical problems. MYCIN was the actualization of their work on inexact reasoning in medicine. This model allowed the researchers to explore the nature of unformalized medical reasoning processes and, more important, to quantify this type of knowledge. Quantification allowed the use of computers to provide expert opinions for nonexpert physicians and other health care professionals about the use of antimicrobial therapy. This attempt at quantification of inexact medical reasoning laid the foundation for future development/exploration of artificial intelligence and its applications for health care.

Ball conducted some of the first surveys of hospital information systems. Her surveys collected data on the functions of the system, the cost, and what each vendor sold in terms of hardware and software.

The creation of smaller computers and the adoption of open system philosophy, which allowed for smaller and more open systems, inspired Paul Allen and Bill Gates. In 1975 they founded Microsoft Corporation. Within the next 10 years this company created and marketed an operating system that became the primary operating system on thousands of personal computers (PCs). The invention and subsequent use of the silicon chip in 1975, coupled with the rapid proliferation of PCs based on the silicon chip, marked the beginning of a worldwide revolution in computer technology.

1980s

International Developments

The spread of information management systems in medicine, nursing, and health care continued rapidly on the international scene. During the MEDINFO 80 Conference held in Tokyo, Japan, a definition for the term *medical informatics* evolved. Collen (1995) defined **medical informatics** as "the application of computers, communications and information technology, and systems to all fields of medicine—to medical care, medical education, and medical research" (p. 41). During this decade Canada continued to expand its health care information systems within its national health care system. In the Soviet Union, 47 additional regional computerization centers governed by the Health Ministry were established. The Soviet countries also developed a book of algorithms and programs for health care information systems. Egypt expanded its pilot program to include two additional geographical areas and also upgraded and expanded its computerized medical information management systems for the initial pilot participants. A hospital information systems project was begun at Obafemi Awolowo University Teaching Hospital in Ile-Ife, Nigeria, in 1988 (Dani, Makanjuola, & Ojo, 1993). Based on MUMPS/Fileman technology from the U.S. Department of Veterans Affairs, it was modified for the Nigerian medical records environment.

Additional internationally hosted MEDINFO conferences held in 1983 and 1989 included significant international paper presentations. The 1983 IMIA Conference in Amsterdam, the Netherlands, established several firsts. It was here that Ball coined the term *nursing informatics*. The first Working Group on Nursing Informatics was also initiated at this conference. In 1989 the IMIA became an organization independent of the IFIP. Included in its membership were international representatives. Dr. Marian Ball, an American, became its first female president in 1992.

In 1983 the Chinese Medical Informatics Association was founded by Z. Ouyang of the People's Republic of China. A year later, in 1984, the creation of the Japanese Association of Medical Informatics occurred. Five years later, in 1989, two additional informatics-focused societies were founded: the Korean Medical Informatics Society and the Hong Kong Society of Medical Informatics (Kaihara, 1999).

Martin Bangemann, the European commissioner for the European Community (EC), released a report entitled "Europe's Way to the Information Society: An Action Plan" that helped initiate the construction of an integrated, broadband network to be implemented in Europe starting in 1988. This network eventually became part of the Internet.

Two other significant events highlight this decade in informatics. In 1989 Mandil coined the term *health informatics.* Of greater importance was the application of work that began in the 1970s at CERN (Conseil Européen pour la Recherche Nucléaire, also called the European Organization for Nuclear Research or the European Laboratory for Particle Physics) in Geneva, Switzerland. This work enhanced the development of file transfer protocols (FTPs). FTPs allowed the movement of documents from one computer to another. In the 1980s, the ability to move documents from one place to another had a significant impact on the rapid adaptation of networked health care information systems. This shift had the potential to change health care delivery through a focus on solutions to problems of health care via a best practice model and the adoption of networked health care information systems worldwide.

Developments in the United States

The 1980s witnessed an explosion of external factors that influenced health care in the United States. Major technological players and events driving this explosion included the following:

- Introduction of the first commercial disk drive by IBM
- The government-ordered split of American Telegraph and Telephone (AT&T)
- The meteoric rise of Microsoft Corporation and its operating system to a position of dominance in the computer and economic fields
- Other legislative efforts that focused on copyright and protection of information

The evolution and development of the computer chip by Intel, along with the subsequent manufacture of PC clones, overtook Apple Computer's personal proprietary computers. The overall shift in computer focus from mainframe architecture to individual machines signaled a shift in power to the user. However, the need to communicate compelled inventors to explore communication among computers and people/users. Examples included the construction of the Defense Agency Research Projects Agency (DARPA) network to cope with communication in the event of an atomic war. This trend toward computer communication, or networks, was pushed along by Metcalf's conception of the ethernet, a form of communication over wires, along with developments in communication protocols such as the transmission control protocol/Internet protocol (TCP/IP). The networks and architectures (such as the client server) using these protocols shaped future health care applications.

One of the more prominent diagnostic expert systems in the early 1980s was Internist-1. Miller, Pople, and Myers (1982) sought to apply symbolic reasoning to develop computer-assisted diagnoses. It was an experimental computer program capable of making multiple and complex diagnoses in internal medicine. The goal of Internist-1, through modeling of physician behavior as a decision support aid, was to (1) keep physicians up-to-date with current knowledge; (2) make experts more available to the community as a whole, and (3) decrease potential medical bias related to fatigue; time; and limited knowledge, education, and/or experience (van Ginneken, 1999). Limitations included the failure by physicians to integrate Internist-1 into their practice patterns, the narrow scope of its database, and the program's inability to explain its conclusions (van Ginneken, 1999). Other systems that emerged as a result of Internist-1 include Quick Medical Reference (QMR) (Internist-1's direct successor), DxPlain, Iliad, and Meditel.

1990s

International Developments

Technology applications exploded in the 1990s with the advent of increasingly sophisticated hardware and software, increased memory and speed, and the decreased cost of digital computer technology. From the development and use of the Internet to satellites and wireless innovations, from mainframes to minicomputers to microcomputers to workstations to global networks, the amount of knowledge generated and the necessity for management of increasingly complex information systems was evident everywhere, especially in the health care arena. Of note was the International Council for Nursing Practice (ICNP), which began its work toward an international standard nursing language early in this decade (Clark, 1998).

Laires, Laderia, and Christensen (1995), Mandil et al. (1993), and Elioutina and Tarasov (1995) have documented the dramatic changes that occurred in the health care informatics field. In 1994 the EC implemented the Good European Health Record (GEHR), a project of the Advanced Informatics in Medicine Project of the European Community (Ingram, 1995). This project used smart card technology to contain

FIGURE 21–1 | Good European Health Record Project

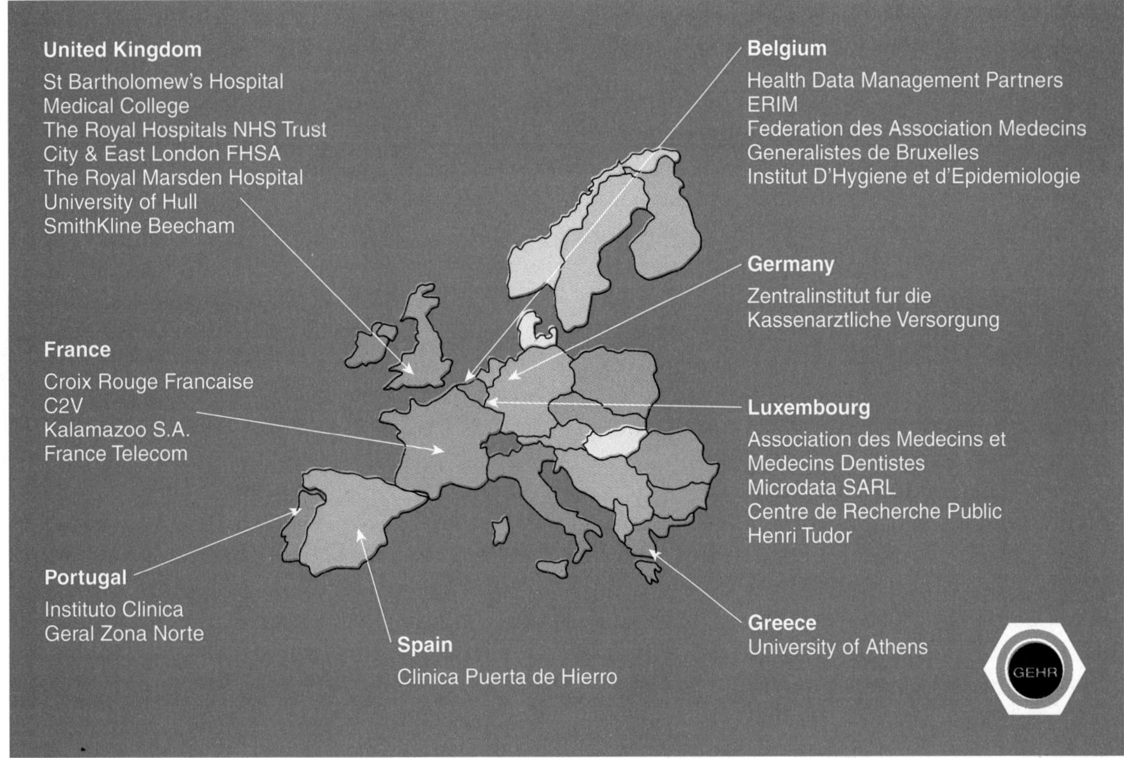

Countries represented in the Good European Health Record Project. *(Reprinted with permission of David Ingram, MD, and Dipak Kalra, MD.)*

health records for consumers in selected EC countries on an experimental basis (Figure 21-1). A year later, the EC developed and implemented DIABCARD: A Smart Card for Patients With Chronic Diseases, as a pilot study in Italy and Spain (Engelbrecht, et al., 1995).

The years 1993 and 1994 witnessed the establishment of 95 additional regional computer informatization sites by the Health Ministry within the Russian federation. However, the introduction of mandatory comprehensive health care insurance virtually halted further creation and adoption of new health care information systems.

In Africa, Musoke (1993) spoke eloquently of the challenges that faced health care professionals in African nations. These professionals managed health care information while confronting, among other things, extremely limited funds, lack of access to data, chronic civil war and internal strife, and limited computerization and access to technologies. Berhanu and Byass (1993) highlighted the implementation of health care information systems at the All-Africa Leprosy and Rehabilitation Training Centre (ALERT) in Addis Ababa, Ethiopia. The initial implementation focused on data analysis for a large, longitudinal field trial for leprosy treatment and use of a financial package. Lisse (1993) described a low-cost wide area networking system that employed computer networking and electronic mail to connect hospital and clinical information systems in Namibia. Rattan and Mienje (1993) presented information from Senegal on the African Regional Centre for Technology and its mission to facilitate support of information technology for health care. Thirty-one member states from across continental Africa participated. A pilot project, HEALTHNET, was implemented in July 1991 to facilitate communication and information sharing among health care professionals in the sub-Saharan African countries of Kenya, Uganda, Tanzania, Zambia, and Zimbabwe.

Braa and Hedberg (2000) have described the results of a longitudinal approach to the planning, implementation, and preliminary evaluation of a country-wide project in South Africa to develop district-based health care information systems. Minimum data sets were adopted and implemented as primary components of the health care information systems framework. These authors discuss the importance of grass root and key stakeholder involvement in all of the decision making and creation steps, as well as the implementation and evaluation of steps of the project. By 2000, three provinces in South Africa had completed integration of a district-based health care information system. The remainder will be phased in depending on "an incremental process of aligning actors" (Braa & Hedberg, 2000, p. 26), which is acknowledged to be a long-term process.

Juxtaposition between Japan and South Africa on developing health care information systems reveals insights about the use of health care information systems in those countries. Kaihara (1999) has suggested that in Japan computers and technology have changed dramatically but that the essence of health care has not been impacted by information technology as much as had been anticipated. With the exception of data processing and laboratory results shown on a monitor, information technology related to health care remains much the same as it was in the 1970s. Health care providers have not been able to apply clinical decision-making systems to the "real world" of practice. Standards remain in the developmental stage, information from distinct computerized patient care records remains incompatible, and there is a paucity of reliable clinical databases available for practicing evidence-based medicine. In Japan, as of 1996, Kaihara reported that two thirds of health care information systems trials had been or were about to be abandoned because of lack of funding and trained personnel. His analysis suggests that the need to make health care information systems applicable to the health care setting (i.e., "the real world") in terms of availability, cost, and ease of operation is very real.

Heeks, Mundy, and Salazar (1999) have discussed the reasons for the success or failure of health care information systems. According to these authors, "Successful health care information systems will be those that match the health care environment with respect to technical, social and organizational factors; most especially the perceptions of key stakeholders" (p. 4). Health care professionals from all disciplines access the health care records of their patients. Administrative and financial personnel also require access to these same records. A variety of health care information systems have been developed worldwide to meet these needs. Systems have been created to store and retrieve financial, administrative, medical, nursing, pharmacy, dental, allied health, and consumer information pertinent to health care. There is a definite demand for patient information, not only for each professional but also for the consumer.

Countries in the international arena have developed and implemented health care information systems that use a **systems approach.** Identification of key **stakeholders** and **working partnerships** has developed among countries that might or might not share common borders, are multilingual, and acknowledge the existence of and need to share scarce resources. These are important components of the systems approach that governs international utilization of health care information systems. Based on computers and networked telecommunication devices such as telephone lines, wireless radio, satellites, and high-speed fiberoptic cable, health care information systems are able to receive, store, and retrieve information generated anywhere, irrespective of time and location. These means of communication and tabulation have great potential for linking best practices, improving the quality of life, and saving lives worldwide. Coupled with the development and adoption of multilingual minimum data sets, health care information may be shared rapidly and in a cost-efficient fashion. In effect, the international community has demonstrated an evolutionary path different from that of the United States. For example, in Europe the adoption of common standards has been necessary for health information access to occur. In the United States, the forces of capitalism and entrepreneurialism have led to a greater degree of disagreement on standards of health information use and access.

Examples of functioning international health care information systems include, but are not limited to, the following:

- The CARE Telematics Project is a consortium of public and private partners led by the World Health Organization Regional Office for Europe (Zollner, 1995). The purpose of this consortium is to "demonstrate the capability of telecommunications in improving the efficiency and effectiveness of national administrations which have a responsibility in health, including disease prevention and control and medical care, as well as related areas such as environmental health, management of emergencies and disasters, statistics and strategic planning and evaluation" (Zollner, 1995, p. 279). The project, with 6 partners, 18 associate partners, and more than 70 user administrations as of 1995, had been deemed a success.
- OPADE: Optimization of Drug Prescription Using Advanced Informatics is a joint venture among individuals from Belgium, France, Italy, Sweden, and the United Kingdom for the purpose of developing and evaluating an intelligent, multilingual computerized drug prescription system (CDPS) from a medical, patient compliance, and economic point of view (deZegher et al., 1995). The alpha version of the project was completed with recommendations for further necessary refinements before the system could be fully implemented in a clinical setting. These refinements included the need for a "structured and coded drug database with standard EDI messages that allow for telemaintenance of the CDPS knowledge base from professional sources, and standard prescription messages to allow for transfer of patient prescription information from the CDPS to various third parties" (deZegher et al., 1995, p. 258). Project teams from participating countries are currently working toward solving these challenges in order for the systems to be implemented in clinical settings.
- OBSQID: Continuous Quality Development in Perinatal Care Through Use of Quality Indicators is a World Health Organization Regional Office for Europe initiative that involves the collection of data on 17 essential quality indicators of perinatal care from 29 countries (Johansen & Roos, 1995). The collection and dissemination of the information gained from these quality indicators will facilitate the exchange of data from regional, national, and transnational perspectives. It also allows

for the identification and monitoring of best practices in perinatal care.

- ORATEL: Telematic Systems for Quality Assurance in Oral Health Care is described as "a telematic system which would facilitate daily monitoring and evaluation of a dental practice; support the transfer of knowledge and goal setting; and stimulate and orient oral health providers towards a quality assurance approach through a proactive clinical/quality assurance reminder system and self-education" (Johansen, Moller, & Petersen, 1995, p. 507). Partners in Denmark, Italy, Sweden, Spain, Germany, and the United Kingdom have conducted this project. The World Health Organization Regional Office for Europe in Denmark contains the database terminal that links the Health for All initiative of this European collective effort.
- TELENURSING is an EC project whose purpose is "to promote standardized and formalized clinical nursing care data based on uniform definitions of data items with the purpose of developing countable and comparable nursing minimum data sets as a means of communicating nursing care information electronically between clinical settings, health care sectors nationally and European-wide and a means of producing Euro-Nursing Health statistics on people's need for nursing care" (Mortensen & Nielsen, 1995, p. 115). Current efforts of this group include Telenurse and TelenurseID-ENTITY (Mortensen, 1999). These projects continue the work of the original project regarding technology and nursing efforts in Europe. This group has also explored the potential of using the ICNP with the nurse record in Europe (Mortensen, 1997).

Box 21–2 Selected Examples of Standardized Languages

ICD: International Classification of Diseases. Started in the mid-1800s in the United Kingdom.
SNOP: Systematized Nomenclature of Pathology. Developed in 1965.
SNOMED: Systematized Nomenclature of Medicine. Started in 1974.
UMLS: Unified Medical Language System. Begun in 1976 by the National Library of Medicine.
NANDA: North American Nursing Diagnoses Association. First issued in 1982.
NILT: Nursing Intervention Lexicon and Taxonomy. First published in 1992.
ICNP: International Classification of Nursing Practice.

South America has begun several health care initiatives (Stammer, 2000). In Peru, "swipe cards" are being implemented. These cards validate the patient's identity and eligibility at any public health center. Both Argentina and Ecuador have instituted the computerized management of pharmacy benefits for all citizens. Uruguay has instituted an online service for physicians called Red Medica (Medical Network) and also employs limited videoconferencing for medical rounds in its large urban hospitals.

Developments in the United States

The early part of the 1990s saw a flurry of development in many areas, ranging from communications to **standardized languages** (Box 21-2). Efforts in nursing from this decade include the Home Health Care Classification, Omaha System, and Nursing Intervention Lexicon and Taxonomy (NILT) (Clark, 1999). The Nursing Interventions Classification (NIC)—a standardized language that describes treatments that nurses perform—and the Nursing Outcomes Classification (NOC)—developed to evaluate the effect of nursing interventions—were released in the mid to late 1990s. Standardized languages in medicine for this decade continued earlier efforts related to the development of ICD, SNOMED, and UMLS, among others.

Organizational development and growth can be considered an indication of acceptance by a profession. Multiple health care information organizations expanded from their roots in the earlier part of this decade (Box 21-3). Of note is the role of the American Nurses Association (ANA) in terms of computer technology. Since the 1980s the ANA has been involved with computer technology and its application for nurses (Saba & McCormick, 1996). A key point was in 1992, when nursing informatics was recognized as a specialty by the ANA with the publication of a handbook describing core competencies within the scope of practice of nursing informatics (ANA, 1994; Young, 2000). In the mid-1990s the ANA also offered a certification process that recognized the uniqueness and value of nursing informatics. These two events marked a significant change in attitude about the legitimacy and recognition of nursing informatics and informatics in general. In addition, in 1995 the ANA established the Nursing Information and Data Set Evaluation Center (NIDSEC) to review, develop standards for information systems, and evaluate systems against those standards. NIDSEC has recognized 12 nursing languages developed to document nursing care (American Nurses Association, 2001).

As the health care market has become increasingly complex, so has health care software. Software application programs for health care number in the thousands with what seem to be programs for any and all purposes. Figures quoted for the number of vendors range from approximately 300 to over 500 vendors. As late as 1996, a source on the Internet reported that the amount spent in the United States on health care information systems was approximately $14 billion with a 5-year growth projection of about $100 billion. Within

Box 21—3 Health Care Information Organizations

IFIP: International Federation for Information Processing. Founded in 1960 and considered to be the origin of many health care information organizations today.

IEEE: Institute of Electrical and Electronics Engineers. Founded in 1963.

IMIA: International Medical Informatics Association. Origin in late 1960s and early 1970s. Formally established in 1979.

AMIA: American Medical Informatics Association. Formed in late 1990. Efforts of the American Association for Medical Systems and Informatics (AAMSI), the American College of Medical Informatics (ACMI), and the Symposium on Computer Applications in Medical Care (SCAMC) helped with its formation.

AMIA-NIWG: Nursing Informatics Working Group. One of the earliest workgroups of the AMIA. Has been involved with many other organizations, especially with the International Medical Informatics Association (IMIA).

IMIA Working Group 11—Dental Informatics: The first official meeting was held on August 22, 1990, in conjunction with the Medical Informatics Europe Meeting in Glasgow, Scotland.

HIMSS: Health Information Management and Systems Society. Founded in 1961 as a professional membership organization.

CPRI and HOST: Computerized Patient Record Institute and Healthcare Open Systems and Trials consolidated in 2000 with a change in focus from the computer-based patient record to the health care information system.

Table 21–2 **Important Legislation Impacting Documentation Requirements**

Legislation	Year
Nursing Training Act	1964
Social Security Amendments (Medicare and Medicaid)	1965
Quality Assurance Program; Professional Standard Review Organizations (PSROs)	1972
Health Services Research, Health Statistics, and Medical Libraries Act	1974
National Health Planning and Resources Development Act	1974
Omnibus Budget Reconciliation Act	1989
Social Security Amendments; Prospective Payment System (DRGs)	1983
Health Insurance Portability and Accountability Act (HIPAA) (contains Administrative Simplification Care requirements)	1996

From Saba, V., & McCormick, K. (1996). *Essentials of computers for nurses* (2nd ed.). New York: McGraw-Hill.
DRGs, Diagnosis-related groups.

the last years of this decade, health care informatics was swept up by the Internet and the potential lure of the World Wide Web (WWW). The increased popularity of electronic data interchange (EDI), with its ability to reduce human errors, has revolutionized the billing end of health care.

A number of health care professionals have realized the potential of the Internet and the WWW. In the early 1990s Lee Hancock and Gary Malet assumed leadership roles. Hancock was an early pioneer of the use of mailing lists as a means of health information distribution. Malet established a resource called the Medical Matrix, which could be thought of as one of the earliest health information portals, or information collections, on the Internet. These early attempts to take advantage of this new mode of communication have evolved into current sites administered by companies such as Healtheon/WebMD, Medscape, and Oncolink. Increased communication among health care professionals and consumers via electronic mail (eMail), hypertext markup language (HTML), and hypertext transfer protocol (HTTP) continue to have an impact on health care. These technologies have revolutionized information provision, access, and availability between the health care provider and the consumer. Technology has changed the traditional concept of the health care provider from a gatekeeper to a facilitator. Table 21-2 lists federal legislation that has influenced health care documentation.

Nationally and internationally, health care informatics was revolutionized during the 1990s by the further development of the file transfer protocol (FTP) and its application to the international telecommunications network. The global network of fiberoptic cables that gird the world provides a vast international telecommunications network that is able to send data, information, knowledge, and potentially, wisdom about health care information anywhere in seconds. Although the capability exists to assess virtually unlimited health care information, there continues to be difficulty with the practical application of this technology in some parts of the world. Issues identified that impact the development of workable health care information systems include (1) the lack of standard nomenclature or language; (2) funding for development of clinically based decision support systems; (3) scarce national resources in terms of money, personnel, electricity, and telephony in developing and Third World countries; and (4) differences in funding for country-specific health care (i.e., national health care, managed care, or limited or no available care).

Slawson, Shaughnessy, and Bennett (1994) questioned the usefulness of available medical information. A formula to assist in determining the usefulness of medical information was developed and consisted of the following three criteria: "(1) it must be relevant to everyday practice, (2) it must be correct, and (3) it must require little work to obtain" (p. 508). The formula was structured as follows:

$$\text{Usefulness of } \textit{medical} \text{ information} = \text{Relevance} \times \text{Validity} \div \text{Work}$$

This formula could also be used to determine the usefulness of *health care* information. Health care providers, policy makers, consumers, and a myriad of other people interested in accurate and useful health care information could also use this formula. Slawson, Shaughnessy, and Bennett (1994) offered a complementary idea that suggested that useful medical or health care information could determine whether a disease-centered or a patient-centered approach would provide the most benefit for a patient requesting care. A well-designed and functional clinical decision support system has the potential to assist the health care practitioner in becoming a better master of health care information. More detailed information about clinical decision support systems can be found in Chapter 5.

HISTORICAL DEVELOPMENT OF EDUCATIONAL PROGRAMS IN HEALTH CARE INFORMATICS

Traditionally, individuals interested in mathematics and engineering were captivated by the idea of creating a machine that would communicate and tabulate information more quickly than a human. Many of these early pioneers had advanced degrees in mathematics or engineering. Hollerith, a prime example, was awarded the doctor of philosophy degree from Columbia University in the late 1800s for his work that led to the Hollerith Tabulating Machine. Although not directly related to health care informatics, this example illustrates the interests of a person attracted to the use of computers and technology for information management.

In the mid-1950s the Russians acknowledged the importance of information management. However, it was not until the mid-1960s that medical informatics became integrated into university curricula as a component of medical education. The first universities that integrated medical informatics education into medical education were located in France, Holland, Belgium, and the USSR (Collen, 1995). The United States quickly followed suit in the late 1960s and early 1970s. Although there were courses in medical informatics at this time, an entire medical informatics program of study still did not exist.

Blum outlined how and why he and his colleagues became proficient in medical informatics (Blum & Duncan, 1990). He attributed the development of their proficiency to the following six factors:

1. A change in the mode of information transfer from rote memorization of facts to the use of problem-solving techniques
2. Curiosity about whether a machine could solve a problem created by humans
3. Generalized curiosity
4. Appreciation and knowledge that there are limits to human performance and that perhaps a machine (computer) may perform better
5. A general interest in technology
6. A mathematics or engineering background (in essence, until the 1970s, much of the learning was "on the job" training because there were no formal programs that addressed education for health care informatics)

The late 1970s through the early 1990s saw the introduction of informatics into disciplines other than medicine. Nurses and other health care providers recognized the importance of informatics and began to include relevant informatics

Table 21–3 Health Care Informatics Specialist Requirements Circa 2000

Computer Science (Knowledge)	Health Care (Knowledge and Experience)	Managerial Skills (Knowledge and Experience)
Theory and practice of hardware and software applications	Hospital administrative experience	Know the basics of acquiring computer equipment, applications, network systems, and other services from a "real world" perspective
Operating systems and compilers	Admission, transfer, and discharge information experience	Have product knowledge, performance, and reputation information available
Database management	Know the jargon of health care	Know the economics of data processing, data mining, nomenclatures, standards, contracts, leasing versus purchasing, and rental agreements
Computer graphics	Ability to assist health care providers with defining, organizing, and analyzing health care problems to permit automation to proceed rationally	Develop positive relationships with vendors of hardware, software, and networking vendors
Artificial intelligence	Knowledge and experience with discipline-specific nomenclatures and standards	Knowledge and application of systems thinking, stakeholder buy-in combined with a behavioral perspective
Human-computer interface		
Network administration	Understand the economics of the health care system	Frequent updating and retraining in managerial applications of technologies
Internet/Web-based applications	Audit courses in health care administration	Application of wisdom to managerial skills
Programming language and techniques	Frequent updating and retraining in the primary care, community-based managed care arena	
Software engineering and development	Application of wisdom to health care	
Economics of computing		
Systems: organizational, learning and information		
Nomenclatures and standards		
Frequent updating and retraining on systems		
Application of wisdom to computer science		

Data based on Covvey, H., Craven, N., & McAlister, N. (1985). *Concepts and issues in health care computing.* St. Louis: Mosby.

content in the curricula of professional education programs. An early example was a curriculum for nursing informatics education in a nursing program developed by Ronald and Skiba in 1977 at the State University of New York at Buffalo. The University of Maryland at Baltimore School of Nursing and the University of Utah School of Nursing, realizing the importance of proper informatics education and training for nurses, started informatics-specific educational programs in the late 1980s and early 1990s, respectively. In 1992 the University of Maryland started, and continues to maintain, the only doctoral program in nursing informatics (Saba & McCormick, 1996). The National Library of Medicine also contributed to the early development of informatics education and continues to contribute through its numerous fellowships, conferences, grant funding, and the Integrated Advanced Information Management Systems (IAIMS) programs.

Covvey, Craven, and McAlister (1985) first articulated the idea of a specialist prepared in health care computing, suggesting that "recent innovations at some universities would support the idea of health care computing as a distinct profession with discernible demands and challenges necessitating the need for appropriate curricula to be developed and taught" (p. 202). Their description of the skills needed by a health care computing specialist includes a background in computer science, health care, and managerial experience.

Covvey, Craven, and McAlister based their recommendations on the premise that computing in the medical arena was vastly different from computing in the business arena. They believed that there was a philosophical difference between what they termed "rational number crunching" for cost and profit purposes by administrators and the orientation of health care providers, who were more behaviorally oriented toward providing care to patients and less concerned about cost and profit. In essence, they believed that there was a disparity in the objectives for managing health care information between the two groups. The thinking of today is not substantially different from that of 1985. The educational preparation of a health care information specialist today requires essentially the same skills with the addition of network, systems, and Internet perspectives. Table 21-3 describes the components required circa 2000.

Disciplines that originally created educational programs in informatics were predominantly computer science, business administration, health care administration, medicine, nursing, and pharmacy. Slowly, dental and allied health programs have created programs or integrated informatics education into their curricula.

CONCLUSION

Computers and technology grew out of mankind's need to communicate, tabulate, and manage information. The early inventions of the abacus, Babbage's Difference Engine, ENIAC, guided missiles, and space exploration moved efforts from computer hardware to software applications. This shift facilitated movement of these systems from business, industry, and the military into health care. Early applications were used predominantly for financial, administrative, and data processing functions. (The term *bioengineering* is used to describe the adaptation of biology and engineering to health care.) The next phase, computer informatics, was a combination of computer science, information science, and engineering. Medical informatics, with its focus on data, information, and knowledge applied to medical care, followed quickly. Nursing informatics, with its focus on cognitive science, information science, and computer science within the realm of nursing science, was developed next. Subsequently, as the concept of health care information systems became more prevalent, the term *health care informatics* was adopted.

The use of health care informatics within health care is occurring worldwide. These changes have occurred in a parallel fashion between the United States and the international community. Although the initial development and implementation were from an administrative perspective, clinical systems have becoming increasingly important. In addition to the development of discipline-specific informatics applications, such as medical and nursing informatics, the development of globally focused health care informatics is also occurring. The use of the term *health care informatics* is indicative of the multidisciplinary nature of managing information within the health care arena.

Although the approach to health care informatics and the application of health care information systems differs between the United States and the international community, there are several similarities. We must target the development of standards for international health care informatics that are applicable for all, because the next generation of health care information systems will operate via a global, networked infrastructure of fiberoptic cables, satellites, and other, as yet undeveloped technology applications. According to Fitzmaurice (1995), "Cooperation among nations that leads to understanding each society's concerns and to sharing research that evaluates the acceptability and costs of potential solutions can speed the development, diffusion and integration of health care information technology advances" (p. 646). The focus will be on the integrated access to patient data with the added benefit of health knowledge and wisdom being accessible to the global community, thus fulfilling the initiatives begun at the 1978 Alma Ata Conference, which identified the goal of *health for all.*

Web Connection

Health care informatics is evolving as the components of informatics, computer science, and information science and the discipline of science continue to innovate. Studying the history of health care informatics not only provides an opportunity to learn from the experiences and interpretations of past and current experts but also gives insight into its progress and future perspectives. The Web Connection activities for this chapter will take you on a journey through time to learn what has contributed to the current views and capabilities of health care informatics. You will examine resources that describe past innovations and see how they apply to technology and its implementation to health care today.

discussion questions

1. Compare and contrast the development of health care informatics in the international community and in the United States.
2. Discuss the educational preparation recommended for those wanting to become health care informatics specialists.
3. Analyze the concepts of data, information, knowledge, and wisdom, and apply these concepts to the construction of international standards for computerized patient records available on a global network.
4. Debate the question "Will there ever exist a standard nomenclature (language) usable by all members of the global community to communicate health care information?" Cite examples to support your statements.

REFERENCES

American Nurses Association. (1994). *The scope of practice for nursing informatics.* Washington, DC: Author.

American Nurses Association. (2001). *Nursing information and data set evaluation center.* Washington, DC: Author. Retrieved July 2, 2001, from the World Wide Web: http://www.nursingworld.org/nidsec/.

Barnett, G., et al. (1989). COSTAR—A computer-based medical information system for ambulatory care. In J. van Bemmel (Ed.), *Yearbook of medical informatics—The promise of medical informatics.*

Berhanu, T., & Byass, P. (1993). The development and support of informatics in an African setting: Experiences at ALERT, Addis Ababa. In S. Mandil et al. (Eds.), *Health informatics in Africa: HELINA 93.* Amsterdam: Excerpta Medica.

Blum, B. (1986). *Clinical information systems.* New York: Springer-Verlag.

Blum, B., & Duncan, K. (1990). *A history of medical informatics.* New York: ACM Press.

Boutros, S. (1993). Egyptian experience with microcomputers in monitoring and evaluating of health care programmes. In S. Mandil et al. (Eds.), *Health informatics in Africa: HELINA 93.* Amsterdam: Excerpta Medica.

Braa, J., & Hedberg, C. (2000). Developing district-based health care information systems: The South African experience. *Proceedings from the IFIP 9.4 International Conference 2000,* May 2000, Cape Town, South Africa.

Brandejs, J. (1976). *Health informatics: Canadian experience.* New York: American Elsevier.

Clark, D. (1998). The international classification for nursing practice project. *Online Journal of Issues in Nursing,* September 30. Available from the World Wide Web: http://www.nursingworld.org/ojin/tpc7/tpc7_3.htm.

Clark, D. (1999). A language for nursing. *Nursing Standard, 13*(31), 420-447.

Collen, M. (1970). General requirements for a medical information system (MIS). *Research, 3,* 393-406.

Collen, M. (1995). *A history of medical informatics in the United States, 1950 to 1990.* Indianapolis: American Medical Informatics Association.

Covvey, H., Craven, N., & McAlister, N. (1985). *Concepts and issues in health care computing.* St. Louis: Mosby.

Dani, O., Makanjuola, R., & Ojo, J. (1993). A hospital information system in a Nigerian university teaching hospital. In S. Mandil et al. (Eds.), *Health informatics in Africa: HELINA 93.* Amsterdam: Excerpta Medica.

deZegher, I., et al. (1995). OPADE: Optimization of drug prescription using advanced informatics in health informatics in health. In M. Laires, et al. (Eds.), *Health in the new communications age: Health care telematics for the 21st century.* Amsterdam: IOS Press.

Elioutina, S., & Tarasov, V. (1995). Current state and perspectives of healthcare informatics in Russia. *International Journal of Bio-Medical Computing, 39,* 163-167.

Engelbrecht, R., et al. (1995). DIABCARD: A smart card for patients with chronic diseases. In M. Laires, et al. (Eds.), *Health in the new communications age: Health care telematics for the 21st century.* Amsterdam: IOS Press.

Farley, B.G., & Clark, W.A. (1954). Simulation of self-organizing systems by digital computer. *IRE Transactions on Information Theory, 4,* 76-84.

Fitzmaurice, J. (1995). The American perspective for the future in health. In M. Laires, et al. (Eds.), *Health in the new communications age: Health care telematics for the 21st century.* Amsterdam: IOS Press.

Graves, J., & Corcoran, S. (1989). The study of nursing informatics. *Image: The Journal of Nursing Scholarship, 21*(4), 227-230.

Hannah, K., Ball, M., & Edwards, M. (1999). *Introduction to nursing informatics* (2nd ed.). New York: Springer-Verlag.

Haux, R., Knaup, P., & Schmucker, P. (1999). Commentary—Medical and health information systems; the boundaries are still fading. In A. McCray & J. van Bemmel (Eds.), *Yearbook of medical informatics 1999* (pp. 235-237). New York: Schattauer.

Heeks, R., Mundy, D., & Salazar, A. (1999). *Why health care information systems succeed or fail.* Working Paper Series No. 9. Manchester, UK: University of Manchester, Precinct Centre, Institute for Development Policy and Management.

Hogarth, M. (1997). *Medical informatics: An introduction.* Retrieved from the World Wide Web: http://informatics.ucdmc.ucdavis.edu/Concepts/Intro.htm.

Ingram, D. (1995). GEHR: The Good European Health Record in health. In M. Laires, et al. (Eds.), *Health in the new communications age: Health care telematics for the 21st century.* Amsterdam: IOS Press.

Johansen, K., Moller, I., & Peter, P. (1995). ORATEL: Telematic systems for quality assurance in oral health care. In M. Laires, et al. (Eds.), *Health in the new communications age: Health care telematics for the 21st century.* Amsterdam: IOS Press.

Johansen, K., & Roos, J. (1995). OBSQID: Continuous quality development in perinatal care through use of quality indicators. In M. Laires, et al. (Eds.), *Health in the new communications age: Health care telematics for the 21st century.* Amsterdam: IOS Press.

Joos, I., et al. (1992). *Computers in small bytes—The computer workbook* (2nd ed.). New York: National League for Nursing Press.

Kaihara, S. (1999). The promise of medical informatics in Asia. In A. McCray & J. van Bemmel (Eds.), *Yearbook of medical informatics 1999* (pp. 61-64). New York: Schattauer.

Laires, M., Ladeira, M., & Christensen, J. (Eds.). (1995). In *Health in the new communications age: Health care telematics for the 21st century.* Amsterdam: IOS Press.

Lisse, E. (1993). Computer networking in developing countries. In S. Mandil et al. (Eds.), *Health informatics in Africa: HELINA 93.* Amsterdam: Excerpta Medica.

Mandil, S., et al. (Eds.). (1993). *Health informatics in Africa: HELINA 93.* Amsterdam: Excerpta Medica.

McDonald, C. (1976). Protocol-based computer reminders, the quality of care and the non-perfectability of man. *New England Journal of Medicine, 295,* 1351-1355.

Miller, R., Pople, H., & Myers, J. (1982). Internist-1: An experimental computer-based diagnostic consultant for general internal medicine. *New England Journal of Medicine, 30,* 468-476.

Mortensen, R. (Ed.). (1997). *ICNP in Europe: Telenurse.* Amsterdam: IOS Press.

Mortensen, R. (Ed.). (1999). *ICNP and telematic applications for nurses in Europe: The telenurse experience.* Studies in Health Technology and Informatics. Amsterdam: IOS Press.

Mortensen, R., & Nielsen, G. (1995). Telenursing. In *Health in the new Communications Age: Health care telematics for the 21st century* (pp. 115-126). Amsterdam: IOS Press.

Musoke, M. (1993). Problems of information flow for health professionals in Africa: Role of computer-based information. In S. Mandil et al. (Eds.), *Health informatics in Africa: HELINA 93.* Amsterdam: Excerpta Medica.

National Library of Medicine. (1999). Biomedical Research in Current Research. Retrieved July 10, 1999, from the World Wide Web: http://lhc.nlm.nih.gov/M3W3/phs_history/phs_history_102.html.

Nelson, R., & Joos, I. (1989). On language in nursing: From data to wisdom. *PLN Visions,* Fall, p. 6.

Payne, L. & Brown, P. (1975). *An introduction to medical automation* (2nd ed.). Philadelphia: J.B. Lippincott.

Rattan, R., & Mienje, S. (1993). The information system of the African Regional Centre for Technology, and its potential applications to Health. In S. Mandil et al. (Eds.), *Health informatics in Africa: HELINA 93.* Amsterdam: Excerpta Medica.

Rautaharju, P. (1999). Commentary—The birth of automatic ECG screening by digital electronic computer. In A. McCray & J. van Bemmel (Eds.), *Yearbook of medical informatics 1999* (pp. 183-185). New York: Schattauer.

Saba, V., & McCormick, K. (1986). *Essentials of computers for nurses.* Philadelphia: J.B. Lippincott.

Saba, V., & McCormick, K. (1996). *Essentials of computers for nurses* (2nd ed.). New York: McGraw-Hill.

Scholes, M., & Barber, B. (1980). Towards nursing informatics. In D.A.D. Lindberg, & S. Kaihara (Eds.), *MEDINFO: 1980* (pp. 7-73). Amsterdam, Netherlands: North-Holland.

Shortliffe, E., & Buchanan, B. (1975). A model of inexact reasoning in medicine. *Math Bioscience, 23,* 351-379.

Slawson, D., Shaughnessy, A., & Bennett, J. (1994). Becoming a medical information master: Feeling good about *not* knowing everything. *Journal of Family Practice, 38* (5), 505-513.

Stammer, L. (2000). Brazil and its neighbors. *Healthcare Informatics,* August, pp. 26-36.

Turley, J. (1996). Toward a model for nursing informatics. *Image: The Journal of Nursing Scholarship, 28*(4), 309-313.

University of St Andrews, Scotland: School of Mathematics and Statistics. (1999). Konrad Zuse. Retrieved July 10, 2001, from the World Wide Web: http://www-history.mcs.st-andrews.ac.uk/history/Mathematicians/Zuse.html.

van Ginneken, A. (1999). Commentary—Diagnostic support: Towards the intelligent integrated reference source. In A. McCray & J. van Bemmel (Eds.), *Yearbook of medical informatics 1999* (pp. 175-179). New York: Schattauer.

Warner, H., Olmsted, C., & Rutherford, B. (1971). HELP—A program for medical decision-making. *Computers and Biomedical Research, 5*(1), 65-74.

Weed, L. (1968). Medical records that guide and teach. *New England Journal of Medicine, 278*(11), 593-600.

Young, K. (2000). *Informatics for healthcare professionals.* Philadelphia: F.A. Davis.

Zollner, H. (1995). The CARE Telematics Project. In M. Laires, et al. (Eds.), *Health in the new communications age: Health care telematics for the 21st century* (pp. 279-289). Amsterdam: IOS Press.

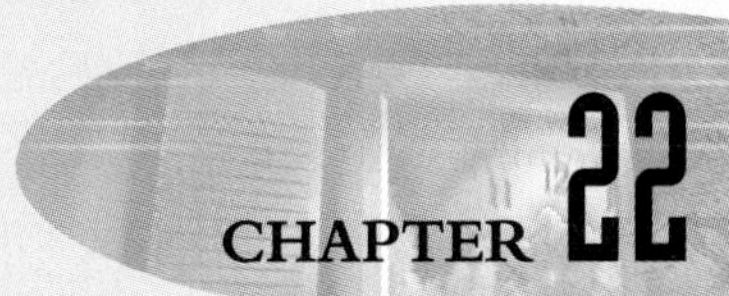

The Future of Health Care Informatics Education

JAMES P. TURLEY

Learning Objectives

Upon completion of this chapter, the reader will be able to:

1. ***Discuss*** the components of health care informatics education.
2. ***Relate*** the components to each other and the underlying sciences.
3. ***Discuss*** the relationship between the components of health care informatics education and different models of health care informatics education.
4. ***Explain*** the impact of educational technology on future trends in health care informatics education.
5. ***Discuss*** future professional trends that will redefine health care informatics education.

Outline

Assumptions, Driving Forces, and Guiding Principles
- *Health Care Informatics*
- *Health Care Informatics as a Science*
- *Health Sciences and the Health Professions*
- *Health Care Delivery*
- *Outcomes Research*
- *Financing Health Care*
- *Educational Trends*
- *Educational Technology*
- *The New Student*

Future Educational Programs and Health Care Informatics
- *Health Care Informatics Curriculum*
- *Developing Process Knowledge*
- *Communication of Knowledge*
- *Decision Making*
- *Technology*

Key Terms

chaordic
computational health care informaticians
computational knowledge
garden path reasoning
Heizenberg Principle
just-in-time learning
net generation, N-Gen students
process-based education
safe classroom

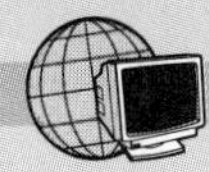

Web Connection

Go to the Web site at http://evolve.elsevier.com/Englebardt/. Here you will find Web links and activities related to the future of health care informatics education.

Health care informatics is a relatively new science and as such is still evolving. Entering into a discussion about a rapidly changing science is fraught with danger. Because the nature of the science changes quickly, the educational process of that science is required to change quickly. The discovery of new applications that have yet to be tested by the practitioners of that science is a challenge in educating new practitioners. The constant development of the science, with new areas of investigation and application, creates ongoing changes in educational demands. The educational methods and strategies needed to make an evolving science useful and applicable to the practice must continuously adapt to the changes in the science. In addition, society and related sciences continue to place new demands on the emerging science. This discussion of the future of health care informatics education is fraught with all of these dangers. Therefore this discussion is meant to suggest possibilities, provoke considerations, and have the reader think broadly about not only the definition of health care informatics but also the future of health care informatics education. This chapter begins with assumptions about the definition of health care informatics. These assumptions underlie the discussion concerning the education of health care informatics specialists or informaticians. Both *health care informatics specialist* and *informatician* are accepted terms for identifying practitioners of this specialty.

Education is in a period of rapid change. The nature of the university and its contract with society are under considerable review. It is becoming clear that not only is the science of education changing, but also the structures that house education are changing. The changing role of education and the changing role of universities are addressed obliquely in this chapter. The issues of technology and education are also discussed in Chapters 11 and 12. However, there are additional assumptions and definitions that are discussed in this chapter as a basis for discussing health care informatics education.

ASSUMPTIONS, DRIVING FORCES, AND GUIDING PRINCIPLES

The following section presents primary assumptions, driving forces, and guiding principles that can be expected to have an impact on the future of health care informatics education. Any or all of these assumptions may prove to be wrong. Some may even prove to be correct. These assumptions are guide points that must be interpreted according to the specific needs and situation of the reader and not as absolutes to be taken without serious reflection.

Health Care Informatics

Health care informatics is an interdisciplinary specialty that has grown primarily out of nursing and medical informatics, as well as other specialty areas in informatics. Nurses have held a number of views of informatics. Early views placed considerable importance on the impact of computers on nursing. Issues of computer literacy and utilization of computer technology were important considerations (Turley, 1996b). The classic definition of nursing informatics by Graves and Corcoran (1989) brought nursing out of the technology view and into a knowledge view. Graves and Corcoran discussed the application of technology to benefit the clinical practice of nursing by making the knowledge of nursing more available and by assisting in the structuring of nursing knowledge. Building on Graves and Corcoran's concepts of data, information, and knowledge, Nelson and Joos (1989) introduced wisdom as the appropriate application of knowledge to meet human needs in health care. A recent approach by Turley (2000a) focuses on the communication aspects of knowledge rather than on the knowledge itself. The focus on communication addresses a more process-embedded type of knowledge, which moves the definition of informatics further from a technology view.

Many informatics definitions are found within nursing itself (Graves & Corcoran, 1989; Turley,

1996b). Other definitions have focused on the inherently interdisciplinary nature of informatics. The question of whether informatics belongs within a discipline of science (such as nursing, medicine, or dentistry) or whether it, by its nature, sits on the boundaries between disciplines is one that will continue to cause debate. This debate was introduced in the preface of this textbook. This chapter assumes that health care informatics is interdisciplinary. The assumption implies that the need for communication of data, information, knowledge, and wisdom underlies the core of health care informatics.

This does not change the need for discussion of informatics issues within a discipline. However, it does consider that the discussion within a discipline has as its goal communication of information across disciplinary lines for the benefit of the recipients of health care. A focus on the communication nature of information creates a different set of priorities and assumptions from when the focus is on the structuring of data, information, and knowledge within a specific health discipline. The different interpretations of the structure of health care informatics requires not only different approaches/strategies for educating students but also a different understanding of the underlying sciences that are represented in the definition.

Health Care Informatics as a Science

The rapidity of change in the field of health care informatics interferes with the formation of a science. It is difficult to both explain existing phenomena and predict future phenomena when the domain being studied is constantly shifting. In physics this is referred to as the Heizenberg principle. The **Heizenberg Principle** states that just the act of observing a phenomenon changes the nature of that phenomenon.

There has been little discussion in the literature as to whether or not health care informatics is a science. The usual understanding of a science is that it defines and structures a unique area of knowledge. The science helps to explain phenomena in the area of concern and provides insight for further research into the knowledge of the domain. This section addresses issues of rapid change, rapid redefinition, and chaordic theory as they relate to the discussion of health care informatics as a science.

What is the domain of health care informatics? In older definitions the domain would be the application of computer technology to health care (Schwirian et al., 1989). Other definitions include the application of information technology to health care (Graves & Corcoran, 1988). Some definitions of health care informatics focus on the nature of data, information, and knowledge (Graves, 1993). Other definitions focus on the nature of communication of data, information, and knowledge (Turley, 2000b). It is clear that all four definitions are related. However, each definition has a different primary focus and, as such, creates a different structure for the science it describes.

The evolving definitions of health care informatics imply that a single formal definition of the science is unlikely to be accepted in the near future. However, health care informatics professionals are continuing to order and organize the domain of knowledge that addresses computational knowledge in health. **Computational knowledge** is knowledge related to the use of computers in analyzing and solving scientific problems. It is distinct from computer science (which is the study of computers and computation) and information science (which focuses on conceptual tools for integrating the technological, behavioral, and contextual knowledge about information processing and communication). As computational knowledge in health becomes ordered, health care informatics will approach the definition of a science (Suppe, 1977, 1989).

Science has historically gone through periods of change and then had time for the integration of the new insights. Traditional work by Suppe (1977, 1989) and others studied the nature of science during less turbulent periods. The rapid evolution of science during the late twentieth century and early twenty-first century is unlike any other period in recorded history. There has been a dramatic shift in what science is able to investigate. Major advances in science have occurred not within discipline boundaries but at the intersections of traditional sciences. The impact of the new knowledge coming at the boundaries of science affects the nature and structure of science as much as it does the nature of the new knowledge. If new knowledge is being generated at the intersection of two traditional sciences, it may be that the traditional structure of science is inadequate to provide the newly required structure and understanding for the new knowledge.

If the very nature of science is undergoing a change, how should the health sciences as a whole, and health care informatics in particular, be understood? Advances in genomic and structural biology areas can lead researchers to wonder whether one is studying chemistry, physics, biology, or mathematics. In such examples it is neither possible nor useful to attempt to organize the phenomena in terms of the traditional sciences because the phenomena do not uniquely belong to a single science. Health care informatics addresses similar issues of "confusion" or "massive reconceptualization." The issues related to data, information, knowledge, and wisdom make it clear that the structure of knowledge does not exist in the abstract. Data, information, knowledge, and wisdom exist in the mental models of the people who use them. Cognitive science has demonstrated that people build models in order to understand the relationships that exist among information elements (Gardner, 1987). Traditionally, data, information, and knowledge are conceptualized as existing independently of the human minds that use them. They are reflected as having a structure based on the science that describes them and thus have a structural independence.

Researchers understand that the mental models people use to organize and store information have as much impact on the structure of data, information, and knowledge as a structure imposed by science (Capra, 1988). As more is learned about cognitive processes, mental models, and decision science, more is understood about the complex interactions between the way people think about knowledge and the knowledge that is thought about (Gardner, 1987).

The science of health care informatics provides new tools and new ways to understand the complex relationships between health-related knowledge and the people who use the data, information, and knowledge. As the science evolves, it will generate new tools for research, new models for the conceptualization of health data, and indeed, eventually a new science.

Chaordic theory provides another vantage point from which to understand new approaches to science. Hock (1999, 2000) coined the term **chaordic** to refer to the combination of chaos and order found in organizations. Chaordic organizations contain the notion of self-regulation, or the generating of order from chaos. Writings by Zukov and Finklestein (1980), Capra (1988), and others have pointed out the need to reconceptualize the current notion of science to combine the notions of chaos and order at the same time. Hock has provided an approach that recognizes the traditional scientific models but also seeks to extend them into new ways of organizing knowledge.

Health care informatics appears to be evolving through such a chaordic period. New components and new aspects of health care informatics are being identified on a regular basis. There are different schools addressing different assets of the domain of knowledge (genomics, proteinomics, critical care, public health). Different groups (clinicians, outcomes managers, financial analysts) structure the knowledge differently. The different disciplines (dentistry, medicine, nursing) use different mental models. The demands placed on the knowledge by different disciplines require different knowledge structures to achieve their goals. Yet, out of this chaos there appears to be a growing sense of order, at a higher level of abstraction, leading to the creation of knowledge typologies and interaction processes between knowledge and mental models, resulting in new forms of order. Currently, health care informatics can be seen as being in a state of chaordic development.

Health Sciences and the Health Professions

The health sciences have not always thought of themselves as sciences or professions. As recognized disciplines, their knowledge was organized into a science rather late. Individual health professions traditionally educate their students in isolation from each other. At the same time, health care practice focuses on the need for team-based delivery of care. The seeming contradiction between the educational structure and the delivery structure warrants comment and investigation.

On June 26, 2000, Francis Collins of the National Genome Research Institute and J. Craig Ventor of Celera Genomics announced that their combined research had resulted in the decoding of the 3 billion chemical bonds of the human genome (Genome, 2000). Although this first analysis of the human genome will not result in immediate changes in the delivery of health care, the long-term impact of understanding the human genome cannot be underestimated. The chemical sequencing of the bonds as well as computational analysis resulted in the derivation of the human genome. Computational analysis has always been important in the delivery of health care. Computations have traditionally occurred at a fairly low level (e.g., calculation of body mass index, drug dosages based on milligrams per kilogram of body weight, etc.). More recently, the development of magnetic resonance imaging (MRI) and positron emission tomography (PET) scans has led to computationally complex abilities for image processing. Continuous monitoring of physiologic variables has brought the need for rapid computations of simple relationships to the bedside. The understanding of the human genome will make all aspects of future health care computationally more complex. When computationally complex relationships that are too complex for human effort are combined with developing mental models, entirely new models of health and disease therapy will be developed. It remains to be seen how the health professions and health care informatics will incorporate the issues related to computational health care into their education and their practice. In some cases new computational health care professions may arise, and some of the traditional health disciplines may disappear.

Health Care Delivery

In addition to the changes in science and the changes in the health care professions, there will be changes in health care delivery. Research in the human genome will result in therapies and pharmaceuticals that will be custom developed for the individual client's genome. Drugs will be custom designed to maximize the drug's effect and minimize side effects with greater sensitivity and specificity. Since diseases can have different proximal causes, it will be possible to construct the exact treatment that is appropriate for each person. Pharmacists, physicians, and nurses will have the ability to customize any set of interventions to have the greatest impact on the client being treated.

The number of possible therapies will expand exponentially. The process of making decisions will become the focus of massive computational effort. Computation will become a core component of health care informatics, not only in structuring and controlling the domain of knowledge but also in the application of the domain of knowledge to practice or wisdom. A clear expectation is that there will be a rapid rise in the number of **computational health care informaticians** in all aspects of health care. Computational health care informaticians will specialize in transforming the data, information, knowledge, and wisdom used in one area by a health care professional into useful knowledge for another health care professional in a different circumstance.

Other new roles or job descriptions suggested by the changing definitions of health care informatics are starting to become clear. In addition to the computational health care informatician, new roles could include those of the *health care information modeler,* who would create computer models of the mental models used by clinicians; the *health care information translator,* who would specialize in converting knowledge used in one situation to knowledge available for other situations; and the *consumer health care informatician,* who would specialize in translating the mental models of the professional to those of the consumer end user. In the Web-based world, consumer health care informaticians are beginning to emerge. However, there is little to no research studying the mental models of the consumer and modeling consumer-based information in a way that truly represents the needs of the consumer.

Each of these roles may generate any number of potential job descriptions. The need for health care informaticians with a strong computationally based understanding of how knowledge is communicated among different groups will form the basis for many of these future jobs. From an educational perspective, it is not fully understood how these jobs or roles will be developed. Therefore it is hard to develop educational programs that prepare students for these anticipated jobs. Educational institutions must maintain a great deal of flexibility for health care informatics degree programs to be able to adapt to future changes in the definition of health care informatics, as well as adapt to changes in technology.

Outcomes Research

In addition to the changes taking place within health care informatics, many changes external to the field are influencing the development of health care informatics. Today, there is a focus on health outcomes. Outcomes research proposes to find the most cost-effective solution to health care problems while maintaining a high level of quality.

The move to outcomes-based research takes many forms. There is discussion about how to research discipline-specific outcomes, such as medical or nursing outcomes. Although discipline-specific approaches are interesting, this approach neglects the fact that health care is becoming increasingly complex. It is delivered by multidisciplinary teams and involves the patient as a team member. The multidisciplinary team–based approach makes it difficult to focus on the outcomes of a single discipline. Research by Horn, Sharkey, and Phillips-Harris (1998), Slater (1999), and others provides insight into the systemic nature of health care delivery. Recent discussion concerning medical and health care errors (Kohn, Corrigan, & Donaldson, 2000) also demonstrates the systemic nature of health care problems. To deal effectively with these problems, the policies and processes involved in delivering care across the total system must be addressed, by looking not at individuals but at the system as a whole. These insights suggest that a focus on discipline-based outcomes will not result in the greatest research benefit.

Outcomes and medical error research provide another area for health care informatics investigation. With the development of data warehouses as part of large-scale clinical information systems, large repositories of clinical health care data are growing at a rapid rate. Hence there is a need for health care informatics specialists who understand and can use large-scale clinical data sets. The growth of large-scale clinical data sets within the health care system is also causing informatics specialists to understand health care practices and the statistical design techniques that are used in large-scale clinical data analysis. These changes have resulted in a need for informatics specialists who have the ability to mine data and create successful studies from large-scale clinical data sets.

Financing Health Care

Another external change is the alteration in health care financing. Recent trends are starting to show that the current model of managed care is entering a failure mode. For example, in Houston, Texas, the fourth-largest city in the United States in the 1999 census, all companies except one have already announced that they will be exiting the market for health maintenance organization (HMO)–based senior care. This approach to the financing of health care may no longer be financially viable (PacifiCare to renew, 2000).

Managed care plans have slowed the rate of health care cost growth during the past few years, but health care costs are now returning to the rate of growth that occurred before managed care became a dominant force in the health care market. In many cases, cost increases for managed health care plans are reaching double-digit annual growth. Many employers indicate that they cannot afford health care plans with this rate of growth. Health care informatics has yet to demonstrate that health care information systems can contain the rise in health care costs.

It is likely that other models for health care financing will soon develop. It is not yet clear what these models will be. The lack of choice has been a major complaint against the existing managed care model. Therefore it is likely that the next scheme for financing health care will allow more choice both by clients and by providers. Increased choice may indeed result in increased cost, and funding schemes may not be totally paid for by employers.

It is clear from the changes in health care financing and the ability to gather large-scale clinical data that there will be major changes in the relationship between the health care system and the people who use it. It may be that with increased data it will be possible to:

- Document the cost-effectiveness of preventive health care measures
- Move to risk-based insurance assessments
- Move to a tiered-based health insurance
- Become more parsimonious in the use of health care services

Any or all of these changes will create new health care delivery models. New health care delivery models will result in major changes in future health care informatics education programs.

Health care informatics will also be affected by many internal and external changes in the health care environment. Reciprocally, health care informatics will act to change that environment. The ability to manipulate large amounts of data, the ability to segment and relate the data to cohorts of people who share similar health care problems, and the link to human genomic data will change the services that health care providers can deliver. Whether these services will be available and affordable will change the way society will view health care. The future will see greater interaction between the work done by health care informaticians and the scope of health care delivery. This scenario forms the background for understanding how health care informatics education should be structured in the future.

Educational Trends

Kovel-Jarboe (1996) addressed four future possibilities for higher education:

1. Higher education would continue to be campus- and classroom-based education.
2. Delivery of higher education would begin to move away from fixed sites and times.
3. Higher-education institutions would be differentiated by their use of distance and instructional techniques.
4. Higher-education consortia will compete with educational entrepreneurs.

For each of these scenarios Kovel-Jarboe examined the drivers, the impact on faculty and students, and institutional roles and requirements. Each perspective generated a different model of what would happen in the future. In establishing these four scenarios, Kovel-Jarboe saw them as a result of a series of changing opportunities and constraints to higher education (Box 22-1).

In addition to these trends, higher education is beginning to see changes in students' entry level knowledge and skills. Students are entering higher education with a level of technological sophistication that rivals or exceeds that of the faculty. Many students have grown up in learning environments. These students may not have the experience of working alone, which has been the traditional core of higher education. The educational experiences of these students will likely differ markedly from that of their instructors.

Cardenas et al. (1997) have listed the following as improvements to students' learning, which will occur as technology innovates the educational system. These are not guaranteed but rather probable results.

- Learning ecosystem, as the walls and classroom are pushed out
- Custom-designed learning
- Student-centered learning
- Redefined, enhanced roles
- Engagement
- Interlinking of the content and the learner
- Empowering skills
- Full inclusion

From elementary school through higher education, the old walls separating the educational/learning environment and the outside world are disappearing. More higher-education students are working at the same time that they are involved in education. In many cases they bring what they have learned from education to the work environment, and they bring the problems and issues of the work environment into the educational setting. As technology allows them access to both environments at the same time, the old boundaries will disintegrate. This is not to say that education should be driven solely by the skill needs of the workplace. Rather, the opportunity for education to leverage the perceived needs of the work environment is created and allows the work environment to use the new skills that the worker/student brings back to it. The integration of work and educational environments creates a possible synergy that institutions of higher education have not traditionally used. At

Box 22–1 Changing Opportunities and Constraints to Higher Education

1. Globalization
2. The changing demographics of longer lives
3. The restructuring of working environments
4. Technological change with the increasing invasion of technology
5. Demand for accountability, including control costs, elimination of duplication, and focus on educational outcomes
6. Consumerism in higher education
7. Raised expectations of employers and businesses
8. The rate of knowledge growth
9. Changing models of teaching and learning
10. Changing campus demographics
11. Concern for community
12. New patterns of decision making in the entire business of education

From Kovel-Jarboe, P. (1996). The changing contexts of higher education and four possible futures for distance education. *Horizon Site.* Retrieved from the World Wide Web: http://horizon.unc.edu/projects/issues/papers/kovel.asp.

the same time, the rise of "universities" solely for the purpose of meeting the skill needs of a single institution or organization is occurring. These range from the McDonald's University, Click2learn, and SmartPlanet to institutes established by high-technology companies.

In the aggregate, these organizations are forming an alternative university structure that is outside the influence of traditional educational organizations. The alternative university structure points to the fact that there is a need for "just-in-time education"—a type of learning in which learners can access what they need to know exactly when they need to know it—that is not being met by traditional universities. If traditional universities do not meet this need, the alternative university structure will continue to grow and thrive.

Educational Technology

Many of the changes in education are made possible by changes in the underlying technology that supports education. First, computers with very fast processors, running at speeds greater than 1 GHz, are proliferating. Computers themselves are being incorporated into a multitude of devices. Second, the increased use of special-purpose devices and the ability of those devices to communicate with each other are increasing the ubiquity of computing resources. In the future the learner will not "sit down to the machine"; rather, ubiquitous Web-interfaced machines will give the student access to learning resources at any time and in any place. The third major technological change is the increasing ubiquity of high-speed network access. It is common for wired areas to offer network access speeds in excess of 100 Mbps. Wireless networks in a confined space (such as within 300 feet of a transceiver) are now seeing constant throughput speeds of 11 Mbps. Sprint has announced a rollout of broad-spectrum (public space use, outdoors, between buildings) wireless networks with speeds of 11 Mbps in several cities. People accustomed to wireless networks in their workplace will now be able to use wireless networks that work between workplaces. Home customers using digital subscriber line (DSL) and cable modem systems are used to throughputs as fast at home as they are in the workplace. The addition of high-speed broadband wireless networks will ensure that people will have access to equal throughputs on the way to home or work, as well as at home and work.

As the use of high-speed machines, ubiquitous access, and high-speed networks merge, people will have access to modes of computing that could only be dreamed of in the past. Standardized high-speed access will allow real-time video to be transmitted to any setting. Learners will be able to enter collaborative learning environments at the time of their choosing. In the same way that eMail and synchronous chat have made message communication virtually instantaneous, high-speed ubiquitous devices will allow teaching and learning to be virtually instantaneous.

It is not yet clear how social systems will adjust to these new modes of education. One of the current advantages of enrolling in an educational program is that the learner is able to step out of the work environment in order to enter the learning environment. By being removed from the workplace for the purpose of education, it is possible for the learner to focus more completely on the learning tasks at hand. Whether the learner will have the same opportunity to shift focus while in the workplace remains to be seen. As the learning environment integrates into the work environment, it is not clear if the learner will be able to adapt to the learning role and at the same time maintain the roles and functions that are necessary for the workplace.

The New Student

The combination of these technologies will allow for an immediacy of learning that would not be possible otherwise. Over the past few years there have been many people who have discussed the notion of **just-in-time learning** (Novicki, 1996). There are two challenges to the notion of just-in-time learning. The first challenge is that just-in-time learning is associated with technical education and not with academic education. The focus on technical skills that can be learned quickly and easily is very different from the academic model concerned with learning a domain of knowledge. The second challenge is that just-in-time learning also focuses on learning small bits of knowledge, rather than a domain of knowledge.

The issues of "bits" and "domains" raise several questions. Is it possible for individuals to independently integrate all of the bits of knowledge into an organized whole? Can education by "continual education" be integrated into the mastery of a knowledge domain? If so, can this integration be done by the learner with or without the assistance of an educator? How will this learning compare with that addressed by traditional block-time concentrations of study with the assistance of an instructor?

The future of just-in-time learning is one that must be studied. Because health care informatics is so technologically driven, the impact of technology on the learning of future health care informatics specialists is likely to accelerate faster than the impact on other areas of health care education. Thus studies of learning behaviors of health care informaticians will have implications for the education of other health care professionals.

Some departments of health care informatics have created special sections or departments to deal with the impact of technology on education. The University of Texas Health Science Center at Houston has proposed such a focus.

The introduction of this technology into the teaching and learning environment will put new demands on both the educator and the learner. Kashmanian (2000) has summarized the ten major characteristics of what are referred to as **net generation,** or **N-Gen students,** as follows:

1. Fierce independence
2. Emotional and intellectual openness
3. Inclusion
4. Free expression and strong views
5. Innovation
6. Preoccupation with maturity
7. Investigation
8. Immediacy
9. Sensitivity to corporate interest
10. Authentication and trust

These characteristics will help to create a more cooperative learning environment. The use of the Web stimulates a more interactive learning environment. This creates a substantial change from the current learning environment, which is based on a television or broadcast mode, where information is broadcast at the front of the room and students are expected to listen. Students will increasingly work in cooperative groups with faculty members acting as guides and facilitators. Classroom study will be project based and have greater application to the work arena. Tapscott (1999) has noted that educational systems will have to radically alter their structure, their use of technology, the way they relate to students, the way they allow students to relate to each other, and the way they value learning. These changes will occur over a period of time as the next generation of students enters the educational process. However, now is the time to begin planning for these changes.

Future education will move away from the notion of content to focus on **process-based education.** It is expected that process-based education will occur more rapidly for health care informatics programs. Health care informatics students need to focus on gathering the latest content and organizing it for their immediate purpose. Technology has a half-life of 12 to 18 months. If these programs focus on teaching the technology, students will have out-of-date information before they graduate. Rather, the educational process for these students must focus on the acquisition of current content, the organization of that content for a specific purpose, and then learning how to apply the content in a team-based context. This approach is not to imply that domain content is unimportant; rather, it recognizes that domain content will be changing quickly and continuously. The critical educational challenge is to teach students to organize new knowledge, integrate it into existing knowledge structures, and then apply that knowledge in solving informatics-related problems. Measures of educational performance will focus on the students' ability to perform by applying their knowledge to problems in structured situations. As students progress through the program, they should increasingly learn how to create knowledge structures around the problems they have solved and apply those knowledge structures to new problems in team- or group-based situations.

The focus will increasingly be on learning how to learn. Learning how to learn implies that the focus is on the use of frameworks to structure learning, including mechanisms to access current data, information, knowledge, and wisdom. This may not be a smooth process. Models of chaordic knowledge acquisition are beginning to appear. The example of hyperlinked knowledge defies the traditional structure of science's hierarchical knowledge yet provides a rich educational environment.

This transition in education will be difficult for faculty and students who were educated when knowledge as content was the core metric for evaluating the quality of the education. As in problem-based education, content does not become unimportant, but the content is so transitional that education must also measure the degree of "forgetting" of old knowledge. It is an unusual concept for education to measure "forgetting" (Bateson, 1979). However, "forgetting" has become an important concept in health care informatics, where information systems are capable of maintaining and presenting outdated data, information, knowledge, and wisdom. The process of gathering or capturing new information, integrating the new information into existing or novel frameworks, and then "forgetting" that information in an appropriate manner forms the overlying structure of process education.

The student will critically monitor the data, information, knowledge, and wisdom flowing through the student's cognitive system. Students and faculty will begin an interesting voyage as they implement this style of education, learn how to value it, and then learn how to evaluate it. The combination of process knowledge and just-in-time education will create a new framework that will become the background for understanding the education of health care informatics specialists.

Professionals in the health disciplines have long recognized that they were in "practice disciplines." They have understood the tension between understanding a domain of knowledge as an academic exercise and then applying that domain of knowledge in the practical arena. Historically, education of health care professionals followed an apprenticeship model. Students learned what they needed to know as they followed an expert practitioner. There was no distinction between the academic knowledge and the applied knowledge. During the twentieth century the health professions entered into programs of education in institutions of higher education. These programs have had a tendency to separate the academic knowledge from the clinical practice. For many of the health disciplines, students spend a number of years understanding the basic sciences (e.g., anatomy, physiology chemistry, and communication science). After they understand the sciences in the abstract sense, the students are then initiated into clinical situations to learn how to apply or practice the sciences. The separation of science into the "science of the abstract" and "science of the concrete" has been investigated and discussed in other works (Levi-Strauss, 1966; Turley, 1996a).

Benner (1984) traced the evolution of clinical expertise from the beginning practitioner to the expert. In doing so, Benner showed how the novice practitioner collects too much information and is unable to organize it efficiently. By contrast, the expert practitioner selects a rather small amount of knowledge. However, the expert collects the critical knowledge for understanding the phenomena presented. Another difference is that the novice practitioner uses a step-by-step process of organizing the information into clinical knowledge, whereas the expert uses a process of heuristic reasoning that appears to jump directly to the conclusion. This process of cognitively integrating information in decision-making processes is well understood but difficult to teach.

The advance of a technologically rich teaching environment will allow students to practice this type of embedded decision making without "real world" consequences, such as hurting patients. Virtual reality and augmented reality technologies will allow students to "play" in virtual clinical settings. This approach possesses several advantages: not only are patients protected, but also the students will be able to review their own interactions with virtual patients and those of the other members of their team. Marshall University School of Medicine uses this approach with its project called The Interactive Patient (Marshall University, 1995).

Marino (1998) has discussed his vision for a **safe classroom** where students could attempt to practice without fear of evaluation retribution. After the students achieved mastery, they would demonstrate their mastery to the instructor. This notion of the safe classroom focuses both on the notion of safety for the patient and on a safe environment for the student.

The concept of a safe classroom requires a high degree of student interaction with course material. As students become more interactive with knowledge, they seek more and varied sources for their course material. They are not limited to the material "inside the course" but have access to reference material from the Web, materials compiled by other students, and online library materials. The most important component is that the student has access to collaborative peers and instructors using a high-speed digital technology. In the future the environment will be increasingly rich, not only in terms of multimedia materials but also in terms of student-to-student, student-to-instructor, and student-to-other communication resources. To the degree that these are achieved seamlessly, the student will not only have a better model for work experience but will also have experience in the educational arena with the technologies used in the work arena.

The most difficult aspect in the use of this technology for education is in understanding how to integrate educational technology with students who have not had prior experience with technology and may not be comfortable with its use. Will higher education implement the same education using multiple forms of delivery, or will higher education "force" faculty and students to use the technology? Institutions may choose multiple ways of addressing these questions, and solutions are likely to occur over time as more technologically literate students enter into the health professions. However, it is also likely that some institutions are ready to make a revolutionary change in the way they teach. Although this may alienate some students, these institutions can become magnet institutions for students interested in new ways of learning. Educational institutions may become stratified on the basis of their degree of educational technology utilization. This is not so much a value statement as it is recognition that there will be multiple types of learners and that not all institutions can compete for all learner types.

As students gather by learning types, the question is further raised as to whether the health professions can continue educating in isolation from each other. The clinical practice arena is moving toward a delivery system that is multidisciplinary and team based. Students usually learn in discipline isolation. How, then, does the transition occur to team-based practice if it is not part of the educational process? During the past 20 years, this question has been discussed but not so eloquently presented as in the recent Institute of Medicine report (2001). However, issues of professional licensing, fiscal constraints on universities, and professional issues of control have kept interdisciplinary education from happening. There are, of course, examples of pilot implementations of interdisciplinary education, but these have hardly evolved into an educational standard. As the new paradigms of knowledge become more prevalent and process-based education moves to the fore, the question of multidisciplinary education will again be addressed. It may become more tolerable in a technology-rich educational environment.

The issues of education are not necessarily the same for new students in the profession as they are for those who have already entered a profession. For people who have already entered a profession, there are issues of retraining and issues of continuing education. Continuing education tends to focus on small bits of education that can be obtained in 1 or 2 days. Continuing education can present an overview of the issues of health care informatics and/or the technologies involved. There is not sufficient time in a continuing education model for students to become conversant and proficient with the components of health care informatics. There are funding sources and opportunities for people in professions to take time out and refocus their careers. Such opportunities, for example, are funded by the National Institutes of Health (e.g., National Research Service Award [NRSA] Training Grants and Fellowship) and other sources (e.g., private foundations).

Although many will become users of what is developed by informaticians, those who are researching and developing the new technologies will need to obtain additional training or retraining to become active health care informaticians. Given the educational needs of professionals, educational programs will have to adapt to the needs of the students while at the same time guaranteeing the educational integrity of the program. This is another consideration to be addressed in conjunction with just-in-time education and technology-mediated education.

The knowledge explosion is particularly acute for health care informaticians. The increase in health care knowledge is extraordinary. Likewise is the increase in the rate of advances in computer technology. Combined with these is the increase in knowledge technology. These are combining to form a discipline with knowledge explosions in multiple directions. The problems of knowledge explosion will not only create a problem for the students but may also create a more complex problem for those who are designing and developing health care informatics curricula. Different programs will balance these components differently, but all programs will need to include each of the components to some degree.

FUTURE EDUCATIONAL PROGRAMS AND HEALTH CARE INFORMATICS

Given the background discussion presented, it is clear that education in health care informatics cannot follow the educational models that have been used in other health professions. Students need to learn the limits of technology used in health care informatics by being immersed in technology as part of the educational process. They need to learn in a technology-rich environment where issues relevant to health care informatics flow from the work arena to the educational arena and vice versa. As noted earlier, the domain content is changing so rapidly that the faculty may not be the most knowledgeable people in the classroom. In this environment it is clear that the educational paradigm will move from teaching to learning. The focus will not be on how to "teach" an area of content but on how to "learn" specific content. Students and faculty will work together in a shared exploration learning how to integrate new domain content and to organize theories and models in order to create real solutions to "real world" problems.

The distinctions between faculty and students will be based on the ability to guide and to integrate. The focus will be on developing cost-effective quality solutions for problems from the clinical arena. Faculty members will be required to create a chaordic model in the classroom where there is sufficient chaos to help the students converge a new sense of order. The sense of order will arise from the proposed solutions to the presented problems. In this model of education, not every solution is a good solution. Hence students will need to be able to not only solve the problem but also evaluate the solution as to its appropriateness and cost-effectiveness. Students will learn to critique each other and evaluate the proposed solutions.

To create this environment, there must be a cooperative venture of students and faculty working toward a common goal: learning how to learn health care informatics. Students and faculty will jointly reflect on each other's work. The learning environment will be a cooperative work environment. So how will these cooperative work environments be constructed? The model comes more from the participants in high-technology think tanks than it does from the purveyors of education.

The goal is to create an environment where adults are free to "play." The model comes from the research and development laboratories created by inventive corporations. The model is that of Xerox's PARC, Hewlett Packard's HP Labs, AT&T's Bell-Labs, and in the educational arena, the Massachusetts Institute of Technology's (MIT's) MediaLab. These learning environments bring together people of great talent with a charge to create new things. The high productivity in these environments is not a guarantee, nor have the companies always understood how to market the products developed. Xerox's PARC developed many of the technologies of the personal computer (PC) age, but the technologies were marketed by other companies such as Adobe, Apple, and 3Com.

This chapter has addressed a number of complex issues relating to changes in education, educational technology, and the definition of health care informatics. Not all of these issues have been resolved. Some of them will not be resolved in the near future. However, despite the instability of the underlying sciences and the issues that health care informatics address, there is a need to focus on issues related to curriculum design for health care informatics. This section of the chapter reflects on these issues and presents a possible model for a health care informatics curriculum. Given the current state of the science, it is unlikely that a single model will suffice for all health care informatics programs. It is clear that some educators will make a decision to put more weight on some components while minimizing others. Others will add unique components to their curriculum model.

Health Care Informatics Curriculum

Although this chapter is not the final word on the health care informatics curriculum, this section outlines key issues to consider in the development of a health care informatics curriculum. A framework that can be used to construct a number of versions of health care informatics curricula is presented. This framework can be used to stimulate productive faculty discussions in the process of developing a health care informatics curriculum. Table 22-1 summarizes the key concepts in the curriculum model. The table has four columns. These columns reflect the main concepts discussed earlier: (1) categories of information, (2) discipline-related issues, (3) the movement toward team-based learning and care delivery, and (4) computational issues. The horizontal rows are grouped into categories that include (1) developing process knowledge, (2) communication of knowledge, (3) decision making, and (4) technology. These categories are discussed in other works (Turley, 2000a, 2000b).

Table 22–1 Component Outline for a Health Care Informatics Curriculum

Category	Discipline Issues	Team Issues	Computational Knowledge
Developing process knowledge			
Workflow	Organizing knowledge for practice	Communicating practice	Just-in-time knowledge
Informed practice	Structures for just-in-time knowledge	Link outcomes to practice and knowledge	Model knowledge for when it is needed as it is needed
Reflective practitioner	Understand how knowledge is used	Contrast client outcomes with the professional's outcomes	Client information model in terms of local cohort and practitioner knowledge model
Team-based knowledge	Define the culture, as well as the domain	Understand cross-cultural knowledge transfer	Automatic "translation" of knowledge into other taxonomies
Communication of knowledge			
Taxonomy and nomenclature	Develop appropriate taxonomies	Link to other taxonomies	Meta-knowledge
Development of minimum data sets	Nursing Minimum Management Data Set (NMMDS)	Coordinate with other data sets (e.g., Uniform Bill 92 [UB-92] Hospital Discharge Data Set, etc.)	Aggregate data into information and knowledge
Knowledge induction	Mental models ARCS Data mining	Compare discipline's information models Coordinate use of data into data warehouses Use aggregate clinical knowledge to create care paths	Data mining Knowledge induction
Consumer knowledge	Translate discipline knowledge to consumer model	Organize team-based knowledge into health plan for consumer	Automated translation of knowledge across models
Creation of meta-knowledge	Hierarchical understanding of discipline knowledge	Meta-concept mapping (e.g., Unified Medical Language System [UMLS] and Systematized Nomenclature of Human and Veterinary Medicine [SNOMED], extensible markup language [XML] technology support)	Computational models of data aggregation and knowledge manipulation

Continued

Table 22–1 Component Outline for a Health Care Informatics Curriculum—cont'd

Category	Discipline Issues	Team Issues	Computational Knowledge
Decision making			
Decision models	Information processing LENS Model Judgment	Apply decision model to unique and cooperative decisions	Develop computational models
Decision support systems	Technology of decision support Examples of decision support	Integrate decision support systems to address all client needs Coordinate decisions for comprehensive care	Monitor decision support systems' effect on cohort care
Federal guidelines	Health Insurance Portability and Accountability Act (HIPAA) Centers for Medicare & Medicaid Services (CMS) (formerly the Health Care Financing Administration [HCFA]) Agency for Healthcare Research and Quality (AHRQ)	Medical/health errors	Error-reporting systems Error solution institutes
Technology			
Database	Relational Network Hierarchical Object oriented	Decide on appropriate technology to achieve project goal Ease of migration to advanced technology	Integration of database and data models Automated translation of data across models
Communication	Technical standards including H 323 Internet video, H 320 interactive TV, T 120 white board, Wireless standards 802.11b, Bluetooth	Determine the impact of communications technology on clinical practice Monitor rapid advances in wireless technology	Automated knowledge models of knowledge display and adaptive knowledge systems
Standards organizations	Health Level Seven (HL-7) Digital Imaging Communication in Medicine (DICOM) Comité Européen de Normalisation-Technical Committee-251 (CEN-TC-251) American Society for Testing and Materials (ASTM)	Be certain that choices address industry standards Monitor evolution of standards	Creation of knowledge model standards for health care

Table 22–1 Component Outline for a Health Care Informatics Curriculum—cont'd

Category	Discipline Issues	Team Issues	Computational Knowledge
Technology—cont'd			
Ubiquitous computing	Personal devices Interface design Imbedded systems Augmented reality	Compare discipline display needs Monitor industry and technology trends Create computationally efficient data	Integration of data flow into work life Data interpreted dynamically in terms of context

The intersections of the rows and columns create cells that serve to focus the content for a health care informatics curriculum. The elements in the table cells are examples only and are not meant to be a comprehensive listing of the domain. Many of these issues are not new and have been discussed by others examining the critical elements for health care informatics. However, the column that focuses on the computational issues in health care informatics generates a new element for curriculum consideration. Although computational knowledge has been implicit in many health care informatics curriculum discussions, it has seldom come forward with this much focus.

Discussions that have attempted to relate traditional views of health care informatics with those of bioinformatics have created a new appreciation for the impact of computational knowledge. Health care informatics must learn to incorporate the insights of computational knowledge in order to help clinicians manage the expansion of knowledge and task complexity that are modifying the health care workplace. Learning to manipulate the additional knowledge will be a survival skill for future clinicians.

Issues related to computational knowledge will likely be the framework for the development of the next generation of health care informaticians and informatics-related areas. The development and modeling of computational knowledge can be applied to multiple health areas from clinical issues, to bioinformatics, to health education. Computational knowledge will generate new priorities and developments for health care informatics. It will require increased standardization at lower levels of knowledge and processes in order to allow for the higher-level computational, efficient processes to occur. Data mining may show how to create health care knowledge from clinical data warehouses, but it may also require a more formal structure for the development of any future data warehouse.

Developing Process Knowledge

The shift in focus from content knowledge to process knowledge will be one of the most difficult transitions for faculties organizing informatics curricula. There are a number of broad issues that come under the area of process knowledge. The detailed example given here is not exhaustive but exemplary. This example demonstrates four of these issues. First, in examining the issue of workflow and health care, the common approach is to use an external functional approach. More important is to look at the flow of data or information in the process of workflow. All health care practitioners are processing and managing large amounts of data at every point in the clinical process. This includes not only the data that represent individual patients but also the information, knowledge, and wisdom that represent norms, references, and background criteria. The mapping of this information is a knowledge map view of the workflow. This mapping creates a very different view of the workflow.

Second, the issue of communicating knowledge and wisdom becomes increasingly complex with the move from the individual person to the discipline to across disciplines. Different disciplines use different knowledge models and knowledge structures. To communicate effectively, each health care provider must have a basic understanding of how other providers will use and map knowledge. It would be very easy to overwhelm any individual provider or group of providers by supplying all of the knowledge that any one provider is using in any given clinical situation. The total number of data points must be reduced, whereas the amount of information must be increased. Third, the data and information must be communicated in ways appropriate for use by other health care providers. This is a process that humans already do and is often demonstrated in the teaching-learning event. The question is whether this process can be automated, thereby using the resources of information systems to decrease the workload of practitioners.

Fourth, this approach will create new mechanisms from which to understand the reflective practitioner (Schon, 1990). The reflective practitioner will examine the knowledge and data models of his or her practice, review the communication of that knowledge to other practitioners, and understand its relationship to outcomes. If this process is successful, there will be greater understanding of the knowledge used by the team of health care providers. This knowledge will require more formal definition, complex understanding, and finally, understanding of how these knowledge models can become automated.

Communication of Knowledge

Data, information, knowledge, and wisdom always exist in a context. It is illogical to attempt to understand data, information, knowledge, and wisdom separate from their context. The result is a misunderstanding of the data, information, knowledge, and wisdom. This creates problems for much of the current research into taxonomy and nomenclature. Discussions concerning taxonomy and nomenclature often approach the topic as if the data were independent of the context. There is some beginning work that attempts to place data, information, and knowledge into context, such as the work done for the Arden Syntax (Hripcsak et al., 1994). Of course, it is important to clearly understand the declarative knowledge while at the same time understanding the contextual nature of the declarative knowledge.

As taxonomy systems are developed, the relationships among them, as well as the common hierarchies that occur within knowledge, will become evident. The commonalties in taxonomy systems will point to areas where meta-knowledge may be available. Not all knowledge will sit in a strict hierarchical format. Some clinical knowledge, particularly knowledge and context, may have a more heuristic model than a hierarchical one. The heuristic model is more obvious, since knowledge overlaps with the concept of wisdom. Knowledge modeling is an increasingly important part of informatics, particularly as the profession seeks ways to automate the structuring of knowledge relationships that occur in clinical health care data.

Understanding of knowledge, and particularly knowledge in context, provides insights on how to develop minimum data sets. Werley and Lang

(1988) have long called for the development of minimum data sets in nursing. Several minimum data sets already exist in health care. Clark (1998) summarized much of this work in nursing. The work in any single discipline needs to be coordinated with the work done in relation to other minimum data sets and aggregated into more complex information-knowledge-wisdom structures.

Another approach to these same issues is the use of knowledge induction approaches. These concepts have come from computer science in the area of artificial intelligence. Graves (1999) has described the development of knowledge bases using ARCS software. ARCS is a research-knowledge system (ARKS) for storing, managing, and modeling knowledge from the scientific literature. Graves' method for creating knowledge bases also allows knowledge bases to be interrelated. Other approaches for automated data mining can be used. These approaches can be statistical or associative. Very little work has been published in the area of data mining in health care. Abbott et al. (1998) have taken the lead in developing and designing techniques for nursing. For additional information on data mining, see Chapter 5, which is written by Dr. Abbott.

One of the areas consistently missing from the development of knowledge and knowledge structures for health care professionals has been the understanding of how professionals' knowledge is mapped to the models used by consumers. In her work with CareLink, HeartCare, and other projects, Brennan (1998) has demonstrated how consumers can be brought into the clinical practice arena using technology. More research needs to be done to understand the knowledge models that consumers bring. It may be possible to create automated devices that can translate professional knowledge into the knowledge models of consumers. As consumers become more equal partners in the design and delivery of health care, the need to model consumer knowledge will become more acute.

Decision Making

As discussed earlier, the function of knowledge in health care is that of "knowledge in use," or wisdom, the appropriate use of knowledge. For the average clinician, the issue of "knowledge in use" will focus on decision making. Decision making is a continuous, iterative process. At certain critical junctions, it is possible to identify specific decisions that affect the future of the clinical process. In many cases there is a complex, ongoing set of small decisions that clinicians make independently of other care providers. These small or minor decisions are often part of what is referred to as **garden path reasoning,** in which each individual, small decision appears correct but does not take into account the larger picture or context in which the decisions need to be made and understood (Johnson, Moen, & Thompson, 1988). Garden path reasoning is a common decision error process. Studying different decision-making models will not guarantee that a decision maker will not be led down the "garden path." This is especially true when the decision area is very comfortable for decision makers and decision makers are not as critical as they should be either in evaluating new data or in placing the decision making in the larger context.

Although understanding decision models cannot protect the decision maker from garden path reasoning errors, understanding these models can alert decision makers to consider the range and complexity of options that are available when making even routine decisions. Decision models can be based on assumptions that can be clearly delineated and tested. Understanding the models creates another approach for the reflective practitioner to use in understanding the scope of health care data and its impact on the decisions that affect patients.

As health care data become more copious and complex, it is unlikely that decision makers will be allotted additional time to understand the complexities of the decisions that are being made. As discussed earlier, changes in the health care system are also putting constraints on the ability of clinicians to make decisions and the amount of time that is available for the decision making. Health care is clearly a data- and knowledge-intensive business. As the complexity of the knowledge increases and the amount of available time decreases, there will be increased need for decision support that is integrated into health care information systems. Decision support systems can occur in a variety of forms. Most students are aware of the formal medical decision support systems such as Iliad or Quick Medical Reference (QMR) (Friedman et al., 1999). These systems have been used both in a teaching frame and in a clinical frame to assist the clinician with medical diagnoses. Weed's problem knowledge coupling (PKC) approach (1991) represents a radically different approach to gathering and displaying knowledge in a decision support environment. The PKC approach is highly documented in terms of the current research but requires that the client answer a wide variety of questions that do not appear to have any immediate rationale. However, the system captures a variety of health-related information, which allows the PKC approach to avoid garden path reasoning errors.

Hirsch, Chang, and Gilbert (1989) have researched the feasibility of decision support systems in nursing diagnoses. Chang has examined the use of decision support in teaching and in the diagnosis of patients with acquired immunodeficiency syndrome (AIDS). The use of decision support has not been widely adopted in health care, but the development of new techniques and the increased burden placed on all health care staff may make the need for such systems more acute in the future. This will be particularly true if the decision support system generated for a single discipline can demonstrate its impact on other decision-making systems and other components of the health care team.

The Agency for Healthcare Research and Quality (AHRQ) has a long history of developing guidelines for evidence-based practice. Many of these guidelines have been incorporated into decision support systems. The AHRQ has used a consensus panel approach that, although slow and time consuming, creates results. With data from the Centers for Medicare & Medicaid Services (CMS) (formerly known as the Health Care Financing Administration [HCFA]) and the new rules required under the Health Insurance Portability and Accountability Act (HIPAA), the data available to researchers may well increase. This may allow a more automated approach to the understanding of guidelines and a resultant decrease in human errors in health care. The National Patient Safety Foundation of the American Medical Association (AMA) is attempting to be a clearinghouse for new knowledge and data that can improve patient safety (AMA, 2000). The approach that this group is taking involves a systems view of knowledge and decisions that affect the health of a patient, recognizing that the last act taken resulting in an error may be the least important in solving the complex set of minor mistakes that led to the identified error. This more ecological approach models the context-based knowledge approach discussed earlier. Information systems will need to have a similar model in order to assist with the process.

Technology

In health care informatics, students do not study technology for its own sake. Rather, technology is seen as an enabling tool that allows the informaticist to create a product or solution. It is easy to forget that paper is a technology because it is so ubiquitous. Paper is used for many different purposes, be it a record of a patient's experience during the past shift, a copy of an electrocardiogram, or a drawing to explain to a patient the site of a surgical incision. Paper is foldable, portable, inexpensive, and available, yet health care providers seldom if ever think of the technology of paper, how it is made, what its tensile strength is, and how it is used by other people in the clinical arena. Until the technology "disappears" as a technology in the same way that paper did, there is a need to understand the characteristics of the technology used in health care. Elliott (1999) has summarized the current trends in technology, at least from one perspective.

As discussed earlier, technology is among the areas with the greatest rate of change. The issue of what elements of technology are most critical depends on the health care informatics focus of the student. However, it is clear that every student should be conversant with each of the major technologies that impact health care informatics. Historically, the focus has been on technologies from computer science and information science. Increasingly, the future will include the areas of computational knowledge and knowledge display. For example, there are fine differences in display between liquid crystal and plasma displays. How these differences influence the decision making of a radiologist reviewing a complex intensive care unit (ICU) display is unclear. The level of color, brightness, and intensity all create subtle shifts in what the eye sees and hence how the data are interpreted in the process of decision making.

Clearly, health care informatics specialists need to be aware of the development of industry standards. Standards have several advantages for interoperability. However, standards are also restrictive in the face of revolutionary technology that does not yet have a standard. People can fail to adopt the new technology when it is appropriate and instead wait for the standards to catch up with the technology. The result creates a dynamic tension for the early adopters of technology.

Standards have both hardware and software components. The adoption of extensible markup language (XML) is a case in point. The basic structure has been developed and adopted by the World Wide Web consortium. XML is now appearing as a standard in products from all of the major database developers and will become increasingly important as a technology that allows materials to be accessed by incompatible systems (e.g., PCs, handheld devices, and Web-enabled telephones). The same data source can deliver data in an appropriate format for each of these products because of the XML standardization. However, by allowing people to create their own tags, XML can create a situation where two customers using the same information system may no longer be able to share information. A detailed discussion of technical standards is presented in Chapter 17.

The true value of a technology is determined by how well it achieves the purposes for which it was developed or implemented. Many interesting technologies will appear that will not initially have an impact on health care informatics. However, like Post-it notes, the innovation can become ubiquitous and used for many new and innovative uses. One of the key roles in health care informatics is finding these new and innovative uses. For health informatics specialists to identify these innovations, they must have a view of the solution and how it would be implemented within the health care arena. Understanding how people think and how they interact with technology is a major area of study. One needs only to review Norman's work (1988) to remember how important the interaction is between the human and the device. Errors are often created by bad interfaces in objects ranging from intravenous (IV) pumps, to medications (shapes and colors), to computer interfaces. These are often issues of improper design of the technology. Chapter 15 provides a discussion of human-computer interactions in health care. Table 22-1 summarizes the discussion elements. As mentioned earlier, the table is not meant to be exhaustive. Rather, it is a way to break out and understand some of the elements that interact with each other in the development of an informatics curriculum. As such, the table should be seen as a starting point for discussion and a mechanism for delineating the complex interactions among the knowledge elements.

Discipline-specific issues will need to be a focus within health care informatics programs for the foreseeable future. At the current time, nursing is the sole profession in the United States that has a certification that recognizes informaticists in health care. The other disciplines may follow nursing's lead, or it may be that there will be a separate certification in health care informatics that is beyond the scope of a single discipline. In 2001 the Health Information and Management Systems Society (HIMSS) began the process of developing certification examinations in health care information management. There is also an initiative to register or certify informatics education programs outside the jurisdiction of the discipline certification. The International Medical Informatics Association Working Group 1: Health and Informatics Education (2001) is currently reviewing this as a possibility.

CONCLUSION

Informatics is in a period of rapid transformation, as is health care itself. The future looks to be even more chaordic than the past. There will be periods of rapid transition and periods of seeming order that will then be followed by another period of rapid transition. This will be seen with the impact of genomics. The technology is creating great stores of new data. It is clear that genomics will have a tremendous impact on the future of health and health care. These changes will impact the delivery of health care, the ethics of health care, and possibly even the definition of health. However, genomics is only one area where health knowledge is growing exponentially. The age of large-scale information systems will allow patients and clinicians to know more about a person's health history, as well as the health history of family members, and place all of that information in the context of similar cohorts of patients.

Currently, how all of the data, information, knowledge, and wisdom will be modeled, stored, or retrieved is not understood. Clearly, there will be questions. For example, who should have access and under what conditions should access be available? Advancements in informatics and information technology will make these questions more acute. Even the questions of taxonomy and the structure of the health care knowledge model will affect the way the model can be used and the purposes for which it can be used. It will be difficult to determine the "best" model as new uses for aggregated health data, information, knowledge, and wisdom continue to be generated in the future, but to some extent that future will be determined by our understanding in the present time. Like Elliott (1999), it is possible to point to some informatics trends. Future informatics trends are shown in Box 22-2.

The future will be a period of continuous change. The exact impact of these trends can only be hinted at; however, the ability to prepare for them must be addressed by today's students and today's practitioners. In many ways the technology changes will be the simplest to address. The more complex areas will focus on the aspects of social change that technology changes will bring about. Health care already accounts

Box 22–2 Future Informatics Trends

- Larger amounts of patient information will be linked.
- Information will be able to be aggregated by several overlapping grouping cohorts: family, geography, workplace, genetics, risk factors, etc.
- Health care will become increasingly targeted to meet the needs of individuals; therapies will be based on one's genetics, lifestyle, preferences, etc.
- The amount of information will be overwhelming and require computational assistance at all levels.
- The professions will either adapt to these changes in health care, or they will be replaced.
- Health care will be increasingly seen as knowledge work.
- Technology will pervade all aspects of health care.

for almost 15% of the goods and services produced in our country. Should more resources be committed? Should the way that health care resources are allocated be changed? Should more resources be put into prevention and less into acute care? How should health care providers be educated? What will be the new responsibilities of the patient or client?

As the knowledge base of health care increases and health care becomes a knowledge-driven industry, future practitioners will be able to address questions that their predecessors could only wonder about. Now is the time to begin to educate health care informatics specialist for the new generation of health care providers.

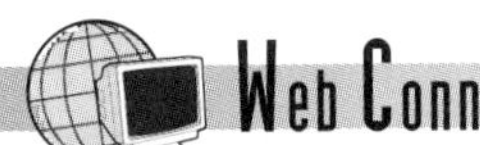

Web Connection

Education is experiencing a period of rapid change. Preparing successful future practitioners requires that educators and learners alike adopt a learning approach that integrates the management and processing of information into their practice area and their personal growth and development. Leveraging the power of Internet technology is one way to provide just-in-time learning and easy, convenient access to information. In the Web Connection activities for this chapter, you will examine types of educational opportunities available on the Internet and analyze how they advance both discipline-specific education and health care informatics education.

discussion questions

1. Is health care informatics a science?
2. What is the appropriate preparation for a student interested in being admitted to a health care informatics program?
3. What concepts or content should be required in all health care informatics curricula?
4. How will technology change health care informatics education?
5. How will health care informatics change the role of health care providers?

REFERENCES

Abbott, P., et al. (1998). Can the U.S. minimum data set be used for predicting admissions to acute care facilities? *Medinfo, 9*(Pt. 2), 1318-1321.

American Medical Association. (2000). *National Patient Safety Foundation.* Chicago: Author. Retrieved from the World Wide Web: http://www.ama-assn.org/med-sci/npsf/about.htm.

Bateson, G. (1979). *Mind and nature: A necessary unity.* New York: Bantam Books.

Benner, P. (1984). *From novice to expert: Excellence in power in clinical nursing practice.* Addison-Wesley.

Brennan, P. (1998). A computer network home care support demonstration: A randomized trial in persons living with AIDS. *Computers in Biology and Medicine, 28*(5), 489-508.

Capra, F. (1988). *The turning point: Science, society and rising culture.* New York: Bantam Doubleday Dell.

Cardenas, V., et al. (1997). New directions: Teachers and technology for the 21st century. *Horizon Site.* Retrieved from The World Wide Web: http://horizon.unc.edu/projects/issues/papers/scheuer.asp.

Clark, J. (1998). The international classification for nursing practice project. *Online Journal of Issues in Nursing,* September 30. Retrieved from the World Wide Web: http://www.nursingworld.org/ojin/tpc7/tpc7_3.htm.

Elliott, J. (1999). Nine hot technology trends. *Healthcare Informatics,* February, pp. 81-110. Retrieved from the World Wide Web: http://www.healthcare-informatics.com/issues/1999/02_99/nine.htm.

Friedman, C., et al. (1999). Enhancement of clinicians' diagnostic reasoning by computer-based consultation. *JAMA, 17*(282), 1851-1856.

Gardner, H. (1987). *The mind's new science: A history of the cognitive revolution.* New York: Basic Books.

Genome: Milestone promises to answer and raise questions. (2000). *Houston Chronicle,* June 27, p. A20.

Graves, J. (1993). Data versus information versus knowledge. *Reflections, 19*(1), 4-5.

Graves, J. (1999). *What is a knowledge base?* Indianapolis: Sigma Theta Tau. Retrieved from the World Wide Web: http://www.stti.iupui.edu/library/kb_what.html.

Graves, J., & Corcoran, S. (1988). Design of nursing information systems: Conceptual and practice elements. *Journal of Professional Nursing, 4*(3), 168-177.

Graves, J., & Corcoran, S. (1989). The study of nursing informatics. *Image: The Journal of Nursing Scholarship, 21*(4), 227-231.

Hirsch, M., Chang, B., & Gilbert, S. (1989). A computer program to support patient assessment and clinical decision-making in nursing education. *Computers in Nursing, 7*(4), 157-160.

Hock, D. (1999). *Birth of the Chaordic Age.* New York: Berrett-Koehler.

Hock, D. (2000). The art of chaordic leadership. *Leader to Leader,* Winter, p. 15. Retrieved from the World Wide Web: http://www.pfdf.org/leaderbooks/L2L/winter2000/hock.html.

Horn, S., Sharkey, P., & Phillips-Harris C. (1998). Formulary limitations and the elderly: Results from the managed care outcomes project. *American Journal of Managed Care, 4*(8), 1105-1113.

Hripcsak, G., et al. (1994). Rationale for the Arden Syntax. *Computers and Biomedical Research, 27,* 291-324

Institute of Medicine. (2001). *Crossing the quality chasm: A new health system for the 21st century.* Washington, DC: National Academy Press.

International Medical Informatics Working Group 1. (2001). *Health and medical informatics education.* Retrieved from the World Wide Web: http://www.rzuser.uni-heidelberg.de/~d16/.

Johnson, P.E., Moen, J.B., & Thompson, W.B. (1988). Garden path errors in diagnostic reasoning. In L. Bolc & M.J. Coombs (Eds.), *Expert system applications.* New York: Springer.

Kashmanian, K. (2000). The impact of computers on schools: Two authors, two perspectives. *Technology Source,* July/August. Retrieved from the World Wide Web: http://horizon.unc.edu/ts/reading/2000-7.asp.

Kohn, L., Corrigan, J., & Donaldson, M. (2000). *To err is human: Building a safer health system.* Washington, DC: National Academy Press.

Kovel-Jarboe, P. (1996). The changing contexts of higher education and four possible futures for distance education. *Horizon Site.* Retrieved from the World Wide Web: http://horizon.unc.edu/projects/issues/papers/kovel.asp.

Levi-Strauss, C. (1966). *The savage mind.* Chicago: University of Chicago Press.

Marino, T. (1998). A vision of safe science classroom. *Technology Source.* Retrieved from the World Wide Web: http://horizon.unc.edu/TS/vision/1998-03.asp.

Marshall University, School of Medicine. (1995). *The interactive patient.* Retrieved from the World Wide Web: http://medicus.marshall.edu/medicus.htm.

Nelson, R., & Joos, I. (1989). On language in nursing: From data to wisdom. *PLN Vision,* Fall, p. 6.

Norman, D. (1988). *The design of everyday things.* New York: Doubleday Currency.

Novicki, C. (1996). Best technology: Just-in-time learning. *Fast Company, 5,* 28.

PacifiCare to renew Medicare pact/Plan's HMO only one left for area seniors. (2000). *Houston Chronicle,* July 6. Business Section, p. 1.

Schon, D. (1990). *Educating the reflective practitioner: Toward a new design for teaching and learning in the professions.* New York: Jossey-Bass.

Schwirian, P., et al. (1989). Computers in nursing practice: A comparison of the attitudes of nurses and nursing students. *Computers in Nursing, 7*(4), 168-177.

Slater, C. (1999). Outcomes research and community health information systems. *Journal of Medical Systems, 23*(4), 335-347.

Smith, A.R., & Chang, B.L. (1996). Nursing diagnoses for hospitalized patients with AIDS. *Nursing Diagnosis, 7*(1), 9-18.

Suppe, F. (1977). *The structure of scientific theories* (2nd ed.). Chicago: University of Illinois Press.

Suppe, F. (1989). *Semantic conception of theories and scientific realism.* Chicago: University of Illinois Press.

Tapscott, D. (1999). *Growing up digital: The rise of the next generation.* New York: McGraw-Hill.

Turley, J.P. (1996a). Decision making and science of the concrete. *Holistic Nursing Practice, 11*(1), 6-14.

Turley, J.P. (1996b). Toward a model for nursing informatics (Review). *Image: The Journal of Nursing Scholarship, 28*(4), 309-313.

Turley, J.P. (2000a). Informatics and education: The start of a discussion. In. B. Carty (Ed.), *Introduction to nursing informatics: Education for practice.* New York: Springer.

Turley, J.P. (2000b). Toward an integrated view of health informatics. *One step beyond: The evolution of technology and nursing. Proceedings of the Seventh International Conference on Medical Informatics,* April/May, Auckland, NZ.

Weed, L. (1991). *Knowledge coupling: New premises and new tools for medical care and education.* New York: Springer.

Werley, H., & Lang, N. (1988). *Identification of the Nursing Minimum Data Set.* New York: Springer.

Zukov, G., & Finklestein, D. (1980). *Dancing Wu Li Masters.* New York: William Morrow & Co.

CHAPTER 23

Future Directions in Health Care Informatics

RAMONA NELSON
SHEILA P. ENGLEBARDT

Learning Objectives

Upon completion of this chapter, the reader will be able to:

1. ***Describe*** various approaches to identifying future directions and trends.
2. ***Identify*** major agencies and organizations predicting future directions and trends.
3. ***Explain*** how and why future directions and trends are used in planning.
4. ***Identify*** future technology trends.
5. ***Identify*** future directions and trends in health care delivery.
6. ***Identify*** future directions and trends in health care informatics.

Outline

What Is Futures Research?
- *Challenges to Thinking About the Future*
- *Time Lags and Future Planning*

Purpose of Futures Studies

Approaches for Predicting
- *Trend Analysis and Extrapolation*
- *Content Analysis*
- *Scenarios*
- *Backcasting*

Trends Influencing Health Care Informatics
- *Societal Trends*
- *Technology Trends*

Future Directions in Health Care Informatics
- *Education*
- *Jobs and Roles*
- *Regulation and the Role of Informatics*

Key Terms

backcasting
content analysis
decision lag
extrapolation
futures research
futurists
information lag
Internet2
megatrends
policy-effect lag
scenarios
trend analysis

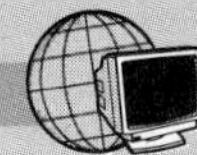

Web Connection

Go to the Web site at http://evolve.elsevier.com/Englebardt/. Here you will find Web links and activities related to future directions in health care informatics.

Health care informatics is a profession grounded in the present while planning for the future. The practitioners of this profession are managing today's health care information systems while designing tomorrow's systems. Planning for tomorrow's systems requires a conceptual framework of the potential future. The goal of this chapter is to provide the context for that framework and introduce the reader to the process for using the framework. The chapter introduces the reader to the concept of rational prediction and **futures research.** Selected tools and methodologies for predicting, managing, and determining the future are presented. The chapter concludes by identifying selected trends in technology, health care delivery, and informatics that have been identified in the current literature. By reviewing current trends and predictions, as well as the tools for predicting, managing, and planning the future, the health care informatics specialist is introduced to his or her leadership role as a predictor, manager, and planner of future health care information systems. With a better understanding of the future, it is possible to make better decisions today.

WHAT IS FUTURES RESEARCH?

Thirty years ago, Alvin Toffler (1971) published the book *Future Shock* about "what happens to people when they are overwhelmed by change. It is about how we adapt or fail to adapt to the future" (p. 1). This book was written before the invention of the personal computer (PC) or the explosive impact of the Internet. Today, the scope of change is growing at an ever-increasing rate of speed. In the practice of health care informatics, the only constant is change. Major innovations are changing health care delivery and computer technology, as well as the knowledge and expectations of health care providers and clients. Changes in each of these areas are reconfiguring the field of health care informatics. At the same time, health care informatics is changing health care delivery and technology practice, as well as the users of both the health care system and technology. As Toffler identified, many people are overwhelmed by the degree and speed of change. "Without a structure, a frame of reference, the vast amount of data that comes your way each day will probably whiz right by you" (Naisbitt & Aburdene, 1990, p. 13). Health care informatics specialists must not only adjust to overwhelming change but must also play a leadership role in interpreting the vast amount of information that comes their way each day while planning for future health care information systems.

Many people assume that there is no credible approach to predicting the future and that, in turn, there are no reliable approaches to planning for the future. It is true that the future cannot be known with absolute certainly. However, when systematic research approaches are used, it is possible to successfully predict future directions and trends. In fact, recognition of these trends allows many different futures to become possible. One example of this can be seen with the publication of the book *Megatrends* by John Naisbitt 20 years ago (1982). **Megatrends** are trends that impact all aspects of society. The ten trends identified by Naisbitt are listed in Box 23-1. Each of these trends continues to have a major influence on health care informatics. The field of futures studies provides a theoretical basis for meeting the challenges of dealing with change and planning for the future. Futures studies, as a research-based discipline, began in the 1950s and 1960s in response to the growing complexity of organizational life and world affairs. The research tools and techniques needed for futures studies were developed to understand and respond to the rapidly changing and largely unpredictable future (University of Houston—Clear Lake, n.d.)

Although health care informatics uses traditional forecasting and planning methods, as well as futures studies, it is important to note that futures studies differ from traditional forecasting and planning disciplines. First, futures studies tend to focus on a longer time horizon, typically

Box 23—1 Naisbitt's Megatrends for the 1980s

From		To
Industrial society	→	Information society
Forced technology	→	High tech/ high touch
National economy	→	World economy
Short term	→	Long term
Centralized	→	Decentralized
Institutional help	→	Self-help
Representative democracy	→	Participatory democracy
Hierarchies	→	Networking
North	→	South
Either/or	→	Multiple options

studying the world 10 to 50 years from now. Supporting futures studies are traditional forecasting and planning researchers who study political, economic, and market trends on a 1- to 3-year horizon. Strategic planning in health care informatics typically projects 1 to 3 years into the future in the context of institutional long-range planning, which looks out over a period of 5 to 10 years. For example, vendor contracts for major health care informatics systems tend to cover a 5- to 10-year period. The combination of findings and predictions from political, economic, and market researchers, along with futures studies, provides a framework for planning these long-term contracts.

Second, forecasters focus on incremental changes from existing trends, whereas **futurists** focus on systemic, transformational change. Both types of change are key to the successful planning of health care informatics systems.

Third, futurists do not offer a single prediction. Rather, they describe alternative, possible, and preferable futures, keeping in mind that the future will be created, for the most part, by decisions made today. The technical infrastructure being built today will have a major impact of the technical choices of tomorrow.

Challenges to Thinking About the Future

People almost always gear their present actions and reactions to their future expectations. They prepare themselves in the present to meet future demands (Rescher, 1998). However, there are factors that influence the way that people think about the future and that, in turn, influence the effectiveness of future planning (May, 1996). First, when thinking about the future, people tend to think about the short term as opposed to the long term. Present issues are usually most important. Tasks that need to be completed today take a higher priority over tasks that can wait until next week. This type of thinking is sometimes referred to as "putting out fires." For example, a health care informatics specialist may spend an afternoon answering users' questions but feel too busy to document the questions as a basis for a new educational/training program or for upgrading functions in the current health care informatics system.

Second, small rates of growth often seem insignificant. However major trends start from small, persistent rates of growth. This is especially true when dealing with exponential growth. Five years ago, very few patients asked for copies of their medical reports, and a very small percentage of those patients would have considered accessing their health care data via the Internet. Today, developing the policies and technologies used to provide clients with access to their health-related data is becoming an important part of the informatics specialist's job.

Third, there are intellectual, imaginative, and emotional limits to the amount of change that individuals and organizations can anticipate and for which they can plan. The future exists only in the imagination. The imagined future is built on assumptions that were developed in the past. An important part of planning for the future involves identifying and evaluating these assumptions. Often the anticipated future is not totally correct. In addition, the mental image of the future may be vague and lack concreteness. The further into the future one plans, the more the disconnection between the present and the future is experienced. However, the intellectual, imaginative, and emotional limits related to future thinking can be decreased in two ways. The first way is by building on the thinking of experts in the field. This book, as well as many others, includes content related to future directions in health care computing. Second, these limitations can be decreased by understanding the tools and techniques used by traditional forecasters and planners, as well as futurists.

Time Lags and Future Planning

Organizations, like individuals, have difficulties dealing with the future. As McMahon has pointed out, governments deal with three distance time lags—the **information lag,** the **decision lag,** and the **policy-effect lag** (McMahon, cited in May 1996). All organizations, including health care organizations, face these same time lags.

Most information is somewhat out of date by the time it is available. Even with automated data collection systems, there is a significant time lag before the data are processed and presented in a usable format. In many cases, data collection systems are not automated, which involves a much longer data collection period. Once information is received, it must be interpreted and evaluated. For example, a health care institution is considering how it might use voice data entry in the future. Will voice entry replace the keyboard or remain a limited-use technology? Finding, interpreting, and evaluating current information is time consuming. Once the information has been interpreted, a decision must be made. Should the institution plan for voice entry to be integrated throughout the system, and if so, how should this be done? The decision-making process is complex. Several levels of personnel need to be involved, including users, technical experts, informatics specialists, and administrators. Reaching a decision will take a significant amount of time. Once the decision is made, additional time can be used to implement the decision. During this time period, the initial information becomes increasingly outdated.

PURPOSE OF FUTURES STUDIES

The health care informatics specialist uses futures studies in three primary ways. The first way these studies are used is in foreseeing or predicting future trends and directions. For example, in the 1970s and 1980s much of health care was financed via fee-for-service funding approaches. Health care information systems were designed to capture charges. The introduction of the prospective payment system and managed care in the 1990s required that health care institutions capture costs rather than charges. Existing information systems were totally ineffective in capturing costs. The ability to predict these kinds of major changes could be a significant advantage to vendors and health care institutions alike.

Foreseeing the future makes it possible to more effectively manage future events. Managing is the second way that health care informatics specialists use futures studies. Cost/benefit analysis is an example of using futures studies for management. Finally, creating the future is a third way that health care informatics specialists use futures studies. By thinking of possible future scenarios, the informatics specialist can work toward creating the environment in which these futures might be possible. Using the work of futurists and the tools of futures studies makes it possible to imagine possible future trends and directions, to determine their probability, and to decide on preferable future directions.

APPROACHES FOR PREDICTING

Qualitative and quantitative methods are used in traditional forecasting and planning and by futurists to foresee, manage, and create the future. The qualitative and quantitative methods are what separate these researchers from the soothsayers. Multiple methods are needed to identify and address future challenges. Selected examples are presented in this chapter to demonstrate the nature of these methods.

Trend Analysis and Extrapolation

Trend analysis involves looking at historical data and identifying trends in the data. The following example illustrates trend analysis. A log of help desk calls demonstrates that over the last 2 months there have been an increasing number of calls from clinical managers and department heads concerning the institution's standard spreadsheet software. Initially there were several calls from three clinical managers who work in the same division. Currently these three managers are making very few of the calls. However, a number of different managers are now calling with questions. Figure 23-1 presents an example of how the increased number of calls might appear on a graph.

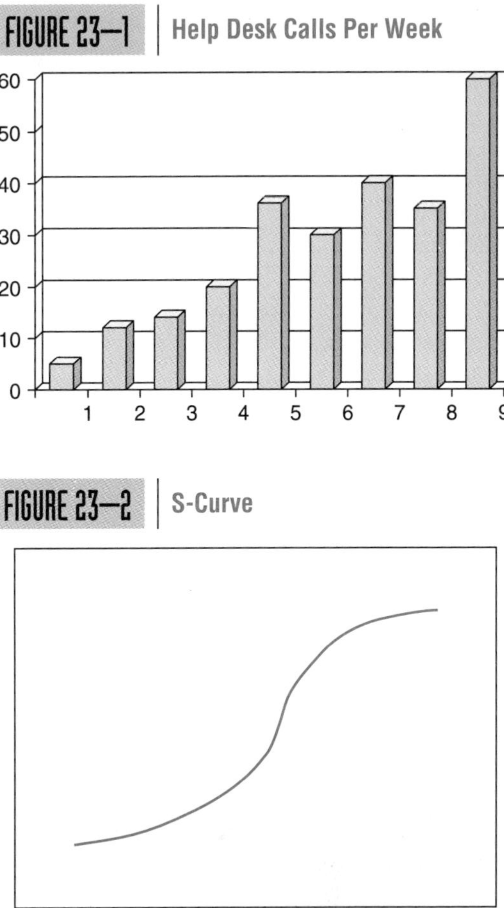

FIGURE 23-1 | Help Desk Calls Per Week

FIGURE 23-2 | S-Curve

Extrapolation consists of taking these historical data and extending them into the future. Needless to say, the upward trend line will not continue forever. Eventually the growth will start to slow, and an S-curve will develop. With an S-curve, the initial growth is slow, but then the growth becomes very rapid. Once the event begins to reach its natural limit, the rate of growth slows again (Figure 23-2). Another example is the pattern of use of the Internet as a source of health information. Initially, only a small number of people used this resource, but the number of Internet users has increased rapidly. In the future the rate of growth is expected to decrease. In the help desk example the expected patterns of growth can be used to plan educational programming, as well as help desk staffing. The need for these educational programs can be expected to grow and then level off. Although trend analysis and extrapolation demonstrate using quantitative methods for foreseeing the future, qualitative methods are also important. One example of qualitative methods is content analysis.

Content Analysis

Content analysis was the major research approach used to identify the trends in the book *Megatrends* (Naisbitt, 1982). Content analysis involves reviewing a number of information resources, noting what topics are discussed, what is being said about these topics, the amount of space allocated to each topic, and what topics are not discussed. Content analysis was also the approach used to identify the trends and future directions included in this chapter. Books, journal articles, conference topics, and Internet sites were reviewed to determine informatics trends and future directions. By its very nature, content analysis includes a certain amount of bias. The assumptions made in identifying topics and trends have a major impact on determining the forecasts produced. This is one of the reasons why it is important to review several different resources from several different perspectives to determine trends.

Scenarios

Scenarios involve asking individuals to envision positive and negative images of a possible future. A well-constructed scenario may be a direct extrapolation or may suggest events and conditions not presently being considered. The envisioned scenarios should be multifaceted and holistic. A scenario should be complete, internally consistent, and free of personal bias. Elements in the scenario should not be contradictory or improbable.

Three major approaches are used by futurists to construct a scenario:

1. The Delphi method can be used to elicit expert forecasts for a specific time frame. A combination or synthesis of opinions is used to develop the scenario.
2. Experts from different disciplines develop scenarios that reflect the viewpoint of their disciplines. These are modified and combined to produce an overall scenario.
3. A cross-impact technique is used to test the effect of one aspect of the scenario on all of its contributing parts.

Scenarios can be used to highlight a range of alternative possible outcomes of events. These can assist the analyst in dealing with events and interactions among events that might otherwise be ignored (Weingand, 1995).

By envisioning possible positive futures, it is possible to plan activities that support the development of that future. On the other hand, envisioning negative futures makes it possible to act now to prevent the negative future. Health care informatics specialists can use this tool in health care settings. For example, asking several different levels and types of health care providers to develop a scenario describing their charting needs in 3 to 5 years may be very useful in planning a system-wide documentation system. Using scenarios for planning usually involves backcasting.

Backcasting

Backcasting is concerned with creating desirable futures. In **backcasting,** one envisions a desired future endpoint and then works backward to determine what activities and policies would be required to achieve that future. Backcasting involves six steps:

1. Determine goals or the desired future state.
2. Specify objectives and constraints.
3. Describe the present system.
4. Specify exogenous variables.
5. Undertake scenario analysis.
6. Undertake impact analysis.

The end result of backcasting is to develop alternative images of the future, thoroughly analyzed as to their feasibility and consequences (Goertzel, n.d.).

TRENDS INFLUENCING HEALTH CARE INFORMATICS

Health care informatics has its roots in health and health care delivery, as well as in computer, information, and cognitive science. Trends and future directions in society, technology, and health care delivery have an impact on both the study and practice of health care informatics. A comprehensive review of these trends and their effects is beyond the scope of this book. In this chapter, selected examples of technological and social trends are presented. In addition, key trends in health care delivery are listed in Box 23-2. The

Box 23–2 Future Trends and Directions in Health Care Delivery

1. The development of information technology will impact all aspects of health care.
2. The rapid pace of introducing new technologies will continue with a significant increase in the number of new technologies available, such as the following:
   - Minimally invasive surgery
   - Genetic mapping, testing, and gene therapy
   - Use of specialized microchips for individualized therapies such as pumps
   - Artificial blood and other body parts
3. Medical technology and the aggressive interventions of health plans will continue to drive health care activity out of the inpatient setting (Institute for the Future, 2000). The continuing oversupply of acute health care capacity and the desire to control costs will increase health-related business consolidations and integration.
4. Changing technologies, settings for health care delivery, and financing of health care, along with the surpluses and shortages of various health care workers, will result in a shift in the traditional health care worker's job skills.
5. Health care costs will continue to grow. Both government and employers will tend to shift the increased expense to the consumer.
6. Increased education and access to information will empower both providers and consumers. Consumers increasingly will engage in shared decision making with their providers.
7. An increased emphasis on guidelines and protocols will lead internal managers in provider organizations and external managers working for intermediaries to assume increased authority for managing physicians' practice behaviors and patients' lifestyle and health behaviors.
8. Community health care challenges such as HIV/AIDS and environmental contamination will result in an increased emphasis on public health measures, including the development of international health-related information systems.

chapter concludes by demonstrating how trends and future directions influence and help to create the future of health care informatics.

Societal Trends

Shifting population demographics, changing cultural and lifestyle trends, and adjustments in the economic climate have implications for the future directions of health care technology.

Aging Population

The average age of the population has increased as mortality and fertility trends have declined in the United States. In addition, the large cohort of people born between 1946 and 1964 (the baby boomers) are now beginning to significantly change the proportion of the population over 55 years of age. The growth in the elderly population is particularly obvious in the older segments of the elderly (over 85 years old) (Deardorff & Montgomery, 2001). This age group uses significantly more health care resources than younger groups.

These demographic changes will increasingly affect the demands made on the Social Security system including Medicare. The number of elderly and the health status of this population will have a major impact on the health care industry.

Changing Racial and Ethnic Demographics

In the United States the growth of the Hispanic population exceeds that of the white, non-Hispanic population. This growth pattern is expected to continue in the foreseeable future. The white population, on the other hand, is expected to be the population group with the slowest growth rate between 1995 and 2025. The Asian population is the fastest-growing group in the United States, with growth occurring as a result of immigration, as well as increases in the birth rate. Other minority groups increasing at a slower rate are black, American Indian, and Eskimo populations (Campbell, 1996).

A major challenge for the health care industry, as well as for software and systems designers, is to recognize and accommodate the needs of an increasingly diverse and global population. For example, attention must be focused on approaches that make access to the Internet available to underserved populations, including the development of culturally sensitive health-related content written in multiple languages. Other population changes, in addition to the aging of the population, are changes in household compositions (e.g., there are fewer children, more single parents, and more single-sex households). The health care system and, in turn, health care information systems must be designed to recognize and support the health and well-being of these populations.

Increased Emphasis on Healthy Lifestyles

An emphasis on the informed consumer who takes responsibility for his or her own health care is the model for the future. Furthermore, there is a growing knowledge of the environmental threats to health and an awareness of the need for the public to be a force to rectify these threats. Increased access to the Internet is providing increased access to health care information, including evidence about lifestyle changes with a positive impact on health, strategies for choosing health care plans, and disease- and condition-specific information. As more full text materials are offered over the Internet, consumers are beginning to read some of the same health care literature as providers. As consumers take more responsibility for their health and health care and have better access to information sources on the Web and via high-definition television (HDTV), the relationship between the client and the provider is changing. This change in relationship will change the practice of health care delivery. Providers will not be expected to be all-knowing but will be called on to be excellent information guides, offering decision support to consumers as well as developers of high-quality electronic consumer information sources.

Technology Trends

The speed of advancement in technology and computing is so rapid that it resembles episodes in science fiction. Therefore predictions about the future of technology trends often simulate crystal ball gazing. One common forecast is that the level of dependence on computers in our society will continue to increase dramatically as changes in the speed, capacity, and complexity of applications continue. According to Moore's law, the processing power of the transistor chip is doubling every 18 months, in turn driving down the costs of hardware; in addition, Gilder's law states that communications costs will halve and speed will double every 18 months for the foreseeable future (Daly, 1999).

In addition to the advances in current computer technology that have been described in this book, other technological advances such as HDTV have implications for the health care industry. HDTV has a resolution that is six times the detail of current television sets. Furthermore, digital broadcasts can be multicast (e.g., offer multiple choices from the same broadcaster), include surround-sound, and be customized or individualized by the viewer (Cringely, n.d.). The possibilities for the use of HDTV for patient and provider education, for transmission of radiological reports, for telehealth consultations, and the like, are endless.

These rapid changes and predictions of ongoing advances in technology create a context for the evolution of health care informatics and for significant changes in the practice of informatics professionals. Predictions of technological changes that are on the horizon are provided here as examples of transformations that will have an impact on health care organizations and on the practice of informatics professionals.

Technology Predictions

Computers will increasingly be woven into our everyday lives. The following are some ideas about coming developments (Future, 1999).

- Embedded processors in home appliances will allow access to home appliances via cell phones.
- High-speed networks will be the norm.
- Image compression and high-speed multimedia applications will transform the Web.
- Software will recognize natural language commands.
- Digital identities (a growing combination of personal information, stored in governmental, hospital, insurance, and other databases) will proliferate.
- Major changes in computer technology will continue to occur at least every 18 months (Moore's law).

Wireless Technology

The popular move toward the increasing use of wireless technology suggests that the norm will be for people to access the Internet using their ubiquitous cell phones, handheld devices, and yet-to-be-developed wireless tools. In other parts of the world, the idea of a Web phone with access to the Web and eMail retrieval has been readily accepted. In Japan, for example, more than 10 million people have adopted Web phone use since 1999 (Alpert & Musser, 2000). In Finland, 67% of teenagers routinely identify their cell phones as extensions of their hands. Nokia, a large manufacturer of cell phones, predicts that 1 billion people (16% of the world's population) will be using cell phones by 2002 (Bloomberg News, 2000). In some countries, cell phones are already being used to make cashless vending machine purchases. This growth in use continues despite concerns about the impact of such phones on health and their unsafe use in automotive vehicles.

Box 23–3 Agencies and Organizations Predicting the Future

Club of Rome
Finland Futures Academy
Finnish Society for Futures Studies (FSFS)
Futures Studies Educational Network (REEF)
Global Discourse (GD) (a Baha'í student association)
International Society for the Systems Sciences (ISSS)
Rand Corporation
Strategic Futures International, Inc.
United Nations Commission on Global Governance
University of Houston—Clear Lake Institute for Futures Research
World Future Society (WFS)
World Futures Studies Federation (WFSF)

Impact on the Health Care Organization

According to Luker (1999), changes in technology are obvious disrupters of the status quo and thus become catalysts for organizational change. Successful organizations will anticipate and manage these disruptions. This is especially true for health care organizations and has important implications for health care informatics professionals (Box 23-3).

PriceWaterhouseCoopers (PWC), one of the largest international accounting firms, addresses the future of technology trends by stressing the impact of information technology on the way that organizations conduct business. The PWC projections are particularly salient for the health care industry, which has placed increased emphasis on business strategies and methods since the 1980s. Coming changes in computer platforms and communications focus on the development of wireless technology, speech and handwriting recognition, smart appliances, Web portals, and virtual reality interfaces. In addition, the evolution of component technologies and the appearance of new computing architectures will affect the way that organizations do business (PriceWaterhouseCoopers, 2000).

Impact on Security of Health Care Data

Research to resolve security problems related to the protection of personal and corporate data is ongoing. Increased use of two-factor authentication, smart cards, and biometric encryption is on the horizon. Two-factor authentication systems require two independent items: something the user knows (e.g., a password or mother's maiden name) and something the user has (e.g., a smart card or key) (Kay, 2000). Smart cards are small electronic devices that contain a processor, systems software and applications software, and electronic memory. Smart cards may be used for storing individual health care records so that the information is available whenever health care is needed (Webopedia, 2001). Biometric encryption is the process of using a physiological or behavioral characteristic to recognize a person. Physical distinctions such as fingerprints, retinas, palm prints, handwritten signature, and voice recognition are some of the methods of biometric encryption (Campbell, Alyea, & Dunn, 1997). Predictions are that biometrics will be widely used for PC, personal digital assistant (PDA), and cell phone authentication and that passwords will become obsolete.

Impact of the Internet

Daly (1999) has described the three driving forces related to the economics of the Internet as technological innovation in hardware and software, economics of networks, and effects of new applications. As the cost of connecting to the Internet decreases and access increases, more people from a variety of backgrounds and experiences will have contact with new sources of information.

Educational uses of the Internet have already expanded to include increased use by businesses for staff development and training, informal (continuing education) learning, and formal (academic) learning. Educational offerings tailored or customized for specific individuals will expand and afford opportunities for self-directed learning. Health care professionals and ancillary workers will obtain required continuing education on the Web. Hospitals and other health care and community agencies will increasingly use new technologies to link current and potential consumers to their institutions via portal applications.

Distance learning is no longer a special service of a teaching institution; it is not just a trend. Distance education is a form of learning in which students and teachers are located in different geographical locations and interact via the use of technology. Students increasingly expect to be able to be "any time, any place" learners. The growing competition in the educational marketplace, in which universities in one geographical area offer their programs to a global audience, has become commonplace. Educators who wish to survive and thrive in the future educational market must ensure that they have the time and resources needed to develop the skills and expertise required to use technology effectively to achieve positive student outcomes. Distance education has transformed into distributed education, which reflects the different geographical locations of instructors, students, and learning materials that allow for learning that is independent of time and place. The term *distributed education* recognizes the quality of the educational experience as well as the format for delivering the education. It includes both distance education and the integration of technology within traditional classrooms. Distributive education encourages interactions between and among faculty and students that ensure the development of learning communities. The future of distributed education is the democratization of educational resources—allowing students in underserved and rural areas to have access to the same quality of education as those in wealthier environments.

More than 180 universities in the United States, in partnership with industry and government, are working on the development of **Internet2**, a collaborative effort to create the Internet of tomorrow. The primary goals of the Internet2 consortium are as follows (Internet2a, 2000):

- To create a leading-edge network capability for the national research community
- To enable revolutionary Internet applications
- To ensure the rapid transfer of new network services and applications to the broader Internet community

This consortium will revolutionize the Internet, making new applications and technologies available to the public. "A key goal is to accelerate the diffusion of advanced Internet technology, in particular into the commercial sector. In this way, Internet2 will help to sustain United States leadership in Internet working technology. Internet2 will benefit non-university members of the educational community as well, especially K-12 and public libraries" (Internet2b, 2000, para 10).

FUTURE DIRECTIONS IN HEALTH CARE INFORMATICS

The following nine trends have been predicted by Healthcare Informatics Online (Trends, 2000):

1. Increased development of application service providers (ASPs)
2. Challenge of complying with privacy and security regulations
3. Impact of extensible markup language (XML) as a new language for defining data so that old and new applications can communicate with each other
4. Use of the Web for purchases and procurement
5. Use of computers to speed up routine operations and decrease costs
6. Increased use of wireless networking technologies
7. Use of voice recognition and other interactive technologies
8. Artificial intelligence
9. Convergence of technologies to unite data, video, and voice

Each of these trends will change the practice of health care informatics. Examples of how these changes will impact health care informatics can be seen in education, in the jobs and roles of health care informatics specialists, and in the regulations concerning the role of informatics.

Education

Access to Web-based interdisciplinary informatics education will contribute to the growth and development of the field of health care informatics. In addition to the continued development of informatics professionals, all health care practitioners will be required to have core skills and knowledge in health care informatics. Increasingly, hybrid academic programs will incorporate computer and information sciences into the curricula for health care professionals. Of note is the University of Pennsylvania School of Nursing's joint program in nursing and technology for undergraduates. This program was planned to accommodate those who wish to combine clinical training with training in engineering and technology (University of Pennsylvania, 2001).

Increased emphases on consumer health informatics, bioinformatics, and security issues will be reflected by changes in the curriculum.

Jobs and Roles

Informatics professionals make up one of the fastest growing specialties in health care (Thornton, 2001). Existing roles in hospitals and other health care settings will grow more complex as institutional clinical information systems are adopted by more agencies and include sophisticated decision support applications.

Existing roles as consultants, programmers, systems developers, and installers will be increasingly available, and new roles will develop as technology changes advance. Roles will require flexibility, commitment to innovation, and a willingness to stay current in the field and adopt new practices as they become available.

Regulation and the Role of Informatics

Health data privacy concerns will continue to drive governmental regulatory efforts. The passage of the Health Insurance Portability and Accountability Act (HIPAA) in 1996 initiated a growing conversation about the role of regulation in data transactions and the confidentiality of medical records. The growing problems associated with industrial espionage and hackers have caused both organizations and the government to take steps to protect their data by developing monitoring systems. Motivation to develop governmental regulations may be driven by growing initiatives against cyber-crime. The increased use of ASPs by health care organizations who use Web-enabled services for functions such as patient registration, scheduling, and claims processing, as well as for case management, leaves the health care industry vulnerable to cyber-crime.

CONCLUSION

Society, technical, and health care delivery trends have both short- and long-term implications for health care informatics professionals. This crystal ball gazing has touched on selected major predictions in the field. The common thread that runs throughout is the vision of increased dependence on computers that will be omnipresent, seamless, and ubiquitous in our society. Change is the only constant. The challenge for the health care informatics professional is to assume the leadership role as a predictor, manager, and planner for future health care information systems. This requires that health care informatics specialists be ready to anticipate trends and plan for advances with the primary goal of having a positive impact on the quality of health care.

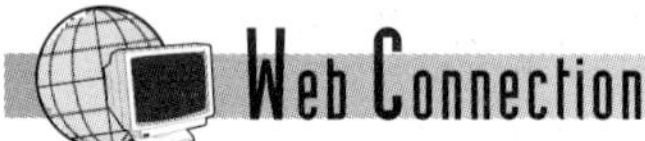

Health care informatics is a profession grounded in the present while planning for the future. Predicting future events makes it possible to more effectively manage them. The ability to analyze, synthesize, and integrate futures research into the clinical, administrative, and educational arenas of health care informatics offers the best preparation for providing safe and effective health care in the new millennium. The Web Connection activities for this chapter focus on the trends that have been identified as setting future directions in health care informatics. You will examine trends that have been identified and explore resources that provide perspectives on these trends.

discussion questions

1. Describe how the tools and techniques used for futures research can be used to develop a strategic plan for an information systems department in a health care institution.
2. Box 23-3 includes several organizations involved in futures research. Select four of these organizations, and search their Web sites to determine major predictions at each site. Analyze

your results to identify both overlapping and contradictory findings. Why do you think you might find both overlapping and contradictory findings?

3. Describe three future population trends, and discuss the potential impact of these trends on the development of new health care information systems.
4. Identify and briefly describe four major technological issues, trends, or developments that are projected to occur by 2010.
5. Consider the following statement: "The aggressive use of new information technology applications is a 'good' thing for health care organizations." Make a cogent argument in support of or in opposition to the statement.

REFERENCES

Alpert, M. & Musser, G. (2000). *The wireless web.* New York: Scientific American. Retrieved June 29, 2001, from the World Wide Web: http://www.sciam.com/2000/1000issue/1000alpert.html.

Bloomberg News. (2000). *Nokia bumps up forecast for spread of cell phones.* Cnet News.com. Retrieved July 3, 2001, from the World Wide Web: http://news.cnet.com/news/0-1006-200-4004361.html?tag=bplst.

Campbell, J.P., Alyea, L.A., & Dunn, J.S. (1997). *Government applications and operations. An introduction to biometrics.* Fort Meade, MD: The Biometric Consortium. Retrieved July 3, 2001, from the World Wide Web: http://www.biometrics.org/REPORTS/CTSTG96/.

Campbell, P.R. (1996). *Population projections for states by age, sex, race, and Hispanic origin: 1995 to 2025* [Report No. PPL-47]. Washington, DC: U.S. Bureau of the Census, Population Division. Retrieved June 29, 2001, from the World Wide Web: http://www.census.gov/population/www/projections/ppl47.html.

Cringely, R.X. (n.d.) *Digital TV: A Cringely crash course. PBS Online.* Retrieved June 29, 2001, from the World Wide Web: http://www.pbs.org/opb/crashcourse/.

Daly, J. (1999). A measure of the impact of the Internet: A tutorial. iMP. *Information Impacts.* McLean, VA: The Center for Information Strategy and Policy, Science Applications International Corporation. Retrieved May 10, 2001, from the World Wide Web: http://www.cisp.org/imp/december_99/daly/12_99daly.htm.

Deardorff, K.E., & Montgomery, P. (2001). *National population trends.* Washington, DC: U.S. Bureau of the Census. Retrieved May 10, 2001, from the World Wide Web: http://www.census.gov/population/www/pop-profile/nattrend.html.

Future. (1999). Future technology. *PC Magazine.* New York: Ziff Davis Media. Retrieved June 29, 2001, from the World Wide Web: http://www.zdnet.com/pcmag/features/future/.

Goertzel, T. (n.d.). *Methods and techniques of futures studies.* Retrieved June 6, 2001, from the World Wide Web: http://crab.rutgers.edu/~goertzel/futuristmethods.htm.

Institute for the Future. (2000). *Health and health care: 2010 The forecast, the challenge.* Princeton, NJ: Jossey-Bass Publishers. Retrieved June 14, 2001, from the World Wide Web: http://www.rwjf.org/rw_publications_and_links/publicationsPdfs/iftf/index.htm.

Internet2a. (2000). *About Internet2. Internet2.* Ann Arbor, MI: University Corporation for Advanced Internet Development. Retrieved July 3, 2001, from the World Wide Web: http://www.internet2.edu/html/about.html.

Internet2b. (2000). *Frequently asked questions about Internet2. Internet2.* Ann Arbor, MI: University Corporation for Advanced Internet Development. Retrieved July 3, 2001, from the World Wide Web: http://www.internet2.edu/html/faqs.html#.

Kay, R. (2000). *Technology quickstudy authentication.* Mt. Morris, IL: Computerworld. Retrieved July 3, 2001, from the World Wide Web: http://134.53.40.1/dms/robbgl/385/Readings/Authentication/Technology%20Quick Study%20Authentication.htm.

Luker, M. (1999). *Marketing views. The Alliance Report Online: Strategies for the healthcare marketplace.* Retrieved May 10, 2001, from the World Wide Web: http://www.alliancehlth.org/publications/0500mktview.htm.

May, G. (1996). *The future is ours.* Westport, CT: Adamantine.

Naisbitt, J. (1982). *Megatrends.* New York: Warner Communication.

Naisbitt, J., & Aburdene, P. (1990). *Megatrends 2000.* New York: William Morrow.

PriceWaterhouseCoopers. (2000). *PriceWaterhouse-Coopers reveals future of technology trends—From wireless communication to computing platforms.* Retrieved May 10, 2001, from the World Wide Web: http://www.pwcglobal.com/852566130069A85B/0/0ADAA7320F43DE028 52568EA006E4A24?Open.

Rescher, N. (1998). *Predicting the future: An introduction to the theory of forecasting.* Albany: State University of New York.

Thornton, J. (2001). Career outlook: Health and medicine: A promising future for health pros. *U.S. News and World Report.* Retrieved June 4, 2001, from the World Wide Web: http://www.usnews.com/usnews/edu/careers/grad/ccmedout.htm.

Toffler, A. (1970). *Future shock.* New York: Bantam.

Trends. (2000). *Hot technology trends. Healthcare Informatics online.* Retrieved July 3, 2001, from the World Wide Web: http://www.healthcare-informatics.com/issues/2000/02_00/cover.htm.

University of Houston—Clear Lake. (n.d.). *Master of science in studies of the future.* Homepage. Retrieved June 4, 2001, from the World Wide Web: http://www.cl.uh.edu/futureweb/program.html.

University of Pennsylvania. (2001). *Joint degree program in nursing and technology. Joint Degrees.* Retrieved July 3, 2001, from the World Wide Web: http://www.nursing.upenn.edu/admissions/programs/undergrad/parts/joint_degree/TECH.asp.

Webopedia. (2001). *Webopedia.* INT Media Group, Inc. Retrieved July 13, 2001, from the World Wide Web: http://webopedia.internet.com/TERM/s/smart_card.html.

Weingand, D. (1995). Futures research methodologies: Linking today's decisions with tomorrow's possibilities. *Conference Proceedings—Sixty-first IFLA General Conference,* August 20-25. Retrieved June 6, 2001, from the World Wide Web: http://www.ifla.org/IV/ifla61/61-weid.htm.

GLOSSARY

A

access The ability to obtain or the procedure for obtaining data and information or resources for specific purposes and by specific users (Chs. 2, 20).

accreditation A process by which a health care entity (organization, discipline) is given official or formal authorization, approval, or recognition for its practice. It generally requires an external review against a set of accepted standards by knowledgeable reviewers (Ch. 19).

ActiveX A loosely defined set of technologies developed by Microsoft. ActiveX is an outgrowth of two other Microsoft technologies called OLE (Object Linking and Embedding) and COM (Component Object Model). ActiveX is not a programming language, but rather a set of rules for how applications should share information (Ch. 13).

adds, moves, and changes This phrase refers to telephone service-related actions: **adds** result in a new phone set being added to the system, **moves** change the location of a phone set, and **changes** modify the type of service that is available on a phone set (e.g., call forwarding or voice mail) (Ch. 6).

administrative simplification Provisions of the Health Insurance Portability and Accountability Act of 1996 (HIPAA) (P.L. 104-191) that were passed to provide standards and a regulatory framework to assist the health care industry in overcoming the multiplicity of proprietary solutions developed by scores of vendors to support the collection, storage, access, transmission, and use of health information in electronic form. The regulations mandate standards for:

- Electronic administrative transactions such as claims, referrals, eligibility, enrollment, and payment
- Codes for medical procedures, diagnosis, devices, drugs, and so forth, such as CPT, ICD, NDC, and HCPCS
- Unique identifiers for providers, health plans, and employers
- Unique identifiers for individuals for precise linking of records, security, and privacy (Ch. 20).

admission, discharge, and transfer (ADT) Admission, discharge, and transfer are basic functions within a health care information system that track patients' encounters across an organization's care area. They are also a repository for patient demographic information and insurance information. *ATD* is another accepted format for this acronym (Ch. 7).

adult learning theories Theories explaining how adults learn. They suggest that adult learning is a discrete domain that differs from childhood or adolescent learning. These learning theories describe a number of similar learning characteristics shared by adult learners (Ch. 1).

Agency for Health Care Policy and Research (AHCPR) Former name of the Agency for Healthcare Research and Quality (Ch. 10).

Agency for Health Research and Quality (AHRQ) The lead federal agency on health and health care quality research (Ch. 10).

agency relationship An agency relationship exists when a person, group, or institution (the agent) acts on the behalf of another person, group, or institution (the principal) because of a contractual or ethical obligation. The principal is bound by the actions of the agent with a third party (Ch. 4).

aggregate The collection or gathering of elements into a mass or whole (Ch. 7).

algorithm A set of rules specifying how to solve a problem or perform a task. The rules are nonviolable, mutually exclusive, and 100% inclusive. They proceed in an orderly fashion to a stated goal (e.g., the steps to follow in alphabetizing a list) (Ch. 3).

American Health Information Management Association (AHIMA) Professional association for health information managers. *Health information managers* is a new term for medical records professionals (Ch. 10).

American Medical Informatics Association (AMIA) A multidisciplinary association made up of individuals, institutions, and corporations interested in developing and using information technologies to improve health care (health informatics) (Chs. 2, 10).

American Society for Testing and Materials (ASTM) A not-for-profit, national standards development organization that provides a forum for the development and publication of voluntary consensus standards for materials, products, systems, and services (Ch. 10).

analog Anything that occurs on a continuum, that is, experienced in infinite increments. An analog system is the opposite of a digital system, which can only make sense of data in finite increments (Ch. 11).

andragogy Initially defined by Dr. Malcolm Knowles as the art and science of helping adults to learn, it has evolved to refer to learner-focused education for people of any age (Chs. 1, 12).

application service provider (ASP) Third-party entities that manage and distribute software-based services and solutions to customers across a wide area network from a central data center. In essence, ASPs are a way for companies to outsource some or almost all aspects of their information technology needs via ASPs that offer software as a service rather than as a product (Ch. 13).

Arden Syntax Defined by Broverman (1999, p. 26) as "a balloted and internally deployed standard that was created with the goal of allowing users to create and share pieces of medical knowledge in a format that can be implemented by computer systems" (Ch. 5).

ASTM Committee E31 The American Society for Testing and Materials committee responsible for health care informatics standards (Ch. 18).

asynchronous Communication between two or more people in which sending and receiving occur at different times; therefore the communication is stored somewhere. Examples include eMail, electronic discussion forums, and listservs (Chs. 11, 12).

atomic-level data The smallest recognizable entity useful in differentiating a characteristic (e.g., systolic blood pressure) (Ch. 3).

attributes The characteristics or properties of a person, place, concept, or thing. For example, 128 RAM may be an attribute of a computer used to describe that computer (Ch. 1).

authentication The identification of an individual with the highest degree of confidence; usually provided through trusted third parties and systems that can vouch for the individual's identity even though the individual may not be physically present. This concept is tied closely to public key infrastructure (PKI) and digital certificates (Ch. 20).

automated decision support system A computer system that uses knowledge and a set of rules for using the knowledge to interpret data and/or information and make *recommendations* (Ch. 1).

automated expert system A computer system that uses knowledge and a set of rules for using the knowledge to interpret data and/or information and make *decisions* (Ch. 1).

automated information system A computer system that takes in data and/or information, processes it, and displays or disseminates it (Ch. 1).

availability The ability of users to easily access data and information appropriate to their authorized needs when they need it (Ch. 20).

B

backcasting A procedure whereby one envisions a desired future endpoint and then works backward to determine what activities and policies would be required to achieve that future (Ch. 23).

behavioral learning theories Theories that explain learning by breaking it into its smallest parts. The smallest unit of learning is the stimulus-response (S-R) unit. The stimulus is the input to the system or learner. The response is the output or behavior exhibited by the learner (Ch. 1).

best of breed This term denotes an information system that is considered the strongest in a particular area. An organization can combine best-of-breed systems from different vendors such as the ADT system, financial system, laboratory system, and radiology system (Ch. 7).

bibliographic managers Software programs that create reference databases, allow search and retrieval, and integrate with word-processing software (Ch. 2).

bioengineering The integration of physical, chemical, or mathematical sciences and engineering principles for the study of biology medicine, behavior, or health (Ch. 21).

bit Abbreviation for binary digit; the smallest unit of measurement in the digital world, having a value of 0 or 1. Larger combinations of bits serve as the building blocks for computer processes (Chs. 2, 11).

Boolean logic A form of logic in which all values are expressed either as true or false. Symbols used to specify the desired operation are often called Boolean operators. They consist of equal to (=), more than (>), less than (<), and any combination of these, plus the use of "and," "or," and "not" (Ch. 3).

Boolean operators Symbols or terms used to express Boolean logic. Boolean operators are used to combine terms in database searching. The three most common Boolean operators are "and," "or," and "not." See Figure 2-2 (Ch. 2).

boundary The demarcation between a system and the environment of the system (Ch. 1).

broken code Programming code that fails to function as expected. The code might not have functioned correctly from the start, or the code could have worked initially but then been broken by the addition of a new release of the product. Either way, the vendor is usually responsible for fixing the broken code as soon as it is reported (Ch. 9).

browser A client program that uses the hypertext transfer protocol (HTTP) to make requests of Web servers throughout the Internet on behalf of that browser. A browser is an application program that provides a way to look at and interact with all the information on the World Wide Web. Netscape and Internet Explorer are leading browser software programs (Ch. 13).

byte Eight bits (binary digits)(Ch. 2).

C

cable modem A modem designed to operate over cable TV lines. Because the coaxial cable used by cable TV provides much greater bandwidth than telephone lines, a cable modem can be used to achieve faster access to the World Wide Web. This, combined with the fact that millions of homes are already wired for cable TV, has made the cable modem something of a holy grail for Internet and cable TV companies (Ch. 13).

carrier signal A signal of a specific frequency that is modulated to transmit information (Ch. 17).

cascade effect This occurs as part of a complex change when a small, early error becomes the basis of large-scale destabilization of the organization due to replication or reverberations related to the error (Ch. 14).

CD-ROM (compact disk, read only memory) A type of optical disk storage system that handles large amounts of data—up to 1 GB (gigabyte)—although the most common size is 650 MB (megabytes) (Ch. 16).

certification A written statement indicating that a particular set of standards or requirements has been met at a particular level of performance (Ch. 19).

certified trainers System trainers who go through a rigorous training process that includes a return demonstration of training on the specific system for which they are to be certified. Quality end-user training is more likely to be provided when system trainers are certified in this manner (Ch. 9).

change theories Theories that explain how systems, including people and organizations, experience and respond to alterations in the environment (Ch. 1).

channel A physical element that carries a message between a sender and a receiver. Examples of channels are sound waves, telephone lines, and paper (Ch. 1).

chaordic Behavior referring to the combination of chaos and order found in organizations (Ch. 22).

chat software A means by which people who are online at the same time can type messages to one another and, almost instantaneously, the message appears on the screens of their co-users. Often referred to as **chatware** to indicate software that allows users to "chat" with each other in real time (Ch. 12).

chatware Another name for chat software (Ch. 12).

chief executive officer (CEO) Often, but not always, the president of an organization and the most important spokesman for the company (Ch. 9).

chief information officer (CIO) The highest ranking executive, often the vice president, of an organization, who is responsible for providing and supporting the appropriate information technology services for the organization in support of its goals (Ch. 9).

chief nursing officer (CNO) The highest ranking nurse executive responsible for nursing services in a health care organization (Ch. 10).

child table A table that is subordinate to a higher level table in a database (Ch. 3). See **detail table.**

circuit-switched network A method of network transmission in which a dedicated connection is established between two points on the network. Most telephone systems use circuit-switched networks (Ch. 11).

classification The process of grouping similar items together according to a specific scheme or model (Ch. 10).

client server A network architecture that splits an application into a front-end client application and a back-end server component as the basis for distributed applications. The front-end application runs on a workstation, collects information from the user, and prepares it for the server. The server receives requests from the client, processes requests, and returns the information to the appropriate clients for presentation to the user (Ch. 7).

client server computing Use of computer resources using a network architecture in which client applications on the user's machine request resources from a central server that provides services to users by managing shared resources. Most Internet applications are built on the client server model (Ch. 11). See **client server.**

clinical data management systems (CDMS) An early term or precursor of electronic health record systems (Ch. 10).

clinical data repository (1) An independent platform that stores clinical data retrieved from legacy, transaction-oriented systems for display and use in formats conducive to clinician query for the support of patient care (Chs. 4, 7). (2) Electronic storage of the data and information from individual client health records. The repository enables an organization to assemble, reorganize, and analyze information from a variety of internal systems, including digital imaging (Ch. 10).

clinical decision support system (CDSS) "In its ideal sense, CDS [clinical decision support] is a set of knowledge-based tools that are fully integrated with both the clinician workflow components of a CPR [computerized patient record] and a repository of complete and accurate clinical data" (Perreault & Metzger, 1999, p. 6) (Ch. 5).

closed systems Systems that are enclosed in an impermeable boundary and do not interact with the environment (Ch. 1).

code A numeric or alphanumeric representation of a data element or classified item (Ch. 10).

code set Any set of codes used for encoding (converting to equivalent cipher text) data elements, such as tables of terms, medical concepts, medical diagnostic codes, or medical procedure codes (Ch. 19).

coercive pressure Requirements for behavior that are based on power (Ch. 14).

cognitive learning theories Theories that use four steps to explain learning. These steps are (1) how the learner takes input into the system, (2) how that input is processed, (3) what type of learned behaviors are exhibited as output, and (4) how feedback to the system is used to change or correct behavior (Ch. 1).

cognitive skills Thinking skills used for critical thinking and problem solving (Ch. 2).

cognitive walk-through A usability assessment method that uses a detailed review of a sequence of real or proposed actions required to complete a task (Ch. 15).

commercial, off-the-shelf (COTS) software Prepackaged software available to any buyer. The software may require differing levels of end-user involvement to implement. Microsoft Office is an example of a COTS software product. Many vendors in the U.S. health care information systems market offer COTS software. Custom-developed software, although popular in the earlier years of hospital information systems, is less likely to be used for large-scale information systems projects (Ch. 8).

Committee E31 Committee of ASTM that addresses health informatics standards (Ch. 10). See **ASTM Committee E31.**

Common Object Request Broker Architecture (CORBA) An architecture that enables pieces of programs, called *objects,* to communicate with one another regardless of what programming language they were written in or what operating system they are running on. CORBA was developed by an industry consortium known as the Object Management Group (OMG) (Ch. 13).

communications Shared understanding, meaning, or information between two or more people (Ch. 11).

companion standards Standards that accompany a primary standard. For example, the standard for the computerized patient record (CPR) is accompanied by companion standards for the use of a CPR in an emergency department; standards for reservation, admission, transfer, and discharge; as well as other companion standards (Ch. 17).

computational health care informaticians Specialists in transforming the data, information, knowledge, and wisdom used in one area by a health professional and converting them into useful knowledge for another health professional in a different circumstance (Ch. 22).

computational knowledge Knowledge related to the use of computers in analyzing and solving scientific problems. It is distinct from computer science, which is the study of computers and computation, and information science, which focuses on conceptual tools for integrating the technological, behavioral, and contextual knowledge about information processing and communication (Ch. 22).

Computer Interface Literacy Measure (CILM) A computer literacy measurement tool that includes both a self-report section and a knowledge application section (Ch. 2).

computer literacy Ability to acquire and apply a basic understanding of current computer hardware systems and software applications to a problem in a particular work setting (Ch. 2).

Computer-based Patient Record Institute (CPRI) An organization of private sector organizations devoted to facilitating the achievement of the vision of the Institute of Medicine's 1991 report on the computer-based patient record. In 2000, CPRI and HOST (Healthcare Open Systems and Trials) consolidated to form CPRI-HOST (Ch. 10).

computer-supported cooperative work (CSCW) CSCW focuses on people as they act in their normal (work) lives. *CSCW* is a generic term that combines the understanding of the way people work in groups with the enabling technologies of computer networking and associated hardware, software, services, and techniques (Ch. 15).

concepts A group of ideas or items. They may represent an abstract idea such as love or a concrete object such as fruit (Ch. 1).

confidentiality (1) The concept that information and data, once disclosed, will not be shared without the permission of the information's originator (the person). Confidentiality describes a health care professional's duty to protect the secrecy of information about a patient's condition, regardless of its source (Chs. 8, 10). (2) A condition in which information is shared or released in a controlled manner (i.e., the expectation of the individual disclosing the private information that the person receiving the information will hold it in confidence). Confidential information is information held under restriction of further disclosure (Ch. 20).

consumer health care informatics A growing segment of health care informatics with a focus on the use of information technology and the Internet for the provision of access to information about health care and wellness for patients and other health care consumers. Also called **consumer informatics.** (Ch. 12).

consumer informatics The study, development, and implementation of computer and telecommunications applications and interfaces designed to be used by health consumers. Also called **consumer health care informatics** (Ch. 12).

contact center A center that provides computer-intermediated services through telephone, eMail, Web-based, and videoconferencing methods (Ch. 11).

content analysis A process that involves reviewing a number of information resources and noting what topics are discussed, what is being said about these topics, how much space is allocated to each topic, and what topics are not discussed in order to identify trends and predict future directions (Ch. 23).

contextual The interrelated conditions in which something exists or occurs; background or environment (Ch. 15).

contextual inquiry A usability method, related to ethnographic techniques, that is a technique in human-computer interaction. This method allows quicker determination of rich details of an activity by observing representative users in work settings (Ch. 15).

controlled vocabulary Standard subject headings or index terms assigned by indexers and organized into a thesaurus of terms (Ch. 2).

core vendor system An information system that is developed and supported by a commercial provider and that serves as the basis for any other systems that are integrated within an organization (Ch. 7).

credentialing A generic term referring to the process involving confirmation of educational preparation, experience, employment history, level of prescriptive authority, certification, or documentation of valid, current professional licenses (Ch. 18).

criterion of rationality A criterion used for decision analysis under conditions of risk by using the expected value criterion after assuming all decision states are equally likely (Ch. 4).

criterion of realism A weighted average computed for each decision alternative by using an "index of optimism." The criterion of realism is used for decision analysis under conditions of uncertainty to represent the middle ground between the maximax criterion and the maximin criterion (Ch. 4).

critical care information systems (CCIS) An automated information system designed specifically to record and evaluate the care of critically ill patients. Such systems are usually used in intensive care units (Ch. 10).

critical care monitoring applications Applications and devices used for electronic monitoring of critically ill patients. These devices are attached to the patient to collect and record specific data (e.g., electrocardiograph data) from the patient on a second-to-second basis. These applications are used to support the care of critically ill patients and may be interfaced with clinical information systems (Ch. 6).

Cumulative Index of Nursing and Allied Health Literature (CINAHL) Bibliographic database of nursing and allied health literature (Ch. 16).

D

data Uninterpreted elements that are not organized, evaluated, analyzed, or synthesized. For example, the number 98 could refer to a test grade, a weight, an age, or a temperature. Because data are uninterpreted, they do not have meaning. The term may also refer to the characters in a database field (e.g., the first name in the first name field) (Chs. 1, 2, 3, 21).

data archive The length of time data is kept (Ch. 7).

data definition language The data definition language provides a link between the user and the physical view of the database (Ch. 4).

data dictionary Information about the data in a database (e.g., what data are contained and where they are located). Sometimes called *metadata,* the data dictionary is a table of tables containing a list of all the tables in the database, as well as the fields in the tables and a description of the fields (Chs. 3, 4).

data element An identifiable representation of facts; the entities in an electronic health record to which values are assigned (Ch. 10).

data manipulation language (DML) A language that allows nonprogrammers to request data from a database management system (DBMS) and perform a variety of operations on the data contained in the database (Ch. 4).

data marts A subject-oriented, integrated collection of data used to support a specific function such as clinical care or the management of a single department. Data marts provide a decentralized approach to data distribution (Ch. 4).

data mining A single step in the knowledge discovery in large databases (KDD) process, in which an analytic algorithm is applied to a data set to "quarry" or search for patterns and trends that exist in the data (Ch. 5).

data purging Decisions about which data should be deleted and when (Ch. 7).

data set A collection of data elements organized for a specific purpose (Ch. 2, 3, 10).

data warehouse A database optimized for long-term storage, retrieval, and analysis of data from multiple sources serving the long-term business and clinical needs of the organization. A data warehouse works retrospectively to report trends, offer comparisons, and provide strategic analyses to manage the health care of groups and support informed decision making using financial administrative and operational data (Chs. 4, 5, 10).

database A structured collection of data elements, associated data values, and data relationships stored on computer-readable media (Chs. 3, 4, 7, 10).

database management system (DBMS) The collection of programs necessary to organize and retrieve information from a database. There are several different models (e.g., relational, hierarchical, and object-oriented) (Chs. 3, 4).

database model The archetype used to plan the storage, retrieval, and management of data in a database management system. Examples include relational, hierarchical, and object-oriented database models (Ch. 3).

date arithmetic A method of using dates for calculations, for example, a box on a computer-based form that automatically adds or subtracts a given number of days, months, or years to a date and inserts the results in a field in a table (Ch. 3).

decision analysis A method for producing consistent and rational decisions, particularly under conditions of risk or uncertainty (Ch. 4).

decision lag The time needed by an organization to make a decision once the information needed to make that decision has been collected (Ch. 23).

decision making A course of action taken in making a choice between alternatives (Ch. 5).

decision support system (DSS) (1) A computer-based tool for helping managers to make decisions by retrieving, summarizing, and analyzing relevant data (Ch. 4). (2) Any "system" that supports the human decision-making process. A DSS can be automated or nonautomated. The reader may also want to review the definition of an **automated decision support system** (Ch. 5).

defacto standard (1) A definition or format, either open or proprietary, that is widely used and accepted in the absence of an official standard (Ch. 11). (2) Standards that have become standard because a large number of companies have agreed to use them (Ch. 17).

deliverable An output from a process. The typical usage refers to an output from a vendor to a client, such as a report or a specification (Ch. 9).

delivery methods Techniques and procedures for delivering information using technology (Ch. 2).

Delphi technique Research method that draws on expert opinions for forecasting without necessarily bringing people together. Uses a consensus-building technique (Ch. 2).

demand management The systematic management of the demand for resources by patients and providers (Ch. 4).

desired health outcomes The desired short- and long-term health status, functional status, and well-being of individuals resulting from an intervention by a health professional (Ch. 14).

detail table The table in a relational database that contains none, one, or an infinite number of records with the same unique identifier as one record in another table in the database (the master table). In other words, in a multitable relationship, a table whose records depend on the records in the master table (Ch. 3).

diffusion of innovation The process by which an innovation is communicated through certain channels over time among members of a social system (Ch. 1).

digital Anything that can be broken down into discrete intervals of measurement or based on discontinuous data or events (Ch. 11).

digital certificates Data that are sent with an electronic message and used to prove the identity of both the sender and receiver of the message. Messages sent with digital certificates are encrypted to ensure that no information is lost or altered in transit. The message may contain the digital signature of the sender (Ch. 20).

digital subscriber line (DSL) A technology that uses existing copper pair wiring and special hardware, attached to both the user and switch ends of the line, to achieve data transmission over the wires at far greater speeds than standard phone wiring (Ch. 13).

distance education A form of education whereby students and instructors are geographically separated (Ch. 12).

distributed education The creation of a learner-centered environment with technology enabling asynchronous and synchronous communication among students and faculty. This can refer to both distance education and the use of technology to enhance a traditional classroom setting (Ch. 12).

dynamic content This concept describes Web pages that automatically update information or generate customized Web pages on the fly in response to user input. Static Web pages, on the other hand, are hard-coded and do not offer interactivity (Ch. 11).

dynamic homeostasis The process used by a system to maintain a steady state or balance (Ch. 1).

E

early adopters Individuals within a social system who adopt new ideas readily and serve as role models for others in the organization. They follow the lead set by innovators (Ch. 1).

early majority Individuals in a social system who are willing to adapt to innovation but who do not lead the process (Ch. 1).

economic order quantity (EOQ) model The simplest deterministic inventory model. It balances ordering costs against the costs of maintaining inventory to produce the optimal ordering quantity (Ch. 4).

eHealth (1) A term that encompasses the wide range of health care activities involving the electronic transfer of health-related information on the Internet. The term connotes the convenience, low cost, and ready accessibility of health-related information and communication using the Internet and associated technologies, such as eMail and the World Wide Web (Chs. 10, 13). (2) A new health care economic model composed of health plans, managed care options, specialists, and pharmacies that increasingly use the Internet and electronic records (Ch. 20).

electronic commerce Conducting business online. This includes, for example, buying and selling of products with digital cash and via electronic data interchange (EDI) (Ch. 17).

electronic data interchange (EDI) EDI refers to the electronic transfer of data from computer to computer, application to application, or process to process (Ch. 4). EDI is the transfer of data between different companies using networks such as the Internet. EDI is becoming increasingly important as an easy mechanism for companies to buy, sell, and trade information (Ch. 17).

electronic health record (EHR) (1) Any information relating to the past, present, or future physical/mental health or condition of an individual that resides in electronic system(s) used to capture, transmit, receive, store, retrieve, link, and manipulate multimedia data for the primary purpose of providing health care and health-related services (Ch. 10). (2) Can also refer to both the data and information as well as the application maintaining the data and information. The systems, data repositories, and technology that support the data and information related to an individual from birth to death and across all health care provider environments (Ch. 7).

electronic health record system (EHRS) An application that functions to add, delete, modify, view, copy, print, transmit, upload, download, and perform other manipulations on the data and information in the electronic health record (Ch. 10).

embedded form A form for a master table on which is placed, or embedded, a form for a detail table or tables. Embedding allows data from a primary key field in the master table to be automatically replicated in the foreign key field of the detail table (Ch. 3).

encoder Converts the content of the message to a code. An encoder can be a person or a software program (Ch. 1).

encryption The encoding of data into a format that is accessible only through the use of a secret key, or password. Encryption is used to secure the transmission of data. There are several commonly used types of encryption (Ch. 11).

end user The person who will use the components of a system (Ch. 7).

enterprise computing Internets or intranets established within an organization that have integrated a variety of legacy systems and applications into a seamless whole (Ch. 11).

entropy A measure of the disorder or unavailability of energy within a system (Ch. 1).

equifinality The tendency of open systems to reach a characteristic final state from different initial conditions and in different ways (Ch. 1).

ergonomics Ergonomics is intertwined with human-computer interaction (HCI) but focuses on the design and implementation of equipment, tools, and machines related to human safety, comfort, and convenience (Ch. 15).

ethnographic techniques Qualitative research methods borrowed from anthropology and sociology and used to conduct investigative fieldwork and analysis of people in cultural social settings. These techniques can be useful as usability methods for assessing groups of users and computers (Ch. 15).

European Committee on Standards (CEN) An organization that organizes and directs the development of standards for electronic health records and EHRSs within Europe (Ch. 10).

evidence-based practice Interventions and treatments based on data and research that are organized into best practices, guidelines, standards, protocols, or clinical pathways to support clinical decision making in health care professional practice (Ch. 14).

expected value (EV) criterion A criterion used for decision analysis under conditions of risk to compute a weighted average for each decision alternative by multiplying the payoff for each alternative associated with a particular decision state by the probabilities associated with those decision states. The alternative with the highest expected value is selected (Ch. 4).

extensible markup language (XML) XML is a pared-down version of standard generalized markup language (SGML), designed especially for Web documents. It allows designers to create their own customized tags, enabling the definition, transmission, validation, and interpretation of data between applications and between organizations (Ch. 13).

extrapolation An estimation process whereby historical data are extended into the future to predict future patterns and trends (Ch. 23).

F

fat-client computing A computing model in which applications reside permanently on a user's personal computer whether they are being used or not (Ch. 11).

field A distinct category of collected data in a database such as personal identification (name), demographic (gender), billing (amount due), or clinical (diagnosis-related group) information. This may be demonstrated as a column in a database that contains pieces of data representing the same characteristic for all the records, such as the birth dates of people in the database (Chs. 3, 4).

field entry The specific datum in a database field (Ch. 3).

field name The name given to the column in a table containing data. It is used to manipulate the data and should depict the data the field contains (e.g., BirthDate would be an appropriate name for a field containing birth dates of people in the database) (Ch. 3).

file A collection of records (Ch. 4).

file transfer protocol (FTP) The protocol used on the Internet for the exchange of files between computers. A protocol is an agreed-upon format for transmitting data between two devices (Ch. 13).

firewall A system of software and hardware devices that functions as a security monitor between an organization's intranet and the Internet. It protects a private network from users from other networks (Ch. 11).

first-generation computer Analog devices that focused on military communication and tabulation for cryptography—missile launch, guidance, and space exploration. The initial focus was on the development of computer hardware, and then expansion included computer applications for business administration and accounting tasks (Ch. 21).

FITness An acronym created by the Computer Science and Telecommunications Board (CSTB) of the National Research Council. CSTB has defined computer literacy for all college graduates as fluency with information technology (FITness) (Ch. 2)

flat database A database that consists of only one table (Ch. 3).

fluid outsourcing A condition in which internal functions of an organization are periodically assessed and then contracted to an external organization when the cost and quality of the internal department's work is not competitive (Ch. 14).

forecasting The science of estimating future events based on past events. Three classes of forecasting methods are extrapolation, causal, and judgmental (Ch. 4).

foreign key A field or fields whose data match a primary key in another table. Foreign keys are not unique for each record in a table (Ch. 3).

form A view of the data in a table that, although derived from the data in a table or tables, can be structured to present specified fields, calculated data based on data in a table, or fields from many tables. The form demonstrates the structure that will be used to format a report. It is this ability that makes possible the data entry concept of "entry once, use many times" (Ch. 3).

framework A conceptual structure for organizing ideas (Ch. 1).

full text Usually applied to digitized documents, as distinguished from citations or abstracts of documents. Full text indicates that the complete document is provided (Ch. 2).

futures research An area of research that uses scientific tools and methodologies for predicting, managing, and determining the potential future (Ch. 23).

futurists Researchers who use a variety of research tools and methods to systematically predict, manage, and plan the potential future (Ch. 23).

G

Gantt chart A list of specific tasks with bars that represent the duration of each task. Named for Henry Gantt, an engineer who designed a horizontal bar chart as a production control tool (Ch. 9).

garden path reasoning A common decision error process in which each individual, small decision appears correct but may be incorrect because it does not take into account the larger picture or context in which the decisions need to be made and understood (Ch. 22).

geographical information systems (GIS) Computer systems that are capable of assembling, storing, manipulating, and displaying geographically referenced information. Use in health care applies mapping software in conjunction with health care demographic and utilization data to demonstrate demographic and utilization patterns related to the health status of populations (Ch. 4).

go-live The moment when a new information system becomes active or live (Ch. 9).

governmental regulation Legislated laws, rules, and regulations that mandate compliance or conformance to a particular set of performance processes or outcomes (Ch. 19).

graph theory Those classes of problems represented by a graph that consists of points (vertices) connected by lines (edges) (Ch. 4).

graphical interface A program interface that takes advantage of the computer's graphics capabilities to make the program easier to use. Well-designed graphical user interfaces can free the user from learning complex command languages. On the other hand, many users find that they work more effectively with a command-driven interface, especially if they already know the command language (Ch. 13).

group decision support systems Computer-based interactive systems that facilitate the solution of unstructured problems by a group of decision makers. The software supports consensus building, usually by facilitating brainstorming, narrowing of alternatives, and voting by group members (Ch. 4).

grouping A type of sorting used in reports to present information from records with an identical characteristic in one field (e.g., the state field) together. Additional groupings can be performed within each group (e.g., the cities within each state and then an alphabetization of all the names within a given city). Calculations can be done for individuals, for any of the groups, or for the entire set of records (Ch. 3).

guideline interchange format (GLIF) An extension of the Arden Syntax that improves the ability of the syntax to represent protocols for care and complex multicomponent guidelines in a temporal fashion (Ch. 5). See **Arden Syntax.**

H

hardware Physical parts of a computer that perform the functions of data processing, storage of data and programs, input of data, and output of processed information (Ch. 2).

health care informatics The study of how health data, information, knowledge, and wisdom are collected, stored, processed, communicated, and used to support the process of health care delivery to clients and for providers, administrators, and organizations involved in health care delivery (see Preface).

health care information system (HIS) The integration and presence of both hardware and software components that support the informatics to carry out all aspects of providing quality patient care and conducting the day-to-day business of health care (Ch. 7).

health information Any information—oral or recorded in any form or medium—that is created or received by a health care provider, health plan, public health authority, employer, life insurer, school or university, or health care clearinghouse and that is related to the past, present, or future physical or mental health or condition of an individual; the provision of health care to an individual; or the past, present, or future payment for the provision of health care to an individual (Ch. 20).

Health Insurance Portability and Accountability Act (HIPAA) An act signed into law in August 1996 as Public Law 104-191. The intent of HIPAA is to improve the efficiency and effectiveness of the health care system. This law amended the Social Security Act to enable the promulgation of administrative simplification regulations that are intended to reduce the costs and administrative burdens of health care by making possible the standardized, electronic transmission of many administrative and financial transactions that are currently carried out manually on paper. Regulations based on this act were established by the federal government and have the objectives of ensuring the availability of health information when and where it is needed (portability) and also ensuring that the information remains secure and confidential so that it is accessed only by those who have appropriate need for the information (accountability). Objectives of the act are (1) guaranteeing health insurance coverage upon job change or loss, (2) reducing fraud and abuse, and (3) encouraging the development of health information systems that use electronic data interchange (EDI) for the administrative and financial transactions specified. In addition, HIPAA seeks to establish the required use of national transaction standards between organizations electronically (Chs. 6, 10, 13, 20).

Health Level Seven (HL7) (1) A messaging standard that enables disparate health care applications to exchange key sets of clinical and administrative data (Ch. 5). (2) One of several accredited standards developing organizations (SDOs) operating in the health care arena. Most SDOs produce standards (sometimes called *specifications* or *protocols*) for a particular health care domain such as pharmacy, medical devices, imaging, or insurance (claims processing) transactions. HL7's domain is clinical and administrative data (Chs. 10, 13).

Health on the Net Foundation (HON) A not-for-profit international Swiss organization created in 1995. Its mission is to guide laypersons or non-medical users and medical practitioners to useful and reliable online medical and health information. HON provides leadership in setting ethical standards for Web site developers (Ch. 12).

Health Plan Employer Data and Information Set (HEDIS) A set of standardized performance measures, related to significant public health issues, designed to ensure that purchasers and consumers of health care have the information they need to reliably compare the performance of managed health care plans. Included in HEDIS is a consumer experience survey. HEDIS is sponsored by the National Committee for Quality Assurance (NCQA) (Ch. 18).

Healthcare Open Systems and Trials (HOST) An enterprise created in 1994 by CPRI and Microelectronics and Computer Technology Corporation to accelerate the deployment of open, interoperable, and integrated information systems in health care. CPRI and HOST consolidated in 2000 as CPRI-HOST (Ch. 10). See **Computer-based Patient Record Institute (CPRI).**

HealthSTAR An online bibliographic database that provides access to health services technology, administration, and research literature. HealthSTAR is produced by the National Library of Medicine (NLM) and the American Hospital Association (AHA) (Ch. 2).

Heizenberg Principle The difficulty involved both in explaining the existing phenomena and in predicting future phenomena when the domain being studied is constantly shifting (Ch. 22).

heuristic evaluations Assessments of a product according to accepted guidelines or published usability principles. Commonsense rules that increase the probability of problem solving (Ch. 15).

homegrown product An information system product that is designed and coded for a particular hospital or system and is usually not for sale by a vendor (Ch. 4).

horizontal integration Corporate systems that include a number of units that have similar organizational structures. For instance, a long-term care corporation made up of multiple skilled nursing facilities or a hospital corporation with ownership of multiple hospitals (Ch. 14).

human factors The scientific study of the interaction among people, machines, and their work environments (Ch. 15).

human-computer interaction (HCI) The study of how people design, implement, and use interactive computer systems and how these systems affect individuals, organizations, and society. It should be noted that *HCI* can refer to either *human-computer interface* or *human-computer interaction* (Ch. 15).

hypertext A term coined by Ted Nelson around 1965 for a collection of documents (or "nodes") containing cross-references or "links," which with the aid of an interactive browser program, allow the reader to move easily from one document to another. The extension of hypertext to include other media—sound, graphics, and video—has been termed *hypermedia* but is usually just called *hypertext,* especially since the advent of the World Wide Web and HTML (Ch. 13).

hypertext markup language (HTML) The authoring language used to create documents on the World Wide Web (Ch. 13).

hypertext transfer protocol (HTTP) The underlying protocol used by the World Wide Web. HTTP defines how messages are formatted and transmitted and what action Web servers and browsers should take in response to various commands. For example, when a URL is entered into a browser, an HTTP command is sent to the Web server directing it to fetch and transmit the requested Web page (Ch. 13).

I

inferencing The process of recognizing the relationship between two terms, concepts, or ideas (Ch. 5).

informatics The scientific discipline that studies the structure and general properties of information and the processes of communication (Ch. 21).

informatics literacy The ability to apply basic informatics concepts and skills within a specific field or discipline (Ch. 2).

information Data that have been organized and processed to produce meaning (Chs. 1, 2, 21).

information competencies Knowledge base that allows one to apply core information skills. Competencies include the ability to recognize the need for information, acquire and evaluate information, organize and maintain information, and interpret and communicate information (Ch. 2).

information lag The time required for an organization to collect, evaluate, and interpret data and information when making a decision (Ch. 23).

information literacy Ability to identify an information need, locate pertinent information, evaluate the information, and apply it correctly. Information literacy and information competency are often interchangeable terms (Ch. 2).

information need Knowledge required for a particular purpose (e.g., related to the problem to be solved or the question to be answered) (Ch. 2).

information services department (ISD) The administrative unit of a health care institution that is responsible for the oversight of telecommunications systems, clinical applications, administrative applications, personal computer and help desk support, systems administration, and network support (i.e., all technical and functional information needs) (Chs. 7).

information systems (IS) The department within a hospital or organization responsible for technical and functional information needs (Ch. 8).

information technology (1) The branch of technology with a focus on the study, application, and processing of data and the development and use of the hardware, software, networks, and procedures associated with data processing (Ch. 8). (2) A particular discipline or sector that develops and sells products related to computers, including hardware, software, system software, network software, and so forth (Ch. 9).

infrastructure The component physical parts of information technology, including hardware, network, and peripheral devices that are used to interconnect computers and users (Ch. 7).

innovators Individuals within a social system who are the first to adopt a new technology (Ch. 1).

input Data and information that are entered into an information system using a variety of input devices (Ch. 7).

input devices Hardware that captures data for processing by a computer. Examples of input devices include keyboards, voice recognition software, and direct system interfaces (Chs. 2, 7).

Institute for Scientific Information (ISI) Scientific organization that publishes the *Web of Science* literature database (Ch. 2).

Institute of Medicine (IOM) An organization within the National Academy of Sciences that undertakes studies related to health care and medicine at the request of government agencies (Ch. 10).

integrated delivery system (IDS) An organizational structure that brings diverse health care delivery organizations into a single multiservice enterprise (Ch. 10).

integration Seamless access to unified data across multiple systems (Ch. 7).

integrity Ensuring the completeness and accuracy of data and information as well as the protection of data and information from processes that would invalidate them (Ch. 20).

intelligent agent architecture A piece of software that can autonomously accomplish a task for a person or other entity. The software has a "trigger" built into it. Once the trigger is executed, the agent can carry out its function without further intervention (Ch. 5).

interface Hardware or software necessary to interconnect components of a computer system or to connect one computer system to another (Ch. 7).

interface engine A computer system or program that translates and formats data for exchange between two or more independent computer applications. The purpose of the interface engine is to ensure that messages are reliably delivered to the receiving application programs (Ch. 6).

International Classification of Diseases, 9th Revision, Clinical Modification **(ICD-9-CM)** A classification system used in the United States to capture the medical reasons for health care. It is used to describe diseases and operations and provides information used for physician reimbursement, hospital payments, quality review, and benchmarking (Ch. 10).

International Classification of Primary Care (ICPC) The ordering principle of the domain of international family practice, providing logically structured classes for this domain's common symptoms, complaints, diagnoses/health problems, and interventions (Ch. 2).

International Medical Informatics Association (IMIA) An independent organization established under Swiss law in 1989. IMIA's mission involves the application of information science and technology in the fields of health care and research in medical and health informatics (Ch. 2).

Internet (1) A global network connecting millions of computers. Unlike online services, which are centrally controlled, the Internet is decentralized by design. Each Internet computer, called a host, is independent. Its operators can choose which Internet services to use and which local services to make available to the global Internet community (Ch. 13). (2) Any collection of networks interconnected by standard protocols like TCP/IP (Ch. 11).

Internet2 A project of a consortium of more than 100 universities with government and industry partners to create a separate Internet to meet academic needs in research, teaching, and learning (Ch. 23).

Internet protocol (IP) This term specifies the format for transmitting packets or blocks of data, also called *datagrams,* and the addressing scheme used in transmission. Most networks combine IP with a higher level protocol called *transmission control protocol* (TCP), which establishes a virtual connection between a destination and a source. IP by itself is something like the postal system. It allows a person to address a package and drop it into the system without a direct link between the sender and the recipient. TCP/IP, on the other hand, establishes a connection between two hosts so that they can send messages back and forth for a period of time. TCP/IP is the set of protocols used on the Internet (Ch. 13). See **transmission control protocol (TCP).**

intranet (1) A private or internal company network that takes advantage of the easy-to-use TCP/IP protocol for file transfer, browsing, and communications (Ch. 13). (2) A TCP/IP Internet that uses systems like firewalls to limit access to those with proper authorization. Generally used to share information within an organization (Ch. 11).

inventory models Models representing several different approaches to managing inventory, ranging from single-product deterministic algorithms reflected by the economic order quantity model, evolving to stochastic variants of the deterministic models, and ending with current just-in-time applications. A technique for managing multiple components used in industrial production is called *manufacturing resource planning* (MRP) (Ch. 4).

IS application portfolio This term connotes the suite of software applications planned, proposed, or implemented in an organization. As a portfolio is built, consideration must be given to the number of high-, medium-, and low-risk applications to be included. Those considerations will include available resource dollars, technical and functional staff to implement and support an application, and the effect the application and/or its implementation will have on meeting the overall strategic goals of the organization (Ch. 8).

J

Java A high-level programming language developed by Sun Microsystems. Java is an object-oriented, general-purpose programming language with a number of features that make it well suited for use on the World Wide Web. Java allows executable programs called *applets* to be distributed on the World Wide Web (Ch. 13).

Joint Commission on the Accreditation of Healthcare Organizations (JCAHO) An independent, not-for-profit organization that is the primary agency for setting standards and accrediting hospitals and other health care organizations (Ch. 10).

just-in-time learning Learning that takes place when a specific learning need is identified and met by an intervention that causes the learner to engage in the learning process. Just-in-time learning is associated with technical education often focused on technical skills that can be learned quickly and easily (Ch. 22).

K

key field Field in a record that holds unique data that differentiate that record from all the other records in the file or database. Account number, product code, and customer name are typical key fields. As an identifier, each key value must be unique in each record (Ch. 3).

knowledge Information that has been organized, analyzed, and synthesized. Knowledge results when data and information are identified and the relationships between the data and information are formalized (Chs. 1, 2, 5).

knowledge discovery The discovery of pieces of knowledge, both known and unknown, generally as a result of the application of knowledge discovery in large data sets (KDD). In other words, the basic task is to extract knowledge from lower level data (Ch. 5).

knowledge discovery in large data sets (KDD) "The melding of human expertise with statistical and machine learning techniques to identify features, patterns, and underlying rules in large collections of healthcare data" (Abbott, 2000, p. 141) (Ch. 5).

knowledge-based systems (KBS) Computer programs that reason with explicitly stated knowledge. Such systems include a database of knowledge and a set of procedures, protocols, and rules for using the database in the process of reasoning (Ch. 5).

L

laggards The last group of individuals within a social system to adopt a new technology (Ch. 1).

late majority The group of individuals within a social system who will adopt a new technology only after most of the uncertainty that is inherent with the new idea has been removed (Ch. 1).

lead part The unit of a system that plays the dominant role in the operation of the system (Ch. 1).

learning An increase in knowledge, a change in attitude or values, or the development of new skills (Ch. 1).

learning styles Individual differences in how people take in and process information when learning (Ch. 1).

legacy system A system in which an organization has made substantial investments over time. The ability to migrate from or interoperate with a legacy system is an important factor when considering new systems and applications (Ch. 11).

lexicon A vocabulary of words used for a specific subject. In the health care informatics industry, the language and terms have special meaning for their users (Ch. 17).

linear programming A mathematical technique for solving problems with finite resources in which both the objective function and the constraints can be expressed as nonnegative equalities or inequalities (Ch. 4).

logic A form of algebra in which all values are reduced to either true or false. Boolean logic is especially important for computer science because it fits nicely with the binary numbering system, in which each bit has a value of either 1 or 0. Another way of looking at it is that each bit has a value of either true or false (Ch. 2).

Logical Observation Identifiers Names and Codes (LOINC) A database that provides a standard set of universal names and codes that identify individual laboratory results (e.g., hemoglobin, serum sodium concentration), clinical observations (e.g., vital signs, hemodynamics, intake/output, electrocardiogram, obstetric ultrasound, cardiac echo, urological imaging, gastroendoscopic procedures, pulmonary ventilator management, discharge diagnosis, diastolic blood pressure, other clinical observations), and diagnostic study observations (e.g., PR interval, cardiac echo left ventricular diameter, chest x-ray impression) (Ch. 18).

look-up table A table of data that provides the entries for another table (e.g., a list of surgical procedures performed in a given hospital) (Ch. 3).

loose coupling A condition in which departments in an organization are given additional autonomy and power of decision making within a reporting structure (Ch. 14).

M

machine learning techniques The study of computer algorithms that improve automatically through experience. Applications range from data mining programs that discover general rules in large data sets, to editing systems that automatically learn the user's common spelling errors (Ch. 5).

master table The table in a relational database that has one record whose unique identifier matches none, one, or many in another table in the database (the detail table) Another term for master table is parent table (Ch. 3).

matrix management A type of management in which professionals are typically assigned, with the approval of their direct manager, to projects that are managed by other managers. Sometimes one professional can be a participant on several projects, none of which involve his or her direct superior. Performance appraisals are usually performed by the direct manager, with input from the appropriate project managers (Ch. 9).

maximally effective care This type of care seeks to produce the maximum improvement in health regardless of cost (Ch. 4).

maximax criterion An optimistic decision analysis criterion, used under conditions of uncertainty, that assumes the maximum payoff for each alternative. The decision maker chooses the alternative representing the "best of the best" payoffs (Ch. 4).

maximin criterion A pessimistic decision analysis criterion, used under conditions of uncertainty, that assumes the minimum payoff for each alternative. The decision maker chooses the alternative representing the "best of the worst" payoffs (Ch. 4).

maximum likelihood criterion This criterion is used for decision analysis to select the decision state of nature with the highest probability of occurrence and then to select the alternative with the highest payoff for that decision state (Ch. 4).

medical informatics "The application of computers, communications and information technology, and systems to all fields of medicine including medical care, medical education, and medical research" (Collen, 1995, p. 41) (Ch. 21).

medical logic modules (MLM) A language for encoding medical knowledge. Each MLM contains sufficient logic to make a single medical decision. MLMs are used to generate clinical alerts, interpretations, diagnoses, screenings for clinical research, quality assurance functions, and administrative support warnings (Ch. 18).

Medical Subject Headings (MeSH) The National Library of Medicine's controlled vocabulary thesaurus. Thesauri are carefully constructed sets of terms often connected by "broader than," "narrower than," and "related" links. Thesauri are also known as *classification structures, controlled vocabularies,* and *ordering systems* (Ch. 2).

MEDLINE The National Library of Medicine's extensive bibliographic database covering the fields of medicine, nursing, dentistry, veterinary medicine, the health care system, and the preclinical sciences (Ch. 10).

megatrends Trends, usually driven by national policy or global economic forces, that have an impact on all aspects of society (Ch. 23).

message-bearing signal A signal that transmits a sequence of characters to convey information or data. The point to modulation is to take a message-bearing signal and superimpose it on a carrier signal for transmission (Ch. 17).

middle-range theory A theory that is applicable only to a specific set of conditions or context (Ch. 14).

mimetic pressure Encouragement to assume a behavior that imitates a popular standard demonstrated by recognized leaders (Ch. 14).

minicomputer A medium-scale, centralized computer that functioned as a multiuser system. Minicomputers are the product of the discovery that transistors could function as their own circuit boards, greatly increasing computational power and diminishing the size and power requirements of computers (Ch. 21).

minimax regret criterion This criterion assesses the opportunity costs (termed *regret*) associated with each decision (demand) state. The maximum regrets associated with each decision alternative are identified, and the alternative with the minimum of these maximum regrets is chosen (Ch. 4).

model A description or image used to help visualize something that cannot be observed directly (Ch. 1).

model library This includes a variety of statistical, graphical, financial, and "what if" models (Ch. 4).

model manager This system accesses and deploys the collection of available models in a model library (Ch. 4).

multimedia The processing and integrated representation of information in more than one format (e.g., video, voice, music, or data, or in a health care record, text, digital radiography, and waveforms such as electrocardiograms) (Ch. 17).

N

National Library of Medicine (NLM) Federally funded library that is a repository for and disseminator of health and health care information (Ch. 10).

National Practitioner Databank–Healthcare Integrity Protection Database (NPD-HIPDB) A federally maintained, restricted-access database of physicians, dentists, and other health care practitioners who have a record of an adverse action or settlement of medical malpractice. Adverse action reports include negative actions concerning licensure, clinical privileges, and professional membership. HIPDB is a national disclosure program for reporting certain adverse actions taken against providers, suppliers, and practitioners. These include licensure and certification actions, exclusion from participation in federal and state health care programs, civil judgments, and criminal conviction related to health care and other adjudicated actions or decisions (Ch. 18).

needs statement Articulation of specific information required to answer a question or solve a problem (Ch. 2).

negentropy A measure of energy that can be used by a system for maintenance as well as growth (Ch. 1).

net generation (N-Gen students) Students who exhibit the following characteristics: fierce independence, emotional and intellectual openness, inclusion, free expression and strong views, innovation, preoccupation with maturity, investigation, sense of immediacy, sensitivity to corporate interest, authentication, and trust (Ch. 22).

network A system that transmits any combination of voice, video, and/or data between computers. The overall design includes sharing hardware, software, information, and rules or protocols for communications (Ch. 7).

network problems A type of optimization problem represented by networks that are defined as graphs whose edges have one or more numbers associated with each edge. These numbers may represent any number of parameters pertinent to the problem to be solved, such as costs, distances, or time. Graphs and networks have desirable properties that permit efficient solution of optimization problems (Ch. 4).

niche software Software that has been developed to meet the specific information needs of a department (Ch. 8).

noise A disturbance that is not part of a message but occupies space on the channel, affects the signal, may distort the information carried by the signal, and is transmitted with the message (Ch. 1).

nomenclature (1)Systematic listing of the proper names for concepts, items, actions, and other aspects of a particular knowledge domain or a particular area of interest (Ch. 10). (2) Standardized language (Ch. 21).

Nonnumerical Unstructured Data Indexing, Searching, and Theorizing (NUD*IST) A software package for thematic evaluation of narrative responses to surveys (Ch. 16).

normative pressure Encouragement to assume a behavior recognized as an accepted expectation of behavior within one's group (Ch. 14).

North American Nursing Diagnosis Association (NANDA) A voluntary organization of individuals and groups within the nursing profession that supports the identification, development, and publication of nursing diagnoses (Ch. 10).

number crunching The performance of considerable mathematical calculations by a computer (Ch. 21).

nursing informatics The integration of information science (a field of study that focuses on the collection, storage, retrieval, and dissemination of data and information), cognitive science (an interdisciplinary field of study that draws on many fields [e.g., psychology, artificial intelligence, linguistics, and philosophy] to develop theories about human perception, thinking, and learning), and computer science (a field of study that focuses on computer hardware and software) within the realm of nursing science (Ch. 21).

Nursing Interventions Classification (NIC) A classification system used to describe treatments that nurses perform in all settings and in all specialties (Ch. 10).

Nursing Management Minimum Data Set (NMMDS) A database composed of 17 data elements organized into 3 categories: environment, nurse resources, and financial resources. The database is used to identify and collect the factors that are needed by nurse administrators and managers to manage nursing care and to describe the health care and nursing environment associated with the diagnosis, intervention, and outcome segments from administrative, management, and resource perspectives (Ch. 18).

Nursing Minimum Data Set (NMDS) Sixteen core data elements brought together to capture nursing practice that define a minimum set of items with uniform definitions that concern professional nursing (Ch. 10).

NURSYS Database of nurse licensure information about nurses in the United States, including personal information, license description, education information, disciplinary action, verification request, fee-tracking information, historical information, and source information. NURSYS was implemented by the National Council of State Boards of Nursing in 1998 (Ch. 18).

O

one-to-many A type of relationship in relational tables in which a record in the master table has one record with the same unique identifier as many in the detail table. It is the most common relationship in databases (Ch. 3).

open source software A program whose source code can be downloaded for free and modified or developed to meet the needs of the user (Ch. 2).

open standards A definition or format that is publicly accessible. Standards developed by official standards organizations are generally open. Open standards help promote interoperability among various software and hardware products (Ch. 11).

open system (1) A system that is enclosed within a semipermeable boundary and interacts with the environment (Ch. 1). (2) A biological metaphor of organizations that emphasizes a holistic view, interdependence of internal elements, dependence on environmental resources, constancy of change, equifinality, and periodic restructuring as organizations grow (Ch. 14).

operating system Software program that manages all other programs on a computer. It controls computer functioning by managing tasks, data, and data devices (Ch. 2).

optimally effective care Care that seeks to produce improvement in health at the point where the greatest difference exists between the benefits and the costs of care (Ch. 4).

oracle A model used for early clinical decision support systems (CDSS). The name of the model is based on the answer given by a Greek god (oracle) to a question asked by a mortal supplicant. The model suggests that the decision support system is prepared to answer any question (Ch. 5).

organization science The scientific study of organizations originating within or integrating across traditional disciplinary perspectives (Ch. 14).

organization theory Conceptual frameworks with a group of interrelated principles that predict the interaction of structure, design of work processes, people, and the environment in organizations (Ch. 14).

organizational behavior The study of individuals, interpersonal interactions, and group dynamics at work (Ch. 14).

organizational culture The norms, values, and informal standards of behavior that develop among people over time in an organization to guide behavior (Ch. 14).

original document A document that is not a copy of another document; this document can serve as the source for copies (Ch. 10).

output Information or data that are generated by computers, such as reports (both printed and onscreen) or field population, from integrated systems (Ch. 7).

output devices Hardware that makes computer-generated information accessible (e.g., printer, display screen, plotter) (Ch. 2).

P

packet-switched network A network that transmits data by dividing them into pieces of information (series of packets). The packets are reassembled on the receiving end and may take different paths to arrive at the final destination. The TCP/IP Internet is the world's largest packet-switched network (Ch. 11).

parent table The table in a relational database that has one record whose unique identifier matches none, one, or many in another table in the database (the detail table) Another term for parent table is *master table* (Ch. 3).

patient data management systems (PDMS) An early term for what have become electronic health record systems (Ch. 10).

pedagogy The art and science of educating children—often used as a synonym for teaching (Ch. 12).

performance indicators The quantitative and qualitative measures chosen to monitor performance of an organization (Ch. 14).

performance management system The organization of information that measures financial, personnel, and clinical processes and outcomes for health care organizations (Ch. 14).

personal digital assistant (PDA) Generic name for a host of portable hand-held devices being used to manage personal information and communications (Ch. 11).

phenomenon An observable fact or event of scientific interest (Ch. 1).

point of care (POC) The area where patient care is provided, often at the bedside or in a clinic room (Ch. 7).

point of service (POS) The area where a service is provided to a patient, for example, the blood-drawing area or the area where an MRI is performed (Ch. 7).

policy-effect lag The time required for an organization to implement a solution and achieve the benefits of that solution (Ch. 23).

pooled interdependence A condition in which units within an organization are each essential and interdependent due to being part of the same organization but do not directly interact. Organizational survival is dependent on adequate performance of each unit (Ch. 14).

portal A Web site that provides access to a variety of services and information. Through proper authentication, many portals can be customized to reflect the personal interests and needs of individual users (Ch. 11).

primary key The field or fields that contain data that uniquely identify a record in a table (Ch. 3).

primary sort A reordering of the records in a database based on criteria applied to the data in a field (e.g., alphabetizing by last name) (Ch. 3).

privacy An individual's desire to limit disclosure of personal information. The concept that control over the disclosure of information known by an individual about himself or herself belongs only to that individual. An individual may share that information with another person but may do so with the expectation that the other person will respect the right of privacy and will not use or further disclose the information without permission (Chs. 8, 10, 20).

process-based education Education focused on teaching students to organize new knowledge, to integrate it into existing knowledge structures, and then to apply that knowledge in solving informatics-related problems (Ch. 22).

product evaluation A process whereby an information system is measured for its value and its expected impacts. A product evaluation determines the worth of an information system after implementation (Ch. 9).

product implementation The installation of the hardware and software components of an information system. The information system must be planned, built, tested, trained, and turned on for installation to be complete (Ch. 9).

product selection A decision by a person or a group of people about the expectations or functions of an information system. The requirements are used to decide which system to select (Ch. 9).

production job A computer program that is run by the computer operations staff on a routine basis to perform some data-processing need of the organization such as producing patient statements or payroll checks (Ch. 6).

Program Evaluation and Review Technique (PERT) Chart A specific chart format for presenting tasks and their interdependencies. It is a project management tool that can be used to schedule and coordinate projects (Ch. 9).

project plan A method for organizing and tracking the goals, milestones, tasks, subtasks, resources, costs, and time frames for a project (Ch. 8).

proprietary standards A definition or format owned and controlled by a private entity (Ch. 11).

protocol A set of agreed-upon rules for transmitting data between networked devices and applications (Ch. 11).

Public Key-Encryption Infrastructure (PKI) A security method that provides encryption of information using randomly generated, electronic "keys" so that the information may be transmitted securely over networks to a designated individual who holds a corresponding digital key that can decrypt the information. The level or complexity of the encryption and decryption algorithms determines the degree of protection obtained and the cost of the technical infrastructure necessary to carry out the desired security plan (Ch. 20).

Purdue Usability Testing Questionnaire A questionnaire for comparing the relative usability of different software systems (Ch. 15).

push technology A distribution technology in which selected data are automatically delivered to a user's computer or based on preset criteria (Ch. 15).

Q

query A question asked of data in a database. Queries produce the requested fields from records that match the criteria requested and can retrieve data from one or many tables (Ch. 3, 7).

query language A variant of the data manipulation language that can be used to directly interact with the database and pose conditions for data retrieval via natural language queries, query-by-example, or structured query language (Ch. 4).

Questionnaire for User Interaction Satisfaction (QUIS) A paper-and-pencil or Web-based product that addresses users' perceptions of the system for areas such as overall reaction, terminology, screen layout, learning, system capabilities, and other subscales such as multimedia applications. The instrument underwent psychometric evaluations, which demonstrated adequate statistical properties (Ch. 15).

queuing theory This theory provides mathematical formulas for the solution of problems related to things that are waiting to be handled (waiting line problems) (Ch. 4).

R

reasoning A systematic thinking process by which one arrives at a conclusion (Ch. 5).

receiver A device or individual that receives a message that has been sent over a channel (Ch. 1).

reciprocal interdependence A condition in which units within an organization rely on feedback loops between professionals, agencies, and/or patients for delivering a service (Ch. 14).

record The collection of data in the fields of a database that belong to one entity. A database record is essentially the digital equivalent of a file folder stored within a traditional filing cabinet; it represents data items stored within a number of fields for a distinct entity such as an individual patient (Chs. 3, 4).

regulation A rule issued by a governmental authority that has the force of the law. Regulations can be issued at the federal, state, or local level (Ch. 19).

relational database A database that is composed of more than one table. The tables are "related" by identical information in a field in each table (Chs. 3, 21).

report writer A software program that formats and produces the written output for a computer system (Ch. 4).

reports A view of the data in a printed table. The data can be structured in any way that is useful to the viewer. Among possibilities, data can come from multiple tables, be grouped by criteria, or be calculated. Because reports are organized to be meaningful for the viewer, they can also be defined as the display of information (Ch. 3).

request for information (RFI) An official, written request of a vendor for general facts about a particular product (Ch. 9).

request for proposal (RFP) An official, written request from a buyer to a vendor to submit a plan for the solution to a problem in the form of a system or service. Vendors submit proposals using the criteria established within the RFP. Often, the vendor is expected to comply with standards of content and form that differ by organization. Requests for information often require a huge investment in time and money by both the requesting organization and the vendor (Ch. 9).

resources Sources of support that provide needed information (e.g., people, databases, books, journals, collections of materials, patient records, or other contacts or materials) (Ch. 2).

return on investment (ROI) A financial analysis that describes the specific costs and benefits of a particular product. For a product to have an ROI, the benefits must outweigh the costs. In other words, does the new product pay for itself in terms of either reduced expenses or increased profits? Benefits and costs must both be quantifiable. The assumptions of the analysis are made up of numbers (Ch. 9).

reverberation The process of change throughout a system in response to change in one part of a system (Ch. 1).

rollout The installation of a product at additional sites. When an information system is implemented at one site, such as a nursing unit or a satellite pharmacy, the site is usually described as the pilot site. When the next sites are installed, the rollout of the product is started. The product is considered "rolled out" when all the sites have had the product installed (Ch. 9).

S

safe classroom Classroom where students can attempt new skills and practice them without fear of evaluation retribution (Ch. 22).

scenarios Envisioned positive and/or negative images of possible futures (Ch. 23).

seamless The effect when hardware components and software applications interact without problems and the information system user is unaware of the interactions (Ch. 10).

secondary sort A reordering of records in a database within the grouping of the primary sort (e.g., the sorting of records by city within the primary sort of "state") (Ch. 3).

second-generation computer The invention of transistors resulted in the second generation of computers. These computers were digital devices that were both smaller and faster than analog computers. Silicon chips that were smaller and more powerful than transistors eventually replaced transistors and advanced the process of miniaturization of computing equipment (Ch. 21).

security Measures implemented to protect information and systems, including efforts to ensure the integrity and availability of the information and the information systems used to access information. The means by which an individual or organization holding confidential information secures it from inadvertent disclosure or access by unauthorized third parties. Security includes physical means and procedures that protect the information. Protection against corruption or loss of the information is included within the security responsibilities expected of the custodian of the information (Ch. 20).

sender The originator of a message to be sent over a channel (Ch. 1).

sequential interdependence A condition in which units within an organization are serially dependent on each other's outcomes to produce a health service (Ch. 14).

simple mail transfer protocol (SMTP) The Internet's standard host-to-host mail transport protocol; a protocol for sending eMail messages between servers (Ch. 13).

simulation Use of computer models to imitate a dynamic system in order to evaluate alternatives and improve system performance (Ch. 4).

software Sets of instructions written in a structured programming language that are essential to make computer hardware functional (Ch. 2).

software applications Programs developed to perform specific tasks using a particular operating system (Ch. 2).

Software Usability Measurement Inventory (SUMI) Commercial product for measuring software quality from the end user's point of view (Ch. 15).

sorting The process of ordering records using a specific criterion or criteria (Ch. 3). See **primary sort, secondary sort,** and **tertiary sort.**

specialization The adaptation of a system component such as a body part, a clinical unit, or a computer program to perform a particular set of functions; a specialist is a person with advanced education or experience in an area who is prepared to function in a specific role (e.g., a family nurse practitioner or surgeon) (Ch. 1).

spreadsheet An electronic ledger that organizes information into columns and rows whose intersections forms cells. Cell content can consist of numbers, text, or the product of functions, formulas, and a variety of analytical tools. Mathematical functions are performed on the data in the cells (Ch. 4).

stakeholders (1) Individuals, organizations, or groups that have a vested interest or share in a particular activity, outcome, or investment and who will benefit from a successful activity (Ch. 9). (2) An important component of the systems approach that governs international utilization of health care information systems (Ch. 21).

stand-alone An information system that does not integrate with other systems. The data collected in the system are entered directly into the system and are retained there. Stand-alone or **stovepipe** systems are developed to operate independently. These systems are developed for a specific application and may or may not use standardized languages, protocols, or data exchange standards (Chs. 7, 17).

standard An agreed-upon definition, procedure, or format that has been approved by an organization recognized for setting standards. Standards exist for programming languages, operating systems, data formats, communications protocols, and electrical interfaces (Ch. 17).

standardized language A common set of terms that has been reviewed and accepted by members of a discipline to communicate concerning the phenomena of interest to that discipline (Ch. 21).

standards development organizations (SDOs) Organizations accredited by the American National Standards Institute for developing standards (Ch. 10).

static information Information that remains the same after publication (Ch. 2).

Statistical Package for the Social Sciences (SPSS) A commonly used quantitative data analysis software program (Ch. 16).

storage devices Peripheral devices that hold data such as magnetic tape, magnetic disk, and optical disk. These devices allow computer users to archive or retain data and programs not in use (Ch. 2).

stored program concepts Storing programs and data in a computer diminishing the need to enter data and also reducing the rewiring of circuits and changing of tubes previously required to run each program (Ch. 21).

stovepipe A system developed to operate independently. Also called a **stand-alone** system. These systems are developed for a specific application and may or may not use standardized languages, protocols, or data exchange standards (Ch. 17).

strategic information plan A vision of how information technology can be used to address the mission and the specific information needs of an organization (Ch. 9).

strategic planning The high-level planning done by management. It answers the question, "Where/what do we, as an organization or department, want to be in X number of years?" The result of strategic planning provides the strategic goals to be obtained by the organization over a number of years (Ch. 8).

strategies Actions, plans, or structured approaches to achieving a goal or solving a problem (Ch. 2).

Strengths, Weaknesses, Opportunities, and Threats (SWOT) methodology A methodology developed to assist organizations to assess their position in an industry. The methodology requires the organization to review its strengths, weaknesses, opportunities, and threats both internal and external to the organization (Ch. 8).

subsystem Any system within the target system (Ch. 1).

supersystem The overall system in which the target system exists (Ch. 1).

superusers Staff members who are given extra training before an information system goes live, for the purpose of preparing them to be resources for their peers once the information system is active. Often, superusers continue to support their peers through future product upgrades and changes to screens and databases as long as they are trained to provide this support (Ch. 9).

synchronous A term used to describe communication that occurs at the same time, or in real time. A telephone conversation is an example of synchronous communication (Chs. 11, 12).

system A set of related interacting parts enclosed in a boundary (Ch. 1).

system architecture How systems are linked together via a structure of networks, interfaces, or input devices that enable data to be communicated and shared (Ch. 7).

system backup Copying of data from computer disk drives to magnetic tape or other storage devices so that a second copy of data will be available in case of a computer failure that would result in the loss of the data (Ch. 6).

Systematized Nomenclature of Medicine Reference Terminology (SNOMED) SNOMED refers to the Systematized Nomenclature of Human and Veterinary Medicine or the Systematized Nomenclature of Medicine. SNOMED is a broadly focused collection of terms that encompasses diagnoses, interventions, outcomes, signs and symptoms, and other aspects of human medicine, nursing, veterinary medicine, and related health care practices. SNOMED is distributed in a variety of formats including SNOMED Clinical Terms (SNOMED CT) and SNOMED Reference Terminology (SNOMED RT) (Chs. 2, 10).

systems approach An approach that considers the context of a problem, the component parts of the problem, and the interrelationships among the component parts (Ch. 21).

T

table (in a database) A structured collection of individual pieces of data organized horizontally by a relationship to an entity and vertically by the same piece of information for the different entities. Each row in the horizontal structure is known as a record, whereas the vertical columns are fields (Ch. 3).

tactical information plan A breakdown of the strategic information plan into workable pieces, such as yearly budget projections, yearly product installation times, and a summary of the resources needed. Tactical plans are often referred to as *action plans* (Ch. 9).

tactical planning The detailed planning required to accomplish the goals in the strategic plan of an organization or department. It answers the question, "How will the goals established in the strategic plan be obtained?" The tactical plan defines the broad scope of each objective, the order in which objectives are to be initiated, the major milestones for each objective, and the project manager and team members for each objective (Ch. 8).

target system The system of interest, as opposed to the supersystem or the subsystem (Ch. 1).

task analysis The use of systematic methods to determine what users are required to do with systems by accounting for behavioral actions between users and computers. It is used to determine the goals of a new system and the role of information technology in user activities (Ch. 15).

technology generation The length of time for a new technology to go from concept definition, through development and testing, to mainstream integration within the industry (Ch. 8).

teleconferencing (also called **videoconferencing**) The use of telecommunications technology to enable groups of people at different locations to communicate with each other and learn together, often with an instructor at another distant location. Teleconferencing can be accomplished with high-speed telephone connections, by using satellite links, or via desktop videoconference packages (Ch. 12).

telemedicine The use of telecommunications to provide for consultations between providers and patients who are separated geographically (Ch. 11).

terms Words or phrases that identify a concept (Ch. 2).

tertiary sort A reordering of records within a secondary sort (e.g., doing a primary sort on a state, a secondary sort on the cities within the state, and then reordering the records so that the zip codes within each city are ordered) (Ch. 3).

textwords Natural language used by an author. These are sometimes referred to as *key terms* (Ch. 2).

theoretical model A description, image, or figure used to help visualize a theory (Ch. 1).

theory A scientifically acceptable explanation of a phenomenon (Ch. 1).

thin client In client/server applications, a client designed to be especially small so that the bulk of the data processing occurs on the server (Ch. 13).

thin-client computing A computing model in which small applications, or applets, are downloaded from a network server to a personal computer on an as-needed basis (Ch. 11).

think aloud A usability assessment method where users talk about what they are doing as they interact with an application. The interaction is recorded and analyzed (Ch. 15).

time line A schedule that delineates tasks, resources, duration of the tasks, dependencies of the tasks, and details of the tasks. The schedule for an information system project is often summarized into super tasks for the benefit of tracking by senior management (Ch. 9).

transaction standards Standards for data transactions including health claims and equivalent encounter information, enrollment and disenrollment in a health plan, eligibility for a health plan, health care payment and remittance advice, health plan premium payments, health claim status, referral certification and authorization, and coordination of benefits (Ch. 19).

transistors Solid-state semiconductors (Ch. 21).

transmission control protocol (TCP) One of the main protocols in TCP/IP networks. Whereas the IP protocol deals only with packets, TCP enables two hosts to establish a connection and exchange streams of data. TCP guarantees delivery of data and also guarantees that packets will be delivered in the same order in which they were sent (Ch. 13).

transmission control protocol and Internet protocol (TCP/IP) The suite of standard protocols used to ensure interoperability and reliable transmission of data between devices on the Internet (Ch. 11).

trend analysis A set of procedures that uses historical data to identify the general direction in which things tend to occur or events tend to move (Ch. 23).

trending data Reports or graphs that display data collected from a variety of sources over time. The information displayed can enable projections to be made based on data reports (Ch. 7).

truncation Using symbols to represent letter(s) in order to search for variations in spelling or forms of a word or for variant endings (e.g, comput*) (Ch. 2).

trusted authority (1) A computer system and its associated organization that is able and authorized to provide designated services. (2) A third-party organization that issues digital certificates used to create digital signatures and public-private keys (Ch. 10).

U

Unified Medical Language System (UMLS) A National Library of Medicine project that develops and distributes multipurpose electronic "Knowledge Sources" and associated lexical programs (Ch. 2).

unified terminology A system of terms in which separate nomenclatures are kept intact but linked together through mapping the relationships between terms (Ch. 10).

uniform hospital discharge data set (UHDDS) A set of data elements used by every acute care hospital to create a summary of a client's hospital stay (Ch. 10).

uniform nomenclature A single set of terms with definitions and codes intended to describe all aspects of a domain (Ch. 10).

unique identifier (1) A field entry in a record that belongs to only one record in the table, that is, another record cannot have an identical entry in that field (e.g., social security number) (Ch. 3). (2) The use of unique identifiers is a standardized method to recognize entities within a specified group. These remain unchanged and are usually in the form of an alphanumeric code of a specified length (Ch. 19).

usability Usability addresses specific issues of human performance during computer interactions within a particular context. The effectiveness, efficiency, and satisfaction with which users achieve their goals using computer applications (Ch. 15).

usability assessment A general term encompassing usability testing as well as other examinations of usability. Usability assessments are systematic and structured examinations of the effectiveness, efficiency, or satisfaction of any health human computer interface (HCI) framework component(s) or their interactions (Ch. 15).

usability questionnaires Tools that measure users' perceptions about system usability. Three examples are the Questionnaire for User Interaction Satisfaction (QUIS), the Purdue Usability Testing Questionnaire, and the software usability measurement inventory (SUMI) (Ch. 15).

user interface (UI) A boundary between a user and a computer, typically a computer screen, that allows a human and a computer to cooperatively perform tasks (Chs. 4, 15).

V

vendor A commercial company that sells products. For example, a company that distributes data structured in a format consistent with other resources it distributes and to which it adds enhanced features (Ch. 2).

vertical integration Corporate health systems that include a number of units within one region that may sequentially provide coordinated health services for a target population. The organization of services whereby one health care organization controls or owns a variety of types of services (e.g., hospital, long-term care facility, home health agency, durable medical equipment service) (Ch. 14).

virtual health record The collection of electronic health information from various sources, times, and locations in a system of computers, conveyed over secure networks, and presented in one view as if the records existed in the same computer system in the viewing location (Ch. 20).

virtual organizations Corporate entities with functions that are not geographically located in one area. They may include organizational relationships that are not wholly owned by the corporation such as consortia, alliances, networks, and limited partnerships (Ch. 14).

vocabulary A list of standard terms with specific definitions that have been accepted by a discipline, group, or organization to express, organize, and index the concepts and phenomena of interest (Ch. 10).

voice recognition The developing technology that allows data to be entered into an information system using verbal interaction with the system (Ch. 7).

W

Web server A computer that delivers Web pages. Every Web server has an IP address and possibly a domain name. For example, insertion of the URL http://www.pcwebopedia.com/index.html in browser software sends a request to the server whose domain name is pcwebopedia.com. The server then fetches the page named index.html and sends it to the browser on the originating computer system (Ch. 13).

wildcard Symbols that are used to represent the characters in the truncation process. In many systems the use of an asterisk (*) denotes any number of and any kind of character, and a question mark (?) denotes one character (Chs. 2, 3).

wisdom The appropriate use of knowledge to manage or solve human problems. Wisdom is knowing when and how to use knowledge to manage a client need or problem (Chs. 1, 21).

work breakdown structure A method for establishing a project plan. In this method, the goals of a project are broken down into manageable tasks and subtasks for execution and tracking (Ch. 8).

working partnerships An important component of the systems approach that governs international utilization of health care information systems (Ch. 21).

World Wide Web A system of Internet servers that support specially formatted documents. The documents are formatted in a language called hypertext markup language (HTML) that enables links to other documents, as well as graphics, audio files, and video files. As a result a user can move from one document to another simply by clicking on hot spots (Chs. 11, 13, 16).

WYSIWYG Abbreviation for "what you see is what you get." This application enables users to see on the display screen exactly what will appear when the document is printed (Ch. 2).

INDEX

B

C

O

X

Z